Human Milk for Preterm Infants: An Issue of Clinics in Perinatology

Human Milk for Preterm Infants: An Issue of Clinics in Perinatology

Edited by Julian Lewis

hayle medical

New York

Hayle Medical,
750 Third Avenue, 9th Floor,
New York, NY 10017, USA

Visit us on the World Wide Web at:
www.haylemedical.com

ISBN: 978-1-64647-547-6

Cataloging-in-Publication Data

Human milk for preterm infants : an issue of clinics in perinatology / edited by Julian Lewis.
p. cm.
Includes bibliographical references and index.
ISBN 978-1-64647-547-6
1. Breast milk. 2. Premature infants--Nutrition. 3. Breastfeeding. 4. Perinatology. I. Lewis, Julian.
RJ216 .H86 2023
649.33--dc23

Table of Contents

Preface

Human milk is considered to be the optimum food for newborn nutrition. It is widely acknowledged as the ideal food for almost all infants due to its proven health advantages for both children and their mothers. It has particularly significant health advantages for preterm infants. Human milk is a very complex composite liquid of nutrients for newborn growth that is predominantly composed of proteins, fats and carbohydrates as well as vitamins, minerals and other nutrients. The fat in human milk promotes the development of baby's neurologic tissues and brain which is crucial for premature infants. This book aims to shed light on the role of human milk for preterm infants. It presents researches and studies performed by experts across the globe. The extensive content of this book provides the readers with a thorough understanding of the subject.

This book unites the global concepts and researches in an organized manner for a comprehensive understanding of the subject. It is a ripe text for all researchers, students, scientists or anyone else who is interested in acquiring a better knowledge of this dynamic field.

I extend my sincere thanks to the contributors for such eloquent research chapters. Finally, I thank my family for being a source of support and help.

Editor

1

The Effect of Human Milk on Modulating the Quality of Growth in Preterm Infants

Pasqua Piemontese[1], *Nadia Liotto*[1*], *Domenica Mallardi*[1], *Paola Roggero*[1,2], *Valeria Puricelli*[1], *Maria Lorella Giannì*[1,2], *Daniela Morniroli*[1,2], *Chiara Tabasso*[1], *Michela Perrone*[1], *Camilla Menis*[1,2], *Anna Orsi*[1], *Orsola Amato*[1] *and Fabio Mosca*[1,2]

[1] Neonatal Intensive Care Unit, Fondazione IRCCS Ca' Granda Ospedale Maggiore Policlinico (IRCCS), Milan, Italy,
[2] Department of Clinical Sciences and Community Health, University of Milan, Milan, Italy

***Correspondence:**
Nadia Liotto
nadia.liotto@policlinico.mi.it;
nadia.liotto@gmail.com

Introduction: Human milk is the optimal nutrition for preterm infants. When the mother's own milk is unavailable, donor human milk is recommended as an alternative for preterm infants. The association among early nutrition, body composition and the future risk of disease has recently attracted much interest. The aim of this study was to investigate the effect of human milk on the body composition of preterm infants.

Materials and Methods: Very low birth weight infants (VLBW: birth weight <1,500 g) with a gestational age (GA) between 26 and 34 weeks were included. Clinical data, anthropometric measurements and nutritional intake in terms of the volume of human milk were extracted from computerized medical charts. The human milk intake was expressed as a percentage of target fortified donor human milk and/or target fortified fresh mother's milk, compared with the total volume of milk intake during the hospital stay. All included infants underwent anthropometric measurements and body composition analysis (expressed as fat-free mass percentage) at term corrected age (CA) by air-displacement plethysmography. A comparison between infants fed human milk at <50% (group 1) and infants fed human milk at ≥50% of the total volume of milk intake (group 2) was conducted. Multiple linear regression analyses were conducted to explore the modulating effect of fortified human milk on fat-free mass at term CA.

Results: Seventy-three VLBW infants were included in the study. The mean weight and GA at birth were 1,248 ± 198 g and 30.2 ± 2.0 weeks, respectively. No differences were found regarding anthropometric measurements at birth, at discharge and at term CA between the two groups. The mean fortified human milk intake was 34.9 ± 12.5 and 80.9 ± 15.5% in groups 1 and 2, respectively ($p < 0.001$).
A multiple regression analysis corrected for sex and birth weight demonstrated that intake of ≥50% fortified human milk was associated with a higher fat-free mass percentage at term CA than intake of <50% fortified human milk.

Conclusion: The use of target fortified human milk modulated growth and improved growth quality in vulnerable preterm infants. Thus, the use of donor human milk should be encouraged when fresh mother's milk is insufficient or not available.

Keywords: human milk, donor human milk, preterm infants, body composition, target fortification

INTRODUCTION

Human milk is the optimal nutrition for preterm infants. Increasing evidence has demonstrated that mother's own milk provides significant benefits for extremely preterm infants, such as the prevention of infection and necrotizing enterocolitis and a reduction in the duration of hospital stay (1). In addition, it has been reported that these benefits are modulated according to the dose of human milk fed during hospitalization (2, 3).

Mother's own milk is at the top of the biological hierarchy; therefore, it is always preferable to other sources of milk (4). Nevertheless, donor human milk can be a bridge until a mother's own milk is available and sufficient to meet her infant's nutritional needs (1, 5). Indeed, in a recent meta-analysis, mother's own milk supplemented with donor human milk was associated with a reduced risk in the development of bronchopulmonary dysplasia in very preterm infants compared with that supplemented with preterm formula (6). In 2014, Quigley and McGuire demonstrated that formula-fed preterm and low birth weight infants had higher rates of short-term growth but also a higher risk of developing necrotizing enterocolitis than those who were fed donor human milk (7).

The association among early nutrition, growth, growth quality, and the future risk of developing noncommunicable diseases has attracted much interest in recent years.

In a recent study on the growth of late preterm infants, we demonstrated that being fed human milk is associated with increased fat-free mass deposition at term corrected age (CA) (8).

It has also been reported that formula-fed very preterm infants show an altered body composition. Specifically, compared with breastfed very preterm infants, formula-fed very preterm infants showed increased fat mass at term CA (9, 10), which decreased toward 6 months CA (11).

Conversely, preterm infants fed fortified mother's own milk showed a higher percentage of fat-free mass than formula-fed infants at term CA (12).

Data regarding the effect of human milk (both fresh mother's milk and/or donor human milk) on the modulation of body composition in preterm infants are scarce. Therefore, the aim of this study was to investigate the effect of human milk (both fresh mother's milk and/or donor human milk) on growth and body composition in preterm infants.

MATERIALS AND METHODS

The Ethics Committee of the Fondazione Istituto di Ricovero e Cura a Carattere Scientifico Cà Granda Ospedale Maggiore Policlinico approved the study, and written informed consent was obtained from the parents. All clinical investigations were conducted according to the principles outlined in the Declaration of Helsinki.

Study Design

A longitudinal observational study was conducted.

Very low birth weight infants (VLBW: birth weight <1,500 g) born between May 2016 and December 2017 at the authors' institution with gestational age (GA) at birth from 26^{+0} to 33^{+6} weeks were included in the study.

The exclusion criteria for all infants screened included the presence of congenital diseases, chromosomal abnormalities or cardiac, brain, renal, endocrine or surgical diseases, which can interfere with growth. In addition, infants who required ventilatory assistance and intravenous nutritional support at term CA were excluded.

GA was based on the last menstrual period and first trimester ultrasonogram. CA was calculated using the chronological age and adjusted for GA, which is the number of additional weeks from term (40 weeks) (13).

Data Collection and Nutritional Practices

Clinical data, anthropometric measurements, and nutritional intake in terms of the volume of human milk intake (both fresh mother's milk and/or donor human milk) during the hospital stay were acquired from computerized medical charts (Neocare®).

Parenteral nutrition was started on the first day of life. The parenteral solutions were prepared by the hospital pharmacy according to the medical prescription. The provided volume increased from 80 to 90 ml/kg on the first day to 150–180 ml/kg on the 7th day of life, with an energy/protein ratio from 20.8–24 kcal/g on the first day up to 23.1–27.7 kcal/g on the 7th day of life.

Weaning from parenteral nutrition was scheduled to obtain a weight velocity >15 g/kg/day. To achieve this goal, the macronutrients were reduced gradually according to weight velocity. **Table 1** shows the parenteral nutrition practices according to the internal procedure.

Enteral feeding was started within 24 h of postnatal life using fresh mother's milk. When fresh mother's milk was unavailable or insufficient, donor human milk was started following the acquisition of written informed consent from the parents. In case of lack of parents' consent, infants were fed with preterm formula (energy: 83 kcal/100 ml; carbohydrates: 8.4 g/100 ml; proteins: 2.7 g/100 ml; fat: 4.1 g/100 ml).

For infants with birth weights less than 1,000 g and/or with severe intrauterine growth restriction (<3th percentile according to INTERGROWTH-21st reference curves) (14), enteral feeding was started at 10 ml/kg/day and remained stable for the first 3 days of life. On the fourth day of life, an increase of 10 ml/kg/day was scheduled.

For infants with birth weights greater than or equal to 1,000 g without severe intrauterine growth restriction (<3th percentile according to INTERGROWTH-21st reference curves) (14), enteral feeding was started at 20 ml/kg/day and remained stable for the first 2 days of life. After the third day of life, an increase of 20 ml/kg/day was scheduled.

Enteral nutrition was stopped in cases of septic shock, needs for exsanguinotrasfusion, abdominal distension with a visible intestinal loop, and gastric residual volumes >2 ml/kg for infants with birth weights <750 g, >3 ml/kg for infants with birth weights ranging from 751 to 1,000 g and >5 ml/kg for infants with birth weights greater than 1,000 g.

When the infants tolerated an enteral intake ≥80 ml/kg, a target human milk fortification was started.

TABLE 1 | Parenteral nutrition practices.

Day of life	1		2		3		4		5		6		≥7	
Birth weight (g)	**<1000 g**	**>1000 g**	**<1000 g**	**>1000 g**	**<1000 g**	**>1000 g**	**<1000 g**	**>1000 g**	**<1000 g**	**>1000 g**	**<1000 g**	**>1000 g**	**<1000 g**	**>1000 g**
Volume (ml/kg)	80–90	80	90–100	90	110–120	100–110	120–140	110–120	140–160	120–130	150–160	140–150	150–160	150–160
Glucose (g/kg)	8	9	8	9	9	10–11	9	10–13	10	10–14	10–13	10–14	10–14	10–14
Lipids (g/kg)	2–2.5	2.5	2.5	2.5	2.5	2.5	3	3	3	3	3	3	3	3
Proteins (g/kg)	2.5–3	3	3.5	3	3–3.5	3.5	3–3.5	3,5	3.5–4	3,5	4	3,5	4	3,5
Sodium (mEq/kg)	0	0	0	0	0	0	3	3	3	3	3,5	3.5	4	3.5–4
Potassium (mEq/kg)	0	0	0	0	0	0	2	2	2	2	2	2	3	2–4
Cloride (mEq/kg)	0	0	0	0	0	0	3	3	3	3	3.5	3.5	3.5-6	3.5–4
Calcium (mg/kg)	0	0	60	60	60	70	70	80	80	80	80	80	80	90
Phosphate (mg/kg)	0	0	30	30	30	40	40	50	50	55	55	60	60	70
Magnesium (mEq/kg)	0	0	0.5	0.5	0.5	1	0.5	1	0,5	1	0,5	1	0,5	1

Parenteral nutrition recommendation according to internal procedure (fluids, macronutrients and micronutrients).

Specifically, both donor pasteurized human milk and fresh mother's milk were analyzed using a mid-ray spectrometry human milk analyzer (Miris AB®).

Pooled donor human milk was created by mixing mature thawed human milk from 1 to 5 donors enrolled at the Human Milk Bank at the authors' institution. Analyses of fresh mother's milk were conducted two times/week using a 10-ml sample from a 24 h fresh milk pool. Analyses of donor human milk were conducted using a 10-ml sample from each pool after Holder pasteurization (62.5°C for 30 min) to account for macronutrient depletion due to storage and pasteurization (15). According to these results, the medical team prescribed individualized fortification to comply with the ESPGHAN nutrient intake guidelines (16).

Human milk fortification was performed using bovine human milk fortifiers: FM85 (Nestlè) or Aptamil BMF (Nutricia) as polymeric fortifiers, Aptamil PS (Nutricia) for protein supplementation, and medium-chain triglyceride (MCT) oil (Medifood) for energy provision.

Human milk intake was expressed as the volume of fortified donor human milk and/or fortified fresh mother's milk.

The percentage of human milk intake was computed from the volume of human milk intake compared with the total volume of milk intake during the hospital stay (fortified donor human milk+fortified fresh mother's milk+formula milk). In addition, the proportion of mothers' own milk within the total volume of human milk intake was computed (fresh mother's milk intake %).

Anthropometric Measurements

Body weight, body length and head circumference of all infants included in the study were assessed at birth and at term CA according to standard procedures (17, 18). In detail, a subject's body weight was measured on an electronic scale accurate to the nearest 0.1 g (PEA POD Infant Body Composition System; COSMED, Italy), body length was measured to the nearest mm using a recumbent infant length board, and head circumference was measured to the nearest 1 mm using a nonstretch measuring tape.

Infants with birth weights below the 10th percentile according to INTERGROWTH-21st reference curves (14) were categorized as small for gestational age (SGA).

The weight z-scores at birth and at discharge were calculated according to INTERGROWTH-21st reference and standard curves, respectively (14, 18).

The daily growth rate was calculated using the exponential regression model described by Patel et al. (19) as follows:

$$[1000 \times ln(W2/W1)]/(D2 - D1) \quad (1)$$

where W = weight in grams; D = day; 1 = beginning of the time interval; and 2=end of the time interval (19).

Body Composition Assessment

Body composition was assessed at term CA for all infants included in the study using an air-displacement plethysmography system (PEA POD Infant Body Composition System; COSMED, Italy) (20, 21). The PEA POD assesses FM and FFM by body mass and body volume measurements via the application of whole-body densitometric principles. Body density was computed from the study subject's measured mass and volume and then converted to indicate the total absolute (g) and percentage (%) of FM and FFM using sex-specific equations developed by Fomon et al. (22). The observers were health professionals trained to perform anthropometric and body composition measurements according to our standard procedure. The interobserver coefficient of variation for the FM percentage estimates was 0.3%.

Statistical Analysis

Continuous variables are reported as the mean and standard deviation (SD). Categorical variables are reported as absolute numbers or percentages. Comparisons between infants fed human milk (fresh mother's milk or donor human milk) at less than 50% of the total volume of milk intake during the hospital stay (group 1) and infants fed human milk at greater or equal to 50% of the total volume of milk intake during the hospital stay (group 2) were conducted using the X^2 test for discrete variables and analysis of variance for continuous variables.

TABLE 2 | Basic characteristics at birth of infants included.

	All infants (*n* = 73)	Group 1 (*n* = 24)	Group 2 (*n* = 49)	*p*
Weight (g)	1248 ± 198	1207 ± 208	1269 ± 193	0.215
Length (cm)	38.3 ± 2.8	37.7 ± 3.3	38.6 ± 2.6	0.278
Head Circumference (cm)	26.8 ± 1.9	26.5 ± 2.3	27.0 ± 1.7	0.358
Gestational age (weeks)	30.2 ± 2.0	30.0 ± 2.4	30.3 ± 1.8	0.632
Males: n (%)	32 (43.9)	10 (41.6)	22 (44.9)	0.797
Twins: n (%)	35 (48.5)	13 (54.1)	22 (44.9)	0.463
SGA infants n (%)	25 (34.2)	9 (37.5)	14 (28.6)	0.305
Antenatal steroids n (%)	70 (95.9)	23 (95.8)	47 (95.9)	0.704
Need of invasive ventilatory assistance n (%)	17 (23.3)	5 (20.8)	12 (24.5)	0.558
Duration of invasive ventilatory assistance (days)	0.88 ± 2.0	0.61 ± 1.7	1.0 ± 2.1	0.446
Need of non-invasive ventilatory assistance n (%)	41 (56.1)	15 (62.5)	26 (53.1)	0.558
Duration of invasive ventilatory assistance (days)	20.94 ± 21.0	19.74 ± 23.7	21.53 ± 19.8	0.741

Data are expressed as mean ± standard deviation or n (%). The duration of ventilatory assistance were expressed as days of treatment.

TABLE 3 | Milk volume intake during hospital stay.

	All infants (*n* = 73)	Group 1 (*n* = 24)	Group 2 (*n* = 49)	*p*
Total Milk volume intake (ml)	10357.1 ± 5871.7	11713.1 ± 7756.7	9692.9 ± 4638.5	0.169
Human milk daily intake (ml/day)	118.2 ± 47.3	65.6 ± 25.9	144.0 ± 31.2	<0.001
Human milk volume intake (ml)	6385.4 ± 3498.9	3998.6 ± 2590.8	7554.4 ± 3302.1	<0.001
Human milk volume intake (%)	65.8 ± 26.1	34.9 ± 12.5	80.9 ± 15.5	<0.001
Fresh mother milk intake (%)	64.7 ± 42.6	41.9 ± 43.7	75.9 ± 37.6	0.001

Data are expressed as mean ± standard deviation. The percentage of human milk intake was computed from the volume of human milk intake compared with the total volume of milk intake during the hospital stay (fortified donor human milk + fortified fresh mother's milk+formula milk). Fresh mother milk intake (%) is the proportion of mothers' own milk within the total volume of human milk.

TABLE 4 | Weight z-score and daily growth rate during hospital stay.

	All infants (*n* = 73)	Group 1 (*n* = 24)	Group 2 (*n* = 49)	*p*
Birth weight z-score	−0.60 ± 0.97	−0.61 ± 1.2	−0.59 ± 0.84	0.941
Weight at discharge z-score	−1.26 ± 1.01	−1.14 ± 1.27	−1.32 ± 0.87	0.504
Daily growth rate during parenteral nutrition (g/kg/day)	20.23 ± 5.38	21.99 ± 4.35	19.4 ± 5.67	0.051
Daily growth rate during full enteral feeding (g/kg/day)	15.32 ± 8.06	18.65 ± 12.24	13.70 ± 4.17	0.013
Total daily growth rate during hospital stay (g/kg/day)	16.07 ± 2.42	17.30 ± 2.74	15.46 ± 2.01	0.002

Data are expressed as mean ± standard deviation. The daily growth rates were calculated during the administration of parenteral nutrition, after reaching full enteral feeding (milk volume intake ≥150 ml/kg/day) and during all the hospital stay.

Multiple linear regression analyses were conducted to explore the role of fortified human milk in modulating fat-free mass at term CA according to sex and birth weight. Indeed, it has been reported that gender can influence body composition at term CA (23).

Statistical significance was set at a level of 0.05. All statistical analyses were performed using SPSS software (SPSS, version 20; SPSS, Chicago, IL).

RESULTS

Seventy-three VLBW infants were included in the study. The basic characteristics at birth are shown in **Table 2.** No differences were detectable at birth between the two study groups.

The infants included in the study received parenteral nutrition for 21.9 ± 9.0 days, and full enteral feeding was achieved at 28.9 ± 9.0 days of life; no differences were found between the two groups.

Data regarding human milk intake (fresh mother's milk and/or pasteurized donor human milk) are shown in **Table 3.**

The mean energy and protein intake were 65.7 ± 16.4 Kcal/kg/day and 2.9 g/kg/day during the first week of life, 124.8 ± 13.8 kcal/kg/day and 3.3 ± 0.7 g/kg/day when full enteral feeding was achieved, and 130.8 ± 14.2 kcal/kg/day and 3.6 ± 0.6 g/kg/day at discharge, respectively. No differences in energy and protein intake between the two study groups were detectable during the hospital stay.

The weight z-score at birth and at discharge and the daily growth rates are shown in **Table 4.**

No differences were found in weight z-score at birth or at discharge between the two groups. Group 1 had a higher growth rate than group 2 both after reaching full enteral feeding (milk volume intake≥150 ml/kg/day) and during the entire hospital stay.

The incidence of comorbidities developed during hospitalization was similar in group 1 and group 2. Among all infants included in the study, none developed NEC, 9.6% had cholestasis, 5.5% had bronchopulmonary dysplasia, 9.6% received treatment for patent ductus arteriosus, and 17.8% had sepsis.

The characteristics at discharge and at term CA according to the mode of feeding are shown in **Tables 5, 6.** No differences were found between the two groups regarding the anthropometric measurements and body composition at discharge or at term CA. The infants included in the study achieved the ability to feed orally beginning at 36.4 ± 1.4 weeks of postmenstrual age. No differences were found between groups.

Multiple logistic regression analysis showed that there was a positive association between the human milk volume intake percentage and fat-free mass percentage after correction for birth weight and gender (β = 0.12 ± 0.05, *p* = 0.01). Specifically, the regression model showed that being fed with human milk at more than or equal to 50% of total milk intake was associated

TABLE 5 | Characteristics at discharge according to mode of feeding.

	All infants ($n = 73$)	Group 1 ($n = 24$)	Group 2 ($n = 49$)	p
Weight (g)	2404 ± 424	2471 ± 514	2371 ± 373	0.349
Length (cm)	45.1 ± 2.2	45.3 ± 2.2	44.9 ± 2.2	0.544
Head Circumference (cm)	32.0 ± 2.0	32.2 ± 1.7	31.9 ± 2.1	0.604
Postmenstrual age (weeks)	37.7 ± 1.5	37.8 ± 1.4	37.6 ± 1.6	0.470
Length of stay (days)	51.9 ± 18.5	52.8 ± 19.4	51.4 ± 18.1	0.763

Data are expressed as mean ± standard deviation.

TABLE 6 | Anthropometric measurements and body composition at term corrected age according to mode of feeding.

	All infants ($n = 73$)	Group 1 ($n = 24$)	Group 2 ($n = 49$)	p
Weight (g)	3088 ± 476	3142 ± 628	3062 ± 386	0.506
Length (cm)	48.5 ± 2.3	48.4 ± 2.7	48.6 ± 2.1	0.774
Head Circumference (cm)	34.6 ± 1.3	34.4 ± 1.7	34.7 ± 1.1	0.346
Fat free mass (%)	82.0 ± 11.1	78.6 ± 18.1	83.7 ± 4.5	0.067

Data were expressed ad mean ± standard deviation.

TABLE 7 | Multiple regression analysis model for fat free mass %.

	Beta coefficients	95% Interval of confidence	p
Intercept	95.518 ± 7.876	79.805; 111.231	<0.001
Being male (no vs. yes)	4.396 ± 2.481	−0.552; 9.345	0.081
Birth weight (g)	−0.01 ± 0.006	−0.028; −0.003	0.016
Being fed human milk ≥50% (no vs. yes)	5.883 ± 2.638	0.621; 11.146	0.029

Multiple regression analysis model corrected by gender and birth weight. Being fed with human milk more than or equal to 50% was positively associated with a significant increase in fat free mass percentage at term CA.

with a significant increase in fat-free mass percentage at term CA (**Table 7**).

DISCUSSION

This study examined the relationship between the type of feeding and body composition in VLBW infants. Specifically, we demonstrated that VLBW infants fed human milk (both fresh mother's milk and/or donor human milk) at more than or equal to 50% of the total milk volume intake during the hospital stay displayed an increased fat-free mass percentage at term CA compared to VLBW infants fed human milk at less than 50% of the total milk intake.

Johnson et al. demonstrated that VLBW infants had a fat-free mass deficit at term CA compared to full-term infants (24). Increasing evidence has demonstrated that greater fat-free mass deposition is associated with an improved neurodevelopmental outcome (25). A study conducted at our center demonstrated that human milk feeding is positively associated with fat-free mass deposition in late preterm infants (8).

Our results showed that infants fed human milk at less than 50% of the total milk intake had a higher growth rate than their counterparts. On the other hand, the weight and weight z-score at discharge were similar between the two groups. It must be noted that most of the infants fed fresh mother's milk were in group 2, and consequently, the higher number of breastfed infants can explain the lower growth rate in these infants than in formula-fed infants. Indeed, after reaching full enteral feeding and, above all, after reaching the ability to feed orally, breastfed infants cannot receive adequate fortification from feedings taken directly from the breast. A similar weight was found at term CA between the two groups. Indeed, considering the weight increase percentage between discharge and term CA, infants in group 2 show a slightly higher value than those in group 1 (+31.4 vs. 28.3%), probably due to better adaptation of group 2 infants than group 1 infants after discharge.

To the best of our knowledge, this was the first study to explore the modulating effect of both fresh mother's milk and donor human milk on body composition. In a previous study conducted in our center, Morlacchi et al. demonstrated that preterm infants fed fortified mother's own milk showed a higher percentage of fat-free mass than formula-fed infants at term CA, which was probably due to the higher nitrogen balance in breastfed infants than in formula-fed infants (12). In our study, we did not evaluate infant nitrogen balance; however, we can speculate that being fed both fortified fresh mother's milk and/or donor human milk can result in a similar metabolic response to that obtained by feeding exclusively fresh mother's milk. In addition, in the univariate regression analysis, the percentage of fresh mother's milk intake was not associated with FFM deposition, whereas the total human milk volume intake was positively associated with the FFM percentage at term CA. This observation can most likely be explained by the relatively low percentage of fresh human milk ingested by infants included in the study.

It has been reported that exclusive breastfeeding is associated with lower growth rates in preterm infants than formula feeding (26), especially with standard fortification of human milk (27). In fact, the mean protein content decreases during lactation, while the nutrient needs of VLBW infants remain high (28, 29). In addition, although it has been reported that donor human milk provides nutrients comparable to mother's milk, preterm infants fed donor human milk fortified similarly to fresh mother's milk according to standard methods showed an increased risk of postnatal growth restriction (30, 31). In contrast, it has been reported that fortification of donor human milk to reach 3.5 g/kg of protein intake is associated with significantly greater weight gain and head growth in VLBW infants than feeding a formula-based diet (30). In addition, targeted fortification of human milk seems to represent an optimal strategy to prevent postnatal growth restriction (32, 33).

According to our internal procedure, when infants tolerated an enteral intake of human milk (both fresh mother's milk and/or donor human milk) ≥80 ml/kg/day, targeted human milk fortification is initiated to meet the ESPGHAN guidelines. Consequently, infants fed fortified human milk at more than or equal to 50% of the total milk volume intake during the hospital stay exhibited similar growth at discharge as infants fed less human milk.

In a recent study of 34 VLBW infants (11 breastfed and 23 formula-fed) compared with a control group of 19 full-term infants, it was demonstrated that formula-fed infants were heavier than breastfed infants at term CA and showed higher amounts of adipose tissue and lower amounts of fat-free mass than full-term infants. However, breastfed preterm infants had a similar body composition as full-term infants (34, 35).

In our study, we did not observe any difference in body weight between the two groups, irrespective of the type of feeding, both at discharge and at term CA. Nevertheless, infants in group 2 who were fed ~81% human milk during their hospital stay had an increased fat-free mass at term CA compared with infants in group 1 who were fed only 35% human milk from birth to discharge.

It has been taken into account that in our study, the donor human milk constituted 58% and 25% of the total amount of human milk intake in group 1 and group 2, respectively. This detail underlines the important effect of fresh mother's milk on growth and quality of growth but suggests that donor human milk is preferred over formula milk when fresh mother's milk is not available or is insufficient to satisfy the infant's nutritional needs. Therefore, the strength of the study was the use of donor human milk to supplement fresh mother's milk and the practice of targeted fortification to achieve the nutritional needs of preterm infants.

It must also be taken into account that the infants included in this study were all clinically stable at term CA during the assessment of body composition, and therefore, the results obtained in this study cannot be applied to sick infants. In addition, a limitation of the study is that it is not a randomized controlled trial, although this type of study design has ethical issues.

In conclusion, the use of target fortified human milk modulated the growth of and improved the quality of growth in vulnerable preterm infants. The use of fortified donor human milk when fresh mother's milk is insufficient or not available should be encouraged.

AUTHOR CONTRIBUTIONS

PP and NL conceived and designed the study and wrote the article. DoM, CT, and MP collected the data and were responsible for database management. MG, CM, AO, DaM, and OA performed the clinical evaluations and contributed to the discussion of the results and PR, VP, and FM provided suggestions concerning the content and concept of the article and were responsible for critically revising the manuscript.

REFERENCES

1. Maffei D, Schanler RJ. Human milk is the feeding strategy to prevent necrotizing enterocolitis! *Semin Perinatol.* (2017) 41:36–40. doi: 10.1053/j.semperi.2016.09.016
2. Cacho NT, Parker LA, Neu, J. Necrotizing enterocolitis and human milk feeding: a systematic review. *Clin Perinatol.* (2017) 44:49–67. doi: 10.1016/j.clp.2016.11.009
3. Miller J, Tonkin E, Damarell RA, McPhee AJ, Suganuma M, Suganuma H, et al. A systematic review and meta-analysis of human milk feeding and morbidity in very low birth weight infants. *Nutrients* (2018) 10:6 doi: 10.3390/nu10060707
4. Committee on nutrition; Section on breastfeeding; Committee on fetus and newborn. Donor Human Milk for the High-Risk Infant: Preparation, Safety, and Usage Options in the United States. *Pediatrics* (2017) 139:1. doi: 10.1542/peds.2016-3440
5. Parker MG, Burnham L, Mao W, Philipp BL, Merewood, A. Implementation of a donor milk program is associated with greater consumption of Mothers' own milk among VLBW Infants in a US, Level 3 NICU. *J Hum Lact.* (2016) 32:221–8. doi: 10.1177/0890334415598305
6. Villamor-Martínez E, Pierro M, Cavallaro G, Mosca F, Kramer BW, Villamor, E. Donor human milk protects against bronchopulmonary dysplasia: a systematic review and meta-analysis. *Nutrients* (2018) 10:2. doi: 10.3390/nu10020238
7. Quigley M, McGuire W. Formula versus donor breast milk for feeding preterm or low birth weight infants. *Cochrane Database Syst Rev.* (2014) 2014:CD002971. doi: 10.1002/14651858.CD002971.pub3
8. Giannì ML, Consonni D, Liotto N, Roggero P, Morlacchi L, Piemontese, P. et al. Does human milk modulate body composition in late preterm infants at term-corrected age? *Nutrients* (2016) 8:E664. doi: 10.3390/nu8100664
9. Huang P, Zhou J, Yin Y, Jing W, Luo B, Wang, J. Effects of breast-feeding compared with formula-feeding on preterm infant body composition: a systematic review and meta-analysis. *Br J Nutr.* (2016) 116:132–41. doi: 10.1017/S0007114516001720
10. Cooke RJ, Griffin IJ, McCormick, K. Adiposity is not altered in preterm infants fed with a nutrient-enriched formula after hospital discharge. *Pediatr Res.* (2010) 67:660–4. doi: 10.1203/PDR.0b013e3181da8d01
11. Gale C, Logan KM, Santhakumaran S, Parkinson JRC, Hyde MJ, Modi, N. Effect of breastfeeding compared with formula feeding on infant body composition: a systematic review and meta-analysis. *Am J Clin Nutr.* (2012) 95:656–69. doi: 10.3945/ajcn.111.027284
12. Morlacchi L, Roggero P, Giannì ML, Bracco B, Porri D, Battiato E, et al. Protein use and weight-gain quality in very-low-birth-weight preterm infants fed human milk or formula. *Am J Clin Nutr.* (2018) 107:195–200. doi: 10.1093/ajcn/nqx001
13. Engle WA. American academy of paediatrics committee on foetus and newborn. Age terminology during the perinatal period. *Paediatrics* (2004) 114:1362–4. doi: 10.1542/peds.2004-1915
14. Villar J, Giuliani F, Fenton TR, Ohuma EO, Ismail LC, Kennedy SH. Intergrowth-21st Consortium. Intergrowth-21st very preterm size at birth reference charts. *Lancet* (2016) 387:844–45. doi: 10.1016/S0140-6736(16)00384-6
15. Vieira AA, Soares FV, Pimenta HP, Abranches AD, Moreira, M.E. Analysis of the influence of pasteurization, freezing/thawing, and offer processes on human milk's macronutrient concentrations. *Early Hum Dev.* (2011) 87:577–80. doi: 10.1016/j.earlhumdev.2011.04.016
16. Agostoni C, Buonocore G, Carnielli VP, De Curtis M, Darmaun D, Decsi, T. et al. Enteral nutrient supply for preterm infants: commentary from the European Society of Paediatric Gastroenterology, Hepatology and Nutrition Committee on Nutrition. *J Pediatr Gastroenterol Nutr.* (2010) 50:85–91. doi: 10.1097/MPG.0b013e3181adaee0
17. Agostoni C, Grandi F, Giannì ML, Silano M, Torcoletti M, Giovannini M, et al. Growth patterns of breast fed and formula fed infants in the first 12 months of life: an Italian study. *Arch Dis Child* (1999) 81:395–9.
18. Villar J, Cheikh IL, Victora CG, Ohuma EO, Bertino, E, Altman DG, et al. International standards for newborn weight, length, and head circumference by gestational age and sex: the Newborn Cross-Sectional Study of the INTERGROWTH-21st Project. *Lancet* (2014) 384:857–68. doi: 10.1016/S0140-6736(14)60932-6

19. Patel AL, Engstrom JL, Meier PP, Jegier BJ, Kimura RE. Calculating postnatal growth velocity in very low birth weight (VLBW) premature infants. *J Perinatol.* (2009) 29:618–22. doi: 10.1038/jp.2009.55
20. Ma G, Yao M, Liu Y, Lin A, Zou H, Urlando A, et al. Validation of a new paediatric air displacement plethysmograph for assessing body composition in infants. *Am J Clin Nutr.* (2004) 79:653–60. doi: 10.1093/ajcn/79.4.653
21. Ellis KJ, Yao M, Shypailo RJ, Urlando A, Wong WW, Heird WC. Body composition assessment in infancy: air-displacement plethysmography compared with a reference 4-compartment model. *Am J Clin Nutr.* (2007) 85:90–5. doi: 10.1093/ajcn/85.1.90
22. Fomon SJ, Haschke F, Ziegler EE, Nelson SE. Body composition of reference children from birth to age 10 years. *Am J Clin Nutr.* (1982) 35:1169–75. doi: 10.1093/ajcn/35.5.1169
23. Liotto N, Roggero P, Bracco B, Menis C, Morniroli D, Perrone M, Giannì ML, Mosca F. Can basic characteristics estimate body composition in early infancy? *J Pediatr Gastroenterol Nutr.* (2018) 66:e76–e80. doi: 10.1097/MPG.0000000000001758
24. Johnson MJ, Wootton SA, Leaf AA, Jackson AA. Preterm birth and body composition at term equivalent age: a systematic review and meta-analysis. *Pediatrics* (2012) 130:e640–9. doi: 10.1542/peds.2011-3379
25. Ramel SE, Gray HL, Christiansen E, Boys C, Georgieff MK, Demerath EW. Greater early gains in fat-free mass, but not fat mass, are associated with improved neurodevelopment at 1 year corrected age for prematurity in very low birth weight preterm infants. *J Pediatr.* (2016) 173:108–15. doi: 10.1016/j.jpeds.2016.03.003
26. Spiegler J, Preuß M, Gebauer C, Bendiks M, Herting E, Göpel W. On behalf of the german neonatal network. does breastmilk influence the development of bronchopulmonary dysplasia? *J Pediatr.* (2016) 169:76–80. doi: 10.1016/j.jpeds.2015.10.080
27. Corvaglia L, Aceti A, Paoletti V, Mariani E, Patrono D, Ancora G, et al. Standard fortification of preterm human milk fails to meet recommended protein intake: bedside evaluation by near-infrared-reflectance-analysis. *Early Hum Dev.* (2010) 86:237–40. doi: 10.1016/j.earlhumdev.2010.04.001
28. Gidrewicz DA, Fenton TR. A systematic review and meta-analysis of the nutrient content of preterm and term breast milk. *BMC Pediatr.* (2014) 14:216. doi: 10.1186/1471-2431-14-216
29. Ziegler EE. Breast-milk fortification. *Acta Paediatr.* (2001) 90:720–3. doi: 10.1111/j.1651-2227.2001.tb02795.x
30. Newkirk M, Shakeel F, Parimi P, Rothpletz-Puglia P, Patusco R, Marcus AF, et al. Comparison of calorie and protein intake of very low birth weight infants receiving mother's own milk or donor milk when the nutrient composition of human milk is measured with a breast milk analyzer. *Nutr Clin Pract.* (2018) 33:679–86. doi: 10.1002/ncp.10060
31. Brownell EA, Matson AP, Smith KC, Moore JE, Esposito PA, Lussier MM, et al. Dose-response relationship between donor human milk, Mother's own milk, preterm formula, and neonatal growth outcomes. *J Pediatr Gastroenterol Nutr.* (2018) 67:90–6. doi: 10.1097/MPG.0000000000001959
32. Ginovart G, Gich I, Gutiérrez A, Verd, S. A fortified donor milk policy is associated with improved in-hospital head growth and weight gain in very low-birth-weight infants. *Adv Neonatal Care* (2017) 17:250–7. doi: 10.1097/ANC.0000000000000387
33. Rochow N, Fusch G, Choi A, Chessell L, Elliott L, McDonald K, et al. Target fortification of breast milk with fat, protein, and carbohydrates for preterm infants. *J Pediatr.* (2013) 163:1001–7. doi: 10.1016/j.jpeds.2013.04.052
34. Morlacchi L, Mallardi D, Giannì ML, Roggero P, Amato O, Piemontese P, et al. Is targeted fortification of human breast milk an optimal nutrition strategy for preterm infants? An interventional study. *J Transl Med.* (2016) 14:195. doi: 10.1186/s12967-016-0957-y
35. Nina M, Magdalena Z, Przemko K. Does type of feeding affect body composition in very low birth weight infants? - A prospective cohort study. *Pediatr Neonatol.* (2018). doi: 10.1016/j.pedneo.2018.04.010. [Epub ahead of print].

2

High Temperature—Short Time Pasteurization has a Lower Impact on the Antiviral Properties of Human Milk than Holder Pasteurization

*Manuela Donalisio [1], Massimo Rittà [1], Rachele Francese [1], Andrea Civra [1], Paola Tonetto [2], Alessandra Coscia [2], Marzia Giribaldi [3,4], Laura Cavallarin [3], Guido E. Moro [5], Enrico Bertino [2] and David Lembo [1]**

[1] Laboratory of Molecular Virology, Department of Clinical and Biological Sciences, University of Turin, Turin, Italy, [2] Neonatal Intensive Care Unit, Department of Public Health and Pediatrics, University of Turin, Turin, Italy, [3] Consiglio Nazionale delle Ricerche-Istituto di Scienze delle Produzioni Alimentari, Bari, Italy, [4] Consiglio per la Ricerca in Agricoltura e l'Analisi dell'Economia Agraria, Centro di Ricerca in Ingegneria e Trasformazioni Agroalimentari, Turin, Italy, [5] Italian Association of Human Milk Banks, Milan, Italy

***Correspondence:**
David Lembo
david.lembo@unito.it

Holder pasteurization (62. 5°C for 30 min) is recommended by all international human milk bank guidelines to prevent infections potentially transmitted by donor human milk. A drawback is that it affects some human milk bioactive and nutritive components. Recently, High Temperature-Short Time (HTST) pasteurization has been reported to be a valuable alternative technology to increase the retention of some biological features of human milk. Nevertheless, to date, few data are available about the impact of pasteurization methods other than Holder on the antiviral activity of human milk. The present study was aimed at evaluating the antiviral activity of human milk against a panel of viral pathogens common in newborns and children (i.e., herpes simplex virus 1 and 2, cytomegalovirus, respiratory syncytial virus, rotavirus, and rhinovirus), and at assessing the effect of Holder and HTST pasteurization on milk's antiviral properties. The results indicate that human milk is endowed with antiviral activity against all viruses tested, although to a different extent. Unlike the Holder pasteurization, HTST preserved the inhibitory activity against cytomegalovirus, respiratory syncytial virus, rotavirus and herpes simplex virus type 2. By contrast, both methods reduced significantly the antiviral activities against rhinovirus and herpes simplex virus type 1. Unexpectedly, Holder pasteurization improved milk's anti-rotavirus activity. In conclusion, this study contributes to the definition of the pasteurization method that allows the best compromise between microbiological safety and biological quality of the donor human milk: HTST pasteurization preserved milk antiviral activity better than Holder.

Keywords: human milk, HTST, Holder, antiviral activity, virus, pasteurization

INTRODUCTION

A mother's own milk is the first choice for improving the short- and long-term outcomes for all newborns, including preterm infants (1, 2). When a mother's own milk is unavailable or in short supply, a common occurrence in Neonatal Intensive Care Units, the World Health Organization and the American Academy of Pediatrics recommend the use of donor milk (DM) as the best alternative (2, 3). Human milk (HM) can be considered a species-specific dynamic biological system, known to encompass many kinds of biological functions, including antimicrobial and antiviral properties (2). It is generally agreed that breastfeeding reduces the rate of serious gastroenteritis, especially caused by rotaviruses (HRoVs), and infant respiratory infections, as well as otitis media. The main viruses involved in infant respiratory and middle ear infections are respiratory syncytial virus (RSV) and rhinoviruses (HRhV) (4–7). Furthermore, most herpetic infections are acquired during childhood and their infection is lifelong. The vast majority of herpes simplex virus 1 (HSV-1) infections are oral-labial herpes and they are mainly transmitted by oral-to-oral contact. By contrast, neonatal herpes can occur when an infant is exposed to herpes simplex virus 2 (HSV-2) in the genital tract during delivery. The risk for neonatal herpes is greatest when a mother acquires HSV infection for the first time in late pregnancy (8). Human cytomegalovirus (HCMV) is another herpesvirus, responsible for the most common congenital infection worldwide, affecting 1 out of every 150 live-born infants worldwide (9).

Several specific bioactive and immunomodulatory factors play a role in the milk-mediated defense system against viral infections, including milk proteins, as lactoferrin, lactadherin, lactoperoxidase, lysozyme, and secretory immunoglobulins A (sIgA), but also mucins, sulfated glycolipids, glycosaminoglycans and vitamin A (6, 10–12). Despite the presence of protective factors in HM, some viruses, as human immunodeficiency virus type 1, human T-lymphotrophic virus, zikavirus, and HCMV, are transmitted from mother to infant thus the heat treatment of DM is mandatory in human milk banks (HMBs) to guarantee microbiological safety (13). The ESPGHAN Committee on Nutrition has recently advised that "future research should focus on the improvement of milk processing in HMBs, particularly of heat treatment" (14). Currently, a pasteurization process at 62.5°C for 30 min (the Holder pasteurization method, HoP) is recommended in all international guidelines for the constitution of HMBs (13, 15). However, literature indicates that HoP affects several milk components to variable degrees, with a marked effect on milk protein content and activity (16, 17). Therefore, HMBs and researchers are committed to developing novel or enhanced methods to process DM that can ensure microbial inactivation, while improving the preservation of its nutritional, immunological, and functional constituents (14). High Temperature Short Time pasteurization (HTST) was the first non-HoP technique tested to improve the nutritional and immunological quality of milk, because it has been established in the dairy industry since the 1930s. HTST in food industry is usually performed by heating thin-layered milk in continuous flow systems at 72°C for 15 seconds, although high variability on the processing equipment and conditions was recently observed for HTST when applied to HM pasteurization (18). On the basis of the existing evidence, a new small-scale continuous-flow HTST pasteurizer was recently designed and validated for treating HM by our group (19).

The present research is aimed at assessing whether and to which extent HoP and HTST have an effect on the antiviral properties of raw HM against a panel of viral pathogens causing diseases in newborns and children, as HSV-1, HSV-2, HCMV, RSV, HRhV, and HRoV.

MATERIALS AND METHODS

HM Samples Collection

HM samples were obtained from the HMB of the Città della Salute e della Scienza of Turin, Italy. An ethical review process was not required for this study, because it was not a clinical trial. Each milk donor involved in this research signed a written consent form, where mother's and infant's data protection was assured. Besides, donors where informed that only milk samples stored in excess to the needs of their infants should have been used for research purposes explaining the study design. Two pools of milk were obtained on two different occasions. Both pools (final volume 250 ml) included colostrum (days 1–5 postpartum), transitional milk (days 6–14 postpartum), and mature milk (beyond day 15 postpartum). Each pool contained milk samples from three donors. The donors of the first pool were different from those of the second pool. The donors cleaned their hands and breasts according to the Italian HMB guidelines (13). The milk specimens were collected in sterile bisphenol-free polypropylene bottles using a breast pump and stored by the HMB at −20°C until processed. The individual specimens were thawed overnight in refrigerated conditions, and then pooled rapidly in the morning in the HMB, and shipped refrigerated within 1 h. Upon arrival, pooled samples were processed according to the appropriate technique, and immediately separated in 10-ml aliquots, which were conveyed to the analyzing laboratory within 1 h. Raw milk was also aliquoted immediately after collection and stored as fresh and/or frozen material, as required.

Milk Pasteurization

The milk samples were processed using either HoP or HTST system. HoP was performed directly in sterile bisphenol-free polypropylene bottles using a standard HM pasteurizer (Metalarredinox, BG, Italy). HTST was performed using a patented proprietary device (European Patent n° 2974603), as previously described (19, 20). HTST-pasteurized milk was collected in sterile bisphenol-free polypropylene bottles. Four mL from each sample were skimmed by centrifugation at 2,000 g for 30 min at 4°C in sterile tubes (Eppendorf S.r.l, Milan, Italy), and then shipped refrigerated within 1 h to the laboratory for antiviral assays.

Cells

African green monkey kidney cells (Vero) (ATCC CCL-81) and human epithelial cells Hep-2 (ATCC CCL-23) were grown as monolayers in Eagle's minimal essential medium (MEM) (Gibco/BRL) supplemented with heat-inactivated 10% fetal calf serum (FCS) (Gibco/BRL) and 1% antibiotic-antimycotic solution (Zell Shield, Minerva Biolab) at 37°C in an atmosphere of 5% of CO_2. Human Foreskin Fibroblasts (HFF-1) (ATCC SCRC-1041) at low-passage-number (<30), African green monkey kidney epithelial cells (MA104) and human epithelial adenocarcinoma HeLa cells (ATCC CCL-2) were propagated in Dulbecco's Modified Eagle's Medium (DMEM) (Sigma-Aldrich) supplemented with FCS and antibiotic-antimycotic solution.

Viruses

The neurovirulent strains LV (21) and MS (ATCC VR-540) of HSV-1 and HSV-2, were propagated in Vero cells at 37°C (22). HRhV 1A (ATCC VR-1559) was propagated in HeLa cells, at 33°C. HSV-1, HSV-2, and HRhV titers were determined by the standard plaque method and expressed as plaque-forming unit (PFU)/ml. A bacterial artificial chromosome (BAC)-derived HCMV strain Towne incorporating the green fluorescent protein (GFP) sequence (23) was propagated on HFF-1 and viral titres were determined by fluorescent focus assay. RSV strain A2 (ATCC VR-1540) was propagated in Hep-2 and titrated by the indirect immunoperoxidase staining procedure using an RSV monoclonal antibody (Ab35958, Abcam) (24). Human HRoV strain Wa (ATCC VR-2018) was activated with 5 μg/ml of porcine pancreatic trypsin type IX (Sigma) for 30 min at 37°C and propagated in MA104 cells by using MEM containing 0.5 μg of trypsin per ml. HCMV, RSV and HRoV titers were expressed as focus-forming units (FFU)/ml. Virus stocks were maintained frozen (-80°C).

Viral Inhibition Assay

Antiviral activity of milk samples was determined by plaque reduction assays for HSV-1, HSV-2, and HRhV and by focus reduction assays for HCMV, RSV, and HRoV. Antiviral assays were performed by incubating serial dilutions of milk (from 1/1 to 1/1024 parts in medium) with virus for 1 h at 37 °C and then the mixtures were added to cells for 2 h at 37°C. After three washings with medium, monolayers were overlaid with 1.2%-methylcellulose medium with 2% FCS. The effect on HSV and HRhV infections was evaluated on pre-seeded Vero or Hela cells (10×10^4) respectively, in 24-well plates infected with 200 PFU/well of HSV or 30 PFU/well of HRhV; after incubation for 24 h (HSV-2 and HRhV) or 48 h (HSV-1) cells were fixed and stained with 0.1% crystal violet in 20% ethanol and viral plaques were counted. The mean plaque count for each sample dilution was expressed as a percentage of the mean plaque count of the control (25). In HCMV inhibition assay, cells pre-seeded in 96-well plates at a density of 5.0×10^3/well, were infected with 140 PFU/well of GFP-coding HCMV. After 5-day-incubation at 37°C 5% CO_2 atmosphere, infected cells were visualized as green fibroblasts using fluorescence microscopy and counted. In RSV and HRoV inhibition assays, Hep-2 cells and MA104 were pre-seeded at a density of 1×10^4/well and 1.4×10^4, respectively, in 96-well plates. Cells were infected with 60 PFU/well of RSV or 200 PFU/well of HRoV and, after 16 h (HRoV) or 3 days post-infection (RSV), infected cells were fixed with cold methanol and acetone for 1 min and subjected to virus-specific immunostaining as described previously (26, 27). Fluorescent and immunostained viral foci were microscopically counted and results were reported as percentages of foci in comparison to controls. The endpoints of the assays were the effective milk dilution that reduced the viral plaque/focus formation by 50% (inhibitory dilution-50, ID50) in comparison to that in the untreated control. The ID50 of milk was calculated by using the program PRISM 4 (GraphPad Software) to fit a variable slope-sigmoidal dose–response curve. All data were generated from duplicate wells in at least three independent experiments on each HM pool.

Cell Viability Assay

Cell viability was measured by the MTS [3-(4,5-dimethylthiazol-2-yl)-5-(3-carboxymethoxyphenyl)-2-(4-sulfophenyl)-2H-tetrazolium] assay. Confluent cell cultures seeded in 96-well plates were incubated with different dilutions of milk in triplicate under the same experimental conditions described for the antiviral assays. Cell viability was determined by the CellTiter 96 Proliferation Assay Kit (Promega) according to the manufacturer's instructions. Absorbances were measured using a Microplate Reader (Model 680, BIORAD) at 490 nm. Their effect on cell viability at different milk dilutions was expressed as a percentage, by comparing the absorbances of treated cells with that of the cells incubated with culture medium alone. The 50%-cytotoxic dilutions (CD50) and 95% confidence intervals (CIs) were determined with Prism 4 software.

Statistical Analysis

Statistical analysis was performed using Extra sum-of-square F test as reported in legends of figures, on GraphPad software. Significance was reported for $p < 0.05$.

RESULTS AND DISCUSSION

Antiviral Activity of HM

This paper reports on the antiviral activity of raw milk and investigates the impact of two pasteurization techniques on such biological property. The first set of experiments was dedicated to assess the antiviral activity of two HM raw milk pools against a panel of viral pathogens causing diseases in newborns and children, and representing different viral structures and families: enveloped DNA viruses, as HSV-1, HSV-2, and HCMV (*Herpesviridae* family); enveloped RNA viruses, as RSV (*Paramyxoviridae* family); naked single strand RNA virus, as HRhV (*Picornaviridae* family); naked double strand RNA virus, as HRoV (*Reoviridae* family). **Figure 1A** reports the antiviral activity of the two HM pools, expressed as ID50, i.e., the dilution of milk sample inhibiting the 50% of infectivity. The results revealed that both pools exhibited antiviral activity against all viruses with ID50 ranging from 0.010 to 0.183. As for the viruses belonging to the *Herpesviridae* family, both pools exhibited a similar antiviral activity against HCMV, whereas a statistically significant difference in anti-HSV-1 and anti-HSV-2 activity was observed ($p < 0.05$). These results confirm previous findings that HM samples were endowed with anti-HCMV activity, although to a different extent from sample to sample and from mother to mother (6, 28). Our data evidenced a high activity against HSV-1 and HSV-2, in contrast with other studies that observed weak or no antiviral effect (29–31) for raw HM, whereas, when HM samples were aspirated from the stomachs of the infants within few hours of feeding, they were reported to reduce HSV-1 titers (31). The observed inhibitory activity of milk pools with ID50 around of 0.01 against RSV and 0.05 against HRhV supports

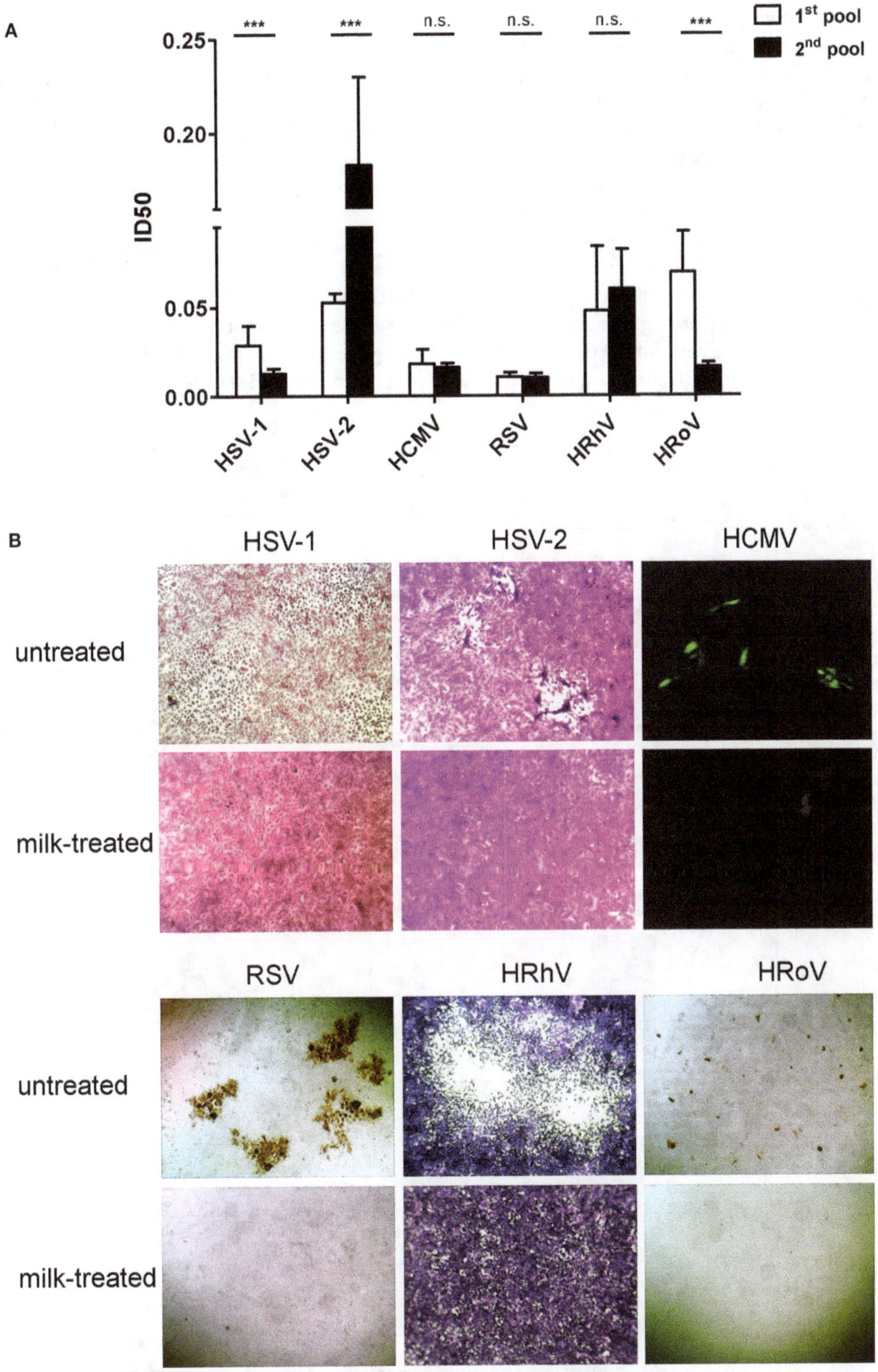

FIGURE 1 | (A) Antiviral activities against HSV-1, HSV-2, HCMV, RSV, HRhV, and HRoV are reported as inhibitory dilution-50 (ID50) values for raw human milk pool #1 (white) and pool #2 (black bar). Data are reported as mean ID50 ± 95% confidence intervals of 4 independent experiments. ID50 values were compared using the sum-of-squares *F*-test. ***$P < 0.001$; n.s., not significant. **(B)** Representative examples of plaque reduction assays and fluorescence foci assays of antiviral assays treating infected cells with raw milk samples at a 1:2 dilution, an inhibitory dilution-100 (ID100) for all viruses. Untreated infected (upper row) and milk-treated infected (lower row) fields are reported for HSV-1, HSV-2, HCMV, RSV, HRhV, and HRoV. HSV-1, HSV-2 and HRhV plaques were visualized after crystal violet staining; RSV and HRoV foci were visualized by ICC (magnification 40X). HCMV fluorescent foci were visually counted as green cells at fluorescence microscopy (magnification 100X). HSV-1, HSV-2, and HRhV plaques are violet; HCMV infected cells are green; RSV and HRoV foci are brown.

clinical observations that maternal milk protects infants against respiratory infections, as bronchiolitis, during the first year of life, and encourages breastfeeding as an effective/inexpensive measure of prevention of lower respiratory tract infections in infancy (32, 33). However, a variable antiviral activity of HM was observed against different HRhV serotypes circulating worldwide (6). Although the anti-HRoV activity of lactoferrin and of milk fat globule membrane components that contains bioactive glycoproteins and glycolipids has been widely reported in the past, Pfaender et al. did not evidence a pronounced reduction in viral titers of HRoV by HM (30, 34). By contrast, our study reports a clear anti-HRoV effect for both milk pools, supporting protection of breastfed children against gastrointestinal viral infection. The differences in the serostatus of the donor mothers for each virus along with the interpersonal variability in the content of antiviral components of HM may explain the different extents of antiviral potencies between the two HM pools, and some inconsistencies with previous literature. **Figure 1B** shows representative images of the total inhibitory effect of raw milk at a 1:2 dilution against all tested viral infections. Of note, all the antiviral activities were not a consequence of cytotoxicity of HM samples, since the CD50 of milk was one or two logarithms greater than the ID50 (data not shown).

Effect of Hop and HTST Methods on Antiviral Activity of HM

The main aim of this work was to assess the impact of two pasteurization methods, HoP and HTST, on the antiviral properties of raw HM. Therefore, in a second set of experiments,

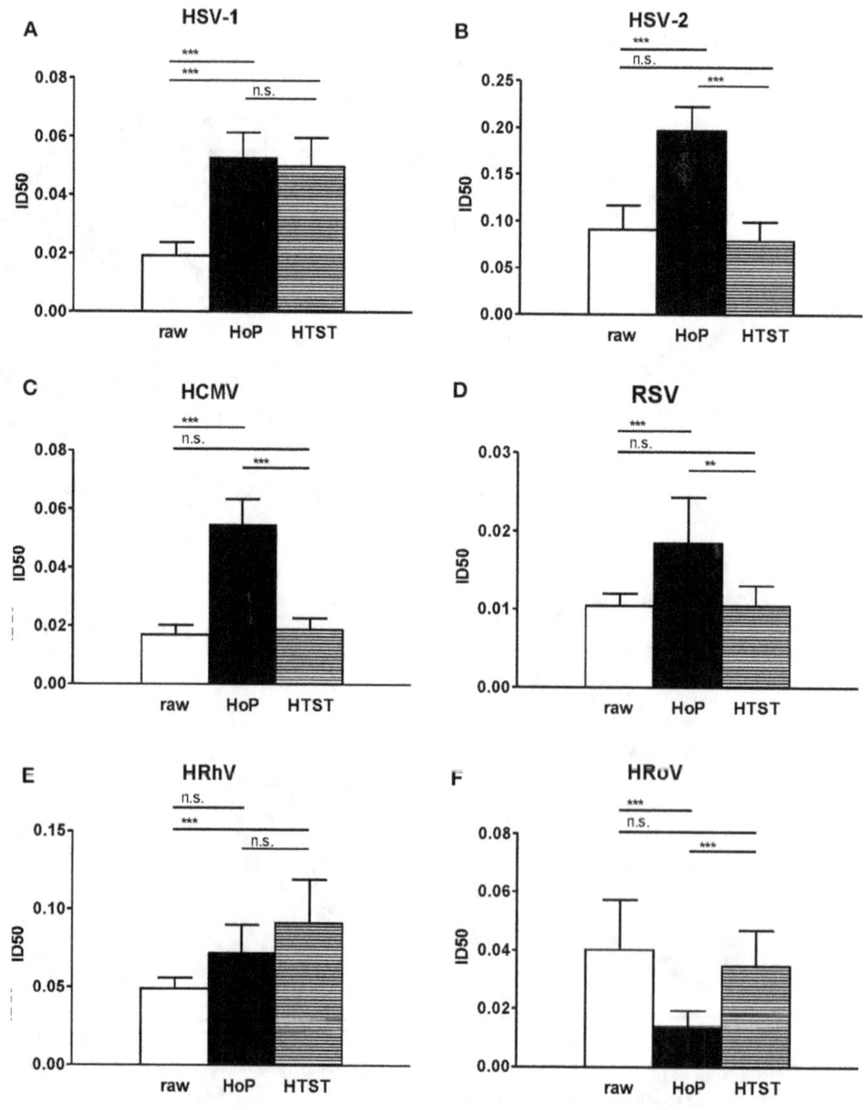

FIGURE 2 | Raw milk (white), Holder pasteurized (HoP, black bar) and HTST pasteurized milk (horizontal striped bar) activities against HSV-1 **(A)**, HSV-2 **(B)**, HCMV **(C)**, RSV **(D)**, HRhV **(E)**, and HRoV **(F)** are reported as a mean ID50 ± 95% confidence intervals of two milk pools. Each pool was tested in 4 independent experiments. ID50 values were compared using the sum-of-squares *F*-test. $^{**}p < 0.01$; $^{***}P < 0.001$; n.s., not significant.

aliquots of the HM pools were pasteurized in parallel or left untreated and their antiviral activity was evaluated. **Figure 2** reports the average of ID50 of the two pools, untreated or pasteurized. The results evidenced a statistically significant reduction of milk antiviral activity following HoP pasteurization against HSV-1, HSV-2, HCMV, RSV, and HRhV infections. These findings may reflect the reduction of specific components with significant immunologic and anti-infective action, such as immunoglobulins and lactoferrin, caused by HoP (16, 17). By contrast, HTST preserved the inhibitory activity of raw milk against most of the tested viruses: no significant difference was evidenced between the ID50 of raw and HTST treated HM samples against HSV-2, HCMV, RSV, and HRoV (**Figure 2**). These data are consistent with previous reports showing that HTST is better than HoP at preserving some biological HM properties, including the antioxidant potential, the lactoferrin content and structure, B and C vitamins, and some cytokines (18). In this experiment, the reliability of such higher biological activity retention is increased by the use of a patented equipment that has a technology readiness level (TRL) of 6, which was directly compared to a commercial HoP device normally used in HMBs. **Figure 2** also showed that HoP and HTST similarly reduced the antiviral activities against HSV-1 and HRhV compared to untreated milk. Unexpectedly, HM anti-HRoV activity was increased by HoP treatment with an ID50 value of 0.014 for pasteurized milk against an ID50 value of 0.04 of raw HM. Although we do not have an explanation for this result, we can speculate that thermal treatment at 62.5°C for 30 min may alter the structure of some HM components thereby increasing their protective activity, such as the release of specific peptides active against HRoV following protein degradation.

CONCLUSION

This study demonstrated that raw HM is endowed with antiviral activity *in vitro* against viral pathogens causing infections in newborns and children. Further studies are needed to investigate the clinical relevance of this activity. HoP method, currently recommended in international guidelines for HMBs, proved to significantly decrease the antiviral activity against HSV-1, HSV-2, HCMV, RSV, and HRhV but not against HRoV. By contrast, HTST preserved antiviral properties of raw HM against four out of six viruses analyzed. These data, along with previous literature, support the HTST as a valid alternative to HoP. Despite the fact that HTST provides a thermal treatment at a higher temperature than HoP (72 vs. 62.5°C, respectively), the far more rapid heating and cooling time of HTST (seconds instead of minutes, respectively) could improve the quality of the final product. This may make HTST suitable for providing the best compromise between microbiological safety and preservation of key biological components and properties of HM, including its antiviral activity.

AUTHOR CONTRIBUTIONS

DL, LC, GM, and EB conceived and designed the study. PT and ACo, collected and pooled the HM samples. MD, MR, RF, and ACi, performed the antiviral assays. LC and MG performed the pasteurizations. MD, LC, and DL analyzed the data. DL, MD, LC, MG, PT, ACo, GM, and EB interpreted the results obtained. MD drafted the manuscript. DL, LC, GM, and EB revised the manuscript. All authors read and approved the final version of the manuscript and agreed to be accountable for all aspects of the work.

REFERENCES

1. Section on Breastfeeding. Breastfeeding and the use of human milk. *Pediatrics* (2012) 129:e827-41. doi: 10.1542/peds.2011-3552
2. WHO/UNICEF. Meeting on infant and young child feeding. *J Nurse Midwifery* (1980) 25:31-8.
3. Horta BL, Victora CG, World Health Organization. Long-term Effects of Breastfeeding: *A Systematic Review*. Geneva:World Health Organization (2013).
4. May JT. Microbial contaminants and antimicrobial properties of human milk. *Microbiol Sci.* (1988) 5:42-6.
5. Yolken RH, Peterson JA, Vonderfecht SL, Fouts ET, Midthun K, Newburg DS. Human milk mucin inhibits rotavirus replication and prevents experimental gastroenteritis. *J Clin Invest.* (1992) 90:1984-91. doi: 10.1172/JCI 116078
6. Clarke NM, May JT. Effect of antimicrobial factors in human milk on rhinoviruses and milk-borne cytomegalovirus in vitro. *J Med Microbiol.* (2000) 49(8):719-23. doi: 10.1099/0022-1317-49-8-719
7. Hanson LA, Lönnroth I, Lange S, Bjersing J, Dahlgren UI. Nutrition resistance to viral propagation. *Nutr Rev.* (2000) 58(2 Pt 2):S31–37. doi: 10.1111/j.1753-4887.2000.tb07801.x
8. Herpes simplex virus [Internet]. World Health Organization. [(Cited Accessed Jun 18, 2018 Jun 18]). Available fromonline at: http://www.who.int/news-room/fact-sheets/detail/herpes-simplex-virus
9. Manicklal S, Emery VC, Lazzarotto T, Boppana SB, Gupta RK. The "silent" global burden of congenital cytomegalovirus. *Clin Microbiol Rev.* (2013) 26(1):86-102. doi: 10.1128/CMR.00062-12
10. Viveros-Rogel M, Soto-Ramirez L, Chaturvedi P, Newburg DS, Ruiz-Palacios GM. Inhibition of HIV-1 infection in vitro by human milk sulfated glycolipids and glycosaminoglycans. *Adv Exp Med Biol.* (2004) 554:481-7.
11. Ng TB, Cheung RCF, Wong JH, Wang Y, Ip DTM, Wan DCC, et al. Antiviral activities of whey proteins. *Appl Microbiol Biotechnol.* (2015) 99(17):6997-7008. doi: 10.1007/s00253-015-6818-4
12. Wakabayashi H, Oda H, Yamauchi K, Abe F. Lactoferrin for prevention of common viral infections. *J Infect Chemother.* (2014) 20(11):666-71. doi: 10.1016/j.jiac.2014.08.003
13. Italian Association of Human Milk Banks Associazione Italiana Banche del Latte Umano Donato (AIBLUD: www.aiblud.com), Arslanoglu S, Bertino E, Tonetto P, De Nisi G, Ambruzzi AM, et al. Guidelines for the establishment and operation of a donor human milk bank. *J Matern-Fetal Neonatal Med.* (2010) 23 (Suppl. 2):1-20. doi: 10.3109/14767058.2010.512414
14. ESPGHAN Committee on Nutrition, Arslanoglu S, Corpeleijn W, Moro G, Braegger C, Campoy C, et al. Donor human milk for preterm infants: current evidence and research directions. *J Pediatr Gastroenterol Nutr.* (2013) 57(4):535-42. doi: 10.1097/MPG.0b013e3182a3af0a
15. Human Milk Banking Association of North America. *Guidelines for the Establishment and Operation of a Donor Human Milk Bank.* Fort Worth, TX, USA. (2018).
16. Peila C, Moro GE, Bertino E, Cavallarin L, Giribaldi M, Giuliani F, et al. The effect of holder pasteurization on nutrients and biologically-active components in donor human milk: a review. *Nutrients* (2016) 8:E477.(8). doi: 10.3390/nu8080477
17. Picaud J-C, Buffin R. Human milk-treatment and quality of banked human milk. *Clin Perinatol.* (2017) 44(1):95–119. doi: 10.1016/j.clp.2016.11.003
18. Peila C, Emmerik NE, Giribaldi M, Stahl B, Ruitenberg JE, van Elburg RM, et al. Human milk processing: a systematic review of innovative techniques to ensure the safety and quality of donor milk. *J Pediatr Gastroenterol Nutr.* (2017) 64(3):353-61. doi: 10.1097/MPG.0000000000001435

19. Giribaldi M, Coscia A, Peila C, Antoniazzi S, Lamberti C, Ortoffi M, et al. Pasteurization of human milk by a benchtop high-temperature short-time device. *Innov Food Sci Emerg Technol.* (2016) 36:228-233. doi: 10.1016/j.ifset.2016.07.004
20. Cavallarin L, Giribaldi M, Antoniazzi S, Bertino E, Coscia A, Gariglio GM. (2015) "*A pasteurizer for continuously treating small volumes of liquid foods*". European Patent n° 2974603, owned by Consiglio Nazionale delle Ricerche, Università degli Studi di Torino, and Giada s.a.s. di Gariglio Gian Marco & C. (Date: Accessed Jan 19.01.17). (2015).
21. Tognon M, Manservigi R, Sebastiani A, Bragliani G, Busin M, Cassai E. Analysis of HSV isolated from patients with unilateral and bilateral herpetic keratitis. *Int Ophthalmol.* (1985) 8(1):13-8.
22. Donalisio M, Quaranta P, Chiuppesi F, Pistello M, Cagno V, Cavalli R, et al. The AGMA1 poly(amidoamine) inhibits the infectivity of herpes simplex virus in cell lines, in human cervicovaginal histocultures, and in vaginally infected mice. *Biomaterials* (2016) 85:40-53. doi: 10.1016/j.biomaterials.2016.01.055
23. Donalisio M, Cagno V, Vallino M, Moro GE, Arslanoglu S, Tonetto P, et al. Inactivation of high-risk human papillomaviruses by Holder pasteurization: implications for donor human milk banking. *J Perinat Med.* (2014) 42(1):1-8. doi: 10.1515/jpm-2013-0200
24. Cagno V, Donalisio M, Civra A, Volante M, Veccelli E, Oreste P, et al. Highly sulfated K5 Escherichia coli polysaccharide derivatives inhibit respiratory syncytial virus infectivity in cell lines and human tracheal-bronchial histocultures. *Antimicrob Agents Chemother.* (2014) 58(8):4782-94. doi: 10.1128/AAC.02594-14
25. Donalisio M, Rusnati M, Cagno V, Civra A, Bugatti A, Giuliani A, et al. Inhibition of human respiratory syncytial virus infectivity by a dendrimeric heparan sulfate-binding peptide. *Antimicrob Agents Chemother* (2012) 56(10):5278-88. doi: 10.1128/AAC.00771-12
26. Donalisio M, Ranucci E, Cagno V, Civra A, Manfredi A, Cavalli R, et al. Agmatine-containing poly(amidoamine)s as a novel class of antiviral macromolecules: structural properties and in vitro evaluation of infectivity inhibition. *Antimicrob Agents Chemother.* (2014) 58(10):6315-9. doi: 10.1128/AAC.03420-14
27. Lembo D, Donalisio M, Laine C, Cagno V, Civra A, Bianchini EP, et al. Auto-associative heparin nanoassemblies: a biomimetic platform against the heparan sulfate-dependent viruses HSV-1, HSV-2, HPV-16 and RSV. *Eur J Pharm Biopharm.* (2014) 88(1):275-82. doi: 10.1016/j.ejpb.2014.05.007
28. Donalisio M, Rittà M, Tonetto P, Civra A, Coscia A, Giribaldi M, et al. Anti-Cytomegalovirus Activity in Human Milk and Colostrum from Mothers of Preterm Infants. *J Pediatr Gastroenterol Nutr.* (2018) doi: 10.1097/MPG.0000000000002071. [Epub ahead of print].
29. Lopez I, Quibriac M, Petitjean J, Bazin M, Duhamel JF, Freymuth F. Neutralizing activity against herpes simplex in maternal milk. *Arch Fr Pediatr.* (1989) 46(4):263-5.
30. Pfaender S, Heyden J, Friesland M, Ciesek S, Ejaz A, Steinmann J, et al. Inactivation of hepatitis C virus infectivity by human breast milk. *J Infect Dis.s* (2013) 208(12):1943-52. doi: 10.1093/infdis/jit519
31. Isaacs CE, Kashyap S, Heird WC, Thormar H. Antiviral and antibacterial lipids in human milk and infant formula feeds. *Arch Dis Child* (1990) 65(8):861-4.
32. Lanari M, Prinelli F, Adorni F, Di Santo S, Faldella G, Silvestri M, et al. Maternal milk protects infants against bronchiolitis during the first year of life. Results from an Italian cohort of newborns. *Early Hum Dev.* (2013) 89(Suppl. 1):S51–57. doi: 10.1016/S0378-3782(13)70016-1
33. Oddy WH. A review of the effects of breastfeeding on respiratory infections, atopy, and childhood asthma. *J Asthma* (2004) 41(6):605-21.
34. van der Strate BW, Beljaars L, Molema G, Harmsen MC, Meijer DK. Antiviral activities of lactoferrin. *Antiviral Res.* (2001) 52(3):225-39. doi: 10.1016/S0166-3542(01)00195-4

3

New Achievements in High-Pressure Processing to Preserve Human Milk Bioactivity

Aleksandra Wesolowska [1,2]*, *Elena Sinkiewicz-Darol* [1,2], *Olga Barbarska* [1,3,4], *Kamila Strom* [3], *Malgorzata Rutkowska* [5], *Katarzyna Karzel* [6], *Elzbieta Rosiak* [7], *Gabriela Oledzka* [3], *Magdalena Orczyk-Pawiłowicz* [8], *Sylwester Rzoska* [5] and *Maria Katarzyna Borszewska-Kornacka* [9]

[1] Laboratory of Human Milk and Lactation Research at Regional Human Milk Bank in Holy Family Hospital, Department of Neonatology, Medical University of Warsaw, Warsaw, Poland, [2] Human Milk Bank, Ludwik Rydygier' Provincial Polyclinical Hospital in Torun, Torun, Poland, [3] Department of Medical Biology, Medical University of Warsaw, Warsaw, Poland, [4] First Department of Obstetrics and Gynecology, Medical University of Warsaw, Warsaw, Poland, [5] High Pressure Physics, Polish Academy of Science, Warsaw, Poland, [6] Faculty of Psychology, Warsaw University, Warsaw, Poland, [7] Department of Food Hygiene and Quality Management, Faculty of Human Nutrition and Consumer Science, Warsaw University of Life Sciences, Warsaw, Poland, [8] Department of Chemistry and Immunochemistry, Wroclaw Medical University, Wroclaw, Poland, [9] Neonatal and Intensive Care Department, University Hospital, Medical University of Warsaw, Warsaw, Poland

Correspondence:
Aleksandra Wesolowska
aleksandra.wesolowska@wum.edu.pl

High-pressure processing (HPP) is a non-thermal technology that is being increasingly applied in food industries worldwide. It was proposed that this method could be used as an alternative to holder pasteurization (HoP; 62.5°C, 30 min) in milk banks but its impact on the immunologic, enzymatic and hormonal components of human milk has not yet been evaluated in detail. The aim of our study was to compare the effects of HPP in variants: (1) 600 MPa, 10 min (2) 100 MPa, 10 min, interval 10 min, 600 MPa, 10 min (3) 200 MPa, 10 min, interval 10 min, 400 MPa, 10 min (4) 200 MPa, 10 min, interval 10 min, 600 MPa, 10 min in temperature range 19–21°C and HoP on the leptin, adiponectin, insulin, hepatocyte growth factor (HGF), lactoferrin and IgG contents in human milk. HoP was done at the Regional Human Milk Bank in Warsaw at the Holy Family Hospital on S90 Eco pasteurizer (Sterifeed, Medicare Colgate Ltd). Apparatus U4000/65 (Unipress Equipment, Poland) was used for pascalization. Milk samples were obtained from women during 2–6 weeks of lactation. Post-treatment culture showed no endogenous bacterial contamination in any tested option. Concentrations of selected components were determined using ELISA tests. The level of all analyzed components were significantly decreased by HoP: leptin 77.86%, adiponectin 32.79%, insulin 32.40%, HGF 88.72%, lactoferrin 60.31@.%, IgG 49.04%. All HPP variants caused an increase in leptin concentration, respectively (1) 81.79% (2) 90.01% (3) 86.12% (4) 47.96%. Retention of insulin after HPP was (1) 88.20% (2) 81.98% (3) 94.76% (4) 90.31% HGF (1) 36.15% (2) 38.81% 97.15% (3) 97.15% (4) 43.02%, lactoferrin (1) 55.78% (2) 57.63% (3) 78.77% (4) 64.75%. Moreover, HPP variant as 200 + 400 MPa preserved IgG (82.24%) better than HoP and resulted not statistically significant change of adiponectin level (38.55%) compare to raw milk. Our results showed that HPP leads to preservation of adipokines, growth factor, and lactoferrin, IgG much better or comparable with HoP.

Keywords: donor milk, high-pressure processing, milk bank, preterm, adipokines, HGF

INTRODUCTION

Mother's milk is a natural first choice feed for every newborn, whether born in term or prematurely. Access to human milk is critical especially for very preterm babies for their current health condition and later life prognosis (1, 2). In those circumstances, human milk has a not only nutritional function but is a source of non-nutritive bioactive compounds. The presumably, cumulative effects of thousands of substance such as anti-inflammatory agents, immunoglobulins, cytokines, growth factors, oligosaccharides, and bioactive peptides from human milk exist in preventing serious complications of prematurity such as necrotizing enterocolitis (NEC) (3–7). Many of these substances such as hormones and cytokines, even have potential for long -term metabolic programming (8).

Hormones as insulin, leptin, adiponectin have impact on infant growth and body composition. **H**epatocyte **G**rowth **F**actor (HGF) and multifunctional milk protein as lactoferrin act in synergy to support the function of the immature gastrointestinal tract of newborns (5, 9–13). Current knowledge about benefit of bioactive factors in breastmilk for infants in early life has results in the increasing number of human milk banks. Therefore, when mother's own milk is unavailable, donor milk is recommended (2, 14). Nearly 80 new units located mostly in hospitals specialized in tertiary neonatal centers and NICU were organized in the last decade in European countries alone (15–17). These professional laboratories operate by screening, collecting, processing, and distributing human milk that has been donated by volunteer nursing mothers unrelated to the recipient infant (18). Although human milk banks are well-equipped and organized, the processing of donor milk needs improvements due to the partial loss of its bioactive properties compared with raw milk (19).

Pasteurization used in mostly human milk banks for microbiological purity consists of heating to 62.5°C for 30 min with obvious side effects for many human milk constituents (20). This approach is especially harmful for non-nutritive elements of human milk such as enzymes, hormones, growth factors and cytokines, leading to their diminished presence and activity. Given this side effect of holder pasteurization, new techniques of processing donated human milk are needed to preserve its bioactivity (19, 21).

In the present research bioactivity of several components of human milk after standard and innovative high pressure processing were evaluated.

MATERIALS AND METHODS

Samples Collection

Milk samples were obtained from 80 donors of the Regional Human Milk Bank in Warsaw at Holy Family Hospital. Donors were given written and verbal instructions on expressing and handling of milk and cleaning of breast pumps. Milk samples were obtained from women (average age was 31 year old) after delivery at term with a surplus of milk during the 2–6 weeks of lactation given informed consent. Samples of ~50 ml of milk were collected at home or in the hospital ward using an electric or manual pump, stored in a refrigerator at temperature 4°C and delivered to human milk bank unit within 24 h while maintaining the refrigeration conditions.

The Bioethics Committee of Warsaw Medical University has accepted the information about conducting this non-interventional study (admission number AKBE/59/15).

Experimental Design and Samples Preparation

The same volume of milk samples from 2 to 4 donors were pooled to achieve the minimum volume of minimum 125 ml necessary for the study. Each batch was divided into aliquots and exposed to 4 variants of **H**igh **P**ressure **P**rocessing (HPP): (1) 600 MPa, (2) 200 + 400 MPa, (3) 100 + 600 MPa, (4) 200 + 600 MPa and holder pasteurization (HoP). The control sample was raw, untreated human milk (**Figure 1**). The experiments were made three times on independent milk batch.

Following the HPP and HoP treatment all samples as well as raw untreated milk were centrifuged at 4,400 rpm for 15 min at 4°C (Centrifuge 5702R, Eppendorf) after which the fat layer and cells were removed and supernatants were aliquoted into Eppendorf tubes prior to freezing at −21°C. Human milk samples were frozen within 48 h of collection.

Microbiological analysis were performed to verify microbiological purity in the case of selected raw and treated milk samples. The analysis were carried out in three replications to the total number of mesophilic aerobic microorganisms (PN-EN ISO 7218: 2008 / A1: 2013, PN-EN ISO 6887-5: 2010) and the number and *Staphylococcus aureus* (PN-EN ISO 6888-1: 2001 / A1: 2004).

Treatment

High Pressure Processing

Human milk samples were exposed to high pressure treatment at the Institute of High Pressure Physics, Polish Academy of Sciences, using U 4000/65 apparatus (designed and produced by Unipress Equipment). The maximum pressure available in the apparatus was 600 MPa, the treatment chamber had a volume of 0.95 L. The pressure-transmitting fluid used was distilled water and polypropylene glycol (1:1). Manufactory designed working temperature of the apparatus ranges from −10°C to +80°C. In our experiments, the temperature of the tested condition was between 19 and 21°C. A pressure of up to 600 MPa was generated in 15–25 s; the release time was 1–4 s.19 and 21°C. Samples were prepared in 4 variants: (1) 600 MPa (2) 200 MPa, 10 min; interval 10 min; 400 MPa, 10 min (3) 100 MPa, 10 min; interval 10 min; 600 MPa, 10 min (4) 200 MPa, 10 min; interval, 10 min; 600 MPa, 10 min.

Holder Pasteurization

Holder Pasteurization (HoP) of human milk samples was done at the Regional Human Milk Bank in Warsaw at the Holy Family Hospital on automatic Human Milk Pasteuriser S90 Eco (Sterifeed, Medicare Colgate Ltd). Samples of 50 ml were treated according to Regional Human Milk Bank standard pasteurization protocol at 62.5°C for 30 min. The correctness of the process

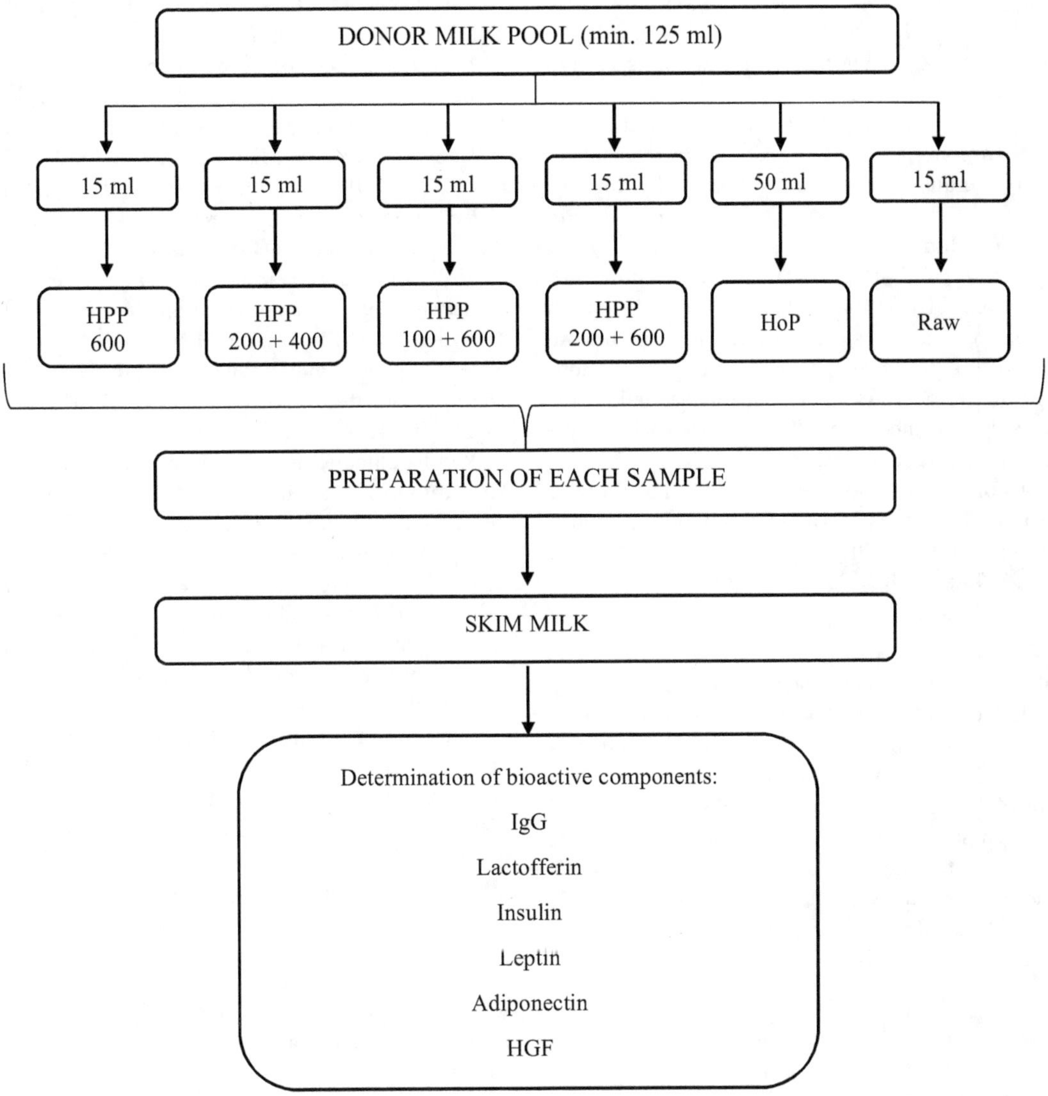

FIGURE 1 | Experimental design of the study.

was confirmed with the data logging system, by recording temperature of the bottle probe every minute.

Determination of Bioactive Components

All of the bioactive components were determined by the ELISA method. The assay detecting particular components in the milk was done at least in three times using milk samples proccesing in independent experiments. The concentration of IgG was determined according to a procedure described earlier (22). Briefly: the $F(ab')_2$ fragment of goat anti human IgG (Jackson ImmunoResearch, USA) was used as a coating agent of the wells of a microtiter plate (Nalge Nunc International, Naperville, IL, USA) to bind IgG from the sample. For testing 100 µl of 100 µl of 100-, 250-, 500-, and 1,000-fold diluted milk and IgG standard preparation from 0.2 to 12.5 ng/100 µl (Jackson ImmunoResearch, USA) were taken. The amount of IgG bound was quantified by phosphatase-labeled rabbit anti-human IgG Fcγ fragment specific antibodies (Jackson ImmunoResearch, USA).

For lactoferrin determination monoclonal anti-human lactoferrin antibody (ABCAM, Cambridge, UK) was used as a coating agent of the wells of a microtiter plate (Nalge Nunc International, Naperville, IL, USA) to bind lactoferrin from the sample. For testing 100 µl of 5 000-, 10 000-, 25 000- and 50 000- fold diluted milk and lactoferrin standard preparation from 0.8 to 25 ng/100 µl (Sigma, St. Louis, MO, USA) were taken. The amount of lactoferrin bound was quantified by phosphatase-labeled rabbit anti-human lactoferrin antibodies (Jackson ImmunoResearch, USA).

The IgG and lactoferrin tests were assayed with 4-nitrophenyl phosphate (SERVA, Heidelberg, Germany) as the enzyme substrate and absorbance was measured in a Stat Fax 2100 Microplate Reader (Awareness Technology Inc., Palm City, FL, USA) at 405 nm with 630 nm as the reference filter. All ELISA immunobinding and washing steps were carried out in a TRIS-buffered saline (TBS, pH 7.5) containing 0.2% Tween 20. All samples were analyzed at four different sample dilutions, each in duplicate.

The concentrations of leptin, adiponectin, HGF, and insulin were analyzed with commercial ELISA kits using microplates pre-coated with a monoclonal antibody specifically for test substances. The following tests were used: Human Leptin (R&D Systems, Inc); Human HMW Adiponectin/Acrp30 (R&D Systems, Inc); Human HGF (R&D Systems, Inc); Insulin ELISA (DRG Instruments GmbH, Germany). For the study, the option for serum/plasma was chosen as the most adequate for human milk. The method was pre-tested on various samples dilutions as proposed in the protocol. As a result of this validation, the final analyses were performed on undiluted milk. Each sample in ELISA assay was measured in duplicate.

The detections of adiponectin, HGF and leptin, insulin were done by microtiter reader (Synergy HTX multimode reader, Biotek®) set to 450 nm with 570 nm as the reference filter. For data analysis Gen5 Data Analysis Software was used.

Statistics

Statistical analysis concerns results obtained for six conditions: raw milk, pasteurized milk (HoP), and milk exposed to four variants of high pressure processing (HPP): 600 MPa, 200 MPa +400 MPa, 100 MPa+ 600 MPa, 200 MPa+ 600 MPa. As a calculation tool MS Excel was used. The results of determined parameters for each sample are showed as a percentage of the initial value observed for raw milk as 100%. Next, means, SD and 95% coefficient intervals (95% CI, which refers to $p \leq 0.05$) were computed. The actual analysis was based on the overview of overlapping of obtained intervals.

RESULTS

The average value of the total viable number of microorganisms in raw milk was determined on the level 3.3 ± 0.90 log cfu / ml. The number of *S. aureus* was determined at 1.57 ± 0.65 log cfu/ml.

Microbiological analyses carried out in pasteurized and pascalised human milk samples did not show the presence of the selected microorganisms (**Supplementary Table 1**).

The concentration of bioactive components in raw milk samples are shown in **Table 1**.

Results of our experiments revealed that HoP caused a statistically significant reduction (49.04%) in IgG content. HPP variants 600 MPa, 100 MPa +600 MPa, and 200 MPa + 600 MPa also decreased statistically significantly the IgG content, 69.68, 69.16, and 68.46%, respectively. The reduction of IgG in 200 MPa +400 MPa (17.76%) was not statistically significant (**Table 2, Figure 2A**).

In the case of lactoferrin HoP caused a statistically significant reduction of this protein (60.31%) in the human milk. HPP variants 600 MPa, 100 MPa +600 MPa, and 200 MPa + 600 MPa also decreased the lactoferrin content statistically significantly, 44.22, 42.37, and 35.25%, respectively. The reduction of lactoferrin in 200 MPa +400 MPa (21.23%) was not statistically significant (**Table 2, Figure 2B**).

Leptin level was significantly reduced by HoP (77.86%) in comparison to the raw milk. In the matter of high—pressure, all HPP variants caused an increase in leptin concentration, (1) 600 MPa; 81.71%, (2) 200 MPa +400 MPa; 86.12%, (3) 100 MPa + 600 MPa; 90.01%, (4) 200 MPa +600 MPa; 47.96%, respectively. Indeed, none of the high pressure variants were significantly different from raw milk (**Figure 2C**).

HoP caused a statistically significant decrease in adiponectin content (31.19%) but not so serious as HPP variants 600 MPa, 100 MPa +600 MPa, and 200 MPa + 600 MPa which reduced the level of protein almost totally: respectively as 97.99, 89.27, and 95.91%. The reduction of adiponectin at 200 MPa +400 MPa was slighter (61.45%), but also statistically significant (**Figure 2D**).

Results obtained for HGF were very similar to adiponectin. HoP caused a statistically significant reduction level of HGF detected in human milk (88.72%). Although the level after HPP treatment by 600 MPa, 100 MPa +600 MPa, and 200 MPa + 600 MPa was decreased not more than 63.85, 61.19, and 56.98%, respectively, it was still significant. Only when it comes to HPP variant 200 MPa +400 MPa was the change in HGF level was almost imperceptible and not statistically significant (2.85%) (**Figure 2E**).

The level of insulin was diminished under the influence of HoP by 32.40% in comparison to raw milk. Among of HPP variants only the treatment of human milk by high pressure as 600 MPa caused statistically significant destruction of protein (11.80%). The reduction in insulin content in human milk after others HPP variants was as following: 200 MPa +400 MPa-−5.24%, 100 MPa + 600 MPa-−18.02%, 200 MPa +600 Mpa-−9.69% but it was not statistically significant (**Figure 2F**).

The content of selected bioactive compounds in raw milk was assumed as 100%, additionally the range of obtained results (minimum-maximum) was presented as an error bar. The asterisks indicate a pair of results that differ statistically significantly with $p \leq 0.05$.

DISCUSSION

The human milk donated for human milk banks needs to be of very high quality concerning microbiological safety, nutritional value, and last but not least, bioactivity. For this reason, an operational procedure has been implemented to monitor the whole process of human milk bank activity. National guidelines have been developed in many countries to improve the standards for recruitment, screen the donors and handle and distribute the collected milk (23–25). There are, many minor differences in operational procedure among milk banks in Europe but the pasteurization stage has a common core process. Holder pasteurization has been a "gold standard" in milk banks worldwide for many years. This process involves heating the milk to 62.5°C within 30 min. The relatively low temperature and long time parameters (for this reason called also Low Temperature Long Time pasteurization, LTLT) was combined to assure microbiological safety and nutritional value

TABLE 1 | Concentration of bioactive components in raw milk.

	IgG (μg/ml)	Lactoferrin (mg/ml)	Leptin (pg/ml)	Adiponectin (ng/ml)	HGF (mIU/ml)	Insulin (pg/ml)
Mean ± SD	11.22 ± 8.83	1.63 ± 0.47	269.97± 56.53	5.30 ± 2.05	1306.15± 956.99	10.24 ± 4.02
Min.	5.74	1.17	226.16	2.94	413.20	6.10
Max.	21.40	2.11	333.78	3.68	2261.00	14.67

The results are presented as mean ± standard deviation with indication on minimum and maximum.

TABLE 2 | Changes in the content of IgG, lactoferrin leptin, adiponectin, HGF, and insulin in human milk after preserving with different methods.

Bioactive components	Raw milk (%)	Holder (%)	High-Pressure Processing			
			600 MPa (%)	100MPa +600 MPa (%)	200 MPa +400 MPa (%)	200 MPa +600 MPa (%)
IgG	100	50.96	30.32	30.84	82.24	31.54
Lactoferrin	100	39.69	55.78	57.63	78.77	64.75
Leptin	100	22.14	181.71	190.01	186.12	147.96
Adiponectin	100	67.21	2.01	10.73	38.55	4.09
HGF	100	11.28	36.15	38.81	97.15	43.02
Insulin	100	67.6	88.20	81.98	94.76	90.31

The results are presented as a retention percentage compare to the content in raw milk (mean values).

(26). Ever since this technique was incorporated into the milk bank system, it has been known to be damaging for many bioactive milk components, such as vitamins: C, folacin, and B6, poly-unsaturated fatty acids and free fatty acid composition (27–30).

The current knowledge of this topic is summarized in a systematic review by Peila et al. (20). The authors distinguished three groups of human milk components according to the influence from holder pasteurization: those significantly affected such as: enzymes, some cytokines, growth factors: IGF, EPO, HGF, GM-GSF, hormones: insulin, adiponectin, vitamins: B6, ascorbic acid, antioxidant capacity, content of nucleotide monophosphate, free amino acid; Those affected but with contradictory results: immunoglobulins S-IgA, IgM, IgG, lactofferin, lysozyme, some cytokines, some vitamins, total fat content including, saturated fatty acid, —mono and polyunsaturated fatty acid. Fortunately there are some thermal resistance components found in human milk such as some cytokines and growth factors, amino acid, some vitamins: D, E, B2, B5, biotin, B3, B12, antioxidant capacity, lipids, total nitrogen content, human milk oligosaccharides. The great heterogeneity in the available data is partially due to a lack of standardized study protocols in this fields. However, the reduced value of pasteurization is great enough to take immediate steps in searching for a technical solution for milk banks.

HPP is one of the most promising alternatives for thermal treatment, but this sophisticated technique has not yet been validated for human milk. For our study we have chosen those components of human milk that were known to be affected by holder pasteurization but hadn't been evaluated in concern on HPP. We focused on biologically active peptides represented by adiponectin, insulin, leptin and HGF because of its impact on metabolism regulation in newborn. In fact the available data concerning preservation of those human milk components are sparing in details. We could only find one study showing the destruction of insulin and adiponectin under the influence of a standard holder treatment (31). However in case of leptin the work has been done on fast—and slow-heat pasteurization 100°C in 5 min and 57°C in 30 min, respectively (32). In all these cases, it was observed that the active peptin level was diminished in the range of 30–40% compared to unpasteurized milk.

Moreover, we included in our research two immunologically important proteins from human milk such as immunoglobulin G (IgG) and lactoferrin. Preservation on immunocomponents in donor milk, are well documented in spite of contradictory results (33–38). Nevertheless, we used those two components as an indicator to compare with trends observed for biologically active peptides of non-nutrition value after thermal and high pressure treated milk.

In our study the mean IgG concentration in untreated milk samples was 11.22 ± 8.83 μg/ml (range 5.74–21.40 μg/ml) **Table 1**. IgG is reported as a very sensitive immunoglobulin with IG4 subclass which was thermal resistance. The loss in the case of holder pasteurization is about 50% relative to untreated milk. Our results are consistent with others, reported by Sousa et al. (38).Only one of the HPP variants (200 MPa +400 MPa) did not statistically significantly decrease the IgG content in milk samples (reduction 17.76%) and gave results better than holder pasteurization (**Figure 2A**).

In the case of lactoferrin the mean concentration detected in raw milk samples was 1.63 ± 0.47 mg/ml (range 1.17–2.11 mg/ml) which is similar to those reported in the literature (39) (**Table 1**) The reduction of lactoferrin level by HoP in current experiments is 60% of the level detected in raw milk samples. The

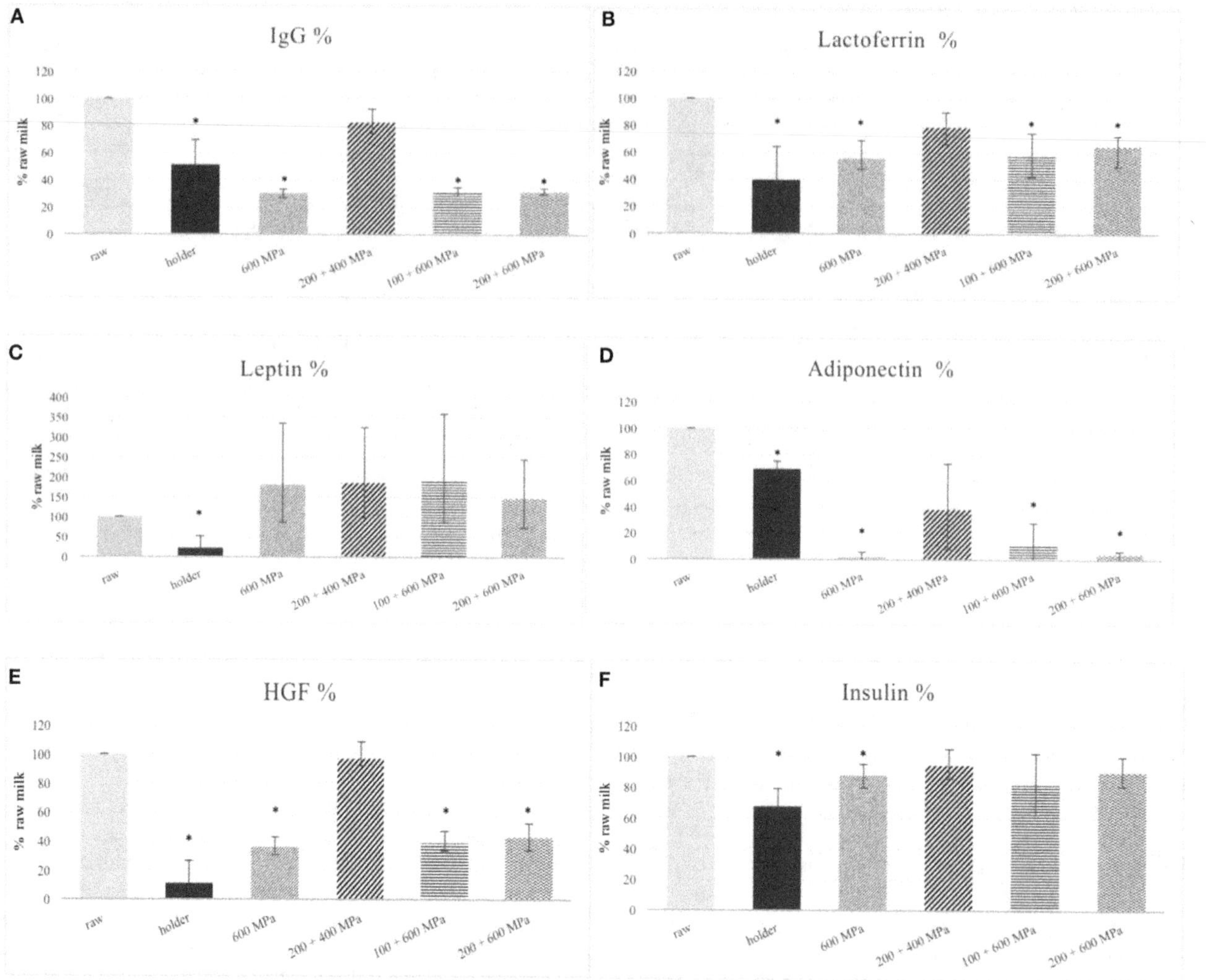

FIGURE 2 | Changes in IgG **(A)**, lactofferin **(B)**, leptin **(C)**, adiponectin **(D)**, HGF **(E)**, insulin **(F)** content in human milk after processing. $^{*}p \leq 0.05$.

difference was statistically significant. It is in the range from 35 to 90% losses observed by others researches. Still it is twice more preserve than was reported by Christen et al. as a 20% retention after HoP (36). All HPP variants used in this study better preserved lactoferrin in human milk than holder pasteurization. Because of the great variance of data the difference was not statistically significant. However, we could see that the best option of HPP is 200 MPa +400 MPa variant, which resulted only 21.23% diminished of lactoferrin level which was not statistically significant comparing to raw milk (**Figure 2B**).

Taking into account the importance of short and long lasting outcome of donor milk nutritional therapy, we decided to extend the research in to evaluate the possibility to preserve the biologically active peptides found in human milk as key metabolism regulation components.

We suspected that HPP variant 200 MPa +400 MPa already tested with success for immunocomponents preservation, will be preferable in comparison to thermal treatment, for hormones such as leptin, adiponectin, insulin, and HGF as well.

As was revealed before, HPP was even most effective as holder pasteurization in the elimination of inoculated microbiological flora of human milk (40). In our current study HPP was able to eliminate commensal bacteria of donors milk successfully (**Supplementary Data**).

The most recent update of Cochrane metaanalysis which evaluated growth and development of preterm born infants fed with formula comparing with donor milk has proven that supplementing mother's milk with pasteurized human milk results in lower rates of weight gain, linear growth and head growth (41). Although it is more important that diet based on solely human milk reduces the NEC risk, hesitation about the consequence of long term under nutrition remains. In this context it seems to be most important to preservation donor milk components with regulation metabolism properties.

Among adipokines derived from human milk, leptin, and adiponectin, have great impacts on the neonatal growth and development. Leptin is a key factor in the regulation of energy balance and appetite (42, 43). Blood leptin concentration in **S**mall for-**G**estational **A**ge (ang. SGA) neonates has been observed to be inversely related to rates of intrauterine growth, suggesting a possible role of leptin in promoting fetus growth (44). Leptin in human milk appears from mammary epithelial cells in milk fat globules as well as being transferred from material blood (45, 46). Leptin receptors have been identified in the human small intestine, which suggests that breast milk leptin could play a role in the short-term control of food intake in neonates (47).

In our experiments, leptin hormone was detected in all analyzed milk samples before and after processing. The mean concentration of leptin in raw milk samples was 269.97 ± 56.53 pg/ml (range 226.16–333.78 pg/ml) which is similar to those reported in the literature (48) (**Table 1**). Leptin seems to be a thermolabile protein, therefore it is not uncommon that treatment in 62.5°C by 30 min decreases the detectable level more than 70%, more slightly sterilization condition as 57°C caused comparable results, as was shown earlier. Surprisingly, after high pressure processing we even detected an increase relative to untreated milk (**Figure 2C**, **Table 2**). This phenomena could be explained by the influence of hydrostatic pressure on the physicochemical property of human milk. Human milk is a very complex biological fluid that could be characterized simply as an emulsion of fat globules in an aqueous liquid with cells components. As was shown leptin is located predominantly in emulsion phase of human milk, which consists of the milk fat droplet or fat-associated proteins. Some portion of human milk leptin is locally synthesized in mammary epithelium cells. In fact documented effects of high pressure on milk lipids have been scarce. However, milk fat globules appear to remain intact under pressure, some alternation in globule size being observed (49). It is not ruled out that pascalization of human milk causes the release of leptin incorporated in milk fat globule or in cellular component of human milk. Indeed, because of high variance, the results after HPP treatment were not statistically significantly different from raw milk.

In the case of adiponectin, the mean concentration detected in raw milk samples was 5.30 ± 2.05 ng/ml (range 2.94–3.68 ng/ml) which was comparable to others findings (**Table 1**). The average quantity of adiponectin in human milk detected by Martin LJ and coworkers was ~19 ng/ml (range 4–88 ng/ml) (50). In another study median adiponectin concentration in human milk was 9.99 ng/ml (range 3.59–20.52 ng/ml). Adiponectin levels remain well detectable throughout the time of breastfeeding with a high level at the beginning of the course of lactation and with a decrease at the time of the introduction of complementary feeding (51). Adiponectin, synthesized by adipocytes, exists in plasma as a several different oligomeric proteins. High-molecular-weight (HMW) adiponectin is a large multimer of 12–18 subunits, thought to be the most biologically active form almost entirely existing in human milk (9). Therefore, we evaluated this particular form of protein in the human milk after processing. We have detected HMV adiponectin in all analyzed human milk samples and we could observed that all methods of treatment significantly decreased the content of adiponectin in milk samples compared to raw milk (**Figure 2D**, **Table 2**). Fortunately, the reduction of adiponectin in HPP variant 200 MPa +400 MPa was not so radical but not very much different from after HoP. As was mentioned earlier, because of the crucial role adiponectin in the regulation of insulin sensitivity in the offspring, reduction of functional hormone in donor milk could be especially problematic for very preterm infants who are at increased risk of insulin resistance and type 2 diabetes later in life (32).

The mean concentration of HGF in raw milk samples was 1306.15 ± 956.99 mlU/ml (range 413.20–2261 mlU/ml) (**Table 1**). In spite of concentrations of HGF in human milk is dependent on many factors including selection of the study group and demographic variables, but the stage of lactation seems to be crucial (52). The HGF level in colostrum is 20–30 higher than in mature milk, which stresses the key role of this growth factor in the development progress of newborns. Moreover, the concentration of HGF in milk from mothers delivered preterm were significantly higher than those from term deliveries. As was speculated earlier, it was finally discovered that trophic action of HGF from human milk occurs by the stimulation of gastrointestinal (GI) epithelial cells (53, 54). In this context, the presence of HGF in donor milk could represent a special benefit in prevention of such serious GI track illnesses such as NEC. As was n in **Figure 2E** the HGF level after treatment by HPP 200 MPa +400 MPa did not significantly differ from the level in raw milk but it was significantly higher than the level of HGF in milk subjected to other high pressure variants or HoP.

Insulin has been detected at very high levels in the human colostrum of healthy mothers (114–306 mU/L) after that decreasing by day 5 postpartum to the physiological levels at the fasting state (55). Insulin seems to be actively transported into milk irrespective of the source because exogenous insulin used for treatment of type 1 diabetes is found in human milk. Surprisingly, that levels of insulin are significantly higher in milk from type 1 diabetic mothers than that of non-diabetic control mothers (56). As has been show earlier, insulin derived from derived insulin could work effectively in newborn exerted hormone dependent effect to glucose homeostasis (57). In addition to the key role of insulin in blood glucose the homeostasis, the properties of dietary hormone in influencing growth and development of the small intestine was postulated (58). Recent studies have shown the link of human milk hormone occurrence, as insulin as well as leptin, with the proper pattern of intestinal microbiome in neonates (59).

In our study the mean insulin concentration in raw milk samples was 10.24 ± 4.02 pg/ml (range 6.10–14.67 pg/ml) which is similar to data reported in the literature (60) **Table 1**. Thermal treatment used in experiments affect significantly the content of insulin in pasteurized human milk compared to raw milk. The pasteurization changes occurred were comparable with the remarkable decreased observed by Ley (32) (**Figure 2F**). In the case of three out of four HPP variants, including HPP 200 MPa +400 MPa, they gave results significantly better than holder pasteurization.

In conclusion, our experiments showed that the 200+400 MPa variant is the best option of high pressure to preserve several metabolic hormones and immunocomponents of human milk. Our findings with persistent bioactive peptides in pascalized human milk is in line with the earliest reports concerning retention of others hormones after HPP with great significance for the infant's health (21, 61, 62).

We showed, for the first time, preservation of several metabolic hormones in donor milk HPP processing. Growing recent studies in nutritional therapy of preterm's have emphasized the role of our discovery (63, 64).

We believed that preservation of important bioactive peptides as hormones and growth factors in human milk is especially important in the context of delivering donor milk for very preterm infants.

LIMITATION OF THE STUDY AND FUTURE DIRECTION

Lack of protocol for evaluation of new techniques was a severe obstacle to improving the pasteurization stage of donor milk. In the next step we would like to follow current expert's recommendation for validation of new method of human milk processing and fit designed methodology for this, especially in the matter of microbiology.

AUTHOR CONTRIBUTIONS

AW: main contributions to the conception and design of the work, analysis and interpretation of data for the work, drafting the work. ES-D and OB: acquisition, analysis and interpretation of data for the work, revising it critically for important intellectual content. KS and MR: acquiring the main part of the data used for the work. KK statistical analysis and interpretation of data for the work. ER: acquiring part of the data for the work. GO, SR, and MB-K: revising it critically for important intellectual content, providing approval for publication of the content. MO-P: acquiring part of the data for the work, revising it critically for important intellectual content. All authors agree to be accountable for all aspects of the work in ensuring that questions related to the accuracy or integrity of any part of the work are appropriately investigated and resolved.

ACKNOWLEDGMENTS

We acknowledge Elzbieta Lodykowska from the Regional Human Milk Bank in Warsaw at Holy Family Hospital for assistance with collecting milk samples and all the mothers who participated the study.

REFERENCES

1. Boyd CA, Quigley MA, Brocklehurst P. Donor breast milk versus infant formula for preterm infants: systematic review and meta-analysis. *Arch Dis Childhood Fetal Neonat Edn.* (2007) 92:F169–75. doi: 10.1136/adc.2005.089490
2. Moro GE, Arslanoglu S, Bertino E, Corvaglia L, Montirosso R, Picaud JC, et al. Human milk in feeding premature infants: consensus statement. *J Pediatr Gastroenterol Nutr.* (2015) 61:S16–9. doi: 10.1097/01.mpg.0000471460.08792.4d
3. Sisk P, Lovelady C, Dillard R, Gruber K, O'shea T. Early human milk feeding is associated with a lower risk of necrotizing enterocolitis in very low birth weight infants. *J Perinatol.* (2007) 27:428. doi: 10.1038/sj.jp.7211758
4. Meinzen-Derr J, Poindexter B, Wrage L, Morrow A, Stoll B, Donovan E. Role of human milk in extremely low birth weight infants' risk of necrotizing enterocolitis or death. *J Perinatol.* (2009) 29:57. doi: 10.1038/jp.2008.117
5. Savino F, Liguori SA, Lupica MM. Adipokines in breast milk and preterm infants. *Early Hum Dev.* (2010) 86(Suppl. 1):77–80. doi: 10.1016/j.earlhumdev.2010.01.011
6. Herrmann K, Carroll K An exclusively human milk diet reduces necrotizing enterocolitis. *Breastfeed Med.* (2014) 9:184–90. doi: 10.1089/bfm.2013.0121
7. Kantorowska A, Wei JC, Cohen RS, Lawrence RA, Gould JB., Lee HC. Impact of donor milk availability on breast milk use and necrotizing enterocolitis rates. *Pediatrics* (2016) 137:e20153123. doi: 10.1542/peds2015-3901
8. Ballard O, Morrow AL. Human milk composition: nutrients and bioactive factors. *Pediatr Clin.* (2013) 60:49–74. doi: 10.1016/j.pcl.2012.10.002
9. Newburg DS, Woo JG, Morrow AL. Characteristics and potential functions of human milk adiponectin. *J Pediatr.* (2010) 156:S41–6. doi: 10.1016/j.jpeds.2009.11.020
10. Garcia C, Duan R-D, Brévaut-Malaty V, Gire C, Millet V, Simeoni U, et al. Bioactive compounds in human milk and intestinal health and maturity in preterm newborn: an overview. *Cell Mol Biol.* (2013) 59:108–31. doi: 10.1170/T952
11. Wada Y, Lönnerdal B. Bioactive peptides derived from human milk proteins—mechanisms of action. *J Nutr Biochem.* (2014) 25:503–14. doi: 10.1016/j.jnutbio.2013.10.012
12. Brunner S, Schmid D, Zang K, Much D, Knoeferl B, Kratzsch J, et al. Breast milk leptin and adiponectin in relation to infant body composition up to 2 years. *Pediatr Obes.* (2015) 10:67–73. doi: 10.1111/j.2047-6310.2014.222.x
13. Fields DA, Schneider CR, Pavela G. A narrative review of the associations between six bioactive components in breast milk and infant adiposity. *Obesity* (2016) 24:1213–21. doi: 10.1002/oby.21519
14. Breastfeeding and the use of human milk. *Pediatrics* (2012) 129:e827–41. doi: 10.1542/peds.2011-3552
15. Arslanoglu S, Corpeleijn W, Moro G, Braegger C, Campoy C, Colomb V, et al. Donor human milk for preterm infants: current evidence and research directions. *J Pediatr Gastroenterol Nutr.* (2013) 57:535–42. doi: 10.1097/MPG.0b013e3182a3af0a
16. Haiden N, Ziegler EE. Human milk banking. *Ann Nutr Metab.* (2016) 69(Suppl. 2):7–15. doi: 10.1159/000452821
17. Moro GE. History of milk banking: from origin to present time. *Breastfeed Med.* (2018) 13:S-16–17. doi: 10.1089/bfm.2018.29077.gem
18. Picaud J-C, Buffin R. Human milk—treatment and quality of banked human milk. *Clin Perinatol.* (2017) 44:95–119. doi: 10.1016/j.clp.2016.11.003
19. Peila C, Emmerik NE, Giribaldi M, Stahl B, Ruitenberg JE, Van Elburg RM, et al. Human milk processing: a systematic review of innovative techniques to ensure the safety and quality of donor milk. *J Pediatr Gastroenterol Nutr.* (2017) 64:353–61. doi: 10.1097/MPG.0000000000001435
20. Peila C, Moro GE, Bertino E, Cavallarin L, Giribaldi M, Giuliani F, et al. The effect of holder pasteurization on *nutrients* and biologically-active components in donor human milk: a review. *Nutrients* (2016) 8:E477. doi: 10.3390/nu8080477
21. Sousa SG, Delgadillo I, Saraiva JA. Human milk composition and preservation: evaluation of high-pressure processing as a nonthermal pasteurization technology. *Crit Rev Food Sci Nutr.* (2016) 56:1043–60. doi: 10.1080/10408398.2012.753402
22. Lis-Kuberka J, Orczyk-Pawiłowicz M, Królak-Olejnik B, Berghausen-Mazur M, Baranska K, Katnik-Prastowska I. Lectin-based analysis of human milk immunoglobulin G fucosylated variants in relation to milk maturation and perinatal risk factors. *J Appl Biomed.* . (2018) 16:232–40. doi: 10.1016/j.jab.2018.02.001
23. Arslanoglu S, Bertino E, Tonetto P, De Nisi G, Ambruzzi AM, Biasini A, et al. Guidelines for the establishment and operation of a donor human milk bank: Italian Association of Human Milk Banks Associazione Italiana Banche

del Latte Umano Donato (AIBLUD: https://www.aiblud.com/). *J Mater Fetal Neon Med.* (2010) 23:1–20. doi: 10.3109/14767058.2010.512414

24. Picaud J-C. VIII. Human milk banks: how to organize the collection of human milk to feed preterm infants. *J Pediatr Gastroenterol Nutr.* (2015) 61:S10–2. doi: 10.1097/01.mpg.0000471456.78296.a6
25. Calvo J, Lara NRG, Gormaz M, Pena M, Lorenzo MJM, Murillo PO, et al. Recommendations for the creation and operation of maternal milk banks in Spain. *An Pediatr.* (2018) 89:65.e1–e6. doi: 10.1016/j.anpede.2018.01.007
26. Wills M, Han V, Harris D, Baum J. Short-time low-temperature pasteurisation of human milk. *Early Hum Dev.* (1982) 7:71–80. doi: 10.1016/0378-3782(82)90009-3
27. Wardell JM, Hill C, Souza S. Effect of pasteurization and of freezing and thawing human milk on its triglyceride content. *Acta Paediatr.* (1981) 70:467–71. doi: 10.1111/j.1651-2227.1981.tb05724.x
28. Van Zoeren-Grobben D, Schrijver J, Van den Berg H, Berger H. Human milk vitamin content after pasteurisation, storage, or tube feeding. *Arch Dis Child.* (1987) 62:161–5. doi: 10.1136/adc.62.2.161
29. Lepri L, Del Bubba M, Maggini R, Donzelli GP, Galvan P. Effect of pasteurization and storage on some components of pooled human milk1. *J Chromatogr B Biomed Sci Appl.* (1997) 704:1–10. doi: 10.1016/S0378-4347(97)00439-8
30. Wight NE. Donor human milk for preterm infants. *J Perinatol.* (2001) 21:249. doi: 10.1038/sj.jp.7200533
31. Resto M, O'Connor D, Leef K, Funanage V, Spear M, Locke R. Leptin levels in preterm human breast milk and infant formula. *Pediatrics* (2001) 108:e15. doi: 10.1542/peds.108.1.e15
32. Ley SH, Hanley AJ, Stone D, O'Connor DL. Effects of pasteurization on adiponectin and insulin concentrations in donor human milk. *Pediatr Res.* (2011) 70:278–81. doi: 10.1203/PDR.0b013e318224287a,
33. Goldsmith SJ, Dickson JS, Barnhart HM, Toledo RT, Eiten-Miller RR. IgA, IgG, IgM and lactoferrin contents of human milk during early lactation and the effect of processing and storage. *J Food Prot.* (1983) 46:4–7. doi: 10.4315/0362-028X-46.1.4
34. Koenig Á, de Albuquerque Diniz EM, Barbosa SF, Vaz FA. Immunologic factors in human milk: the effects of gestational age and pasteurization. *J Hum Lact.* (2005) 21:439–43. doi: 10.1177/0890334405280652
35. Baro C, Giribaldi M, Arslanoglu S, Giuffrida MG, Dellavalle G, Conti A, et al. Effect of two pasteurization methods on the protein content of human milk. *Front Biosci.* (2011) 3:818–29. doi: 10.2741/289
36. Christen L, Lai CT, Hartmann B, Hartmann PE, Geddes DT. The effect of UV-C pasteurization on bacteriostatic properties and immunological proteins of donor human milk. *PLoS ONE* (2013) 8:e78586. doi: 10.1371/journal.pone.0085867
37. Mayayo C, Montserrat M, Ramos S, Martínez-Lorenzo M, Calvo M, Sánchez L, et al. Kinetic parameters for high-pressure-induced denaturation of lactoferrin in human milk. *Int Dairy J.* (2014) 39:246–52. doi: 10.1016/j.idairyj.2014.07.001
38. Sousa SG, Delgadillo I, Saraiva JA. Effect of thermal pasteurisation and high-pressure processing on immunoglobulin content and lysozyme and lactoperoxidase activity in human colostrum. *Food Chem.* (2014) 151:79–85. doi: 10.1016/j.foodchem.2013.11.024
39. Villavicencio A, Rueda MS, Turin CG, Ochoa TJ. Factors affecting lactoferrin concentration in human milk: how much do we know? *Biochem Cell Biol.* (2016) 95:12–21. doi: 10.1139/bcb-2016-0060
40. Windyga B, Rutkowska M, Sokołowska B, Skapska S, Wesołowska A, Wilinska M, et al. Inactivation of Staphylococcus aureus and native microflora in human milk by high pressure processing. *High Press Res.* (2015) 35:181–8. doi: 10.1080/08957959.2015.1007972
41. Quigley M, Embleton N, McGuire W. Formula versus donor breast milk for feeding preterm or low birth weight infants. *Cochr Database Syst Rev.* (2018) 6:CD002971. doi: 10.1002/14651858.CD002971.pub4
42. Palou A, Picó C. Leptin intake during lactation prevents obesity and affects food intake and food preferences in later life. *Appetite* (2009) 52:249–52. doi: 10.1016/j.appet.2008.09.013
43. Langhans W, Geary N, editors. *Frontiers in Eating and Weight Regulation. Forum of Nutrition,* Vol. 63. Basel: Karger (2010), p. 84–93. doi: 10.1159/000264396
44. Koistinen HA, Koivisto V, Andersson S, Karonen S-L, Kontula K, Oksanen L, et al. Leptin concentration in cord blood correlates with intrauterine growth. *J Clin Endocrinol Metab.* (1997) 82:3328–30. doi: 10.1210/jc.82.10.3328
45. Casabiell X, Pineiro V, Tome M, Peino R, Dieguez C, Casanueva F. Presence of leptin in colostrum and/or breast milk from lactating mothers: a potential role in the regulation of neonatal food intake. *J Clin Endocrinol Metab.* (1997) 82:4270–3. doi: 10.1210/jcem.82.12.4590
46. Bonnet M, Delavaud C, Laud K, Gourdou I, Leroux C, Djiane J, et al. Mammary leptin synthesis, milk leptin and their putative physiological roles. *Reprod Nutr Dev.* (2002) 42:399–413. doi: 10.1051/rnd:2002034
47. Barrenetxe J, Villaro AC, Guembe L, Pascual I, Munoz-Navas M, Barber A, et al. Distribution of the long leptin receptor isoform in brush border, basolateral membrane, and cytoplasm of enterocytes. *Gut* (2002) 50:797–802. doi: 10.1136/gut.50.6.797
48. Kugananthan S, Lai CT, Gridneva Z, Mark PJ, Geddes DT, Kakulas F. Leptin levels are higher in whole compared to skim human milk, supporting a cellular contribution. *Nutrients* (2016) 8:E711. doi: 10.3390/nu8110711
49. Huppertz T, Kelly AL, Fox PF. Effects of high pressure on constituents and properties of milk. *Int Dairy J.* (2002) 12:561–72. doi: 10.1016/S0958-6946(02)00045-6
50. Martin LJ, Woo JG, Geraghty SR, Altaye M, Davidson BS, Banach W, et al. Adiponectin is present in human milk and is associated with maternal factors. *Am J Clin Nutr.* (2006) 83:1106–11. doi: 10.1093/ajcn/83.5.1106
51. Bronsky J, Mitrova K, Karpisek M, Mazoch J, Durilova M, Fisarkova B, et al. Adiponectin, AFABP, and leptin in human breast milk during 12 months of lactation. *J Pediatr Gastroenterol Nutr.* (2011) 52:474–7. doi: 10.1097/MPG.0b013e3182062fcc
52. Munblit D, Treneva M, Peroni DG, Colicino S, Chow L, Dissanayeke S, et al. Colostrum and mature human milk of women from London, Moscow, and Verona: determinants of immune composition. *Nutrients* (2016) 8:695. doi: 10.3390/nu8110695
53. Yamada Y, Saito S, Morikawa H. Hepatocyte growth factor in human breast milk. *Am J Reprod Immunol.* (1998) 40:112–20. doi: 10.1111/j.1600-0897.1998.tb00399.x
54. Itoh H, Itakura A, Kurauchi O, Okamura M, Nakamura H, Mizutani S. Hepatocyte growth factor in human breast milk acts as a trophic factor. *Hormone Metab Res.* (2002) 34:16–20. doi: 10.1055/s-2002-19961
55. Kulski J, Hartmann P. Milk insulin, GH and TSH: relationship to changes in milk lactose, glucose and protein during lactogenesis in women. *Endocrinol Exp.* (1983) 17:317–26.
56. Whitmore T, Trengove N, Graham D, Hartmann P. Analysis of insulin in human breast milk in mothers with type 1 and type 2 diabetes mellitus. *Int J Endocrinol.* (2012) 2012:296368. doi: 10.1155/2012/296368
57. Koldovsky O. Hormones in milk. In: Litwack G, editor. *Vitamins and Hormones,* Vol. 50. 1st ed. (1995). p. 77–149.
58. Shehadeh N, Sukhotnik I, Shamir R. Gastrointestinal tract as a target organ for orally administered insulin. *J Pediatr Gastroenterol Nutr.* (2006) 43:276–81. doi: 10.1097/01.mpg.0000226377.03247.fb
59. Gotteland M, Magne F. Alterations in human milk leptin and insulin are associated with early changes in the infant intestinal microbiome. *Am J Clin Nutr.* (2017) 105:234–234. doi: 10.3945/ajcn.116.140129
60. Shehadeh N, Khaesh-Goldberg E, Shamir R, Perlman R, Sujov P, Tamir A, et al. Insulin in human milk: postpartum changes and effect of gestational age. *Arch Dis Child Fetal Neonat Edn.* (2003) 88:F214–6. doi: 10.1136/fn.88.3.F214
61. Viazis S, Farkas BE, Allen JC. Effects of high-pressure processing on immunoglobulin A and lysozyme activity in human milk. *J Hum Lact.* (2007) 23:253–61. doi: 10.1177/0890334407303945
62. Permanyer M, Castellote C, Ramirez-Santana C, Audi C, Perez-Cano FJ, Castell M, et al. Maintenance of breast milk Immunoglobulin A after high-pressure processing. *J Dairy Sci.* (2010) 93:877–83. doi: 10.3168/jds.2009-2643
63. Hair AB, Peluso AM, Hawthorne KM, Perez J, Smith DP, Khan JY, et al. Beyond necrotizing enterocolitis prevention: improving outcomes with an exclusive human milk-based diet. *Breastfeed Med.* (2016) 11:70–4. doi: 10.1089/bfm.2015.0134
64. Miller J, Tonkin E, Damarell RA, McPhee AJ, Suganuma M, Suganuma H, et al. A systematic review and meta-analysis of human milk feeding and morbidity in very low birth weight infants. *Nutrients* (2018) 10:E707. doi: 10.3390/nu10060707

Feeding Practices in Very Preterm and Very Low Birth Weight Infants in an Area where a Network of Human Milk Banks is in Place

Elettra Berti[1], Monia Puglia[2], Silvia Perugi[3], Luigi Gagliardi[4], Cristiana Bosi[5], Anna Ingargiola[1], Letizia Magi[6], Elena Martelli[7], Simone Pratesi[3], Emilio Sigali[8], Barbara Tomasini[9] and Franca Rusconi[1,2] on behalf of the TIN Toscane on-line group*

[1] Anna Meyer Children's University Hospital, Florence, Italy, [2] Health Agency of Tuscany, Florence, Italy, [3] Careggi University Hospital, Florence, Italy, [4] Versilia Hospital, Viareggio, Italy, [5] San Giovanni di Dio Hospital, Florence, Italy, [6] San Donato Hospital, Arezzo, Italy, [7] Santo Stefano Hospital, Prato, Italy, [8] University Hospital of Pisa, Pisa, Italy, [9] University Hospital of Siena, Siena, Italy

***Correspondence:**
Elettra Berti
elettra.berti@gmail.com

Background: Great variability in enteral feeding practices for very preterm (<32 weeks gestational age-GA) and very low birth weight infants (VLBW; ≤1,500 g) have been reported. We aimed to describe data on enteral feeding in Tuscany (Italy), where a network of 6 donor milk banks is in place.

Methods: A 4-years (2012–2015) observational study was performed analyzing the database "TIN Toscane online" on very preterm and VLBW infants. The database covers all 25 hospitals with a neonatal unit.

Results: Data concerning the beginning of enteral nutrition were available for 1,302 newborns with a mean (standard deviation) GA of 29.3 (2.9) weeks, while information at the time of full enteral nutrition was available for 1,235 and at discharge for 1,140. Most infants (74.1%) started enteral feeding during the first 24 h of life. Overall, 80.1% of newborns were fed exclusive human milk, donor milk having the larger prevalence of use (66.8%). Few infants (13.3%) started with exclusive mother's milk. Full enteral feeding was achieved using exclusive human milk in most cases (80%). Full enteral feeding was reached earlier in newborns who were fed human milk than in those fed formula, regardless of GA. Sixty-four percent of infants were still fed with any human milk at discharge. When data at the achievement of full enteral nutrition and at discharge were analyzed stratified by the type of milk used to start enteral feeding, newborns initially fed donor milk presented the highest prevalence (91.3%) of exclusive human milk at full enteral feeding, an important period to prevent necrotizing enterocolitis, while no differences were observed at discharge.

Conclusions: Donor milk was widely used for newborns during the first hours of life, when mother's milk availability may be quite challenging. Starting enteral nutrition with donor milk was associated with early start of enteral feeding and early achievement of full enteral nutrition without affecting mother lactation. The overall prevalence of human milk at discharge (when donor milk is not available anymore) was high (64%), irrespective of the type of milk used to start nutrition.

Keywords: donor milk, human milk, mother's own milk, complementary milk, full enteral feeding, preterm, very low birth weight

INTRODUCTION

Perinatal interventions and care practices have improved survival and long-term outcomes for very preterm (<32 weeks of gestation) and very low birth weight (VLBW: birth weight ≤1,500 g) infants over the last two decades (1, 2). Nutrition is a major element of care for these infants; nevertheless, great variability in enteral feeding practice (3–5) has been reported. A debate is still underway in the scientific community on the best feeding strategy, including time of initiation and the rate of incrementing feeding. Mother's own milk is recommended as the best feeding for all newborns, including preterm and VLBW infants, for its multiple short- and long-term health benefits (6–9). Donor human milk represents the best alternative whenever breastfeeding is impossible, or mother's own milk is unavailable, as commonly occurs in neonatal intensive care units (NICUs) in the very 1st days of infant life (6–9).

To date, only few studies have reported feeding practices adopted for very preterm and VLBW infants during their hospitalization, and little is known on the use of donor human milk in NICUs.

A very recent observational study in 162 Neonatal Units in England showed a low prevalence of use of donor milk in newborn infants <32 weeks gestation, with wide variations (2–61%) across networks. Networks without donor milk availability possibly choose to wait for mother's milk rather than administer formula milk because of the increased perceived risk of NEC; this resulted in newborns fed at a later postnatal age (10). On the other hand, a large study conducted by the Center for Disease Control and Prevention in the US reported that the percentage of neonatal care facilities using donor milk increased 74% between 2011 and 2015. Donor human milk use was more likely in facilities with higher breast-feeding rates and in a state with a milk bank (11).

The aim of the present study is to describe feeding practices currently adopted for very preterm and VLBW infants born in Tuscany, a region of central Italy where a network of donor milk banks is in place and where there is an area-based, web-based registry (TIN Toscane on-line).

We describe feeding practices during NICU hospitalization, focusing on the prevalence of use of mother's own milk, donor human milk and formula feeding at three different time points of enteral nutrition: the beginning of enteral feeding, the achievement of full enteral nutrition, and discharge.

METHODS

A 4 years (2012–2015) observational study was performed based on "TIN Toscane online," an official web-based registry of the Tuscany Regional Health Service. Since 2009, the registry covers all 25 hospitals with delivery units and NICUs in the region and prospectively collects information on maternal and neonatal characteristics of all infants under 32 weeks of gestational age (GA) or with a birth weight under 1,500 g. Since 2012, data concerning feeding practices have also been registered. Written consent for the data collection was obtained from parents. In each unit, a doctor or a nurse directly accesses the registry using a personal ID and password and completes standardized structured forms for each newborn who meets inclusion criteria. Personal health information collected in the registry are de-identified.

TABLE 1 | Principal characteristics of the 1,398 newborn infants <32 weeks gestation or <1,500 g included in the registry from 1-01-2012 to 31-12-2015.

Population characteristics	*n* (%) or mean ± *SD*
Gestational age <32 weeks	1,142 (81.7)
22–25 weeks	186 (13.3)
26–28 weeks	258 (18.5)
29–31 weeks	698 (49.9)
Birth weight<1,500 g and gestational age ≥32 weeks	256 (18.3)
Gestational age (weeks)	29.3 ± 2.9
Weight (grams)	1,204.5 ± 373.5
Males	717 (51.3)
Singleton	863 (61.8)
Vaginal delivery	293 (21.0)
Antenatal steroids	1,179 (84.6)
Apgar score V minute	7.9 ± 1.6
Ventilation and/or oxygen support	1,266 (91.1)
Patent ductus arteriosus	538 (38.9)
Bacterial late onset sepsis	55 (4.0)
Major birth defects	56 (4.0)
Deaths	157 (11.2)
Necrotizing enterocolitis	40 (2.9)
Surgery for necrotizing enterocolitis	36 (2.6)
Focal gastrointestinal perforation	35 (2.5)

Data are collected from neonatal admission until discharge or death, and include demographic characteristics of the mother, obstetric history, and information on delivery, clinical characteristics of the newborn at birth and during the hospital stay, as well as medical or surgical treatments received. Data quality is checked centrally every 2–3 months. Details about perinatal organization in Tuscany and "TIN Toscane online" are reported elsewhere (12).

Types of feeding included mother's own milk, either suckled directly at the breast or freshly expressed and administered by bottle, syringe, or naso/orogastric tube; donor human milk, and formula. For this study, we define as exclusive human milk either exclusive mother's milk, or donor milk, or a mix of the two regardless of the addition of milk's fortifier; "any human milk" refers to the use of human milk (mother's own milk or donor milk) alone or combined with formula; complementary milk is human milk (donor and/or mother's own milk) plus formula.

Feeding practices during NICU hospitalization were analyzed at three different time points: at the beginning of enteral feeding, including minimal enteral feeding; at the achievement of full enteral nutrition—defined as the total daily intake requirement administered via enteral nutrition only, without any parenteral nutrition—and at discharge home.

RESULTS

A total of 1,398 infants were included in the registry in the study period. Their main characteristics are summarized in **Table 1**. Congenital anomalies were considered present if the infant had a major birth defect (from a pre-specified list) recorded.

Beginning of Enteral Nutrition

Information concerning the beginning of enteral nutrition were available for 1,302 cases of 1,398 born in the study period (**Figure 1**).

Most of the infants (74.1%) started enteral feeding during the first 24 h of life. Infants with a lower GA started enteral feeding later than peers with higher GA (**Figure 2**). Mean (SD) age at start of enteral nutrition was 3.7 (7.7) days in infants younger than 25 weeks GA, 1.5 (3.3) days in infants 26–28 weeks GA, 0.6 (2.1) days in infants 29–31 weeks GA and 0.5 (2.4) in those >31 weeks GA and <1,500 g.

Human milk—more frequently, donor milk—was widely used to start enteral nutrition (80.9% of cases) (**Table 2**). In infants who received donor milk, enteral nutrition started very early, at a mean age of 0.4 ± 1.6 days.

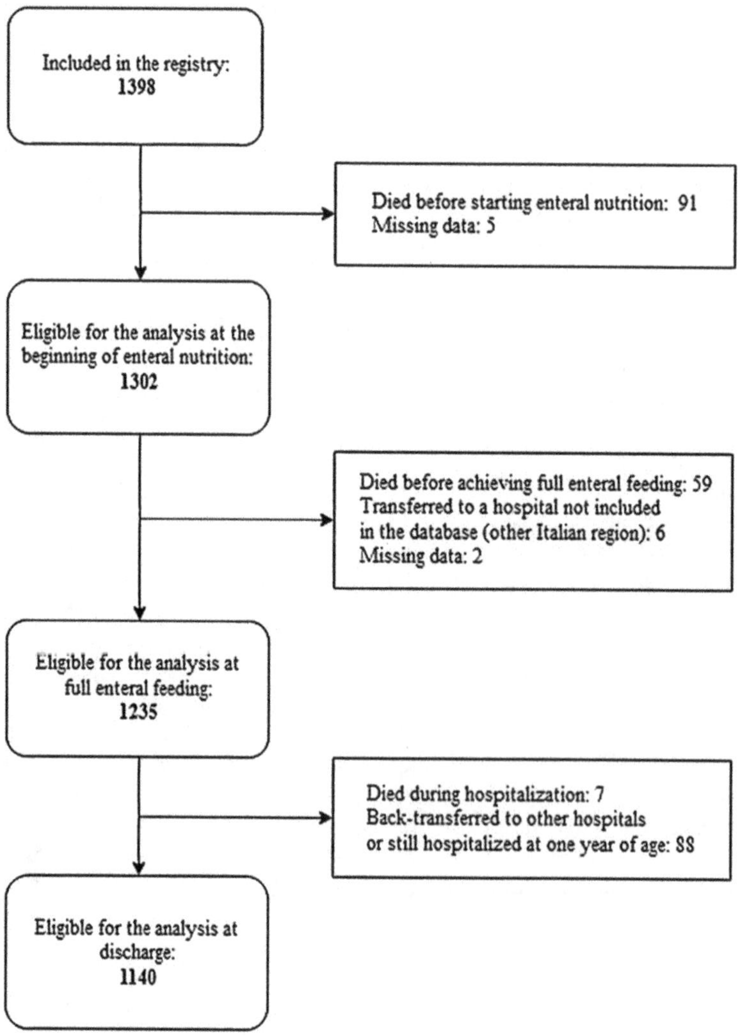

FIGURE 1 | Study population.

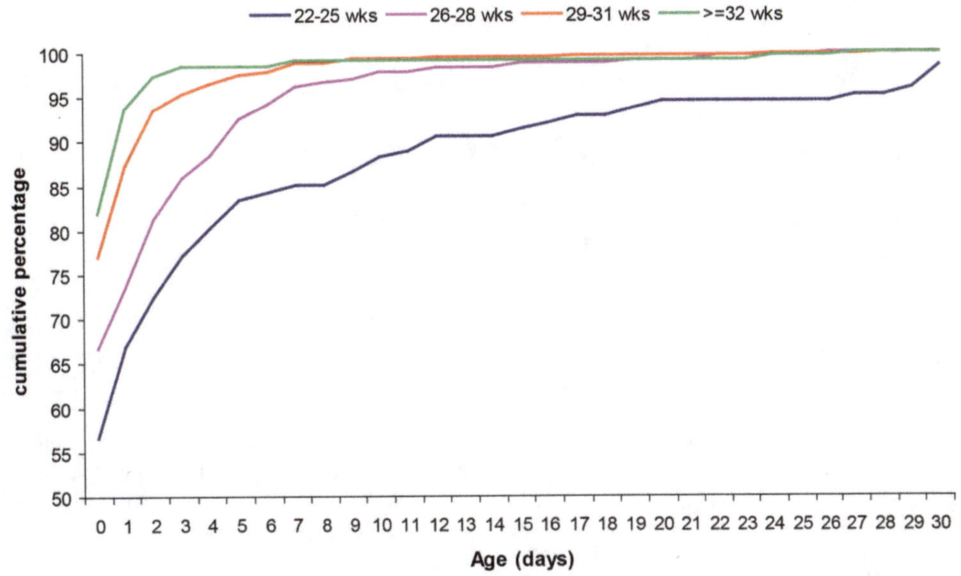

FIGURE 2 | Postnatal age at the beginning of enteral feeding by GA classes.

TABLE 2 | Feeding type at different times during hospitalization.

Feeding type	At the beginning of enteral nutrition		At full enteral feeding		At discharge	
	n	%	*n*	%	*n*	%
Mother's own milk	173	13.3	426	34.5	319	28.0
Donor milk	870	66.8	308	24.9	–	–
Mother's own milk + donor milk	–	–	255	20.6	–	–
Complementary milk	10	0.8	147	12.0	411	36.0
Formula	249	19.1	99	8.0	410	36.0
Total	1,302		1,235		1,140	

Two-hundred fifty nine infants were fed formula or complementary milk at the beginning of enteral nutrition, and most of them (86.9%) were born in the same NICU. The remaining infants initially fed with formula were distributed in 7 centres.

Full Enteral Feeding

Data on feeding at the time of full enteral nutrition were available for 1,235 newborns (**Figure 1**). Full enteral feeding was achieved using any human milk in most cases (92%), and mother's own milk had the highest prevalence of use (**Table 2**).

The median age at the achievement of full enteral nutrition was 11 days (interquartile range-IQR: 7–20 days). Full enteral feeding time was reached earlier in newborns who were fed human milk than in those fed formula, regardless of GA. Mean time ± SD to full enteral feeding was 34.7 ± 14.2 vs. 54.5 ± 47.2 days in infants 22–25 weeks GA; 20.4 ± 10.0 vs. 40.2 ± 32.7 days in those 26–28 weeks; and 10.9 ± 8.3 vs. 18.8 ± 15.3 days in those 29–31 weeks GA; all $P < 0.001$). When feeding type at time of full enteral nutrition was stratified by the type of milk at the start of enteral feeding, newborns who were fed donor milk at the beginning presented a very high prevalence (91.3%) of exclusive human milk at full enteral feeding (**Table 3**).

Feeding at Discharge Home

The median age at discharge home was 49 days (IQR: 36–71). Feeding data at discharge home were available for 1,140 infants (**Table 2**). Sixty four percent of infants were still fed any human milk at discharge. Extremely preterm newborns below 26 weeks of GA presented a higher prevalence of use of formula (70.2%) compared to infants with higher GA (42.5% at 26–28 weeks; 31.18% at 29–31 weeks; 30.4% at ≥32 weeks) ($P < 0.001$). The type of milk at the start of enteral nutrition did not influence the type of feeding at discharge (**Table 4**).

DISCUSSION

The present study gives a picture of enteral feeding practices for very preterm and VLBW infants in Tuscany, a region of central Italy where a network of six donor human milk banks is in place in order to ensure donor human milk provision to all the NICUs in the Region. In our population, the early introduction of enteral feeding was largely performed using exclusive human milk, and primarily donor milk. Full enteral feeding was achieved using exclusive human milk in more than 90% of cases and among these mother's own milk had the highest prevalence of use. Full enteral feeding was reached earlier in newborns fed exclusive human milk, and infants initially fed donor milk presented the highest prevalence of exclusive human milk at full enteral feeding. The type of milk at start of enteral nutrition did not influence that at discharge home.

TABLE 3 | Type of milk at full enteral feeding stratified by type of milk at start of enteral nutrition.

Milk at the start of enteral nutrition	Milk at full enteral nutrition				
	Mother's own milk	**Donor milk**	**Mother's own milk and donor milk**	**Formula**	**Complementary milk**
Mother's own milk	57 35.2%	2 1.2%	28 17.3%	20 12.3%	55 34.0%
Donor milk	273 32.9%	279 33.6%	206 24.8%	18 2.2%	54 6.5%
Complementary milk	0	0	0	2 22.2%	7 77.8%
Formula	94 40.7%	26 11.3%	21 9.1%	59 25.5%	31 13.4%

$P < 0.001$ (Pearson chi-square).

TABLE 4 | Type of milk at discharge home by type of milk at the start of enteral nutrition.

Milk at the start of enteral nutrition	Milk at discharge		
	Mother's own milk	**Complementary milk**	**Formula**
Mother's own milk	41 25.8%	54 34.0%	64 40.2%
Donor milk	224 28.5%	296 37.6%	267 33.9%
Complementary milk	2 22.2%	4 44.5%	3 33.3%
Formula	51 28.0%	57 31.3%	74 40.7%

$P = 0.503$ (Pearson chi-square).

Donor milk is often necessary in very premature infants to start enteral feeding during the first 24–48 h of life, since mother's own milk availability may be quite challenging in this period. In infants who received donor milk, enteral nutrition started very early. The availability of donor milk allowed the double benefit of safe early enteral feeding, particularly in the lower GA classes, and of a full enteral feeding with any human milk in almost all newborns (92%), mostly (80%) with exclusive human milk. Most newborns were fed exclusive human milk for at least 11 days of life, and this aspect is noteworthy, especially for extremely low birth weight infants in order to prevent late-onset sepsis and necrotizing enterocolitis. For these outcomes several authors have reported a protection when human milk is introduced up to >50 ml/kg/day (13–18). Several positive aspects are in fact associated to a fast achievement of full enteral feeding with human milk: bioactive (anti-infective, growth factors) substances in human milk, better digestibility, and shorter exposure to central vascular lines (6, 18–20). On the other hand, a recent double-blind randomized control trial found no significant effect of pasteurized donor milk during the first 10 days of life in preventing serious infections and NEC in VLBW infants when donor milk was used as a supplemental feeding whenever own mother's milk was insufficiently available during the first 10 days of life (21).

Despite the large number of newborn infants who started enteral nutrition with human milk, a consistent proportion (19.9%) was fed milk formula or complementary milk. This practice was almost entirely attributable to a single NICU with no milk bank in the hospital and that must therefore refer to the neighboring banks. In this NICU the use of formula to start enteral nutrition has been gradually decreasing over the study period, possibly related to the implementation of the milk banks' network and the improvement of donor milk availability in the Region. The characteristics (e.g., gestational age, birth weight) of neonates fed formula were not different from those of neonates who were fed human milk. A large observational study in England showed that a wide variation of donor milk use among networks could not be explained by differences in patients characteristics or presence of human milk bank within the network. According to the authors this indicates uncertainty about optimal clinical practice in relation to the use of pasteurized donor milk (10) and the need to have randomized controlled trials on this topic.

Interestingly, having started enteral feeding with donor milk did not adversely affect the proportion of infants fed mother's own milk when full enteral feeding was achieved. This confirms that a breastfeeding support in very preterm infants is part of a wider culture within the neonatal intensive care units and the early use of bank human milk is an integral part of this culture (22, 23).

The overall prevalence of mother's milk was quite elevated even at discharge, although the discontinuation of donor milk before discharge led to an increase of formula fed infants. Proportion of infants fed mother's own milk at discharge (27%) is superimposable to that reported in a previous investigation in neonatal intensive care units in Italy (24).

CONCLUSIONS

This study confirms the importance of having an organized network of human milk banks throughout the territory to start enteral feeding early in very preterm infants and thus allowing a rapid achievement of full enteral feeding safely, particularly in the lower GA groups.

It also demonstrates the need to implement more effective strategies from the moment of achieving full enteral feeding to discharge to support the use of mother's own milk and succeed in obtaining better rates of breastfeeding at discharge.

The Tuscany region has established the Regional Network of Donor Human Milk Banks in 2008 (ReBLUD) and is actively engaged in the promotion of the culture of donor human milk, indicating the adequate availability of donor milk as an element of essential strategic value to support the care of critical newborn infants.

AUTHOR CONTRIBUTIONS

FR, EB, MP, SP, and LG: Conception and design of the study; CB, AI, LM, EM, SP, ES, and BT: Collection of data and critical revision of the manuscript; FR, EB, and MP: Analysis and interpretation of the data; FR, EB, SP, and LG: Drafting of the manuscript and critical revision.

ACKNOWLEDGMENT

We would like to thank the **TIN Toscane online group**: Roberto Banchini, Maria Celeste Papi, Debora Pecori, SP, Carlo Dani (Careggi University Hospital, Florence); AI, EB, FR, Patrizio Fiorini (Anna Meyer Children's University Hospital, Florence); ES, Gianluca Petrillo, Paolo Ghirri (University Hospital of Pisa, Pisa); Giorgio Panariello, BT (University Hospital of Siena, Siena); Armando Giovannoni [Azienda Unita Sanitaria Locale [AUSL] 1, Massa]; Francesca Nardini, Riccardo Moschetti (Ospedale del Cuore Fondazione Toscana G. Monasterio, Massa); Simona Tognetti (AUSL 2, Lucca); Leila Capuzzo (AUSL 3, Pescia); Ugo Gasperini (AUSL 3, Pistoia); Alessandra Brioschi, EM, Pier Luigi Vasarri (AUSL 4, Prato); Carla Carlotti (AUSL 5, Pontedera); Roberto Danieli (AUSL 6, Livorno); Gian Luca Benetti (AUSL 6, Piombino); Monica Tiezzi (AUSL 7, Poggibonsi); Flavio Civitelli (AUSL 7, Montepulciano); LM, Laura Valdambrini, Marco Martini (AUSL 8, Arezzo); Antonio Cardinale (AUSL 8, Montevarchi); Marcello De Filippo (AUSL 9, Grosseto); Leonardo Cafaggi (AUSL 10, Ospedale Santa Maria Annunziata, Bagno a Ripoli); CB, Beatrice Gambi, Marco Pezzati (AUSL 10, Ospedale S Giovanni di Dio, Florence); Rosalia Di Silvio (AUSL 10, Borgo San Lorenzo); Stefania Toti (AUSL 11, Empoli); Giulia Placidi, LG (AUSL 12, Viareggio); MP, Roberto, Berni, Emiliano Sessa, Fabio Voller (Health Agency of Tuscany, Florence).

REFERENCES

1. Fellman V, Hellstrom-Westas L, Norman M, Westgren M, Kallen K, Lagercrantz H, et al. One-year survival of extremely preterm infants after active perinatal care in Sweden. *JAMA* (2009) 301:2225–33. doi: 10.1001/jama.2009.771
2. Smith PB, Ambalavanan N, Li L, Cotton CM, Laughon M, Walsh MC, et al. Approach to infants born at 22 to 24 weeks' gestation: relationship to outcomes of more-mature infants. *Pediatrics* (2012) 129:e1508–16. doi: 10.1542/peds.2011-2216
3. Hans DM, Pylipow M, Long JD, Thureen PJ, Georgieff MK. Nutritional practices in the neonatal intensive care unit: analysis of a 2006 neonatal nutrition survey. *Pediatrics* (2009) 123:51–7. doi: 10.1542/peds.2007-3644
4. Klingenberg C, Embleton ND, Jacobs SE, O'Connell LA, Kuschel CA. Enteral feeding practices in very preterm infants: an international survey. *Arch Dis Child Fetal Neonatal Ed.* (2012) 97:F56–61. doi: 10.1136/adc.2010.204123
5. Bonet M, Forcella E, Blondel B, Draper E, Agostino R, Cuttini M, et al. Approaches to supporting lactation and breastfeeding for very preterm infants in the NICU: a qualitative study in three European regions. *BMJ Open* (2015) 5:e006973. doi: 10.1136/bmjopen-2014-006973
6. American Academy of Pediatrics section on Breastfeeding. Breastfeeding and the use of human milk. *Pediatrics* (2012) 129:e827–41. doi: 10.1542/peds.2011-3552
7. Horta BL, Victora CG, World Health Organization. *Long-Term Effects of Breastfeeding: A Systematic Review*. Geneva: WHO Library (2013).
8. Underwood MA. Human milk for the premature infant. *Pediatr Clin N Am.* (2013) 60:189–207. doi: 10.1016/j.pcl.2012.09.008
9. Moro GE, Arslanoglu S, Bertino E, Corvaglia L, Montirosso R, Picaud JC, et al. European Society for Pediatric Gastroenterology, Hepatology, and Nutrition. Human milk in feeding premature infants: consensus statement. *J Pediatr Gastroenterol Nutr.* (2015). 61:S16–19. doi: 10.1097/01.mpg.0000471460.08792.4d
10. Battersby C, Marciano Alves Mousinho R, Longford N, Modi N, UK Neonatal Collaborative Necrotising (UKNC-NEC) Study Group. Use of pasteurised human donor milk across neonatal networks in England. *Early Hum Dev.* (2018) 118:32–6. doi: 10.1016/j.earlhumdev.2018.01.017
11. Perrin MT. Donor human milk and fortifier use in United States Level 2,3 and 4 Neonatal care Hospitals. *J Pediatr Gastroenterol Nutr.* (2018) 66:664–6. doi: 10.1097/MPG.0000000000001790
12. Gagliardi L, Amador C, Puglia M, Mecacci F, Pratesi S, Sigali E, et al. Area-based study identifies risk factors associated with missed antenatal corticosteroid prophylaxis in women delivering preterm infants. *Acta Paediatr.* (2017) 106:250–5. doi: 10.1111/apa.13563
13. Sullivan S, Schanler RJ, Kim JH, Patel AL, Trawöger R, Kiechl-Kohlendorfer U, et al. An exclusive human milk-based diet is associated with a lower rate of necrotizing enterocolitis than a diet of human milk and bovine milk-based products. *J Pediatr.* (2010) 156:562–7. doi: 10.1016/j.jpeds.2009.10.040
14. Meinzen-Derr J, Poindexter B, Wrage L, Morrow AL, Stoll B, Donovan EF. Role of human milk in extremely low birth weight infant' risk of necrotizing enterocolitis or death. *J Perinatol.* (2009) 29:57–62. doi: 10.1038/jp.2008.117
15. Menon G, Williams TC. Human milk for preterm infants: why, what, when and how? *Arch Dis Child Fetal Neonatal Ed.* (2013) 98:F559–62. doi: 10.1136/archdischild-2012-303582
16. Sisk PM, Lovelady CA, Dillard RG, Gruber KJ, O'Shea TM. Early human milk feeding is associated with a lower risk of necrotizing enterocolitis in very low birth weight infants. *J Perinatol.* (2007) 27:428–33. doi: 10.1038/sj.jp.7211758
17. Schanler RJ, Hurst NM, Lau C. The use of human milk and breastfeeding in premature infants. *Clin Perinatol.* (1999) 25:379–97. doi: 10.1016/S0095-5108(18)30058-7
18. Schanler RJ, Lau C, Hurst NM, Smith EO. Randomized trial of donor human milk versus preterm formula as substitutes for mother's own milk in the feeding of extremely premature infants. *Pediatrics* (2005) 116:400–6. doi: 10.1542/peds.2004-1974
19. Edmond K, Bahl R, World Health Organization. *Optimal Feeding of Low-Birth-Weight Infants*. Geneva: WHO (2006).
20. Corpeleijn WE, de Waard M, Christmann V, van Goudoever JB, Jansen-van der Weide MC, Kooi EM, et al. Effect of donor milk on severe infections and mortality in very low birth weight infants: the early nutrition study randomized clinical trial. *JAMA Pediatr.* (2016) 70:654–61. doi: 10.1001/jamapediatrics.2016.0183
21. Kantorowska A, Wei JC, Cohen RS, Lawrence RA, Gould JB, Lee HC. Impact of donor milk availability on breast milk use and necrotizing

enterocolitis rates. *Pediatrics* (2016) 137:e20153123. doi: 10.1542/peds.2015-3123

22. Williams T, Nair H, Simpson J, Embleton N. Use of donor human milk and maternal breastfeeding rates: a systematic review. *J Hum Lact.* (2016) 32:212–20. doi: 10.1177/0890334416632203
23. Wilson E, Edstedt Bonamy AK, Bonet M, Toome L, Rodrigues C, Howell EA, et al. Room for improvement in breast milk feeding after very preterm birth in Europe: results from the EPICE cohort. *Matern Child Nutr.* (2018) 14:e12485. doi: 10.1111/mcn.12485
24. Davanzo R, Monasta L, Ronfani L, Brovedani P, Demarini S. Breastfeeding at NICU discharge: a multicentre Italian study. *J Hum Lact.* (2013) 29:374–80. doi: 10.1177/0890334412451055

5

Fortification of Human Milk for Preterm Infants: Update and Recommendations of the European Milk Bank Association (EMBA) Working Group on Human Milk Fortification

Sertac Arslanoglu [1*†], Clair-Yves Boquien [2†], Caroline King [3†], Delphine Lamireau [4†], Paola Tonetto [5†], Debbie Barnett [6], Enrico Bertino [5], Antoni Gaya [7], Corinna Gebauer [8], Anne Grovslien [9], Guido E. Moro [10], Gillian Weaver [11], Aleksandra Maria Wesolowska [12] and Jean-Charles Picaud [13,14†]

[1] Division of Neonatology, Department of Pediatrics, Istanbul Medeniyet University, Istanbul, Turkey, [2] PhAN, Institut National de la Recherche Agronomique (INRA), Université de Nantes, CRNH-Ouest, Nantes, France, [3] Department of Nutrition and Dietetics, Imperial College Healthcare NHS Trust, London, United Kingdom, [4] Lactariums de Bordeaux-Marmande, Pôle Pédiatrique, Centre Hospitalo-Universitaire (CHU) de Bordeaux, Bordeaux, France, [5] Neonatal Unit of Turin University, City of Health and Science of Turin, Turin, Italy, [6] Greater Glasgow and Clyde Donor Milk Bank, Royal Hospital for Sick Children, Glasgow, United Kingdom, [7] Banc de Teixits, Fundaciò Banc Sang i Teixits de les Illes Balears, Palma de Mallorca, Spain, [8] Abteilung Neonatologie Klinik und Poliklinik für Kinder und Jugendliche, Leipzig, Germany, [9] Neonatal Unit, Milk Bank, Oslo University Hospital, Oslo, Norway, [10] Associazione Italiana Banche del Latte Umano Donato (AIBLUD), Milan, Italy, [11] Hearts Milk Bank, Rothamsted Research Institute, Harpenden, United Kingdom, [12] Department of Neonatology, Faculty of Health Science, Medical University of Warsaw, Warsaw, Poland, [13] CarMeN Unit, INSERM U1060, INRA U1397, Claude Bernard University Lyon 1, Pierre Bénite, France, [14] Division of Neonatology, Hôpital de la Croix-Rousse, Lyon, France

***Correspondence:**
Sertac Arslanoglu
sertacarslanoglu@gmail.com*

† European Milk Bank Association (EMBA) Working Group on Human Milk Fortification

Evidence indicates that human milk (HM) is the best form of nutrition uniquely suited not only to term but also to preterm infants conferring health benefits in both the short and long-term. However, HM does not provide sufficient nutrition for the very low birth weight (VLBW) infant when fed at the usual feeding volumes leading to slow growth with the risk of neurocognitive impairment and other poor health outcomes such as retinopathy and bronchopulmonary dysplasia. HM should be supplemented (fortified) with the nutrients in short supply, particularly with protein, calcium, and phosphate to meet the high requirements of this group of babies. In this paper the European Milk Bank Association (EMBA) Working Group on HM Fortification discusses the existing evidence in this field, gives an overview of different fortification approaches and definitions, outlines the gaps in knowledge and gives recommendations for practice and suggestions for future research. EMBA recognizes that "Standard Fortification," which is currently the most utilized regimen in neonatal intensive care units, still falls short in supplying sufficient protein for some VLBW infants. EMBA encourages the use of "Individualized Fortification" to optimize nutrient intake. "Adjustable Fortification" and "Targeted Fortification" are 2 methods of individualized fortification. The quality and source of human milk fortifiers constitute another important topic. There is work looking at human milk derived fortifiers, but it is still too early to draw precise conclusions about their use. The pros and cons are discussed in this Commentary in addition to the evidence around use of fortifiers post discharge.

Keywords: nutrition, prematurity, human milk, adjustable fortification, individualized fortification, growth, protein

INTRODUCTION

Inadequate nutrition during the critical periods of brain development alters the growth trajectory of the brain and can have permanent negative consequences. The most critical period of brain growth and development for humans corresponds to the third trimester of pregnancy and for very low birthweight (VLBW) infants these developmental processes take place in the neonatal intensive care unit (NICU) environment (1, 2). Inadequate nutrition and/or poor postnatal growth during the NICU stay has been associated with neurocognitive impairments (3–11) and poor renal function (12) in preterm infants. Recent studies suggest that not only the growth *per se*, but also the quality of growth counts. Better linear growth and early gains in fat-free body mass have been found to be associated with improved neurodevelopment in VLBW preterm infants (13, 14). Thus, optimization of the nutritional care for the preterm infants has a key role in improving neurodevelopmental outcomes and has become a priority.

Despite the advancements in nutritional support over 20 years and current focus on "early intense nutrition" in NICU, undernutrition and extrauterine growth restriction (EUGR) are still important problems for VLBW infants (15–18).

Evidence indicates that human milk (HM) is the best source of nutrition for both term and preterm infants conferring health benefits both in the short and long-term (19, 20). Unfortified HM however does not provide sufficient nutrition to VLBW infants when fed at the usual feeding volumes. Human milk should be supplemented (fortified) with the nutrients in short supply, particularly with protein, calcium, and phosphate to meet high requirements of this group of tiny preterm infants as discussed in the next sections. Although HM fortification is widely adopted in the NICUs all over the world, there is still much inconsistency and variability and even some skepticism around this practice. During the last decade optimization of HM fortification- mainly individualization, and the quality of the fortifiers have been the hot topics of discussion.

The European Milk Bank Association (EMBA) Working Group on HM Fortification aims to document the existing evidence on this field, overviews different fortification approaches, clarifies the terminology and definitions, outlines the gaps in knowledge, and gives recommendations for practice and suggestions for future research.

METHODS

European Milk Bank Association (EMBA) Working Group (WG) on HM Fortification was formed by a group of experts on this field in 2013. In 2016 WG planned to review the related research and to write a position paper with recommendations on HM fortification for preterm infants. The first face-to-face meeting in Milan resulted in organizing the paper into 10 different sections. These sections were then assigned to working subgroups within the WG. The literature review included electronic searches of MEDLINE (1966-30 June 2018), EMBASE (1980-30 June 2018), CINAHL (1981-30 June 2018), the Cochrane Library, and conference proceedings. The electronic search used the following key words: human milk fortification, breast milk fortification, donor milk fortification, banked milk fortification, [human milk OR breast milk] AND [fortification]. All types of articles, including original papers, reviews, and recommendations were considered. Furthermore, the reference lists of the previous reviews and relevant studies were examined. The searches were limited to human studies, and to the published articles written in English. Trials that had been reported only as abstracts were eligible for inclusion if sufficient information was available from the report.

Following the first meeting, a total of 4 face-to-face meetings were held in Milan, Lyon, and Glasgow to formulate and agree on all of the recommendations. All group members interacted during these face-to-face meetings, and by iterative e-mails between them. All conclusions and recommendations were discussed until a full consensus was achieved for each statement.

THE RATIONALE FOR HUMAN MILK FEEDING AND HUMAN MILK FORTIFICATION

Human Milk as the Best Feeding Option for Preterm Infants

Evidence-based data show that HM is the best nutritional and normative standard for infant nutrition (19, 20). Its particular composition—"nutrients with optimal bioavailability, hormonal and enzymatic components, anti-infective, trophic and growth factors, stem cells, prebiotics and probiotics and a myriad of bioactive proteins" -makes HM suited not only to term but also to preterm infants (21–26). Feeding preterm infants with HM, indeed, confers protection against the most important NICU challenges such as necrotizing enterocolitis (NEC) and sepsis (27–33), retinopathy of prematurity (ROP) (34–36), bronchopulmonary dysplasia (BPD) (37, 38) and decreases mortality in a dose-dependent manner (31). Human milk feeding improves long-term neurocognitive development (39–41) and cardiovascular health outcomes (29). Studies comparing solely donor human milk vs. formula show that donor human milk confers protection against NEC (27, 29) and improves feeding tolerance (29). That is why HM is the recommended feeding for all neonates including premature infants. The European Society for Pediatric Gastroenterology Hepatology and Nutrition (ESPGHAN) (29), American Academy of Pediatrics (AAP) (19), and Milan EMBA/ESPGHAN/AAP Joint Meeting Consensus (42) in their most recent recommendation papers stated that "mother's own milk (MOM) is the first choice in the feeding of preterm infants. When mother's milk is not available, pasteurized donor human milk (DHM) should be used."

The Rationale for Human Milk Fortification

Infants born early in the third trimester miss the placental transfer of nutrients which would create stores for use in the postnatal period. Human milk while acting as "a preventive therapeutic drug," doesn't provide sufficient amounts of many nutrients for premature infants when fed at the usual feeding volumes. The main challenge is to meet the high and variable nutrient requirements of these preterm infants during the whole hospitalization period. Insufficient nutrient intakes place the infant at risk of impaired neurodevelopment. To prevent EUGR, which is associated with poor neurocognitive outcome, and to avoid specific nutrient deficiencies, nutrient fortification of HM is necessary (19, 29, 42–46).

The consequences of intakes falling short of requirements vary from nutrient to nutrient. Evidence suggests that inadequate intake of protein is important for slow growth and it is particularly responsible for decreased fat-free mass (FFM) gains which are directly related to poor neurocognitive outcomes (14, 47). Intake of energy is also clearly important. In a single blinded randomized clinical trial, Bellagamba et al. (48) showed that increasing only protein intake by 1 gram during parenteral and enteral nutrition did not improve growth and neurodevelopment of preterm infants with a birthweight 500–1,249 g. Insufficient intake of some nutrients leads to specific deficiency states, such as osteopenia (due to insufficient intake of calcium and phosphorus) and to various micronutrient deficiencies, such as zinc deficiency. It is important that VLBW infants receive adequate amounts of iron, zinc, copper, selenium, and iodine. The need of fortification is less clear with regard to manganese, chromium, and molybdenum (49). For the great majority of other nutrients, small shortfalls may have less serious effects, especially when they are temporary. With protein however, any shortfall is prone to affect growth and carries the risk of neurocognitive impairment. Thus, protein supply needs special attention in early life and meeting the requirements should be the goal (43, 44).

The objective of fortification is to increase the concentration of nutrients to the levels that at the recommended feeding volumes (135–200 ml/kg/d) preterm infants receive amounts of all nutrients that meet requirements (43, 50). Nutrient requirements of preterm infants are defined as intakes that enable the infant to grow at the same rate as a fetus (44). Requirements for most nutrients have been derived from accretion rates of protein, fat and minerals obtained by the analysis of fetal body composition at various stages of gestation (44, 50, 51). Additionally, empirical methods have been employed to define requirements including those for nutrients such as vitamins (44, 51) (**Tables 1, 2**). However, these requirements are variable depending on the

TABLE 1 | Requirements for protein and energy; best estimates by factorial and empirical methods (44).

Body weight, g	500–1,000	1,001–1,500	1,501–2,000
Weight gain of fetus, g/kg/d	19.0	17.4	16.4
Protein, g/kg/d	4.0	3.9	3.7
Energy, Kcal/kg/d	106	115	123
Protein/energy, g/100 kcal	3.8	3.4	3.0

clinical condition and characteristics of each infant either present at birth or evolving during NICU stay (such as IUGR or severe BPD). Therefore, HM fortification needs to be adapted to the specific needs of each infant at each time.

The EMBA Working Group on HM Fortification summarizes the latest recommended intakes for protein, carbohydrates, lipids, and energy in **Table 3**. This table comprises the recommendations of the experts and expert panels (50, 52, 53).

CURRENT HUMAN MILK FORTIFIERS AND SUPPLEMENTS

There are a number of products available for fortifying human milk for preterm babies which differ by the origin of milk used (bovine, human or donkey), and by nutrient composition (multi-nutrient fortifiers or supplements of protein, lipids, carbohydrates).

Multi-Nutrient Fortifiers

Bovine-based multi-nutrient fortifiers contain varying amounts of protein, energy, minerals, trace-elements, vitamins, and electrolytes (**Table 4**). The addition of lipids to multi-nutrient fortifiers with a concomitant reduction in carbohydrate content has allowed a reduction in osmolality of these products (54). In addition, lipids provide a source of essential fatty acids (EFA) which has been shown to improve EFA status in preterm infants (55). As indicated, standard fortification using previously available products was unable to support a satisfactory postnatal growth (See Current Fortification Practices in Neonatal Intensive Care Units: Terminology-Definitions). New fortifiers with higher protein content have been shown to improve short term weight gain (56). Most multi-nutrient fortifiers contain bovine milk protein. Donkey milk was more recently proposed as its composition is very close to human milk (57).

During the past 15 years, some for-profit companies have been set up to collect and buy HM, to manufacture and to sell HM-based products. Prolacta Bioscience is the only one which produces pasteurized HM and HM-based fortifiers. They adhere to the Human Milk Banking Association of North America (HMBANA) guidelines, but test also bacterial content before heat treatment (including pathogens, such as *Bacillus cereus*,

TABLE 2 | Requirements for major minerals and electrolytes determined by factorial method, listed by body weight (51).

	500–1,000 g		1,001–1,500 g		1,501–2,000 g	
	Accretion	**Requirem.**	**Accretion**	**Requirem.**	**Accretion**	**Requirem.**
Ca (mg)	102	184	99	178	96	173
P (mg)	66	126	65	124	63	120
Mg (mg)	2.8	6.9	2.7	6.7	2.5	6.4
Na (meq)	1.54	3.3	1.37	3.0	1.06	2.6
K (meq)	0.78	2.4	0.72	2.3	0.63	2.2
Cl (meq)	1.26	2.8	0.99	2.7	0.74	2.5

TABLE 3 | Recommended enteral protein and energy intakes for clinically stable very low birthweight infants (50, 52, 53).

	Munich consensus 2014	ESPGHAN 2010	Ziegler et al.
Energy (kcal/kg/d)	110–130	110–135	105-127
Protein (g/kg/d)	3.5–4.5	4.0–4.5 (<1 kg) 3.5–4.0 (1–1.8 kg)	3.9-4.0
Protein/Energy (g/100 kcal)	3.2–4.1	3.2–4.1	3.1–3.8
Lipids (g/kg/d)	4.8–6.6	4.8–6.6	–
Carbohydrates (g/kg/d)	11.6–13.2	11.6–13.2	–

Escherichia. coli, Pseudomonas aeruginosa, Salmonella spp., yeast and mold), recreational drugs, nicotine, prescription drugs, milk adulteration and breast milk DNA fingerprint for donor identification. To treat huge volumes of HM (1,200 L from 250 donors) they use Vat pasteurization (63°C, ≥ 30 min). Vat differs from Holder pasteurization which is the commonly used method in non-profit HM banks. Meredith-Dennis et al. (58) showed that Vat pasteurization significantly reduced lactoferrin and total HM oligosaccharide concentrations when compared to Holder pasteurization. Human milk-based fortifier is obtained by concentrating heat-treated donor HM and then adding vitamins and minerals. Various caloric densities of this fortifier allow for individual adjustment based on growth or blood urea nitrogen (BUN). More recently, a novel HM derived cream supplement has been produced by the same company (59, 60).

Although some studies suggested a benefit in terms of morbidity and mortality when babies are fed an exclusively human milk based diet including HM-based fortifier, leading to a reduction of costs (33, 61), much of the work is observational (62–64), and there are still concerns about the efficacy of these products (65). For example, Sullivan et al. (33) showed a significant reduction in NEC rates from 16 to 6%, but this needs to be confirmed in large, independent randomized control trials conducted in units where baseline NEC rates are lower. Sullivan et al. evaluated an exclusive HM-based diet, which consisted of donor HM if no mother's own milk was available and a HM-based fortifier in place of bovine-based formulas and fortifiers. However, the HM-based fortifier was never directly compared with the bovine based fortifier and many of the babies who developed NEC on the bovine fortifier were also on the bovine formula. The OptiMoM study, recently published by O'Connor et al. (66), is the first trial comparing the efficacy of HM-based fortifier to bovine-based fortifier in the absence of formula. There was no difference in feeding tolerance, postnatal growth and morbidity, including NEC ≥ grade 2 (4.7 vs. 4.9%). In 2015, most facilities in US fortified human milk, and approximately one out of five used a HM-based fortifier (67). In summary, HM-based products have been adopted in neonatal care despite being costly and supported by limited efficacy data. Some aspects have not been fully investigated yet, such as metabolic effects and body composition, which are needed before considering these products to be totally safe and effective. It is essential to evaluate the benefit-risk ratio, particularly as these products are very expensive and use large amounts of donated milk to make the fortifier which could be used more directly to feed preterm babies. At the present time these products are available mainly in North America. According to regulations in some European countries, only HM banks in each country are authorized to collect, treat and distribute HM or HM-based products (68, 69). Finally, there could be some ethical concerns. According to available information ethical concerns seem to be well-controlled by present manufacturers but, if the evidence confirms a benefit, the need for these products could increase sharply and ethical questions related to the origin of HM could become a major concern.

In some fortifiers, manufacturers used a hydrolyzed protein source (**Table 4**). There is no evidence supporting the use of such a protein source. It has been shown that preterm infants fed a formula with partially hydrolyzed protein have a shorter transit time, but also a reduced intestinal absorption (70). The rationale cannot be related to the hypothetical prevention of allergy. Indeed, no increased risk of allergy was detected with preterm infants fed on formulas based on cow's milk even those with a high protein content. It has even been suggested that preterm birth reduces the chances of the subsequent development of severe atopic disease (71). Nevertheless, the use of a hydrolyzed protein source is a response to clinicians' preferences, as a lot of professionals are reluctant to add whole bovine protein to HM. This current opinion of professionals comes from a study suggesting that, in a subgroup of preterm infants with a family history of atopy, early exposure to cow's milk increased the risk of

TABLE 4 | Nutrient composition of selected fortifiers and supplements.

	Bovine-based products (per gram of powder)										Human milk-based fortifier (per volume)			
	Multicomponent fortifiers					Protein supplements								
Fortifier	A	B	C	D	E	F	G	H	I	J	K	L	M	N
Volume (ml)	/	/	/	/	/	/	/	/	/	/	20	30	40	50
Energy (kcal)	4.4 (L)	3.5	3.6	4.9 (L)	3.9 (L)	3.4	3.6	3.6	4	3.7	28	42	56	71
Protein (g)	0.36^{PH}	$0{,}25^{EH}$	0.2^{EH}	0.4	0.3	0.82^{EH}	0.72^{EH}	0.86^{W}	0.8^{W}	0.9^{W}	1.2	1.8	2.4	3
Na (mg)	9.2	8,0	5.4	5.6	4.2	7.8	8.2	2.1	2	0	20	40	42	45
Ca (mg)	18.9	14.9	10	32	33	5.2	12.8	0	4	0	103	106	108	111
P (mg)	11	8.7	7	18	19	5.2	0.73	0	3	0	53.8	54.9	56	57.5
Iron (mg)	0.5	0	0	0.5	0.1	0	0.007	0	0	0	0.1	0.15	0.2	0.25

L, lipids; PH, partially hydrolyzed; EH, extensively hydrolyzed; W, whole protein; HMBF, human milk-based fortifier. A-Fortipré®, Nestle; B-Fortema®, Danone; C-FM85®, Nestle; D-Enfamil®, Mead Johnson; E-Similac®, Ross; F-Aptamil PS®, Danone; G-Preemie®, Nestle; H-Beneprotein®, Nestle; I-Pro-Mix®, Corpak; J-Protein instant®, Resource; K- HMBF+4®, Prolacta; L- HMBF+6®, Prolacta; M- HMBF+8®, Prolacta; N- HMBF+10®, Prolacta.

allergic reaction (72). However, more recent studies showed that, compared to exclusively breastfed, preterm infants supplemented with HMF or fed exclusively a preterm formula for 4 months after discharge did not have an increased risk of developing allergic diseases during the first year of life (73). Furthermore, it was previously shown that protein supplementation using whole-protein is efficient (43, 74, 75). In summary, there is no strong evidence to support the use of hydrolyzed protein source in fortifiers, but it is current practice.

Single-Nutrient Supplements

Other products containing only protein, lipids, or carbohydrates are also available. They are useful when individualizing fortification (74–76). Usually, carbohydrate supplements are composed of dextrin maltose, and lipids are composed of medium chain triglycerides. More recently, a novel HM-derived cream supplement has been produced to enhance the energy density of feeds. Infants were supplemented with the 2.5 kcal/ml cream supplement whenever their mother's own milk or donor HM was found to be below 67 kcal/dl (20 kcal/oz) (60). When compared to the control group these infants had improved weight and length growth rates and were discharged slightly earlier. This reduction in length of stay was greater in the subgroup of preterm infants with bronchopulmonary dysplasia (59, 60). However, this finding needs to be replicated in other settings to ensure that this can be done without compromising protein to energy ratio.

Protein supplements have been available for years in some countries, but are not specifically designed for neonates (74–77). One of them contained extensively hydrolyzed protein source (56). Recently a new protein supplement—including partially hydrolyzed protein source-specifically designed for preterm infants, became available in most European countries (54) (Product G, **Table 4**). There is no consensus about how to use these products as studies are scarce. That being said, protein supplements are essential to enable individualized fortification, particularly for Adjustable (ADJ) fortification which has been shown to be associated with clinical benefits (74) (see Individualized Fortification).

CURRENT FORTIFICATION PRACTICES IN NEONATAL INTENSIVE CARE UNITS: TERMINOLOGY-DEFINITIONS

Following the first introduction of the commercial HM fortifiers in the 1980s, HM fortification has become part of the standard nutritional care for preterm infants in most NICUs. The quality of the fortifiers and the methods of HM fortification have improved over time but nutrient fortification remains suboptimal. An optimal approach to fortification is to provide each individual baby with her/his needs, which might be different from the average of the group (44).

Most of the available commercial fortifiers contain varying amounts of protein, carbohydrate, calcium, phosphate, other minerals, trace elements (zinc, manganese, magnesium, copper), vitamins, and electrolytes and are defined as "multi-nutrient HM fortifiers" (see Current Human Milk Fortifiers and Supplements) (43).

In an attempt to clarify the terminology regarding HM fortification practices, in 2010, World Association of Perinatal Medicine (WAPM) Working Group on Nutrition defined the fortification methods in current practice as follows (43):

1. Standard (STD) HM fortification
2. Individualized HM fortification:
   a. Adjustable (ADJ) HM fortification (74, 77, 78)
   b. Targeted HM fortification (76, 79–81)

The EMBA Working Group on HM Fortification adopts this terminology and **Table 5** summarizes the characteristics of these methods.

STANDARD (STD) FORTIFICATION

This is the most widely used fortification method. The standard practice is to add a fixed amount of multinutrient fortifier per 100 ml of HM to achieve the recommended nutrient intakes. This fixed amount has been calculated and determined by the manufacturer assuming a fixed protein content for

TABLE 5 | Current human milk fortification methods (43, 74, 76–79).

Fortification method	Principle	Advantages disadvantages
1. Standard (STD) Fortification	Fortification method currently in use in most of the neonatal units. A fixed amount of fortifier is added to a fixed volume of HM according to the manufacturers' instructions.	Practical. But has not solved the problem of protein undernutrition for VLBW infants. Despite STD fortification many VLBW infants continue to have suboptimal growth.
2. Individualized HM Fortification Methods		
a. Adjustable (ADJ) Fortification	Protein adequacy is monitored by BUN twice weekly, cut-off levels of BUN are 10–16 mg/dl*. If the level is <10 mg/dl extra protein is added to the STD fortification.	Practical, not labor intensive. Doesn't need expensive devices. Monitors protein intake of each infant. Safeguards also against excessive protein intake. Proven to be effective in optimizing growth and protein intake with a RCT. A real individualization method taking into consideration each infant's protein requirement.
b. Targeted Fortification	Macronutrient concentrations in HM are analyzed and based on the results milk is supplemented with extra protein and/or fat.	All macronutrients can be supplemented. Bedside HM analyzers are required. May be labor intensive. Supplementation is done according to the population recommendations, does not take into consideration that each individual infant's requirement may be different.

HM, human milk; VLBW, very low birth weight; BUN, blood urea nitrogen; RCT, randomized controlled trial. **BUN levels of 10–16 mg/dl correspond to blood urea concentrations of 21.40–34.24 mg/dl (3.57–5.71 mmol/l).*

all milk samples without considering intra-, inter-individual and temporal variations. Standard fortification is initiated usually when the fed milk volume is 50–100 ml/kg. Milan EMBA/ESPGHAN/AAP Joint Meeting Consensus recommends fortifying HM for preterm infants with a birthweight <1,800 g (42).

The updated Cochrane review (82) addressed the impact of STD multi-nutrient fortification of HM on growth, development, feeding tolerance and NEC in preterm infants. The systematic review evaluated 1,071 infants in 14 trials. The trials were generally small and weak methodologically. Meta-analyses provided low-quality evidence that STD multi-nutrient fortification of HM, in comparison to the unfortified HM, improved in-hospital weight gain, linear growth, and head circumference growth. Only very little data were available for growth and developmental outcomes beyond infancy and these did not show long-term advantage.

However, when comparisons are made between fortified HM in STD fashion and preterm formula (PF) (83–85) the findings indicate that despite fortification, HM fed preterm infants continue to grow more slowly than PF fed infants. Henriksen et al. (86) reported that 58% of VLBW infants fed predominantly fortified HM had EUGR at discharge. Maas et al. (87) evaluated in-hospital growth of 206 very preterm infants and found that standard deviation score for weight from birth to day 28 decreased more in infants with a cumulative milk intake >75% of all enteral feeds compared to those <25% HM intake. The trend toward poorer weight gain with higher proportions of HM intake persisted also at the time of discharge. Of course these findings cannot be a reason to favor preterm formula vs. HM to promote growth of VLBW infants. Considering all the clinical benefits deriving from the use of HM as already stated in the previous Sections, fortified HM should be the first feeding option for these infants. However, HM fortification should be optimized.

Shortfalls With "Standard Fortification"

The reasons for the limited success with STD fortification include:

Undernutrition, particularly protein undernutrition: STD fortification does not take into account the variability of HM macronutrient content and variability of the infants' requirements. Preterm infants fed fortified HM in STD fashion receive less protein than they need due to "customary assumptions" as explained in the following paragraph. Protein is essential for tissue and organ development, and is a rate limiting factor for growth. A rate of postnatal growth similar to the intrauterine growth can be reached only with adequate protein and energy intakes (3.5–4.5 g/kg/d, 110–130 kcal/kg/d, respectively, **Table 3**). Standard fortification usually provides the recommended energy intakes, but cannot provide the adequate protein intakes for many VLBW infants (actual protein intake 2.8–2.9 g/kg/day) (88). Arslanoglu et al. (88) compared the assumed protein content of fortified HM samples and derived protein intakes to actual (measured) protein content/intakes in a group of preterm infants. Actual protein intakes were consistently and significantly lower than assumed when fortification was performed in STD fashion (range of discrepancy between 0.5 and 0.8 g/kg/day). On the other hand, the differences in energy intake were small and not consistently significant. This observation was important, because it provided a rational basis for simply adding more protein to milk in those infants whose enteral diet came from milk, especially over long periods after birth (89). Similar findings have been reported in the following years by other researchers (75, 90, 91). Picaud et al. (75) showed that one third of extremely low birth weight infants (ELBW) infants needed supplementary protein to reach the expected weight gain. In the recent systematic review and meta-analysis regarding the macronutrient and energy composition of preterm human milk, Mimouni et al. (92) stated that protein content decreased massively (by one-half) and significantly from day 1–3 at week 10–12. During the same time frame; fat, lactose and energy content showed a significant linear increase. Very recently in PREMATURE MILK study Maly et al. (91) reported that protein content decreased during the first 3 weeks of lactation and the recommended protein intakes couldn't be reached with STD fortification in the majority of the infants.

The main reason for ongoing protein undernutrition despite HM fortification is that the STD regimen is based on assumptions about the protein content of the milk. Usually the assumed protein concentration by the manufacturers is 1.4–1.5 g/dl which only occurs during the first 2–3 weeks of lactation. HM protein concentration decreases with the duration of lactation and drops to around 1 g/dl by week 4–6 (43, 91). Thus, the protein intake would be inadequate most of the time throughout the fortification period (43, 44, 93).

Optimization of HM fortification is being widely studied. Improvement of the quality and source of the fortifiers, increasing the protein content of the products, early initiation of fortification are all efforts to improve STD fortification. An attempt at earlier initiation of fortification has resulted in better in-hospital head growth and weight gain in a very recent pre-, post- implementation study (94). However, a systematic review and meta-analysis aiming to ascertain whether randomized controlled trials determined the efficacy of early vs. late initiation of fortification on clinical outcomes gave inconclusive results. In this review Mimouni et al. (95) concluded that there is little evidence that early introduction of human milk fortification affects important outcomes.

Individualization of fortification is believed to be a solution to the problem of protein undernutrition with STD fortification and is currently the recommended method by scientific authorities and expert panels (29, 42, 43). The two methods of individualized fortification (**Table 5**); Adjustable and Targeted methods are discussed in the following Sections separately.

INDIVIDUALIZED FORTIFICATION

Adjustable (ADJ) Fortification

ADJ method was designed specifically to avoid both protein undernutition and overnutrition. With this method, protein intake is adjusted on the basis of each infant's metabolic response. Human milk fortification is initiated with a multi-nutrient fortifier in a STD fashion and as soon as full strength fortification is tolerated, it is guided by blood urea nitrogen (BUN) levels as a surrogate for assessing protein adequacy. If BUN level is below a pre-defined threshold value (<10 mg/dl according to 2012 protocol) (77), extra protein is added in the form of protein supplement. If BUN level is above a specified value suggesting excessive protein (>16 mg/dl), the level of fortification is reduced (**Tables 6, 7**) (74, 77).

This model was evaluated in a randomized controlled trial (RCT) by Arslanoglu et al. (74) and was found practical, feasible and effective to provide the preterm infants with adequate protein intakes approximating intrauterine protein intakes and better in-hospital growth compared to STD fortification. In this study the mean actual (measured) protein intakes reached 3.5 g/kg/d in ADJ group in the second week of the study, while it remained 2.8–2.9 g/kg/d in the STD group. During the 3 weeks intervention period the infants in ADJ group had better weight and head circumference gains compared to STD group (17 vs. 14 g/kg/d and 1.0 vs. 0.7 cm/wk, respectively).

ADJ fortification; i.e., adding extra protein on the basis of BUN measurements, has been in use since this publication with the protocol being refined in 2012 (77).

The Updated Protocol for ADJ Fortification

The threshold range of BUN used to adjust protein supply was selected arbitrarily in the first study (9–14 mg/dl) (74). Adjusting the protein intake according to these values (74), the investigators observed that there was the need to increase the level of fortification during most of the fortification period; and the protein intakes could not reach the recommended intakes at the first week of the fortification. There was need to refine the protocol, and to be cautious only a small increase has been suggested. The threshold values for BUN were modified as 10–16 mg/dl (77, 78). **Tables 6, 7** show the details of the current ADJ fortification regimen.

ADJ fortification starts as STD fortification when the fed milk volume reaches 50–80 ml/kg/d with multi-nutrient fortifier (Level 0). Protein adequacy is evaluated by twice weekly BUN determinations. Extra-protein is added in the form of protein supplement according to the protocol in 3 levels up to 1.2 g per 100 ml of HM (**Table 7**).

In 2013, Alan et al. (96) utilized a slightly modified form of ADJ fortification in their observational study and compared protein intakes and growth in VLBW infants fed HM fortified according to ADJ regimen to those fed in STD fashion (historical controls). The study replicated similar results in terms of higher protein intake and better in-hospital growth including linear growth with ADJ fortification.

Picaud et al. (75) in their recent retrospective study conducted on the preterm infants weighing <1,250 g at birth reported that 1/3 of extremely low birth weight infants required additional protein to supplement the standard fortification to achieve satisfactory weight gain. According to the practice in their NICU they used weekly measured urea levels and growth together to determine the need for extra protein. They confirmed the findings of Arslanoglu et al. (74) that extra protein supplementation not only improved weight gain but also head circumference gain.

In two observational studies, slightly modified forms of ADJ fortification were associated with both better growth and better neurodevelopmental outcomes. Ergenekon et al. in their retrospective study (97) reported better head growth and weight gain in NICU with ADJ fortification in very preterm infants.

TABLE 6 | The products required and the threshold values of the metabolic marker used for the Adjustable (ADJ) fortification method (77).

Fortifier/supplement required	
1. A multi-nutrient fortifier	
2. A protein supplement	
Metabolic marker and threshold values used to adjust protein supply	
Blood urea nitrogen (BUN)	<10 mg/dl–increase the fortification to the next level 10–16 mg/dl–no change >16 mg/dl–decrease the fortification by one level

TABLE 7 | The scheme for adjustable fortification (updated in 2012) (77).

Fortifier/supplement	**Fortification levels and the amount of fortifier/supplement to be added (g per 100 ml HM)**					
	−2	**−1**	**0 Standard (STD)**	**+1**	**+2**	**+3**
Multi-nutrient HM fortifier	1/4 strength	Half strength	Full strength	Full strength	Full strength	Full strength
Protein supplement	–	–	–	0.4	0.8	1.2

This improvement in growth was associated with significant improvement of Bayley scores at 18 months corrected age. Also, in the observational study of Biasini et al. (98), the improved growth with higher protein intakes in ELBW infants was associated with better neurodevelopment evaluated by Griffiths Mental Development Scores at corrected 12 months of age. At 24 months, small for gestational age (SGA) preterm infants having higher protein intake had higher scores.

Very recently, Mathes et al. (99) showed a highly positive correlation between plasma urea concentrations and actual protein intakes and urinary urea-creatinine ratio. They suggest that urinary urea-creatinine ratio, just like plasma urea concentrations may help to estimate the actual protein supply in preterm infants.

TARGETED FORTIFICATION

The concept of targeted fortification is to analyze macronutrient composition of HM and to fortify it in such a way that each infant always receives the amount of nutrient that is suggested in population-based recommendations. This method was proposed and studied first by Polberger et al. in 1999 (79) named as "individualized protein fortification of HM." In this study, protein was the only nutrient considered for supplementation in addition to STD fortification. The milk was analyzed periodically and a target nutrient intake (protein) was delivered, which was 3.5 g/kg/day.

Parallel to the introduction of bedside human milk analyzers it has become possible for the researchers and neonatologists to analyze and tailor the macronutrient content based on real-time analysis of HM. In an observational study de Halleux et al. (81) compared standard vs. targeted (mentioned as "individualized" by the authors) fortification approaches; daily breastmilk composition was measured with a mid-infrared milk analyzer. They added modular fat to HM to reach a target fat content of 4 g/dl. A fortifier was added to reach a protein intake of 4.3 g/kg/day. As a result, the variability of macronutrients in the individualized approach was significantly decreased, but the average fat intake was 8.6 g/kg/day which exceeded the recommendations (see **Table 3**). Weight gain was superior to the STD fortification group and was similar to the formula fed group. Data regarding head circumference gain and linear growth were not shown.

Using a different approach, Hair et al. (59) in a two-center RCT measured breast milk energy density with a near-infrared analyzer. Infants received HM derived cream in addition to HM derived fortifier if energy density was <20 kcal/oz (67 kcal/100 mL). The HM derived cream was standardized to 25% lipids and contained 2.5 kcal/ml. Infants randomized to the HM derived cream group showed superior weight and length gain vs. the control group without cream. However, the validation studies with infrared analyzers have determined that the measurement of calories is not precise because of the inability to accurately measure lactose with these devices (80).

A pilot study conducted by Rochow et al. (76) has been the first to show the feasibility of targeted fortification of all macronutrients through twice daily breast milk analysis (near-infrared), using modular products to bring levels of fat to 4.4 g/dl, protein to 3 g/dl and carbohydrates to 8.8 g/dl. Matched pair analysis of 20 infants fed STD fortified milk was performed. Growth rates of the infants with targeted fortification were similar to the group with STD fortification (~20 g/kg/d). However, the authors showed a high correlation between volume of fed HM and weight gain only in the targeted group. They calculated an additional workload of 5–10 min per milk batch. The similar growth rate could be due to the fact that the STD group had higher milk intake than the targeted group (155 + 5 vs. 147 + 5 ml/kg/d). Another limitation to be improved was the 24 h delay between the milk analysis and the addition of the macronutrients.

Targeted fortification requires a milk analyzer, which is an expensive device, requiring careful calibration. Fusch et al. (100) draw attention to the need of recalibration of these analyzers since they were originally developed for use in the dairy industry and HM has a different matrix and optical characteristics from cow's milk. They conclude infrared analysis seems to be a promising tool for fat and protein with calibration, but lactose and therefore energy cannot be assessed with the current state of technologies.

Buffin et al. (101) compared fat and protein concentrations using two infrared analyzers and reference laboratory methods indicating the same important finding that bedside HM analyzers require recalibration before their use in practice.

In a recent RCT comparing targeted fortification to standard, McLeod et al. (102) did not find any improvement in growth and nutrition in a group of preterm infants born below 30 weeks of gestation. Interestingly, mean measured protein content in the targeted group was higher than the assumed value (1.6 vs. 1.4 g/100 ml), leading to lower amounts of fortifier added to the milk in the intervention group. The authors concluded that targeting fortification on measured composition is labor intensive requiring frequent milk sampling and precision measuring equipment.

POST DISCHARGE FORTIFICATION

There is no consensus about post discharge nutrition, however there is a position paper from ESPGHAN (103) and recent reviews (104–106), including one focusing on HM supplementation (106). The ESPGHAN position paper evaluated randomized trials published before 2004 and proposed fortifying HM up to at least 40 and possibly up to 52 weeks postconceptional age when infants were small for gestational age at discharge. However, the definition of being small for gestational age was not presented: bodyweight at discharge below 10th (moderate growth restriction) or 3rd percentile (severe growth restriction)? Meta-analysis and reviews suggested that there was evidence to use enriched nutrition [preterm formula (PF) rather than post discharge formula (PDF)] after discharge for formula fed babies. But this evidence was not strong enough to recommend fortification of HM after discharge (105, 106).

The last decade was marked by two trends. Firstly, a decrease in the incidence of extra-uterine growth restriction (16, 17, 107). Secondly, an increase in breastfeeding rates at discharge in these infants, despite significant heterogeneity between different neonatal units suggesting that there is room for improvement (108). Post discharge studies comparing enriched vs. standard nutrition highlighted the ability of some preterm infants -like term counterparts- to regulate their intake volume to compensate for differences in energy density between formulas (109–111). However, this is only true for preterm babies reaching term due date and beyond as it has been reported that many less mature preterm babies are not able to compensate for a low nutrient intake feed due to immature feeding skills (112). Therefore, there is a window of opportunity to optimize nutrition post discharge, which might explain why few studies reported a benefit for growth and mineralization of enriched post discharge nutrition.

Despite the widespread use of human milk fortifiers (HMF) for preterm babies on neonatal units there has been little reporting of its use post discharge. It might seem best practice to mirror the principle behind the use of post discharge formulas for formula fed babies, i.e., the bridge between a nutrient dense milk to one of lower density. In accordance with this there have been recommendations that fortifier is continued in preterm breast fed babies either to term or around 52 weeks post conceptional according to their growth trajectory (103, 113). Although the practicality of putting this into practice has been questioned by some reviewers because of the availability of HMF in different countries and the perceived, but not proven, problems with practicability (106), evidence is accruing that it is possible using many different methods (114).

It is known that babies exclusively breastfed post discharge can have reduced bone mineral density and lower lean body mass than formula fed babies (115), although this may have improved with more recent feeding practices on neonatal units. But it does suggest that some fortification of breast milk post discharge will help nutritional status as well as growth.

There have been 3 reports of randomized controlled trials fortifying breast milk post discharge, to 4 months corrected age (116), for around 5–6 months after discharge (117), and to around 12 weeks after discharge (118). Two used commercial HM fortifiers (116, 118) and one (117) a powdered preterm formula. **Table 8** shows the nutrient intervention and numbers of infants in these trials. No difference in growth was found by Zachariassen et al. (116). However, this group did find better lung function in the fortification group at 6 years old (119). O'Connor et al. (118) found better weight, length and bone mineral density and better head growth in babies <1,250 g birth weight, all of which were maintained to 1 year (120). There is also evidence of better visual function (121). Neurodevelopmental outcome at 12–18

TABLE 8 | Nutrient interventions in the randomized controlled trials addressing the effects of fortifying human milk post discharge (116–118).

	O'Connor et al. (118)	Zachariassen et al. (116)	Da Cunha et al. (117)
Additional Protein (g)	0.8/kg	1.37/day	0.5/day
Additional energy (kcal)	~10–15/kg	17/day	20/day
Numbers assessed–intervention	19	102	26
Numbers assessed-Control	20	105	27
Outcomes	Growth at 4,8,12 weeks after discharge Energy and some nutrient intakes (diaries)	Growth at 2,4,6,12 months corrected age Blood urea nitrogen, phosphorus, hemoglobin levels	Neurodevelopment assessed by Bayley III Scale at 12 months corrected age

months was not found to be different between groups (117, 120). In these studies there may not have been sufficient protein given to achieve an optimal growth and possibly neurodevelopmental outcome. In contrast energy should not be a limiting nutrient for a baby feeding fully responsively at the breast as they will access all the energy rich hind milk they require.

All studies found the HMF to be well-tolerated however each used a different method to administer the fortifier, one adding the entire dose into one bottle per day (116) with no adverse gastrointestinal symptoms reported. Another was by bottle but given spread out over the day (117) and the third by cup twice a day (118). None reported any adverse effect on breast feeding rates in the fortified group. A finger feeding device to administer fortifier has recently been evaluated and was well-accepted (122). Technical improvements are required and a large randomized study will be necessary to evaluate the benefits of such a strategy.

There are 2 reports looking at the effect of fortifier post discharge on breastfeeding. One is a case study where breastfeeding was maintained by the addition of fortifier post discharge rather than formula in a baby failing to thrive on the breast (123). A second suggests an improvement in breastfeeding rates at 6 weeks post conceptional age in a group of babies discharged on fortifier compared to a group on breast milk alone (124).

In theory, a gradual step down from full fortification would seem appropriate for breastfed babies to allow adaption to the lower nutrient intake of unfortified breast milk and to support the rapid growth that occurs around term due date.

As studies that evaluated post discharge HM fortification showed no deleterious effect on breastfeeding rates, it is proposed that HMF post discharge is considered in breastfed babies where a post discharge formula would be used were they formula fed, particularly if they have not grown well while on the neonatal unit. One group who might benefit being babies with bronchopulmonary dysplasia BPD (125). More work is needed to assess an optimal amount, length of time and method of administering fortifier in a breast feeding baby post discharge.

CONCLUSIONS-COMMENTS, RECOMMENDATIONS

Conclusions-Comments

- Evidence indicates that HM is the best nutrient uniquely suited not only to term but also to preterm infants conferring health benefits at short and long-term including protection against NICU challenges such as NEC, ROP, BPD sepsis and neurocognitive improvement. Therefore, it is the first choice in preterm feeding.
- Unfortified HM doesn't provide sufficient amounts of nutrients to tiny preterm infants when fed at usual feeding volumes. To prevent EUGR which is associated with poor neurocognitive outcome and to avoid specific nutrient deficiencies, nutrient fortification of HM is necessary.
- The fortification methods in current use are: **1.** Standard fortification, **2.** Individualized fortification: "Adjustable fortification" and "Targeted fortification."
- Despite STD fortification many VLBW infants continue to have suboptimal growth. Optimization of HM fortification is necessary.
- ADJ fortification has been shown to improve protein intakes, somatic and head growth and seems to be a practical method to optimize HM fortification.
- Targeted fortification, being feasible and effective in some trials, needs to be improved.
- Improvement of the quality of HMF is another important issue. Although HM-based fortifier seemed to be promising and some studies suggested a benefit in terms of morbidity and mortality when babies are fed an exclusively human milk based diet using these products, there are still concerns about the efficacy, safety and ethical issues.
- There is no strong evidence to support the use of hydrolyzed protein source in fortifiers.
- There is no consensus about post discharge nutrition. Studies that evaluated post discharge HM fortification showed no deleterious effect on breastfeeding rates, and suggested some advantages.

Recommendations

- Given the solid evidence, HM feeding has become a basic right for preterm infants. Mother's own milk is the first choice in preterm infant feeding and strong efforts should be made to promote lactation. When mother's milk is not available, donor human milk is the best alternative.
- EMBA WG on HM Fortification, in parallel with Milan Consensus (42) recommends fortification of HM for preterm infants with a birthweight <1,800 g.
- Human milk fortification can be started safely with multi-nutrient fortifiers when the milk volume reaches 50–80 ml/kg/d.
- Optimization of HM fortification is required. Individualized fortification (Adjustable or Targeted) is the recommended method for HM fortification. Targeted Fortification may need some fine tuning.
- Quality improvement of the fortifiers is an ongoing process. Because of the limited efficacy and safety data and ethical concerns, it is too early to draw conclusions about the use of HM-based fortifiers.

FUTURE RESEARCH DIRECTIONS

- Research addressing the nutritional management in specific groups of preterm infants (such as BPD, IUGR)
- Randomized controlled trials assessing the efficacy and safety of HM fortification after discharge in different groups depending on their status at discharge
- Randomized trials comparing the efficacy and safety of ADJ vs. Targeted Fortification
- Defining the reasonable and replicable study endpoints including neurocognitive outcomes, body composition in large cohorts
- Optimization of the quality of fortifiers (amount and quality of protein, source of energy, EFA content) while considering ethical dilemmas

AUTHOR CONTRIBUTIONS

SA is leading the EMBA WG on Human Milk Fortification. J-CP, C-YB, CK, DL, and PT are the components of the WG. All contributed to the construction and writing of the manuscript. GM, EB, GW, AW, AGa, AGr, CG, and DB commented on the manuscript as the components of the EMBA Board.

ACKNOWLEDGMENTS

The authors thank the Italian Association of Human Milk Banks (Associazione Italiana Banche del Latte Umano Donato = AIBLUD) for its continuous efforts to promote research in the field of donor human milk and human milk banks, and for the financial support given to the publication of this manuscript.

REFERENCES

1. Stephens BE, Vohr BR. Protein intake and neurodevelopmental outcomes. *Clin Perinatol.* (2014) 41:323–29. doi: 10.1016/j.clp.2014.02.005
2. Belfort MB, Ehrenkranz RA. Neurodevelopmental outcomes and nutritional strategies in very low birth weight infants. *Semin Fetal Neonatal Med.* (2017) 22:42–8. doi: 10.1016/j.siny.2016.09.001
3. Lucas A, Morley R, Cole T. Randomised trial of early diet in preterm babies and later intelligence quotient. *BMJ.* (1998) 317:1481–7. doi: 10.1136/bmj.317.7171.1481
4. Latal-Hajnal B, von Siebenthal K, Kovari H, Bucher HU, Largo RH. Postnatal growth in VLBW infants: significant association with neurodevelopmental outcome. *J Pediatr.* (2003) 143:163–70. doi: 10.1067/S0022-3476(03)00243-9
5. Ehrenkranz RA, Dusick AM, Vohr BR, Wright LL, Wrage LA, Poole WK. Growth in the neonatal intensive care unit influences neurodevelopmental and growth outcomes of extremely low birth weight infants. *Pediatrics.* (2006) 117:1253–61. doi: 10.1542/peds.2005-1368
6. Isaacs EB, Gadian DG, Sabatini S, Chong WK, Quinn BT, Fischl BR, et al. The effect of early human diet on caudate volumes and IQ. *Pediatr Res.* (2008) 63:308–14. doi: 10.1203/PDR.0b013e318163a271
7. Belfort MB, Rifas-Shiman SL, Sullivan T, Collins CT, McPhee AJ, Ryan P, et al. Infant growth before and after term: effects on neurodevelopment in preterm infants. *Pediatrics.* (2011) 128:e899–906. doi: 10.1542/peds.2011-0282
8. Guellec I, Lapillonne A, Marret S, Picaud JC, Mitanchez D, Charkaluk ML, et al. Étude Épidémiologique sur les Petits Âges Gestationnels (EPIPAGE; [Epidemiological Study on Small Gestational Ages]) study group. effect of intra- and extrauterine growth on long-term neurologic outcomes of very preterm infants. *J Pediatr.* (2016) 175:93–99.e1. doi: 10.1016/j.jpeds.2016.05.027
9. Stephens BE, Walden RV, Gargus RA, Tucker R, McKinley L, Mance M, et al. First-week protein and energy intakes are associated with 18-month developmental outcomes in extremely low birth weight infants. *Pediatr Clin North Am.* (2009) 56:631–46. doi: 10.1016/j.pcl.2009.03.005
10. Ong KK, Kennedy K, Casta-eda-Gutiérrez E, Forsyth S, Godfrey KM, Koletzko B, et al. Postnatal growth in preterm infants and later health outcomes: a systematic review. *Acta Paediatr.* (2015) 104:974–86. doi: 10.1111/apa.13128
11. Chan SH, Johnson MJ, Leaf AA, Vollmer B. Nutrition and neurodevelopmental outcomes in preterm infants: a systematic review. *Acta Paediatr.* (2016) 105:587e99. doi: 10.1111/apa.13344
12. Bacchetta J, Harambat J, Dubourg L, Guy B, Liutkus A, Canterino I, et al. Both extrauterine and intrauterine growth restriction impair renal function in children born very preterm. *Kidney Int.* (2009) 76:445–52. doi: 10.1038/ki.2009.201
13. Ramel SE, Demerath EW, Gray HL, Younge N, Boys C, Georgieff MK. The relationship of poor linear growth velocity with neonatal illness and two-year neurodevelopment in preterm infants. *Neonatology.* (2012) 102:19–24. doi: 10.1159/000336127
14. Ramel SE, Gray HL, Christiansen E, Boys C, Georgieff MK, Demerath EW. Greater early gains in fat-free mass, but not fat mass, are associated with improved neurodevelopment at 1 year corrected age for prematurity in very low birth weight preterm infants. *J Pediatr.* (2016) 173:108–15. doi: 10.1016/j.jpeds.2016.03.003
15. Stoll BJ, Hansen NI, Bell EF, Shankaran S, Laptook AR, Walsh MC, et al. Eunice kennedy shriver national institute of child health and human development neonatal research network. Neonatal outcomes of extremely preterm infants from the NICHD Neonatal Research Network. *Pediatrics.* (2010) 126:443–56. doi: 10.1542/peds.2009-2959
16. Horbar JD, Ehrenkranz RA, Badger GJ, Edwards EM, Morrow KA, Soll RF, et al. Weight growth velocity and postnatal growth failure in infants 501 to 1500 grams: 2000-2013. *Pediatrics.* (2015) 136:e84–92. doi: 10.1542/peds.2015-0129
17. Griffin IJ, Tancredi DJ, Bertino E, Lee HC, Profit J. Postnatal growth failure in very low birthweight infants born between 2005 and 2012. *Archs Dis Childh Fetal Neonatal Ed.* (2016) 101:F50e5. doi: 10.1136/archdischild-2014-308095
18. Cole TJ, Statnikov Y, Santhakumaran S, Pan H, Modi N. Neonatal data analysis unit and the preterm growth investigator group. Birth weight and longitudinal growth in infants born below 32 weeks' gestation: a UK population study. *Arch Dis Child Fetal Neonatal Ed.* (2014) 99:F34–40. doi: 10.1136/archdischild-2014-306237.81
19. Eidelman AI. Breastfeeding and the use of human milk: an analysis of the American Academy of Pediatrics 2012 Breastfeeding Policy Statement. *Breastfeeding Med.* (2012) 7:323e4. doi: 10.1089/bfm.2012.0067
20. Victora CG, Bahl R, Barros AJ, França GV, Horton S, Krasevec J, et al. Lancet breastfeeding series group. breastfeeding in the 21st century: epidemiology, mechanisms, and lifelong effect. *Lancet.* (2016) 387:475–90. doi: 10.1016/S0140-6736(15)01024-7
21. Lönnerdal B. Bioactive proteins in human milk-potential benefits for preterm infants. *Clin Perinatol.* (2017) 44:179–91. doi: 10.1016/j.clp.2016.11.013
22. Koletzko B. Human Milk Lipids. *Ann Nutr Metab.* (2016) 69(Suppl. 2):28–40. doi: 10.1159/000452819
23. Hernell O, Timby N, Domellöf M, Lönnerdal B. Clinical benefits of milk fat globule membranes for infants and children. *J Pediatr.* (2016) 173(Suppl.):S60–5. doi: 10.1016/j.jpeds.2016.02.077
24. Bode L. The functional biology of human milk oligosaccharides. *Early Hum Dev.* (2015) 91:619–22. doi: 10.1016/j.earlhumdev.2015.09.001
25. McGuire MK, McGuire MA. Got bacteria? The astounding, yet not-so-surprising, microbiome of human milk. *Curr Opin Biotechnol.* (2017) 44:63–8. doi: 10.1016/j.copbio.2016.11.013
26. Bode L, McGuire M, Rodriguez JM, Geddes DT, Hassiotou F, Hartmann PE, et al. It's alive: microbes and cells in human milk and their potential benefits to mother and infant. *Adv Nutr.* (2014) 5:571–3. doi: 10.3945/an.114.006643
27. Quigley M, McGuire W. Formula versus donor breast milk for feeding preterm or low birth weight infants. *Cochr Database Syst Rev.* (2014) 22:CD002971. doi: 10.1002/14651858.CD002971
28. Maffei D, Schanler RJ. Human milk is the feeding strategy to prevent necrotizing colitis. *Semin Perinatol.* (2017) 41:36–40. doi: 10.1053/j.semperi.2016.09.016
29. Arslanoglu S, Corpeleijn W, Moro G, Braegger C, Campoy C, Colomb V, et al. ESPGHAN Committee on Nutrition. Donor human milk for preterm infants: current evidence and research directions. *J Pediatr Gastroenterol Nutr.* (2013) 57:535–42. doi: 10.1097/MPG.0b013e3182a3af0a
30. Corpeleijn WE, Kouwenhoven SM, Paap MC, van Vliet I, Scheerder I, Muizer Y, et al. Intake of own mother's milk during the first days of life is associated with decreased morbidity and mortality in very low birth weight infants during the first 60 days of life. *Neonatology.* (2012) 102:276–81. doi: 10.1159/000341335
31. Meinzen-Derr J, Poindexter B, Wrage L, Morrow AL, Stoll B, Donovan EF. Role of human milk in extremely low birth weight infants' risk of necrotizing enterocolitis or death. *J Perinatol.* (2009) 29:57–62. doi: 10.1038/jp.2008.117

32. Schanler RJ, Lau C, Hurst NM, Smith EO. Randomized trial of donor human milk versus preterm formula as substitutes for mothers' own milk in the feeding of extremely premature infants. *Pediatrics.* (2005) 116:400e6. doi: 10.1542/peds.2004-1974
33. Sullivan S, Schanler RJ, Kim JH, Patel AL, Trawoger R, Kiechl-Kohlendorfer U et al. An exclusively human milk-based diet is associated with a lower rate of necrotizing enterocolitis than a diet of human milk and bovine milk-based products. *J Pediatr.* (2010) 156:562e7. e561. doi: 10.1016/j.jpeds.2009.10.040
34. Maayan-Metzger A, Avivi S, Schushan-Eisen I, Kuint J. Human milk versus formula feeding among preterm infants: short-term outcomes. *Am J Perinatol.* (2012) 29:121e6. doi: 10.1055/s-0031-1295652
35. Hylander MA, Strobino DM, Pezzulo JC, Dhanireddy R. Association of human milk feedings with a reduction in retinopathy of prematurity among very low birth weight infants. *J Perinatol.* (2001) 21:356e62. doi: 10.1038/sj.jp.7210548
36. Bharwani SK, Green BF, Pezzullo JC, Bharwani SS, Bharwani SS, Dhanireddy R. Systematic review and meta-analysis of human milk intake and retinopathy of prematurity: a significant update. *J Perinatol.* (2016) 36:913–20. doi: 10.1038/jp.2016.98
37. Spiegler J, Preuß M, Gebauer C, Bendiks M, Herting E, Göpel W. German Neonatal Network (GNN).; German Neonatal Network GNN does breastmilk influence the development of bronchopulmonary dysplasia? *J Pediatr.* (2016) 169:76–80. doi: 10.1016/j.jpeds.2015.10.080
38. Dicky O, Ehlinger V, Montjaux N, Gremmo-Féger G, Sizun J, Rozé JC, et al. EPIPAGE 2 nutrition study group.; EPINUTRI Study Group. Policy of feeding very preterm infants with their mother's own fresh expressed milk was associated with a reduced risk of bronchopulmonary dysplasia. *Acta Paediatr.* (2017) 106:755–62. doi: 10.1111/apa.13757
39. Rozé JC, Darmaun D, Boquien CY, Flamant C, Picaud JC, Savagner C, et al. The apparent breastfeeding paradox in very preterm infants: relationship between breast feeding, early weight gain and neurodevelopment based on results from two cohorts, EPIPAGE and LIFT. *BMJ Open.* (2012) 2:e000834. doi: 10.1136/bmjopen-2012-000834
40. Vohr BR, Poindexter BB, Dusick AM, McKinley LT, Higgins RD, Langer JC, et al. National institute of child health and human development national research network. persistent beneficial effects of breast milk ingested in the neonatal intensive care unit on outcomes of extremely low birth weight infants at 30 months of age. *Pediatrics.* (2007) 120:e953e9. doi: 10.1542/peds.2006-3227
41. Lechner BE, Vohr BR. Neurodevelopmental outcomes of preterm infants fed human milk: a systematic review. *Clin Perinatol.* (2017) 44:69–83. doi: 10.1016/j.clp.2016.11.004
42. Moro GE, Arslanoglu S, Bertino E, Corvaglia L, Montirosso R, Picaud JC, et al. American academy of pediatrics; european society for pediatric gastroenterology, hepatology, and nutrition. XII. Human milk in feeding premature infants: consensus statement. *J Pediatr Gastroenterol Nutr.* (2015) 61(Suppl. 1):S16–9. doi: 10.1097/01.mpg.0000471460.08792.4d
43. Arslanoglu S, Moro GE, Ziegler EE, The WAPM Working Group On Nutrition. Optimization of human milk fortification for preterm infants: new concepts and recommendations. *J Perinat Med.* (2010) 38:233–8. doi: 10.1515/jpm.2010.064
44. Ziegler EE. Human milk and human milk fortifiers. *World Rev Nutr Diet.* (2014) 110:215–27. doi: 10.1159/000358470
45. Radmacher PG, Adamkin DH. Fortification of human milk for preterm infants. *Semin Fetal Neonatal Med.* (2017) 22:30–35. doi: 10.1016/j.siny.2016.08.004
46. Hay WW, Ziegler EE. Growth failure among preterm infants due to insufficient protein is not innocuous and must be prevented. *J Perinatol.* (2016) 36:500–502. doi: 10.1038/jp.2016.85
47. Senterre T, Rigo J. Reduction in postnatal cumulative nutritional deficit and improvement of growth in extremely preterm infants. *Acta Paediatr.* (2012) 101:e64–70. doi: 10.1111/j.1651-2227.2011.02443.x
48. Bellagamba MP, Carmenati E, D'Ascenzo R, Malatesta M, Spagnoli C, Biagetti C, et al. One extra gram of protein to preterm infants from birth to 1800 g: A single-blinded randomized clinical trial. *JPGN.* (2016) 62: 879–84. doi: 10.1097/MPG.0000000000000989
49. Domellöf M. Nutritional care of premature infants: microminerals. *World Rev Nutr Diet.* (2014) 110:121–39. doi: 10.1159/000358462
50. Ziegler EE. Meeting the nutritional needs of the low-birth-weight infant. *Ann Nutr Metab.* (2011) 58(suppl. 1):8–18. doi: 10.1159/000323381
51. Ziegler EE, Thureen PJ, Carlson SJ. Aggressive nutrition of the very low birthweight infant. *Clin Perinatol.* (2002) 29:225–44. doi: 10.1016/S0095-5108(02)00007-6
52. Agostoni C, Buonocore G, Carnielli VP, De Curtis M, Darmaun D, Decsi T, et al. ESPGHAN Committee on Nutrition. Enteral nutrient supply for preterm infants: commentary from the European Society of Paediatric Gastroenterology, Hepatology and Nutrition Committee on Nutrition. *J Pediatr Gastroenterol Nutr.* (2010) 50:85–91. doi: 10.1097/MPG.0b013e3181adaee0
53. Koletzko B, Poindexter B, Uauy R. Recommended nutrient intake levels for stable, fully enteral fed very low birth weight infants. *World Rev Nutr Diet.* (2014) 110: 297–99. doi: 10.1159/isbn.978-3-318-02641-2
54. Kreins N, Buffin R, Michel-Molnar D, Chambon V, Pradat P, Picaud JC. Individualized fortification influences the osmolality of human milk. *Frontiers Pediatr.* (2018) 6:322. doi: 10.3389/fped.2018.00322
55. Billeaud C, Boué-Vaysse C, Couëdelo L, Steenhout P, Jaeger J, Cruz-Hernandez C, et al. Effects on fatty acid metabolism of a new powdered human milk fortifier containing medium-chain triacylglycerols and docosahexaenoic acid in preterm infants. *Nutrients.* (2018) 10:E690. doi: 10.3390/nu10060690
56. Rigo J, Hascoët JM, Billeaud C, Picaud JC, Mosca F, Rubio A, et al. Growth and nutritional biomarkers of preterm infants fed a new powdered human milk fortifier: a randomized trial. *J Pediatr Gastroenterol Nutr.* (2017) 65:e83–93. doi: 10.1097/MPG.0000000000001686
57. Coscia A, Bertino E, Tonetto P, Peila C, Cresi F, Arslanoglu S, et al. Nutritional adequacy of a novel human milk fortifier from donkey milk in feeding preterm infants: study protocol of a randomized controlled clinical trial. *Nutr J.* (2018) 17:6. doi: 10.1186/s12937-017-0308-8
58. Meredith-Dennis L, Xu G, Goonatilleke E, Lebrilla CB, Underwood MA, Smilowitz JT. Composition and variation of macronutrients, immune proteins, and human milk oligosaccharides in human milk from nonprofit and commercial milk banks. *J Hum Lact.* (2018) 34:120–9. doi: 10.1177/0890334417710635
59. Hair AB, Blanco CL, Moreira AG, et al. Randomized trial of human milk cream as a supplement to standard fortification of an exclusive human milk-based diet in infants 750–1250 g birth weight. *J Pediatr.* (2014) 165:915–20. doi: 10.1016/j.jpeds.2014.07.005
60. Hair AB, Bergner EM, Lee ML, Moreira AG, Hawthorne KM, Rechtman DJ, et al. Premature infants 750–1,250 g birth weight supplemented with a novel human milk-derived cream are discharged sooner. *Breastfeed Med.* (2016) 11:133–7. doi: 10.1089/bfm.2015.0166
61. Cristofalo EA, Schanler RJ, Blanco CL, Sullivan S, Trawoeger R, Kiechl-Kohlendorfer U, et al. Randomized trial of exclusive human milk versus preterm formula diets in extremely premature infants. *J Pediatr.* (2013) 163:1592–5.e1. doi: 10.1016/j.jpeds.2013.07.011
62. Abrams SA, Schanler RJ, Lee ML, Rechtman DJ. Greater mortality and morbidity in extremely preterm infants fed a diet containing cow milk protein products. *Breastfeed Med.* (2014) 9:281–5. doi: 10.1089/bfm.2014.0024
63. Ganapathy V, Hay JW, Kim JH. Costs of necrotizing enterocolitis and costeffectiveness of exclusively human milk based products in feeding extremely premature infants. *Breastfeed Med.* (2012) 7:29–37. doi: 10.1089/bfm.2011.0002
64. Assad M, Elliott MJ, Abraham JH. Decreased cost and improved feeding tolerance in VLBW infants fed an exclusive human milk diet. *J Perinatol.* (2016) 36:216–20. doi: 10.1038/jp.2015.168
65. Embleton ND, King C, Jarvis C, Mactier H, Pearson F, Menon G. Effectiveness of human milk-based fortifiers for preventing necrotizing enterocolitis in preterm infants: case not proven. *Breastfeed Med.* (2013) 8:421. doi: 10.1089/bfm.2013.0049
66. O'Connor DL, Kiss A, Tomlinson C, Bando N, Bayliss A, Campbell DM, et al. OptiMoM feeding group. Nutrient enrichment of human milk with human and bovine milk-based fortifiers for infants born weighing <1250 g: a randomized clinical trial. *Am J Clin Nutr.* (2018) 108:108–16.

67. Perrin MT. Donor human milk and fortifier use in United States Level 2:3, and 4 neonatal care hospitals. *J Pediatr Gastroenterol Nutr.* (2018) 66:664–9. doi: 10.1097/MPG.0000000000001790
68. Arslanoglu S, Bertino E, Tonetto P, Italian Association of Human Milk Banks, De Nisi G, Ambruzzi AM. Guidelines for the establishment and operation of a donor human milk bank. *J Mater Fetal Neonatal Med.* (2010) 23:1–20. doi: 10.3109/14767058.2010.512414
69. French Human Milk Bank Association. *The Good Pratice Rules for the Collection, Preparation, Qualification, Treatment, Storage, Distribution and Dispensing on Medical Prescription of Human Milk by the Milk Banks.* Available online at: http://association-des-lactariums-de-france.fr/wp-content/uploads/lactarium_guide_bonnes_pratiques_5_janvier_2008_traduction_anglais.pdf
70. Picaud JC, Rigo J, Normand S, Lapillonne A, Reygrobellet B, Claris O, Salle BL. Nutritional efficacy of preterm formula with a partially hydrolyzed protein source: a randomized pilot study. *J Pediatr Gastroenterol Nutr.* (2001) 32:555–61. doi: 10.1097/00005176-200105000-00012
71. David TJ, Ewing CI. Atopic eczema and preterm birth. *Arch Dis Child.* (1988) 63:435–6. doi: 10.1136/adc.63.4.435
72. Lucas A, Brooke OG, Morley R, Cole TJ, Bamford MF. Early diet of preterm infants and development of allergic or atopic disease: randomized prospective study. *Br Med J.* (1990) 300:837–40. doi: 10.1136/bmj.300.6728.837
73. Zachariassen G, Faerk J, Esberg BH, Fenger-Gron J, Mortensen S, Christesen HT, et al. Allergic diseases among very preterm infants according to nutrition after hospital discharge. *Pediatr Allergy Immunol.* (2011) 22:515–20. doi: 10.1111/j.1399-3038.2010.01102.x
74. Arslanoglu S, Moro GE, Ziegler EE. Adjustable fortification of human milk fed to preterm infants: does it make a difference? *J Perinatol.* (2006) 26:614–21. doi: 10.1038/sj.jp.7211571
75. Picaud JC, Houeto N, Buffin R, Loys CM, Godbert I, Haÿs S. Additional protein fortification is necessary in extremely low-birth-weight infants fed human milk. *J Pediatr Gastroenterol Nutr.* (2016) 63:103–5. doi: 10.1097/MPG.0000000000001142
76. Rochow N, Fusch G, Choi A, Chessell L, Eliott L, McDonald K, et al. Target fortification of breast milk with fat, protein and carbohydrates for preterm infants. *J Pediatr.* (2013) 163:1001–7. doi: 10.1016/j.jpeds.2013.04.052
77. Arslanoglu S, Bertino E, Coscia A, Tonetto P, Giuliani F, Moro GE. Update of adjustable fortification regimen for preterm infants: a new protocol. *J Biol Regul Homeost Agents.* (2012) 26(3 Suppl.):65–7.
78. Arslanoglu S. IV. Individualized fortification of human milk: adjustable fortification. *J Pediatr Gastroenterol Nutr.* (2015) 61(Suppl. 1):S4–5. doi: 10.1097/01.mpg.0000471452.85920.4d
79. Polberger S, Raiha NCR, Juvonen P, Moro GE, Minoli I, Warm A. Individualized protein fortification of human milk for preterm infants: comparison of ultrafiltrated human milk protein and a bovine whey fortifier. *J Pediatr Gastr Nutr.* (1999) 29:332–8. doi: 10.1097/00005176-199909000-00017
80. Rochow N, Landau-Crangle E, Fusch C. Challenges in breast milk fortification for preterm infants. *Curr Opin Clin Nutr Metab Care.* (2015) 18:276–84. doi: 10.1097/MCO.0000000000000167
81. de Halleux V, Rigo J. Variability in human milk composition: benefit of individualized fortification in very-low-birth-weight infants. *Am J Clin Nutr.* (2013) 98:529s—35s. doi: 10.3945/ajcn.112.042689
82. Brown JV, Embleton ND, Harding JE, McGuire W. Multi-nutrient fortification of human milk for preterm infants. *Cochr Database Syst Rev.* (2016) 8:CD000343. doi: 10.1002/14651858.CD000343.pub3
83. O'Connor DL, Jacobs J, Hall R, Adamkin D, Auestad N, Castillo M, et al. Growing and development of premature infants fed predominantly human milk, predominantly premature infant formula, or a combination of human milk and premature formula. *J Pediatr Gastr Nutr.* (2003) 37:437–46. doi: 10.1097/00005176-200310000-00008
84. Olsen IE, Richardson DK, Schmidt CH, Ausman LM, Dwyer JT. Intersite differences in weight growth velocity of extremely premature infants. *Pediatrics.* (2002) 110:1125–32. doi: 10.1542/peds.110.6.1125
85. Pieltain C, deCurtis M, Gerard P, Rigo J. Weight gain composition in preterm infants with dual energy X-ray absorptiometry. *Pediat Res.* (2001) 49:120–4. doi: 10.1203/00006450-200101000-00023
86. Henriksen C, Westerberg AC, Rønnestad A, Nakstad B, Veierød MB, Drevon CA, et al. Growth and nutrient intake among very-low-birth-weight infants fed fortified human milk during hospitalization. *Br J Nutr.* (2009) 102:1179–86. doi: 10.1017/ S0007114509371755.
87. Maas C, Wiechers C, Bernhard W, Poets CF, Franz AR. Early feeding of fortified breast milk and in-hospital-growth in very premature infants: a retrospective cohort analysis. *BMC Pediatr.* (2013) 13:178. doi: 10.1186/1471-2431-13-178
88. Arslanoglu S, Moro GE, Ziegler EE. Preterm infants fed fortified human milk receive less protein than they need. *J Perinatol.* (2009) 29:489–92. doi: 10.1038/jp.2009.50
89. Hay WW Jr. Optimizing protein intake in preterm infants. *J Perinatol.* (2009) 29:465–6. doi: 10.1038/jp.2009.53
90. Corvaglia L, Aceti A, Paoletti V, Mariani E, Patrono D, Ancora G, et al. Standard fortification of preterm human milk fails to meet recommended protein intake: bedside evaluation by Near-Infrared-Reflectance-Analysis. *Early Hum Dev.* (2010) 86:237–40. doi: 10.1016/j.earlhumdev.2010.04.001
91. Maly J, Burianova I, Vitkova V, Ticha E, Navratilova M, Cermakova E. PREMATURE MILK study group. Preterm human milk macronutrient concentration is independent of gestational age at birth. *Arch Dis Child Fetal Neonatal Ed.* (2018) 104:F50–6. doi: 10.1136/archdischild-2016-312572
92. Mimouni FB, Lubetzky R, Yochpaz S, Mandel D. Preterm human milk macronutrient and energy composition: a systematic review and metaanalysis. *Clin Perinatol.* (2017) 44:165–172. doi: 10.1016/j.clp.2016.11.010
93. Kumar RK, Singhal A, Vaidya U, Banerjee S, Anwar F, Rao S. Optimizing nutrition in preterm low birth weight infants- Consensus Summary. *Front Nutr.* (2017) 26:20. doi: 10.3389/fnut.2017.00020
94. Ginovart G, Gich I, Gutiérrez A, Verd S. A fortified donor milk policy is associated with improved in-hospital head growth and weight gain in very low-birth-weight infants. *Adv Neonatal Care.* (2017) 17:250–7. doi: 10.1097/ANC.0000000000000387
95. Mimouni FB, Nathan N, Ziegler EE, Lubetzky R, Mandel D. The use of multinutrient human milk fortifiers in preterm infants: a systematic review of unanswered questions. *Clin Perinatol.* (2017) 44:175–8. doi: 10.1016/j.clp.2016.11.011
96. Alan S, Atasay B, Cakir U, Yildiz D, Kilic A, Kahvecioglu D, et al. An intention to achieve better postnatal in-hospital-growth for preterm infants: adjustable protein fortification of human milk. *Early Hum Dev.* (2013) 89:1017–23. doi: 10.1016/j.earlhumdev.2013.08.015
97. Ergenekon E, Soysal ş, Hirfanoğlu I, Baş V, Gücüyener K, Turan Ö, et al. Short- and long-term effects of individualized enteral protein supplementation in preterm newborns. *Turk J Pediatr.* (2013) 55:365–70.
98. Biasini A, Monti F, Laguardia MC, Stella M, Marvulli L, Neri E. High protein intake in human/maternal milk fortification for $\leq$1250 gr infants: intrahospital growth and neurodevelopmental outcome at two years. *Acta Biomed.* (2018) 88:470–6. doi: 10.23750/abm.v88i4.5316
99. Mathes M, Maas C, Bleeker C, Vek J, Bernhard W, Peter A, et al. Effect of increased enteral protein intake on plasma and urinary urea concentrations in preterm infants born at $<$ 32 weeks gestation and $<$ 1500 g birth weight enrolled in a randomized controlled trial - a secondary analysis. *BMC Pediatr.* (2018) 18:154. doi: 10.1186/s12887-018-1136-5
100. Fusch G, Kwan C, Kotrri G, Fusch C. "Bed Side" human milk analysis in the neonatal intensive care unit: a systematic review. *Clin Perinatol.* (2017) 44:209–67. doi: 10.1016/j.clp.2016.11.001
101. Buffin R, Decullier E, De Halleux V, Loys CM, Hays S, Studzinsky F, et al. Assessment of human milk composition using mid-infrared analyzers requires calibration adjustment. *J Perinatol.* (2017) 37:552–7. doi: 10.1038/jp.2016.230
102. McLeod G, Sherriff J, Hartmann PE, Nathan E, Geddes D, Simmer K. Comparing different methods of human breast milk fortification using measured v. assumed macronutrient composition to target reference growth: a randomised controlled trial. *Br J Nutr.* (2016) 115:431–9. doi: 10.1017/S0007114515004614
103. Aggett PJ, Agostoni C, Axelsson I, De Curtis M, Goulet O, Hernell O, et al. Feeding preterm infants after hospital discharge: a commentary by the ESPGHAN Committee on Nutrition. *J Pediatr Gastroenterol Nutr.* (2006) 42:596–603. doi: 10.1097/01.mpg.0000221915.73264.c7

104. Teller IC, Embleton ND, Griffin IJ, van Elburg RM. Post-discharge formula feeding in preterm infants: a systematic review mapping evidence about the role of macronutrient enrichment. *Clin Nutr.* (2016) 35:791–801. doi: 10.1016/j.clnu.2015.08.006
105. Young L, Embleton ND, McGuire W. Nutrient-enriched formula versus standard formula for preterm infants following hospital discharge. *Cochr Database Syst Rev.* (2016) 12:CD004696. doi: 10.1002/14651858.CD004696.pub5
106. Young L, Embleton ND, McCormick FM, McGuire W. Multinutrient fortification of human breast milk for preterm infants following hospital discharge (Review). *Cochr Database Syst.*(2013): CD004866. doi: 10.1002/14651858.CD004866.pub4
107. Lapointe M,Barrington KJ, Savaria M, Janvier A. Preventing postnatal growth restriction in infants with birthweight less than 1300 g. *Acta Paediatr.* (2016) 105:e54–9. doi: 10.1111/apa.13237
108. Wilson E, Edstedt Bonamy AK, Bonet M, Toome L, Rodrigues C, Howell EA, et al. EPICE Research Group. Room for improvement in breast milk feeding after very preterm birth in Europe: Results from the EPICE cohort. *Matern Child Nutr.* (2018) 14. doi: 10.1111/mcn.12485
109. Fomon S, Bell E. Energy. In: Book MY, editor. Nutrition in Normal Infants.St Louis: Mosby (1993). p. 103–20.
110. Carver JD, Wu PY, Hall RT, Ziegler EE, Sosa R, Jacobs J, et al. Growth of preterm infants fed nutrient-enriched or term formula after hospital discharge. *Pediatrics.* (2001) 107:683–9. doi: 10.1542/peds.107.4.683
111. Cooke RJ, Griffin IJ, McCormick K, Wells JC, Smith JS, Robinson SJ, et al. Feeding preterm infants after hospital discharge: effect of dietary manipulation on nutrient intake and growth. *Pediatr Res.* (1998) 43:355–60. doi: 10.1203/00006450-199804001-01528
112. Picaud JC, Decullier E, Plan O, Pidoux O, Bin-Dorel S, van Egroo LD, et al. Growth and bone mineralization in preterm infants fed preterm formula or standard term formula after discharge. *J Pediatr.* (2008) 153:616–21. doi: 10.1016/j.jpeds.2008.05.042
113. Borkhardt A, Wirth S. Nutrition of premature infants after discharge. Consensus paper of the Austrian Society for Pediatric and Adolescent Medicine. *Monatsschr Kinderheilkd.* (2012) 160:491–8. doi: 10.1007/s00112-011-2618-9
114. Marino LV, Fudge C, Pearson F, Johnson MJ. Home use of breast milk fortifier to promote postdischarge growth and breastfeeding in preterm infants : a quality improvement project. *Arch Dis Child.* (2018) doi: 10.1136/archdischild-2018-315951. [Epub ahead of print].
115. Wauben IPM, Atkinson SA, Shah JK Paes B. Growth and body composition of preterm infants: influence of nutrient fortification of mother's milk in hospital and breastfeeding post-hospital discharge. *Acta Paediatr.* (1998) 87:780–5. doi: 10.1111/j.1651-2227.1998.tb01747.x
116. Zachariassen G, Faerk J, Grytter C, Esberg BH, Hjelmborg J, Mortensen S, et al. Nutrient enrichment of mother's milk and growth of very preterm infants after hospital discharge. *Pediatrics.* (2011) 127:e995. doi: 10.1542/peds.2010-0723
117. da Cunha RD, Lamy Filho F, Rafael EV, Lamy ZC, de Queiroz AL. Breast milk supplementation and preterm infant development after hospital discharge: a randomized clinical trial. *J Pediatr.* (2016) 92:136–42. doi: 10.1016/j.jped.2015.
118. O'Connor DL, Khan S, Weishuhn K, Vaughan J, Jefferies A, Campbell DM, et al. Growth and nutrient intakes of human milk-fed preterm infants provided with extra energy and nutrients after hospital discharge. *Pediatrics.* (2008) 121:766–76. doi: 10.1542/peds.2007-0054
119. Toftlund LH, Agertoft L, Halken S, Zaccariassen G. Improved lung function at age 6 in children born very preterm and fed extra protein post-discharge. *Pediatr Allergy Immunol.* (2018) 30:47–54. doi: 10.1111/pai.129.81
120. Aimone, A, Rovet J, Ward W, Jefferies A, Campbell DM, Asztalos E, et al. Growth and body composition of human milk-fed premature infants provided with extra energy and nutrients early after hospital discharge: 1-year Follow-up. *J Pediatr Gastroenterol Nutr.* (2009) 49:456–66. doi: 10.1097/MPG.0b013e31819bc94b
121. O'Connor DL, Weishuhu K, Rovet J, Mirabella G, Jefferies A, Campbell DM, et al. Visual development of human milk–fed preterm Infants Provided With Extra Energy and Nutrients after Hospital Discharge . *JPEN.* (2012) 36:349–53. doi: 10.1177/0148607111414026
122. Thanhaeuser M, Kreissl A, Lindtner C, Brandstetter S, Berger A, Haiden N. Administration of fortifier by finger feeder during breastfeeding in preterm infants. *J Obstet Gynecol Neonatal Nurs.* (2017) 46:748–54. doi: 10.1016/j.jogn.2017.05.005
123. King CL, Winter R. Use of breast milk fortifier in a preterm baby post discharge to avoid use of formula. *Arch Dis Ch F&N.* (2014): 99(Suppl. 1):A80. doi: 10.1136/archdischild-2014-306576.229
124. King CL. Three year experience of using breast milk fortifer post discharge in preterm babies. *Arch Dis child F&N.* (2014):99(Suppl. 1): A47. doi: 10.1136/archdischild-2014-306576.136
125. Theile AR, Radmacher PG, Anschutz TW, Davis DW, Adamkin DH. Nutritional strategies and growth in extremely low birth weight infants with bronchopulmonary dysplasia over the past 10 years. *J Perinatol.* (2012) 32:117–22. doi: 10.1038/jp.2011.67

6

Best Practices for Handling and Administration of Expressed Human Milk and Donor Human Milk for Hospitalized Preterm Infants

_Caroline Steele_*

Children's Hospital of Orange County, Orange, CA, United States

***Correspondence:**
Caroline Steele
csteele@choc.org

The importance of human milk for the preterm infant is well established (1–3). However, the feeding of human milk to preterm infants is typically much more complicated than the mere act of breastfeeding (3, 4). The limited oral feeding skills of many preterm infants often results in human milk being administered via an enteral feeding tube (4). In addition, fortification is commonly required to promote optimal growth and development—particularly in the smallest of preterm infants (2, 4, 5). Consequently, a mother's own milk must be pumped, labeled, transported to the hospital, stored, tracked for appropriate expiration dates and times, thawed (if previously frozen), fortified, and administered to the infant with care taken at each step of the process to avoid microbial contamination, misadministration (the wrong milk for the wrong patient), fortification errors, and waste (1–5). Furthermore, the use of pasteurized donor human milk (DHM) for preterm infants when a mother's own milk is not available has been endorsed by many organizations (1). Therefore, appropriate procurement, storage, thawing (if received frozen), fortification, labeling, and administration must occur with the same considerations of preventing contamination and fortification errors while ensuring the correctly prepared final product reaches the correct patient (1). Many professional organizations have published best practices to provide hospitals with guidelines for the safe and accurate handling and preparation of expressed human milk (EHM) and DHM feedings for preterm infants (1–5). These best practices emphasize the importance of preparation location, trained staff, proper identification of human milk to prevent misadministration, and strategies to prevent fortification errors (1–6). The purpose of this mini-review article is to summarize current published best practices for the handling of human milk for preterm infants within the hospital setting (1–6). Emphasis will focus on the use of aseptic technique with proper sanitation and holding times/temperatures to limit microbial growth; use of technology to prevent misadministration of human milk and fortification errors as well as for tracking of expiration dates/times and lot numbers; and workflow strategies to promote safety while improving efficiencies (1–7).

Keywords: human milk handling, infant feeding preparation, human milk bar code scanning, aseptic technique feeding preparation, safety and human milk

INTRODUCTION

The importance of human milk for the preterm infant is well established (1–3). However, the feeding of human milk to preterm infants is typically much more complicated than the mere act of breastfeeding (3, 4). The limited oral feeding skills of many preterm infants often results in human milk being administered via an enteral feeding tube (4). In addition, fortification is commonly required to promote optimal growth and development—particularly in the smallest of preterm infants (2, 4, 5). Consequently, a mother's own milk must be pumped, labeled, transported to the hospital, stored, tracked for appropriate expiration dates and times, thawed (if previously frozen), fortified, and administered to the infant with care taken at each step of the process to avoid microbial contamination, misadministration (the wrong milk for the wrong patient), fortification errors, and waste (1–5).

Furthermore, the use of pasteurized donor human milk (DHM) for preterm infants when a mother's own milk is not available has been endorsed by many organizations including the World Health Organization (WHO), the Academy of Breastfeeding Medicine (ABM), the European Milk Bank Association, the Human Milk Banking Association of North America (HMBANA), the European Society for Pediatric Gastroenterology, Hepatology, and Nutrition (ESPGHAN), the American Society for Parenteral and Enteral Nutrition (ASPEN), the United States Surgeon General, the Academy of Nutrition and Dietetics, and the American Academy of Pediatrics (AAP) (1). Therefore, appropriate procurement, storage, thawing (if received frozen), fortification, labeling, and administration must occur with the same considerations of preventing contamination and fortification errors while ensuring the correctly prepared final product reaches the correct patient (1).

Many professional organizations, including the Academy of Nutrition and Dietetics, ASPEN, the National Association of Neonatal Nurses (NANN), and HMBANA, have published best practices to provide hospitals with guidelines for the safe and accurate handling and preparation of expressed human milk (EHM) and DHM feedings for preterm infants (1–5). These best practices emphasize the importance of preparation location, trained staff, proper identification of human milk to prevent misadministration, and strategies to prevent fortification errors (1–6).

The purpose of this mini-review article is to summarize current published best practices for the handling of human milk for preterm infants within the hospital setting (1–6). Emphasis will focus on proper sanitation, use of technology for tracking and error prevention, and workflow strategies to promote safety while improving efficiencies (1–7).

LOCATION

For handling of human milk, fortifiers, and feeding systems, preparation location and practices that minimize microbial growth (such as adherence to good hand-hygiene practices and use of "no touch" preparation and administration techniques) are critical (1). A location dedicated for the purpose of handling human milk feedings that is separate from patient care areas reduces risk of contamination and is considered a best practice (1, 2, 8, 9). EHM or DHM feedings should not be prepared in *any* patient care area, including the patient's bedside, due to risk of contamination (1, 2, 5, 7, 9).

EQUIPMENT AND SUPPLIES

Sinks and Dishwashers

The preparation area should contain a handwashing sink with hands-free controls (1). Unless all preparation items are disposable, a three-compartment sink or commercial dishwasher is needed to ensure proper cleaning and sanitizing of all reusable items (1, 10, 11). The dishwasher should reach a wash temperature of 66°C (150°F) and a rinse temperature of 82°C (180°F) (10, 11).

Refrigerators and Freezers

Although not required, dedicated human milk refrigerators and freezers are preferred. Adequate space to store human milk while allowing for appropriate airflow is important to ensure proper temperatures. Refrigeration guidelines for the storage of human milk for healthy infants at home have been described (12). Within the health care setting, refrigerators for human milk storage must be able to maintain temperatures between 2–4°C (35–39°F); freezers must allow for temperatures at or below −20°C (−4°F) to long-term storage (1, 13). A reliable method of temperature monitoring is imperative to prevent loss and promote safety (1). Use of automated systems that alarm when temperatures exceed desired ranges may be beneficial. Location of refrigeration units in areas with limited access, may help prevent tampering and waste.

Laminar Flow Hoods

While laminar flow hoods provide an additional barrier against contaminants, they are typically used in the preparation of sterile products (including medications and processing/packaging of pasteurized donor human milk) (1, 14). However, use of a flow hood does not result in a sterile finished product when used during the preparation of non-sterile feedings (such as unpasteurized EHM and/or non-sterile fortifiers or additives) (1, 15). Furthermore, use of a flow hood should not be a replacement for good handing practices and aseptic technique.

Measuring/Mixing Devices and Storage Containers

All preparation and storage items should be made of stainless steel or food grade plastic that is free of bisphenol A (BPA) and Di(2-ethylhexyl) phthalate (DEHP) (11). Glass items (such as graduated cylinders or beakers) are not generally used for routine handling of human milk in the health care setting due to risk of exposure to glass particles should the glass crack or break (11).

Single-use, disposable items are often selected for human milk collection and feeding preparation due to their convenience and sanitation. Such items may be sterile or non-sterile as there is no evidence that use of non-sterile items results in higher bacterial loads in collected human milk or prepared feedings (1, 16). If reusable items are selected, they must be cleaned and appropriately sanitized between uses to prevent cross contamination.

Human milk and other liquid ingredients should be measured using containers with precise graduations such as graduated cylinders, beakers, liquid measuring cups, or syringes (1). Powdered fortifiers and additives should be measured on a gram scale accurate to a tenth of a gram (1). Scales should undergo regular calibration to ensure accuracy and promote safety (1).

STAFFING AND STAFF HYGIENE

Use of dedicated staff for the handling and preparation of human milk feedings within the health care setting is considered a best practice and has been shown to reduce risk of misadministration errors (1–3, 5). Staff should be well trained in aseptic technique and demonstrate proper steps for handling human milk and fortifiers. Hand hygiene is critical in the handling of human milk to prevent introduction of exogenous microbial contamination (17, 18).

Use of disposable gowns and other personal protective items including a bonnet or hairnet and gloves are recommended (1). Artificial nails and long natural nails have been associated with a *Pseudomonas aeruginosa* outbreak in a neonatal intensive care unit (18, 19). Therefore, it is recommended that staff nails should be short, neatly groomed, and unpolished (17–21).

HUMAN MILK STORAGE

Stored milk should be rotated using first-in-first-out (FIFO) principles with the oldest milk being used first. Storage times and temperatures impact nutritional quality, biologically active components in human milk, and rate/incidence of microbial growth (12, 22–26). Within the acute care setting when human milk is used for immunocompromised patients, storage recommendations are more conservative than for the healthy infant at home (1, 12). Therefore, it is generally recommended (1, 13, 16, 22, 27):

TABLE 1 | Steps for human milk feeding preparation within the acute care setting (1, 13, 28–32).

Don personal protective items per facility policy (may include disposable gowns and bonnets/hairnets)
Perform hand hygiene upon entry into the preparation area, after sanitizing work surfaces, and between each individual patient feeding preparation
Sanitize work space using a facility-approved sanitizing solution appropriate for food contact surfaces upon entry, between each individual patient feeding preparation, and as required to support aseptic technique
Thaw milk if needed using water bath or commercial warmer
Perform a two-person double check of a minimum of two-patient identifiers or use bar code scanning technology to confirm that all bottles of human milk belong to the same patient before combining
Following hand hygiene, don gloves prior to initiating the actual preparation
Measure appropriate volume of human milk using measuring container with 1 mL graduations
Add fortifiers, if appropriate • Ensure accuracy with calculations and measurements to avoid over or under fortification • Consider systems such as a two-person double check or bar code scanning to confirm appropriate fortifier is used • Use pre-portioned fortifiers when available • If not pre-portioned, measure liquid fortifiers using graduated cylinders, beakers, liquid measuring cups, or syringes and weigh powders using a gram scale
Gently mix ingredients in clean disposable or cleaned and sanitized reusable container
Place finished product in a clean disposable or cleaned and sanitized reusable closed container • Prepare no more than 24-h volumes • Finished product may be unit dosed for individual feedings or in bulk volumes
Label each container Recommended components include: • Patient name • Identification number (such as medical record number) • Contents (human milk plus any fortifiers or additives) • Caloric density • Volume in container • Volume per feeding and frequency or rate of administration • Administration route • Expiration date and time • "For enteral use only" or "Not for intravenous use" • "Refrigerate until use"
Refrigerate final product until used
Perform a two-person double check of a minimum of two-patient identifiers or use bar code scanning technology to verify the feeding label against the patient armband to confirm correct identity prior to administration
Monitor time for prepared feedings at room temperature • Decant no more than 4-h volumes for continuous enteral feedings • For oral feeding, discard any milk remaining in the bottle 1 h after initiating feeding due to potential for bacterial contamination from oral flora that may colonize the milk remaining in the bottle

- Fresh milk be stored in the refrigerator (≤4°C or ≤39°F) for a maximum of 48 h
- Thawed unpasteurized milk be stored in the refrigerator (≤4°C or ≤39°F) for a maximum of 24 h
- Thawed pasteurized DHM be stored in the refrigerator (≤4°C or ≤39°F) for a maximum of 48 h
- Fortified milk be stored in the refrigerator (≤4°C or ≤39°F) for a maximum of 24 h
- Hang time for continuous feedings at room temperature for a maximum of 4 h
- Frozen human milk be stored in the freezer for 6–12 months at ≤−20°C (≤−4°F) or beyond 12 months at −70 to −80°C (−94 to −112°F).

PREPARATION AND ADMINISTRATION OF HUMAN MILK FEEDINGS IN THE HEALTH CARE SETTING

Handling of human milk and preparation of individual feedings within the health care setting requires strict adherence to guidelines to ensure the preservation of nutrients and bioactive compounds while reducing risk of harmful microbial growth (1). Fortification accuracy is imperative to prevent feeding intolerance and promote optimal health and growth. Steps for human milk feeding preparation within the acute care setting are outlined in **Table 1** (1, 13, 28–32).

Sterile liquid fortifiers and additives are preferred over powdered products (which are not sterile) to reduce the risk of microbial contamination; sterile options should be used for human milk fortification whenever possible (1, 13). At present, the optimal length of time between preparation and feeding of fortified human milk is unknown (13). Research has shown that over time, the osmolality of fortified human milk increases (by up to 4%) and the size of milk fat globules may become altered (possibly impacting fat digestion) (33). While shortening the storage time for fortified human milk may be advantageous, there is not enough published evidence to suggest a revision of the current recommendations for a maximum of 24 h (1, 13). Centralized fortification of human milk is a best practice and has been shown to improve patient safety (1–8, 13). However, centralized handling processes often preclude the ability to prepare each individual feeding immediately prior to use. Based on current evidence, the benefits of centralized handling appear to outweigh the risks of potential changes to human milk when feedings are prepared in advance (1–8, 13, 34, 35). Facilities may want to consider the shortest amount of time realistically feasible while still utilizing centralized handling processes. To this end, some organizations have opted to prepare 12-h volumes instead of 24-h volumes which also may be beneficial in more quickly implementing feeding order changes and preventing waste (1).

In addition to safe handling practices, processes must be in place to ensure safe administration of human milk and prevent inadvertent infusion via intravenous (IV) lines (1, 13). Enteral feeding misconnections, which may result in death, have been reported in the literature (36). The International Standards Organization (ISO) has set a standard for enteral devices to provide a female (administration set or syringe) to male (feeding tube) orientation known as ISO 80369-3 (37). Feeding connection sets with this unique configuration are known as ENFit® systems (1, 37). Adoption of ENFit® compatible connectors for all enteral infusions promotes patient safety by preventing enteral feedings from being accidentally connected to IV lines or other medical device ports (1, 13, 37).

USE OF BAR CODE SCANNING TECHNOLOGY TO IMPROVE SAFETY

Bar code scanning technology is commonly used in the health care setting to promote patient safety by reducing the risk of misadministration (providing the wrong product to the wrong patient) for processes such as medication, blood, and human milk administration (3–5). Bar code scanning is often used in lieu of a two-person double check to reduce risk of human error and confirmation bias which may occur when a manual check is used (3–5). Such systems have been shown to reduce errors and improve efficiencies (3–5). Scanning technology can assist with monitoring expiration dates and times. Human milk that is beyond its expiration is at greater risk for excessive microbial growth which could be particularly devastating in the critically ill neonate. Consequently, scanning systems may add a layer of patient safety by alerting the clinician if an attempt is made to use an expired feeding. Furthermore, some systems offer the ability to automate fortification calculations and scan fortifiers or additives to reduce risk of fortification errors (3–5). Automatically tracking lot numbers for pasteurized DHM and fortifiers or additives is more efficient than having staff track such information manually and provides a faster method of identifying exactly which patients received a particular product in the event of a product recall. Therefore, bar code scanning technology with human milk preparation and feeding is considered a best practice and is endorsed by many organizations (1–5).

SUMMARY

Human milk in the health care setting, particularly the neonatal intensive care unit, is often viewed as "medicine" or an adjunct therapy. Some of the most fragile patients are those premature or critically ill infants receiving human milk feedings. Therefore, every precaution must be taken with human milk handling to ensure safety. Aseptic technique with proper sanitation and holding times/temperatures to limit microbial growth; use of technology to prevent misadministration of human milk and fortification errors as well as for tracking of expiration dates/times and lot numbers; and workflow strategies to promote safety while improving efficiencies are worthy endeavors of all facilities (1–7).

AUTHOR CONTRIBUTIONS

The author confirms being the sole contributor of this work and approved it for publication.

REFERENCES

1. Steele C, Collins E, eds. *Infant and Pediatric Feedings: Guidelines for Preparation of Human Milk and Formula in Health Care Facilities.* 3rd ed. Chicago, IL: Academy of Nutrition and Dietetics (2018). p. 1–248.
2. Moro GE, Arslanoglu S, Bertino E, Corvaglia L, Montirosso R, Picaud JC, et al. Human milk in feeding premature infants: from tradition to bioengineering. Proceedings of a consensus development conference—EXPO 2015. *J Ped Gastroenterol Nutr.* (2015) 61:S1–19. doi: 10.1097/MPG.0000000000000897
3. Oza-Frank R, Kachoria R, Dail J, Green J, Walls K, McClead RE Jr. A quality improvement project to decrease human milk errors in the NICU. *Pediatrics* (2017) 139:e2–7. doi: 10.1542/peds.2015-4451.
4. Steele C, Czerwin A, Bixby C. Breast milk bar code scanning results in time savings and staff efficiency. *J Acad Nutr Diet.* (2015) 115:23–6. doi: 10.1016/j.jand.2014.06.360
5. Steele C, Bixby C. Centralized breastmilk handling and bar code scanning improve safety and reduce breastmilk administration errors. *Breastfeed Med.* (2014) 9:426–9. doi: 10.1089/bfm.2014.0077
6. Barbas KH. Mother's milk technicians: a new standard of care. *J Hum Lact.* (2013) 29:323–27. doi: 10.1177/0890334413492910
7. Perkey K. Delivering results: Opening an infant nutrition center. *Future Dimens Clin Nutr Pratc.* (2016) 8–12.
8. National Association of Neonatal Nurses. *The Use of Human Milk and Breastfeeding in the Neonatal Intensive Care Unit.* Position statement #3065 (2015). Available online at: http://nann.org/uploads/About/PositionPDFS/1.4.3_Use%20%20of%20Human%20Milk%20and%20Breastfeeding%20in%20the%20NICU.pdf (Accessed May 3, 2017).
9. The Facilities Guidelines Institute. *Guidelines for Design and Construction of Hospital and Health Care Facilities.* Washington, DC: American Institute of Architects (2014). p. 91–2. Standard A2.1-7.2.3.2(3) and Standard 2.1-7.2.3.3(5).
10. NSF International Standard/American National Standard for Food Equipment. *Commercial Warewashing Equipment.* Ann Arbor, MI: NSF International (2012).
11. NSF International Standard/American National Standard for Food Equipment. *Food Equipment Materials.* Ann Arbor, MI: NSF International (2015).
12. Eglash A, Simon L, The Academy of Breastfeeding Medicine. ABM clinical protocol #8: human milk storage information for home use for full-term infants, revised 2017. *Breastfeed Med.* (2017) 12:390–5. doi: 10.1089/bfm.2017.29047.aje
13. Boullata JI, Carrera AL, Harvey L, Escuro AA, Hudson L, Mays A, et al. ASPEN safe practices for enteral nutrition therapy. *JPEN J Parenter Enteral Nutr.* (2017) 41:15–103. doi: 10.1177/0148607116673053
14. The United States Pharmacopeial Convention. USP 797 pharmaceutical compounding—sterile preparations. In: *USP Compounding Compendium 2016.* Rockville, MD: The United States Pharmacopeial Convention (2016) p. 39–84.
15. The United States Pharmacopeial Convention. USP 795 pharmaceutical compounding—nonsterile preparations. In: *USP Compounding Compendium 2016.* Rockville, MD: The United States Pharmacopeial Convention (2016). p. 31–9.
16. Jones F. *Best Practice for Expressing, Storing and Handling Human Milk in Hospitals, Homes, and Child Care Settings.* 3rd ed. Fort Worth, TX: Human Milk Banking Association of North America, Inc. (2011).
17. Centers for Disease Control and Prevention. *Hand hygiene in Healthcare Settings* (2017). Available online at: https://www.cdc.gov/handhygiene/providers/index.html (Accessed May 24, 2017).
18. Association of Perioperative Registered Nurses. *Hand Hygiene.* Available online at: http://www.aorn.org/guidelines/clinical-resources/clinical-faqs/hand-antisepsis-hygiene (Accessed May 3, 2017).
19. Moolenaar RL, Crutcher JM, San Joaquin VH, et al. A prolonged outbreak of *Pseudomonas aeruginosa* in a neonatal intensive care unit: did staff fingernails play a role in disease transmission? *Infect Control Hosp Epidemiol.* (2000) 21:80–5. doi: 10.1086/501739
20. Centers for Disease Control and Prevention. Guideline for hand hygiene in health-care settings. *MMWR Morb Mortal Wkly Rep.* (2002) 51:1–56. Available online at: https://www.cdc.gov/mmwr/PDF/rr/rr5116.pdf (Accessed July 16, 2018).
21. Hedderwick SA, McNeil SA, Lyons MJ, Kauffman CA. Pathogenic organisms associated with artificial fingernails worn by health care workers. *Infect Control Hosp Epidemiol.* (2000) 21:505–9. doi: 10.1086/501794
22. Yuen JW, Loke AY, Gohel MDI. Nutritional and immunological characteristics of fresh and refrigerated stored human milk in Hong Kong: a pilot study. *Clinica Chimica Acta* (2012) 413:1549–54. doi: 10.1016/j.cca.2012.03.018
23. Takci S, Gulmez D, Yigit S, Dogan O, Dik K, Hascelik G. Effects of freezing on the bactericidal activity of human milk. *J Pediatr Gastroenterol Nutr.* (2012) 55:146–9. doi: 10.1097/MPG.0b013e31824f7889
24. Chang JC, Chen CH, Fang LJ, Tsai CR, Chang YC, Wang TM. Influence of prolonged storage process, pasteurization, and heat treatment on biologically-active human milk proteins. *Pediatr Neonatol.* (2013) 54:360–6. doi: 10.1016/j.pedneo.2013.03.018
25. Raoff NA, Adamkin DH, Radmacher PG, Telang S. Comparison of lactoferrin activity in fresh and stored milk. *J Perinatol.* (2016) 36:207–9. doi: 10.1038/jp.2015.186
26. Grazziotin MC, Grazziotin AL, Vidal NM, Freire MH, DaSilva RP. Analysis of the storage methods for raw human milk from mothers with infants admitted to a neonatal intensive care unit, according to Brazilian regulations. *J Hum Lact.* (2016) 32:446–54. doi: 10.1177/0890334416647710
27. Hamosh M, Ellis LA, Pollock DR, Henderson TR, Hamosh P. Breastfeeding and the working mother: effect of time and temperature of short-term storage on proteolysis, lipolysis, and bacterial growth in milk. *Pediatrics* (1996) 97:493–8.
28. Hurrell E, Kucerova E, Loughlin M, et al. Neonatal enteral feeding tubes as loci for colonisation by members of the Enterobacteriaceae. *BMC Infect Dis.* (2009) 9:146. doi: 10.1186/1471-2334-9-146
29. American Academy of Pediatrics Committee on Nutrition. Formula feeding of term infants. In: Kleinman RE, Greer FR, editors. *Pediatric Nutrition.* 7th ed. Elk Grove Village, IL: American Academy of Pediatrics (2014). p. 66–8.
30. United States Department of Agriculture. *Feeding Infants: A Guide for Use in the Child Nutrition Programs.* Available online at: https://www.fns.usda.gov/sites/default/files/feeding_infants.pdf (Accessed April 13, 2018).
31. Petersen S, Greisen G, Krogfelt K. Nasogastric feeding tubes from a neonatal department yield high concentrations of potentially pathogenic bacteria - even 1 day after insertion. *Pediatric Res.* (2016) 80:395–400. doi: 10.1038/pr.2016.86
32. Perry J, Stankorb S, Salgueiro M. Microbial contamination of enteral feeding products in thermoneutral and hyperthermal ICU environments. *Nutr Clin Pract.* (2015) 30:128–33. doi: 10.1177/0884533614541680
33. Takahashi K, Mizuno K, Itabashi K. The freeze-thaw process and long intervals after fortification denature human milk fat globules. *Am J Perinatol.* (2012) 29:283–8. doi: 10.1055/s-0031-1295659
34. Choi A, Fusch G, Rochow, Fusch C. Target fortification of breast milk: predicting the final osmolality of the feeds. *PLoS ONE* (2016) 11:e0148941. doi: 10.1371/journal.pone.0148941
35. Kreissl A, Zwiauer V, Repa A, Binder C, Haninger N, Jilma B, et al. Effect of fortifiers and additional protein on the osmolarity of human milk: is it still safe for the premature infant? *J Pediatr Gastroenterol Nutr.* (2013) 57:432–7. doi: 10.1097/MPG.0b013e3182a208c7
36. Guenter P, Hicks RW, Simmons D, Crowley J, Joseph S, Croteau R, et al. Enteral feeding misconnections: a consortium position statement. *Jt Comm J Qual Patient Saf.* (2008) 34:285–92. doi: 10.1016/S1553-7250(08)34035-5
37. GEDSA. *GEDSA Guidance Supporting ISO 80369-3 ENFit®* (2017). Available online at: http://stayconnected.org/wp-content/uploads/2017/11/GEDSA-ENFit-Guidance-Nov-1.finalv2.pdf (Accessed July 16, 2018).

7

Individualized Fortification Influences the Osmolality of Human Milk

*Nathalie Kreins [1], Rachel Buffin [1,2], Diane Michel-Molnar [3], Veronique Chambon [3], Pierre Pradat [4] and Jean-Charles Picaud [1,2,5,6]**

[1] Neonatal Intensive Care Unit, Croix Rousse University Hospital, Hospices Civils de Lyon, Lyon, France, [2] Regional Human Milk Bank, Croix Rousse University Hospital, Hospices Civils de Lyon, Lyon, France, [3] Centre de Biologie, Hôpital de la Croix Rousse, Hospices Civils de Lyon, Lyon, France, [4] Center for Clinical Research, Croix Rousse University Hospital, Hospices Civils de Lyon, Lyon, France, [5] CarMeN Unit, Inserm U1060, INRA U1397, Claude Bernard University Lyon 1, Pierre Bénite, France, [6] Faculté de Médecine Lyon Sud Charles Merieux, Université Claude Bernard Lyon 1, Pierre Bénite, France

***Correspondence:**
Jean-Charles Picaud
jean-charles.picaud@chu-lyon.fr

Background: Fortification of human milk (HM) increases its osmolality, which is associated with an increased risk of necrotizing enterocolitis. The impact of new fortifiers on osmolality is not well-known, nor are the kinetics regarding the increase in osmolality.

Aim: To determine the optimum fortifier composition for HM fortification by measuring the osmolality of fortified HM made with three powder multicomponent fortifiers (MCFs) and a protein fortifier (PF).

Methods: The osmolality of HM was assessed at 2 (H2) and 24 (H24) h after fortification to compare the effects of MCF (MCF1–3) and PF used in quantities that ensured that infants' nutrient needs would be met (MCF: 4 g/100 ml HM; PF: 0.5 g or 1 g/100 ml HM). To evaluate the early kinetics associated with the osmolality increase, the osmolality of HM fortified with MCF1 or MCF2 was also measured at 0, 1, 5, 10, 15, 20, 30, 40, 50, 60, 90, and 120 min after fortification.

Results: The osmolality increased significantly immediately after fortification, depending on the type of fortification used and the quantity of MCF and PF used, rather than the time elapsed after fortification. The maximum value at H24 was 484 mOsm/kg. The mean increase in osmolality between H2 and H24 was 3.1% ($p < 0.01$) (range: 0.2–10.8%). Most of the increase (>70%) occurred immediately after fortification.

Conclusion: When choosing a fortifier, its effect on HM osmolality should be considered. As most of the increase in osmolality occurred immediately, bedside fortification is not useful to prevent the increase in osmolality, and further research should focus on improving fortifier composition.

Keywords: fortifier, growth, nutrition, prematurity, protein, necrotizing enterocolitis, breastmilk, energy

INTRODUCTION

Human milk (HM) is the gold standard for premature infants' nutrition during hospitalization, but it needs to be fortified to support postnatal growth. Standard fortification with a multicomponent fortifier (MCF) cannot always provide breastfed preterm infants with sufficient amounts of nutrients (1–5). Individualized fortification (adjustable or targeted) has been proposed to improve nutritional support (6, 7). Adjustable fortification relies on monitoring blood urea nitrogen. Protein is added when urea is low (8). This improves the ratio of protein-to-energy intake, which can support gains in weight and head circumference (2, 6, 9, 10). Targeted fortification relies on the analysis of HM composition followed by the addition of protein and/or energy to reach a target composition for covering the theoretical needs of the infant (3.5–4.5 g protein/kg/d and 110–135 kcal/kg/d) (11). However, targeted fortification has been shown to improve only weight gain (not length and head circumference) (2, 7), and a randomized trial failed to show a benefit in growth (12). New MCFs and a specifically designed protein fortifier (PF) powder were recently made commercially available in Europe, allowing better individualization of HM fortification.

Similar to the milk of most mammalian species, the osmolarity of unfortified HM is around 300 mOsm/l (approximately an osmolality of 338 mOsm/kg) (13–15). The presence of micro- and macro-nutrients in MCFs increases the total osmolality (14, 16, 17). Fortification has been thought to lead to an increase in osmolality because HM amylase activity induces hydrolysis of the dextrin (polysaccharides) content of fortifiers, leading to the production of small osmotically active mono- or di-saccharides (5, 13, 16). Glucose polymers are the main source of carbohydrate in most fortifiers because of their lower osmotic activity per unit weight compared to lactose or monosaccharides. High osmolality significantly alters gut mucosal integrity in animals and has been suspected to increase the risk of digestive intolerance and necrotizing enterocolitis in infants (5, 13, 14). Although the evidence is not that strong, it is often considered that the osmolality of fortified HM should remain below 450 mOsm/kg (an osmolarity of 400 mOsm/l) (13). As previous studies showed that the osmolality of HM fortified with older fortifiers increased when it is prepared 24 h before administration, it has been suggested that HM should be fortified at the patient's bedside (16, 18).

We aimed to evaluate the osmolality of HM fortified with available products, from fortification to 24 h after adding the fortifier. We assessed the impact of each fortifier on the osmolality and whether or not bedside fortification is useful for preventing osmolality increase.

MATERIALS AND METHODS

HM Samples

The study involved the regional Auvergne-Rhone-Alpes Milk Bank in Lyon, France. The HM used for the study was unsuitable for use by premature babies due to significant bacteriological contamination (revealed by pre-pasteurization bacteriological testing). Donors provided written consent for use of their milk for research purposes. The HM came from three different donors because we aimed to select HM samples with a wide range of protein and energy contents. According to analysis using infrared spectroscopy (Miris® Uppsala, Sweden), protein and energy concentrations ranged from 1 to 1.6 g/dl and from 60 to 101 kcal/dl, respectively.

TABLE 1 | Composition of the multicomponent fortifiers (MCFs) and protein fortifier (PF) (per gram of powder).

	Multicomponent fortifiers			Protein fortifier
	MCF1 Suppletine® (Lactalis)	MCF3 Fortipre® (Nestle)	MCF2 Fortema® (Bledina)	PF Nutriprem® (Bledina)
Energy (kcal)	3.5*	3.5*	3.5*	3.4*
Protein (g)	0.23**	0.20**	0.25**	0.82**
Na (mg)	7.5	5.2	8.0	7.8
K (mg)	4.5	13.2	5.3	12.3
Ca (mg)	13	15	14.9	5.2
Ph (mg)	8.7	9.0	8.7	5.2
Iron (mg)	0	0.3	0	0

*Energy source: carbohydrates.
**Partially hydrolyzed source.

Preparation of Fortified HM

The preparation of food for hospitalized preterm infants is performed by dedicated staff in a dedicated room close to the regional HM bank that is in the same building as the neonatal intensive care unit at Croix Rousse University Hospital. The milk is stored in a freezer (−20°C) and thawed during preparation. To explore different types of fortifier with different compositions, we prepared samples of fortified HM using the three MCFs available in France in 2016: Suppletine®, which is produced by Lactalis (Laval, France), Fortema® (also called Aptamil® in other European countries), which is produced by Bledina (Villefranche-sur-Saône, France), and Fortipré®, which is produced by Nestlé (Marne la Vallée, France), which were designated MCF1, MCF2, and MCF3, respectively. These samples were prepared with or without the PF Nutriprem®, which is produced by Bledina (Villefranche-sur-Saône, France) (**Table 1**). We added a quantity of each MCF sufficient to cover the protein and energy needs that allowed an enteral intake of 160 ml/kg/day (11). This quantity amounted to 4 g of MCF1, MCF2, or MCF3 in 100 ml HM. The amount of PF added to the HM was either 0.5 g or 1 g per 100 ml HM, which were designated PF1 and PF2, respectively. The recently commercialized PF was specifically designed to increase the protein-to-energy ratio of milk ingested by poorly growing infants or to allow targeted fortification, a strategy that has been shown to be efficient for short-term growth (2, 6, 7). The amount of each fortifier added to the HM was weighed by a precision balance to the nearest 0.1 g, as done routinely by the dedicated staff.

Measurement of Osmolality

Osmolality is a measure of osmolar concentration and is defined as the number of osmoles of solute per kilogram of solvent, expressed as mOsm/kg. It was blindly assessed using the freezing point technique [micro-osmometer automatic ADVANCED 3300, Radiometer S.A.S (Neuilly-Plaisance, France) France]. The freezing point of a solution is altered in direct relation to the amount of solute in solution. The reproducibility of the

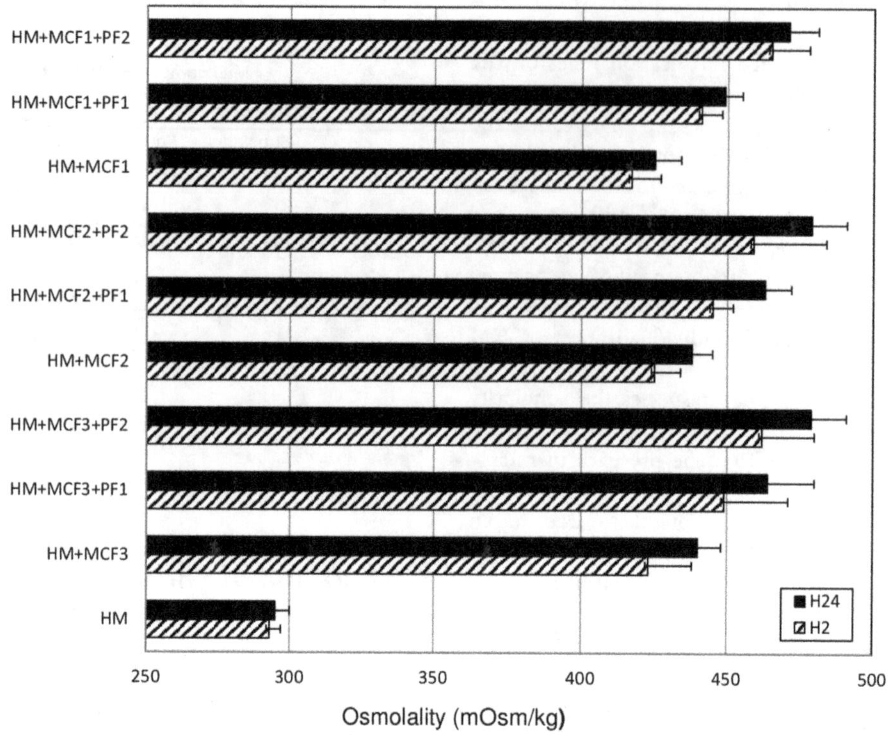

FIGURE 1 | Mean osmolality of human milk assessed at 2 (H2) and at 24 (H24) hours after the addition of three different multicomponent fortifiers: MCF1 (Suppletine®, Lactalis), MCF2 (Fortema®, Bledina), or MCF3 (Fortipré®, Nestlé) at 4 g per 100 ml of human milk, with or without protein fortifier (Nutriprem®, Bledina) at 0.5 g (PF1) or 1 g (PF2) per 100 ml of human milk. HM: unfortified human milk. No significant difference between H2 and H24 (Wilcoxon test).

osmolality assessment based on 11 successive measurements in two HM samples was 0.75%.

First Experiment: Evaluation of Osmolality Due to Fortifier Addition to HM Under Routine Conditions.

We assessed the osmolality at 2 (H2) and 24 (H24) h after the addition of each MCF with or without PF, which reflected routine practices. Indeed, as fortified HM is prepared in the dedicated room close to the HM bank, preterm infants generally receive their first meal no earlier than 2 h after its preparation. Between H2 and H24, the milk was stored at 4°C, just as it is in routine practice, prior to dispensation to premature infants. We calculated the percentage of increase in osmolality between H2 and H24.

Second Experiment: Early Osmolality Kinetics

To precisely investigate the early evolution of osmolality between H0 and H2, we fortified HM with MCF1 or MCF2 and measured the osmolality after fortification at 0, 1, 5, 10, 15, 20, 30, 40, 50, 60, 90, and 120 min. A sample of each preparation was stored at 4°C and the osmolality was measured 24 h later to calculate the proportion of the increase that occurred early after fortification.

Statistics

Osmolality values were presented as mean and one standard deviation. Comparison between H2 and H24 were performed using a Wilcoxon test.

RESULTS

Osmolality was assessed in 30 samples of unfortified or fortified HM. The mean (SD) osmolality of unfortified HM ($n = 3$) was 293 ± 4 mOsm/kg at H2 and it did not increase significantly by H24 (295 ± 5 mOsm/kg, i.e., +0.8%).

The mean (±SD) osmolality of fortified HM ($n = 27$) increased significantly between H2 (443 ± 21 mosm/kg) and H24 (457 ± 20 mosm/kg). The mean increase in osmolality was 3.1% ($p < 0.01$) (range: 0.2–10.8%). However, at H24, the osmolality was over 400 mOsm/kg for all samples and over 450 mOsm/kg for 17 out of the 27 samples (63%) (**Figure 1**).

The increase in osmolality was significant and was of similar amplitude for different types of fortification. When adding an MCF alone ($n = 9$ samples), the osmolality increased from 422 ± 11 mosm/kg at H2 to 434 ± 10 mosm/kg at H24 ($p < 0.01$). When using MCF+PF1 ($n = 9$), it increased from 443 ± 6 to 458 ± 10 mosm/kg ($p < 0.01$), and when using MCF+PF2 ($n = 9$), in increased from 462 ± 17 to 476 ± 11 mosm/kg ($p < 0.01$) (**Figure 1**).

Regarding the kinetics analysis, during the first 2 h after the addition of MCF1 or MCF2, the osmolality increased very rapidly. The increase occurred immediately (during the first minute after fortification) and was similar for both fortifiers tested: +119 mOsm/kg (+40%) for MCF1 and +110 mOsm/kg (+37%) for MCF2. This represented 79 and 76% of the total increase for MCF1 and MCF2, respectively **Figure 2**.

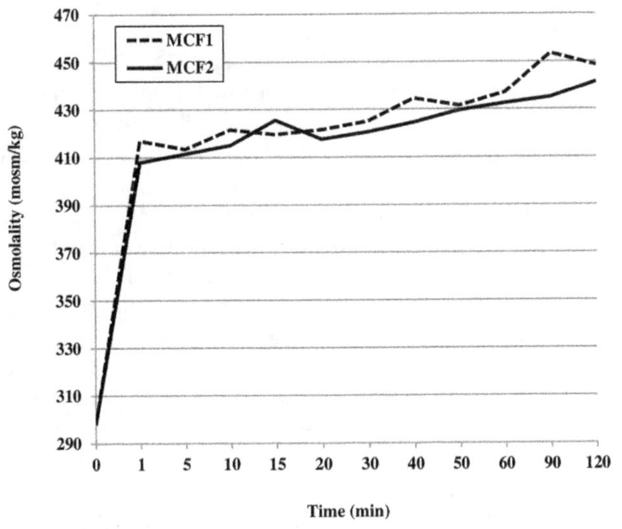

FIGURE 2 | Mean osmolality of human milk assessed during the first 2 h after the addition of two different multicomponent fortifiers: MCF1 (Suppletine®, Lactalis) or MCF2 (Fortema®, Bledina).

DISCUSSION

HM fortification induces an immediate and significant increase in osmolality. Depending on the type of fortification and amount of fortifier added to HM, the osmolality can reach values previously associated with an increased risk of digestive intolerance or necrotizing enterocolitis. A major part of that increase occurred within the first minute after addition of each fortifier.

We observed a slight increase in osmolality (+3.1%) between 2 and 24 h after the addition of MCFs. This is consistent with the previous studies, which showed that storage of HM fortified with first-generation MCFs increased osmolality by 4 and 5–10%, respectively (7, 16, 17). Such a slight increase in osmolality (+14 mosm/kg) during storage was also reported for new products available to improve the nutritional value of HM (14). Rosas et al. more recently reported a slightly greater increase in osmolality (+13–15%) (18). The increase in osmolality during storage was originally thought to be mainly attributable to the amylase in HM that breaks down the polysaccharides in the fortifier to produce molecules with higher osmolality (mono- or di-saccharides) (16, 19). The similar increase in osmolality during storage reported in the 1990s and nowadays is probably related to the similar proportion of carbohydrate (around 70/100 g) and composition (mainly or exclusively dextrin) in fortifiers.

Based on these previously reported results, Choi et al. recently wrote that osmolality was increased by 2.5–5.0% within 10 min after standard fortification, with a further 4% increase after storage at 4°C for 24 h (15). However, this key message is not fully in-line with the reality. Indeed, in all the relevant studies, the time of the initial osmolality assessment was either unreported or was at least 5–10 min after the addition of the fortifier (14, 16–18). The "baseline" osmolality values were already at very high levels. Kriessl et al. presented median "baseline" values—measured "immediately" after fortification—that were already between 475 and 691 mOsm/kg (14). These authors reported a slight but significant increase of 14 mOsm/kg after 24 h of storage at 4°C, which was considered to be of negligible clinical relevance (14). Rosas et al. presented mean "Time 0" values—actually measured at 5 min after fortification—that were between 384 and 486 mOsm/kg (18). Because the increase between the basal value and the value at 5 min after addition of the fortifier represented 59–72% of the total increase in osmolality, Rosas et al. suggested that infant feeding should occur within 5 min after the addition of the fortifier. By measuring the osmolality very early after addition of the fortifier, we were able to show that >70% of the increase occurs during the first minute. Thus, it is clear that the major part of the osmolality increase was not related to the progressive transformation of carbohydrates during the 24-h storage at 4°C prior to administration to infants (16). Instead, it was due to the instant addition of solutes (osmoles) to the HM. Therefore, the main factor explaining the osmolality increase was the amount of fortifier added, as previously suggested by Choi et al. (15). This implies that efficient prevention of increased osmolality should not rely on carrying out bedside fortification to shorten the time between fortifier addition and administration of fortified HM. Furthermore, the recommendation regarding bedside fortification could be deleterious because not all neonatal intensive care units have a dedicated room and dedicated staff to precisely weigh the fortifier and add it in safe hygienic conditions, and fortification should only be considered "safe" when the amount of fortifier can be precisely weighed and added to milk in hygienic conditions.

Notably, the osmolality values reported by previous studies were higher than our values, which could be due to the amount or type of fortifier used. The amount of fortifier tested by other researchers was sometimes greater than the amount recommended by the manufacturer, which was probably done to determine the upper limit that should not be exceeded (14, 18). However, when, in previous studies, the highest dose of protein supplement (4 g) was added to MCF-fortified HM containing 1.8 g protein/dL, it would have led to a protein intake of 7.1 g protein/kg/day for an enteral intake of 160 ml/kg/day (13, 14). Even if this type of fortification (4 g protein supplement) was added to HM containing only 1 g protein/dL, protein intake would have been 5.6 g/kg/day, which is fairly high. Furthermore, such fortification was associated with osmolality values above 600 mOsm/kg (14). These results show that it is crucial to use protein supplements very carefully. Rosas et al. also reported that very high amounts of fortifier increased osmolality up to 500–550 mOsm/kg (18). In our study, we measured HM protein and energy contents and fortified the HM with quantities of MCF and PF required to cover protein and energy needs according to current recommendations (11). This explains why we observed lower osmolality values than those reported by previous studies.

As fortifiers are considered to be food rather than health products, manufacturers are not obliged to provide clinical evaluation before launching these products. However, it should be mandatory to provide clinicians with a precise evaluation of the impact of each new product on the osmolality HM. Choi et al. recently showed that the osmolality fortified HM has a linear relationship with the quantity macronutrients added. These authors proposed a prediction model to predict the osmolality of HM fortified using targeted fortification (16). HM was fortified with North American MCFs (including lipids as an energy source) and supplementary nutrients (protein and/or lipids and/or glucose polymer). The model was validated using specific products available in Canada at that time. However, the model is product-specific and therefore not transferable to neonatal intensive care units that use different products or different fortification strategies. Therefore, evaluating the osmolality of fortified HM is necessary to ensure that safe food is prepared for preterm infants. Such an evaluation should be performed independently from the manufacturer, as Kriessl et al. reported a greater increase in osmolality compared to the values provided by the manufacturer (14).

A limitation of our study is that we did not test cow milk-based fortifiers that use lipids together with carbohydrates as an energy source or HM-based fortifiers. These cow milk-based fortifiers were available only in North America at the time of the study and HM-based fortifier is still not currently available in France. Cowmilk-based fortifiers containing lipids are interesting as they could help to reduce the osmolality of fortified HM. However, Rochow et al. reported that an MCF containing lipids enhanced the osmolality of HM from 295 to 405 mOsm/kg, and to 436 mOsm/kg after targeted fortification (12). In contrast, it has been nicely shown by Choi et al. that the addition of a fat supplement to HM minimally decreased the osmolality (15). The partial replacement of carbohydrates by fat in an MCF may help to reduce the osmotic load and thus the osmolality of fortified HM. The first cow milk-based fortifier containing lipids was evaluated by Rigo et al. (20) and became available for European users in 2017. As expected, the osmolality (390 mOsm/kg) was reduced when compared to previous cow milk-based products and the control MCF (which led to an osmolality of 441 mOsm/kg) (20). Although the study's main objective was to evaluate the effect of the cow milk-based fortifier on growth, digestive tolerance was also evaluated and was similar to that for the control MCF (20). Further investigations are needed to evaluate the osmolality effects of such products under routine conditions, and whether or not they could have an impact on digestive tolerance. Regarding HM-based fortifiers, it has been shown that they lead to a lower osmolality (391–412 mosm/kg) than cow milk-based products (431 mosm/kg) (21). In settings with a high prevalence of necrotizing enterocolitis (16%), HM-based fortifiers have a beneficial preventive effect against necrotizing enterocolitis among preterm infants (22). However, the reality of this benefit is still debated, notably when the prevalence is close to the common level (3–5%) (23).

Another study limitation is that we evaluated osmolality, focusing on the level of 450 mOsm/kg that was proposed as an upper limit by the American Academy of Pediatrics (AAP) in 1976, despite the fact that there is no strong evidence regarding the benefit of this limit (14, 24), Furthermore, there is a difference between the measured osmolality and the effective osmolality *in vivo* because not all substances create an osmotic gradient *in vivo* (25). Molecules that do not lead to an osmotic gradient across the intestinal membrane *in vivo* are not likely to increase the risk of necrotizing enterocolitis due to osmolality (25). Moreover, when particles contributing to osmolality are present in the gut lumen, the normal physiological response is the secretion of hypo-osmolar fluid to reduce the osmolality of the luminal content (13, 26). However, necrotizing enterocolitis is a multifactorial complication of prematurity, and each risk factor, such as using high-osmolality products for enteral nutrition, should be avoided. It is notable that the studies on which the AAP recommendations were based did not take important confounding variables, such as hyperosmolar therapeutic additives and oral drugs, into account (13). Furthermore, the formulas used in the studies reviewed by the AAP had an osmolality in excess of 500 mOsm/kg. A recent meta-analysis of 11 trials (882 infants) of nutrient fortification have not shown evidence of an increase in necrotizing enterocolitis associated with fortification (3). Despite this, while waiting for more precise data, the limit of 450–500 mOsm/kg could be considered appropriate. Our results contribute to improving clinicians' knowledge about the effects of HM fortification, and how to avoid increased osmolality.

In conclusion, the available fortifiers induce a significant increase in osmolality to levels usually considered to be associated with an increased risk of necrotizing enterocolitis. As there are differences in the effect of each type of fortification on HM osmolality, the choice of fortifier should be carefully analyzed. The increases in osmolality occurred immediately after the addition of fortifiers, suggesting that bedside fortification is not the key factor to be taken into account to reduce osmolality of fortified HM. Further research should focus on improving fortifier composition to cover infants' nutritional needs while also keeping osmolality as low as possible.

AUTHOR CONTRIBUTIONS

J-CP, RB, and PP designed and directed the project, and wrote the paper with input from all authors. NK, DM-M, and VC measured the osmolality. DM-M, VC, J-CP, RB, PP, and NK analyzed the data.

ACKNOWLEDGMENTS

We are indebted to Jocelyne Trompette and the teams at the Rhône-Alpes Human Milk Bank for their help in collecting and handling the human milk samples.

REFERENCES

1. Henriksen C, Westerberg AC, Rønnestad A, Nakstad B, Veierød MB, Drevon CA, et al. Growth and nutrient intake among very-low-birth-weight infants fed fortified human milk during hospitalisation. *Br J Nutr.* (2009) 102:1179–86. doi: 10.1017/S0007114509371755
2. Picaud JC, Houeto N, Buffin R, Loys CM, Godbert I, Haÿs S. Additional protein fortification is necessary in extremely low-birth-weight infants fed human milk. *J Pediatr Gastroenterol Nutr.* (2016) 63:103–5. doi: 10.1097/MPG.0000000000001142
3. Brown JV, Embleton ND, Harding JE, McGuire W. Multi-nutrient fortification of human milk for preterm infants. *Cochrane Database Syst Rev.* (2016) 8:CD000343. doi: 10.1002/14651858.CD000343.pub3
4. Corvaglia L, Aceti A, Paoletti V, Mariani E, Patrono D, Ancora G, et al. Standard fortification of preterm human milk fails to meet recommended protein intake: bedside evaluation by near-infrared-reflectance-analysis. *Early Hum Dev.* (2010) 86:237–40. doi: 10.1016/j.earlhumdev.2010.04.001
5. Koo W, Tice H. Human milk fortifiers do not meet the current recommendation for nutrients in very low birth weight infants. *J Parenter Enteral Nutr.* (2018) 42:813–20. doi: 10.1177/0148607117713202
6. Arslanoglu S, Moro GE, Ziegler EE. Adjustable fortification of human milk fed to preterm infants: does it make a difference? *J Perinatol.* (2006) 26:614–21. doi: 10.1038/sj.jp.7211571
7. Polberger S, Räihä NC, Juvonen P, Moro GE, Minoli I, Warm A. Individualized protein fortification of human milk for preterm infants: comparison of ultrafiltrated human milk protein and a bovine whey fortifier. *J Pediatr Gastroenterol Nutr.* (1999) 29:332–8.
8. Arslanoglu S, Moro GE, Ziegler EE, The Wapm Working Group On Nutrition. Optimization of human milk fortification for preterm infants: new concepts and recommendations. *J Perinat Med.* (2010) 38:233–8. doi: 10.1515/JPM.2010.073
9. Alan S, Atasay B, Cakir U, Yildiz D, Kilic A, Kahvecioglu D, et al. An intention to achieve better postnatal in-hospital-growth for preterm infants: adjustable protein fortification of human milk. *Early Hum Dev.* (2013) 89:1017–23. doi: 10.1016/j.earlhumdev.2013.08.015.13
10. Morlacchi L, Mallardi D, Giannì ML, Roggero P, Amato O, Piemontese P, et al. Is targeted fortification of human breast milk an optimal nutrition strategy for preterm infants? An interventional study. *J Transl Med.* (2016) 14:195. doi: 10.1186/s12967-016-0957-y
11. Agostoni C, Buonocore G, Carnielli VP, De Curtis M, Darmaun D, Decsi T, et al.; ESPGHAN Committee on Nutrition. Enteral nutrient supply for preterm infants: commentary from the European Society of Paediatric Gastroenterology, Hepatology and Nutrition Committee on Nutrition. *J Pediatr Gastroenterol Nutr.* (2010) 50:85–91. doi: 10.1097/MPG.0b013e3181adaee0
12. Rochow N, Landau-Crangle E, Fusch C. Challenges in breast milk fortification for preterm infants. *Curr Opin Clin Nutr Metab Care* (2015) 18:276–84. doi: 10.1097/MCO.0000000000000167
13. Pearson F, Johnson MJ, Leaf AA. Milk osmolality: does it matter? *Arch Dis Child Fetal Neonatal Ed.* (2013) 98:F166–9. doi: 10.1136/adc.2011.300492
14. Kreissl A, Zwiauer V, Repa A, Binder C, Haninger N, Jilma B, et al. Effect of fortifiers and additional protein on the osmolarity of human milk: is it still safe for the premature infant? *J Pediatr Gastroenterol Nutr.* (2013) 57:432–7. doi: 10.1097/MPG.0b013e3182a208c7
15. Choi A, Fusch G, Rochow N, Fusch C. Target fortification of breast milk: predicting the final osmolality of the feeds. *PLoS ONE* (2016) 11:e0148941. doi: 10.1371/journal.pone.0148941
16. De Curtis M, Candusso M, Pieltain C, Rigo J. Effect of fortification on the osmolality of human milk. *Arch Dis Child Fetal Neonatal Ed.* (1999) 8:F141–3.
17. Jocson MA, Mason EO, Schanler RJ. The effects of nutrient fortification and varying storage conditions on host defense properties of human milk. *Pediatrics* (1997) 100:240–3.
18. Rosas R, Sanz MP, Fernández-Calle P, Alcaide MJ, Montes MT, Pastrana N, et al. Experimental study showed that adding fortifier and extra-hydrolysed proteins to preterm infant mothers' milk increased osmolality. *Acta Paediatr.* (2016) 105:e555–60. doi: 10.1111/apa.13522
19. Jones JB, Mehta NR, Hamosh M. Alpha-amylase in preterm human milk. *J Pediatr Gastroenterol Nutr.* (1982) 1:43–8.
20. Rigo J, Hascoët JM, Billeaud C, Picaud JC, Mosca F, Rubio A, et al. Growth and nutritional biomarkers of preterm infants fed a new powdered human milk fortifier: a randomized trial. *J Pediatr Gastroenterol Nutr.* (2017) 65:e83–93. doi: 10.1097/MPG.0000000000001686
21. Thomaz DM, Serafim PO, Palhares DB, Melnikov P, Venhofen L, Vargas MO. Comparison between homologous human milk supplements and a commercial supplement for very low birth weight infants. *J Pediatr.* (2012) 88:119–24. doi: 10.2223/JPED.2166
22. Sullivan S, Schanler RJ, Kim JH, Patel AL, Trawöger R, Kiechl-Kohlendorfer U, et al. An exclusively human milk-based diet is associated with a lower rate of necrotizing enterocolitis than a diet of human milk and bovine milk-based products. *J Pediatr.* (2010) 156:562–7.e1. doi: 10.1016/j.jpeds.2009.10.040
23. Embleton ND, King C, Jarvis C, Mactier H, Pearson F, Menon G. Effectiveness of human milk-based fortifiers for preventing necrotizing enterocolitis in preterm infants: case not proven. *Breastfeed Med.* (2013) 8:421. doi: 10.1089/bfm.2013.0049
24. Barness LA, Mauer AM, Holiday MA, Anderson AS, Dallman PR, Forbes GB et al. Commentary on breast-feeding and infant formulas, including proposed standards for formulas. *Pediatrics* (1976) 57:278–85.
25. Fenton TR, Belik J. Routine handling of milk fed to preterm infants can significantly increase osmolality. *J Pediatr Gastroenterol Nutr.* (2002) 35:298–302.
26. Norris HT. Response of the small intestine to the application of a hypertonic solution. *Am J Pathol.* (1973) 73:747–64.

8

High-Temperature Short-Time Treatment of Human Milk for Bacterial Count Reduction

Daniel Klotz[1], Marie Schreiner[1], Valeria Falcone[2], Daniel Jonas[3], Mirjam Kunze[4], Andrea Weber[5], Hans Fuchs[1] and Roland Hentschel[1]*

[1] Center for Pediatrics, Department of Neonatology, Faculty of Medicine, Medical Center - University of Freiburg, Freiburg, Germany, [2] Institute of Virology, Faculty of Medicine, Medical Center - University of Freiburg, Freiburg, Germany, [3] Institute for Infection Prevention and Hospital Epidemiology, Faculty of Medicine, Medical Center - University of Freiburg, Freiburg, Germany, [4] Department of Obstetrics and Gynecology, Faculty of Medicine, Medical Center - University of Freiburg, Freiburg, Germany, [5] Institute of Medical Microbiology and Hygiene, Faculty of Medicine, Medical Center - University of Freiburg, Freiburg, Germany

***Correspondence:**
Daniel Klotz
daniel.klotz@uniklinik-freiburg.de

Background: Human milk (HM) for preterm infants will often be pasteurized for cytomegalovirus (CMV) inactivation and reduction of its bacterial count. High-temperature short-time (HTST) treatment compared to standard Holder pasteurization (HoP) reduces the impact of heat treatment on bioactive HM proteins while effectively inactivating CMV. No data are available for the efficacy of bacterial count reduction using HTST treatments that are available for clinical use.

Objective: To test the antiviral and antibacterial efficacy of HTST treatment protocols in HM using a modified HTST treatment device compared to standard HoP.

Methods: Holder pasteurized 95 mL HM samples were inoculated with *Staphylococcus aureus* (ATCC 6538), *Enterococcus faecalis* (ATCC 29212), *Pseudomonas aeruginosa* (ATCC 27853), *Serratia marcescens* (Smarc 00697), two different strains of *Klebsiella pneumoniae* (ATCC 700603 and Kpn 01605) or spiked with 2×10^5 50% tissue culture infective dose of CMV (AD169) and subsequently subjected to HoP (62.5°C/30 min) or HTST treatment (62°C/5 s, 62°C/15 s, 72°C/5 s, 72°C/15 s, 87°C/2 s, and 87°C/5 s). Bacterial count was determined after treated HM was cultured for 24 h. CMV infectivity was determined by the number of specific CMV immediate early antigen stained nuclei after inoculating human fibroblasts with appropriately prepared HM samples.

Results: Holder pasteurized samples revealed no growth after 24 h incubation. Viable bacterial cultures were retrieved from all tested strains after HTST treatment with the default HTST protocol (62°C/5 s) that is available for clinical use. Using other time-temperature combinations, growth rates of *S. aureus*, *E. faecalis*, *P. aeruginosa*, *K. pneumoniae*, *K. pneumonia,* and *S. marcescens* were depending on treatment time, treatment temperature, bacterial genera and strain. Only after treatment temperatures above 72°C no bacterial growth was observed. CMV was inactivated by any tested time-temperature combination.

Conclusions: HTST treatment inactivates CMV in 95 mL HM samples but is less effective than HoP in bacterial count reduction at a time-temperature combination of 62°C/5 s. For a reliable bacterial count reduction HTST treatment at 87°C was required in this study.

Keywords: bacteria, human milk, cytomegalovirus, holder pasteurization, high-temperature short-time, HTST treatment, preterm

INTRODUCTION

Human milk (HM) is naturally colonized with various microbiota but its content may increase and diversify during HM handling routines in a neonatal intensive care setting (1). HM may also serve as a vector for cytomegalovirus (CMV) which is frequently reactivated in the mammary gland of the CMV seropositive lactating mother and transmitted via HM (2). HM acquired bacterial sepsis and postnatal CMV infection has been observed in preterm infants, displaying various degrees of illness from clinically unapparent infection to septicaemia and death (3). Hence, screening of maternal CMV serostatus and bacterial HM content is performed in many neonatal units (4–7). In case of suspected CMV shedding, HM for preterm infants may either be freeze-thawed or pasteurized for CMV inactivation, temporarily withheld or even discarded within some neonatal units (7). Similar strategies are pursed for bacterial HM content that is exceeding certain threshold levels or includes certain bacterial genera or species (6). Holder pasteurization (HoP, 62.5°C/30 min) which has shown to eliminate most life forms of HM microbiota will be applied by most neonatal units (6–8). However, HoP has an adverse effect on bioactive HM content and may adversely influence the immunocompetence of the preterm infant (9). In contrast, high-temperature short-time treatment (HTST, e.g., 62°C/5 s) preserves bioactive HM proteins compared to Holder pasteurization while effectively inactivating CMV (10). However, data to support the use of HTST treatment to reduce the bacterial HM content are limited and mostly generated by experimental pasteurizers that are not available for practical clinical use (10–13). The aim of this study was to test the antimicrobial efficacy of a HTST treatment system that is available for clinical use compared to standard HoP in artificially inoculated HM.

MATERIALS AND METHODS

Human Milk Sampling

We obtained HM samples from three mothers whose infants were treated in a German tertiary neonatal care unit, written informed consent was obtained from the donating mothers. Two of the donors were CMV seronegative as documented in their prenatal care documentation, one was CMV seropositive. Their expressed HM exceeded their infant's enteral nutrition requirements and was stored frozen in our institutional milk bank. Donors did not receive any antibiotics for at least 4 weeks prior expressing their HM.

Human Milk Preparation for Bacterial Inoculation

HM samples from the CMV seropositive donor, frozen at −22°C, were thawed overnight at 4°C and Holder pasteurized for 30 min holding time in a water bath at a plateau temperature of 62 ± 0.5°C using a LABU Muttermilchpasteur 40 (Labu Buchrucker, Ottensheim, Austria) to eliminate any potentially colonizing HM bacteria. Immediately after the heat treatment, samples of 95 mL were prepared, and microbial cultures were performed as detailed below.

Bacteria for artificial inoculation of HM were cultured on blood agar at 36 ± 0.5°C overnight (Thermo Fisher, Waltham, MA). Thereafter colonies were suspended in 0.9% sodium chloride and enumerated using the optical density method with a turbidity meter at 620 nm (Dade Behring, Sacramento, CA). Concentration of the bacterial suspension was 1×10^8 cfu/mL of which 95 μl was added to a 95 mL HM sample resulting in an inoculation dose of 1×10^5 cfu/mL. Seventy-six HM samples of 95 mL were subsequently inoculated with either *Staphylococcus aureus* (ATCC 6538, $n = 16$), *Enterococcus faecalis* (ATCC 29212, $n = 16$), *Pseudomonas aeruginosa* (ATCC 27853, $n = 12$), *Klebsiella pneumoniae* (ATCC 700603, $n = 11$), *Serratia marcescens* (Smarc 00697, $n = 12$) or *Klebsiella pneumoniae* (Kpn 01605, $n = 9$). Those aliquots were then subjected to heat treatment immediately after inoculation.

The selection of tested bacterial genera and species was based on culture results from the routine HM surveillance screening of our institutional milk bank or based on clinical isolates (Smarc 00697, Kpn 01605) obtained at our neonatal unit.

Human Milk Preparation for Viral Inoculation

HM samples of the two CMV seronegative donors, frozen at −22°C, were thawed overnight at 4°C. All samples were pooled, and one unpasteurized aliquot of the pooled samples was analyzed by CMV-PCR (RealStar, altona Diagnostics, Hamburg, Germany) to confirm that donors did not excrete CMV via HM and one further unpasteurized aliquot of the CMV seropositive donor was accordingly analyzed. Sixteen aliquots of 95 mL milk were prepared and spiked with 2×10^5 50% tissue infective doses per mL/HM of cell-free culture supernatant of CMV laboratory strain AD169. An unpasteurized CMV spiked HM aliquot and an unpasteurized sample of the CMV seropositive donor served as positive reference samples for the CMV cultures. One aliquot of the seronegative donors that was not inoculated

Abbreviations: ATCC, American type culture collection; HM, human milk; cfu, colony-forming unit; CMV, Cytomegalovirus; HoP, Holder pasteurization; HTST, High-temperature short-time; PCR, polymerase chain reaction

with CMV served as an unpasteurized negative reference sample for the CMV cultures. Positive and negative control samples were equally subjected to milk processing for viral analysis (**Figure 1**).

High-Temperature Short-Time Treatment

High-temperature short-time treatment was performed using a Virex II (Lauf, Tübingen, Germany) as described in detail elsewhere (13). For this study this machine was modified to allow heat treatment not only at the usually non-adjustable default setting (62°C/5 s) but also at various adjustable temperatures (62, 72, and 87°C) and time (2, 5, and 15 s) combinations. To increase the applicability of HTST treatment in a human milk bank setting, the bulk volume was increased from the default volume (50 mL) to 95 mL.

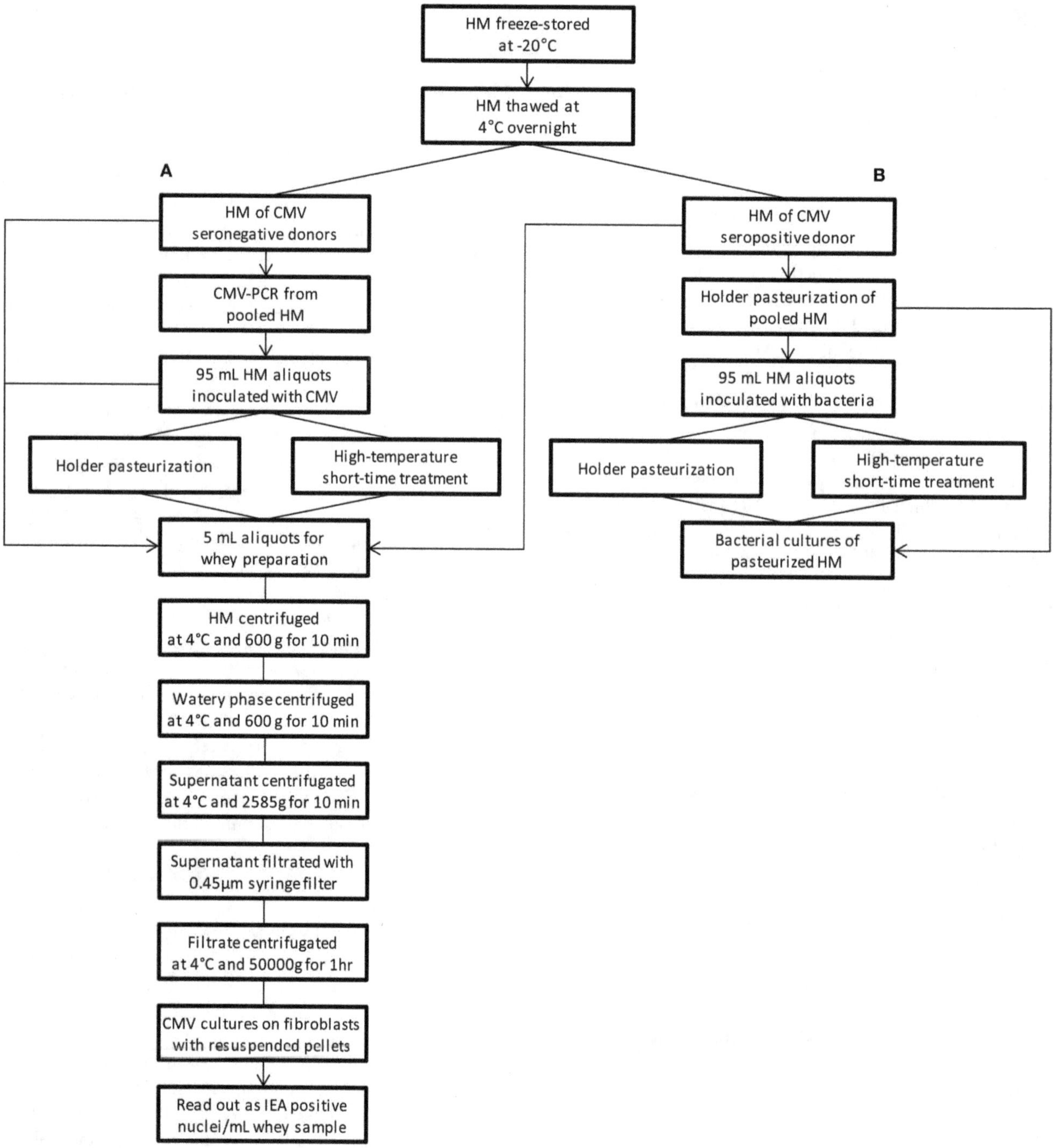

FIGURE 1 | Flowchart of the study procedure. **(A)** viral studies, **(B)** bacterial studies. PCR-Studies of CMV the seropositive donor are not depicted. *HM* human milk, *CMV* cytomegalovirus, *IEA* immediate early antigen.

The 95 mL HM samples that were inoculated with bacteria or spiked with CMV were successively placed in a rotating glass flask. The resulting thin milk layer was heated by hot air to a plateau temperature of either 62°C for a holding time of 2 s (CMV only), 5 s and 15 s or heated to 72°C for 5 and 15 s or to 87°C for 2 and 5 s (CMV not tested at 87°C), respectively (**Table 1**). Afterwards, the glass flask was rapidly cooled with water at 14°C.

Each HTST treatment for a tested time-temperature combination and for a given bacterial species as well as the CMV spiked samples was repeated two fold. Time-temperature curves of every HTST cycle were measured with a sample-frequency of 10 Hz and digitally recorded on an external hard drive. The device was cleaned according to the manufacturer's specification in between the treatments to avoid cross-contamination. Immediately after completion of the heat treatment two agar discs were inoculated with 100 μL pasteurized HM of each sample. The viral samples were stored at 4°C until further processing.

Holder Pasteurization

Three of each 95 mL HM samples that were incubated with different bacterial strains or spiked with CMV as detailed above were subjected to Holder pasteurization at 62.5 ± 0.5°C/30 min using the clinitherm Pasteur 40 (Barkey, Leopoldshöhe, Germany). Immediately after completion of the pasteurization process 100 μL of the HM samples were inoculated onto agar disks, the CMV spiked samples were stored at 4°C until further processing.

Human Milk Processing for Viral Analysis

From each of the three Holder pasteurized CMV spiked samples, 12 HTST pasteurized CMV samples, the unpasteurized CMV spiked samples and the donors' unpasteurized positive and negative reference samples, two 5 mL aliquots (n = 36) were prepared using a Falcon test tube (BD, New Jersey, NJ). To separate the milk fractions aliquots were centrifuged at 4°C and 600 g for 10 min (Centrifuge 5810 R, Eppendorf, Hamburg, Germany). The resulting aqueous layer was centrifuged at 4°C and 600 g for 10 min and the subsequently resulting whey supernatant was further centrifuged at 4°C and 2585 g for 10 min. The resulting whey supernatant was filtrated with the Arodisc Syringe Filter 0,45 μm with Supor Membrane (Pall, NY, NY) and then subjected to ultracentrifugation 4°C and 50,000 g for 60 min (Optima MAX XP, Beckmann Coulter, Brea, CA). The resulting pellet was resuspended in 250 μl tissue culture medium and used to quantify CMV infectivity.

Detection of CMV Infectivity

Human foreskin fibroblasts were seeded into 24 well plates (Falcon, BD, New Jersey, NJ) and were maintained in minimal essential medium until further use (Gibco MEM supplemented with 5% fetal calf serum, Thermo Fischer). The medium was removed before inoculation and 100 μL of processed HM specimen was added to each well. Inoculated plates were centrifuged at 4°C and 900 g for 50 min (Centrifuge 5810 R, Eppendorf, Hamburg, Germany).

TABLE 1 | Concentration and log reduction of HM bacterial content pre and post heat treatment.

		Staphylococcus aureus **(ATCC 6538)**		***Enterococcus Faecalis*** **(ATCC 29212)**		***Pseudomonas aeruginosa*** **(ATCC 27853)**		***Klebsiella Pneumonia*** **(ATCC 700603)**		***Klebsiella pneumonia*** **(Kpn 01605)**		***Serratia marcescens*** **(Smarc 00697)**	
		cfu/mL	Log reduction	cfu/mL	Log reduction	cfu/mL	Log reduction	cfu/mL	Log reduction	cfu/mL	Log reduction	cfu/mL	Log reduction
Pre pasteurization		7.9×10^4	n.a.	1.16×10^5	n.a.	1×10^5	n.a.	5.7×10^4	n.a.	3.6×10^4	n.a.	1.04×10^5	n.a.
Plateau- temperature	Plateau-time												
62.5°C	30 min	$0 \pm 0^{\#}$	>4.9	$0 \pm 0^{\#}$	>5.1	$0 \pm 0^{\#}$	5	$0 \pm 0^{\#}$	> 4.8	$0 \pm 0^{\#}$	> 4.6	$0 \pm 0^{\#}$	> 4.9
62°C	5 s	350 ± 150^b	2.4	$1x10^4 \pm 0^b$	1.1	$7x10^3 \pm 3.6^b$	1.1	–	–	–	–	90 ± 112^d	3.1
62°C	15 s	20 ± 14^c	3.6	$1x10^4 \pm 0^b$	1.1	20 ± 16^a	3.7	0.5 ± 1^a	4.5	$3.6x10^3 \pm 0.5^b$	1.1	$0 \pm 0^{\#a}$	> 4.9
72°C	5 s	40 ± 60^a	3.3	20 ± 20^a	3.8	$0 \pm 0^{\#a}$	5	$0 \pm 0^{\#a}$	>4.8	$0 \pm 0^{\#a}$	>4.6	$0 \pm 0^{\#a}$	> 4.9
72°C	15 s	10 ± 15^a	3.9	20 ± 15^a	3.8	–	–	$0 \pm 0^{\#a}$	>4.8	$0 \pm 0^{\#a}$	>4.6	–	–
87°C	2 s	$0 \pm 0^{\#a}$	>4.9	$0 \pm 0^{\#a}$	>5.1	–	–	$0 \pm 0^{\#a}$	>4.8	–	–	–	–
87°C	5 s	$0 \pm 0^{\#a}$	>4.9	$0 \pm 0^{\#a}$	>5.1	$0 \pm 0^{\#a}$	5	–	–	–	–	$0 \pm 0^{\#a}$	> 4.9

[#] Not detected (lower limit of detection: <10 cfu/mL).
Time-temperature combinations that were not analyzed were marked -
HTST treatment vs. Holder pasteurization: [a] n.s, [b] $p < 0.0001$, [c] $p = 0.0034$, [d] $p = 0.002$
ATCC, American type culture collection; cfu, colony forming units; HTST, high-temperature short-time treatment; n.a., not applicable.

After centrifugation virus inoculum was removed, 1 mL of minimal essential medium was added to each well and the cultures were incubated at 37°C and 5% carbon dioxide for 18 h. Afterwards, monolayers were washed twice in phosphate-buffered saline and fixed with ice-cold acetone for 20 min. Cell monolayers were then incubated with an anti-CMV immediate early antigen (IEA) monoclonal antibody (bioMérieux, Lyon, France) and, after washing, with a fluorescein isothiocyanate-labeled goat anti-mouse immunoglobulin G conjugate (Agilent, Santa Clara, CA). Read-out was the number of CMV specific IEA stained nuclei/mL whey. Duplicates for each sample were analyzed.

Bacterial Count Analysis

We inoculated Columbia blood agar with 5% sheep blood (Thermo Fisher) with 100 μL of the pasteurized whole milk samples. Duplicate plates for each sample were inoculated and counted in all instances. The agar were incubated for 24 h at 36 ± 0.5°C and 5% carbon dioxide in a Heracell incubator (Thermo Fisher) before colony-forming units per milliliter (cfu/mL) were determined with a lower limit of detection of < 10 cfu/mL.

Data Analysis and Statistics

Bacterial HM concentration was determined as cfu/mL; antibacterial efficacy is reported as raw values and log reduction rates. Bacterial counts were transformed to $\log_{10}$ values for statistical analysis. A one-sample *t*-test was employed to compare the reduction in the HTST treatment with the complete reduction observed in the HoP treatment. Statistical analyses were performed using GraphPad Prism (V5.02, GraphPad, San Diego, CA). A *p*-value < 0.05 was considered significant.

RESULTS

A flowchart summarizing the study procedure is given in **Figure 1**. Characteristic time-temperature curves of the HTST pasteurization process at of 62 and 72°C/15 s are shown in **Figure 2**.

No bacterial growth could be detected in any of the pooled and Holder pasteurized HM samples before experimental bacterial inoculation.

Bacterial concentrations in the inoculated 95 mL HM samples after culturing for 24 h were 7.9×10^4 cfu/mL for *S. aureus*, 1.16×10^5 cfu/mL for *E. faecalis*, 1×10^5 cfu/mL for *P. aeruginosa*, 1.04×10^5 cfu/mL for *S. marcescens*, 3.6×10^4 cfu/mL for *K. pneumoniae* (Kpn01605), and 5.7×10^4 cfu/mL for *K. pneumoniae* (ATCC 700603). Again, following HoP no bacterial growth for any of the tested bacterial species or strains could be detected (**Table 1**).

Viable cultures were retrieved from all tested strains after HTST pasteurization with the default HTST protocol of 62°C/5 s of *S. aureus*, *E. faecalis*, *P. aeruginosa* ($p < 0.0001$), and *S. marcescens* ($p = 0.002$). In general, growth rates after HTST pasteurization compared to HoP depended on treatment time, treatment temperature, bacterial genera, species and strain (**Table 1**). Positive bacterial cultures could be retrieved for any tested plateau temperature of <87°C for the cultures incubated with *S. aureus* and *E. faecalis* albeit differences compared to HoP were not consistently statically significant (**Table 1**). The samples incubated with *P. aeruginosa*, *K. pneumoniae* and *S. marcescens* remained without detectable growth after pasteurization of at least 72°C/5 s. The two tested strains of Klebsiella did exhibit differing heat susceptibility ($p = 0.029$). All positive cultures revealed monomicrobial growth consisting of the respective incubated strain.

Number of CMV copies obtained by PCR from the CMV seropositive donors' milk was 7,000 IE/mL and mean (SD) number of IEA positive cells in the positive control sample from the CMV seropositive donor was 20 ± 0/mL. No CMV copies were obtained by PCR and no IEA positive cells could be detected in the negative control samples from the CMV seronegative donor. After experimental CMV spiking a mean (SD) of 32 ± 5.6 IEA positive cells/mL were detected before pasteurization. CMV was inactivated by HoP and HTST pasteurization at all tested time-temperature combinations, no IEA positive cells were found.

DISCUSSION

This HTST treatment system was not as effective in bacterial count reduction as standard HoP at a time-temperature combination of 62°C/5 s. Colony counts of *E. faecalis* and *P. aeruginosa* were still present in abundance and counts of *S. aureus* and *S. marcescens* were reduced by more than two orders of magnitude but were still cultivable after exposure to 62°C/5 s. Only after an being exposed to 87°C all culture remained without growth.

Antibacterial efficacy of different types of HTST pasteurizers have been tested before at temperatures above 70°C and the choice of plateau temperatures within our study was modeled on these observations. Bacterial counts of naturally colonizing HM treated at 72 and 87°C for 1, 3, and 15 s was reduced by 83% to more than 99% (cfu/mL), respectively (12). Heating HM to 71°C/5.75 s, 71°C/9 s or 71°C/18.5 s in a continuous flow pasteurizer revealed more than 5 log reduction in HM artificially inoculated with *S. aureus* or *E. coli*, respectively (11). These observations are in line with our results, while temperatures as low as 62°C for bacterial count reduction in HM were not tested before.

The tested microbiota exhibited variable susceptibility to heat treatment, even between strains (8). This may explain the divergent results from previous studies where HTST treatment at 62°C/5 s of naturally colonized human milk was nearly as effective as HoP (10). Furthermore, this may result in less predictable pasteurization results if bacterial count reduction is pursued.

HTST treatment is currently applied in some neonatal units for CMV inactivation and bacterial count reduction while applying widely differing cut off values for HM microbiota content indicating pasteurization (4–7). Neonatologists that are intending to reduce bacterial HM content need to be aware of the potential limitation of HTST treatment systems in regard of their antibacterial efficacy compared to HoP. However, bacterial

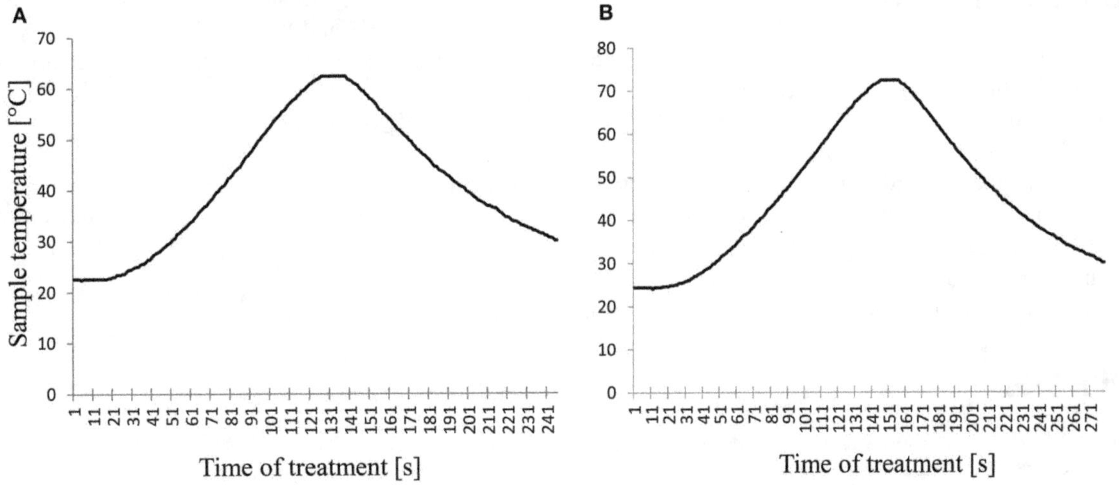

FIGURE 2 | Characteristic time-temperature curves of the high-temperature short-time pasteurization processes. **(A)** time-temperature combination of 62°C/15 s; **(B)** time-temperature combination of 72°C/15 s.

HM count reduction to decrease morbidity in preterm infants–namely from late-onset-sepsis and necrotising enterocolitis–remains debated because sound data to prove a beneficial influence of bacterial count reduction by pasteurization are missing (14–16).

Furthermore, any kind of heat treatment indiscriminately degrades cellular and non-cellular content of HM to a variable degree (17). Affected are both naturally colonizing HM bacteria and biologically active components that are involved in gut maturation and digestion, in shaping the infants immune system as well as its intestinal microbiome (18).

HTST has been shown to increase the retention rate of immunoglobulin A (10), lactoferrin (12, 19), and growth factors (20) amongst other proteins (21) compared to HoP. Therefore, HTST treatment as opposed to HoP of milk for preterm infants may be beneficial to improve neonatal outcome but clinical data are lacking so far. Nevertheless, HM should be subjected to the lowest energy intake possible to achieve a pursued aim, i.e., reducing bacterial count, inactivating virus or both.

CMV inactivation in HM for preterm infants is performed in many neonatal units to prevent HM acquired postnatal CMV infection (5–7). The original purpose of this tested HTST system with a non-adjustable default setting of 62°C/5 s is to inactivate CMV (13, 20). Viral inactivation is facilitated by rapidly heating a thin layer of HM within a rotating glass flask. We increased the default bulk of HM from 50 to 95 mL to advance the feasibility of HTST pasteurization in a human milk bank setting. Because of the resulting increase in thickness of the resulting fluid layer CMV inactivation had to be retested under this condition resulting in an effective CMV inactivation in 95 mL batches.

The apparent desire by some neonatologists to control bacterial content of HM should be considered when developing HM pasteurizers (22). Temperature-time combinations and modes of operation should be tested for its antibacterial efficacy (21) and guided by official regulations concerning pasteurization requirements (23). However, if exclusively CMV inactivation is pursued, a much lower energy intake may be used to treat HM and those requirements may not fit to the current definition of pasteurization of non-human milk (24).

Our study has some limitations. HTST pasteurizers utilized in previous studies were experimental prototypes with different modes of action (continuous flow vs. bulk pasteurization) and different modes of heating (plate heater exchanger vs. heating thermostat), this must be considered when comparing our findings to previous observations. We were not able to test all time-temperature combinations for every bacterium due to limited HM supply. Genera, species and strains other than those tested in our study may be present in HM. Heat susceptibility of those microbiota may be different than the ones tested, and the choice of different strains might have influenced our results. Within the study we exclusively tested HM inoculated with single strains of bacteria, but clinical HM isolates may contain multiple strains. We can only speculate if inoculation with multiple strains could have influenced our results. As different cultural agars exhibit varying recovery rates of heat-processed bacteria the choice of agar might have influenced our results (25). We chose to apply those agars used in the routine HM screening program of our neonatal unit. We did not test HM samples for the presence of bacterial growth inhibitors. Furthermore, different HM concentrations of antimicrobial proteins e.g., lactoferrin or immunoglobulins between donors could have influenced our results. However, there was no history of recent antibiotic treatment of donors and since HM was pooled results for both modes of pasteurization would have been equally affected.

CONCLUSIONS

This HTST treatment procedure inactivates CMV in 95 mL HM samples but is not as effective as standard HoP in bacterial count reduction at a time-temperature combination of 62°C/5 s.

AUTHOR CONTRIBUTIONS

DK conceived and designed the study, participated in the acquisition of the HM samples, performed the pasteurization process, analyzed the data, and wrote the first draft of the manuscript. MS designed the study, performed the pasteurization process, and contributed to drafting the manuscript. VF designed the study, performed the viral assays, and contributed to data analysis and interpretation. DJ designed the study, supervised the bacterial studies, and contributed to data analysis. MK contributed to acquisition of the HM samples and drafting of the manuscript. AW contributed to the study design and reviewed the manuscript. HF and RH contributed to the study design and drafting of the manuscript. All authors reviewed the manuscript.

ACKNOWLEDGMENTS

The authors are indebted to Sabine Weber and Doris Scheibert for their assistance in performing the bacterial cultures and to Ariane Kaiser for her assistance in performing the viral assays.

REFERENCES

1. Fitzstevens JL, Smith KC, Hagadorn JI, Caimano MJ, Matson AP, Brownell EA. Systematic review of the human milk microbiota. *Nutr Clin Pract.* (2017) 32:354–64. doi: 10.1177/0884533616670150
2. Hamprecht K, Maschmann J, Vochem M, Dietz K, Speer CP, Jahn G. Epidemiology of transmission of cytomegalovirus from mother to preterm infant by breastfeeding. *Lancet* (2001) 357:513–8. doi: 10.1016/S0140-6736(00)04043-5
3. Lanzieri TM, Dollard SC, Josephson CD, Schmid DS, Bialek SR. Breast milk-acquired cytomegalovirus infection and disease in VLBW and premature infants. *Pediatrics* (2013) 131:e1937–45. doi: 10.1542/peds.2013-0076
4. Omarsdottir S, Casper C, Akerman A, Polberger S, Vanpée M. Breastmilk handling routines for preterm infants in Sweden: a national cross-sectional study. *Breastfeed Med.* (2008) 3:165–70. doi: 10.1089/bfm.2007.0033
5. Cossey V, Johansson A-B, de Halleux V, Vanhole C. The use of human milk in the neonatal intensive care unit: practices in Belgium and Luxembourg. *Breastfeed Med.* (2012) 7:302–6. doi: 10.1089/bfm.2011.0112
6. Klotz D, Jansen S, Gebauer C, Fuchs H. Handling of breast milk by neonatal units: Large differences in current practices and beliefs. *Front Pediatr.* (2018) 6:235 doi: 10.3389/fped.2018.00235
7. Buxmann H, Falk M, Goelz R, Hamprecht K, Poets CF, Schloesser RL. Feeding of very low birth weight infants born to HCMV-seropositive mothers in Germany, Austria and Switzerland. *Acta Paediatr.* (2010) 99:1819–23. doi: 10.1111/j.1651-2227.2010.01954.x
8. *Scientific Evaluation of Pasteurisation for Pathogen Reduction in Milk and Milk Products Scientific Evaluation.* Available online at: https://www.foodstandards.gov.au/code/proposals/documents/Scientific%20Evaluation.pdf (Accessed November 16, 2017)
9. Ewaschuk JB, Unger S, O'Connor DL, Stone D, Harvey S, Clandinin MT, et al. Effect of pasteurization on selected immune components of donated human breast milk. *J Perinatol.* (2011) 31:593–8. doi: 10.1038/jp.2010.209
10. Klotz D, Joellenbeck M, Winkler K, Kunze M, Huzly D, Hentschel R. High temperature short time pasteurisation of human breast milk is efficient in retaining protein and reducing the bacterial count. *Acta Paediatr.* (2017) 106:763–7. doi: 10.1111/apa.13768
11. Dhar J, Fichtali J, Skura B j., Nakai S, Davidson A. Pasteurization efficiency of a HTST system for human milk. *J Food Sci.* (1996) 61:569–73. doi: 10.1111/j.1365-2621.1996.tb13160.x
12. Goldblum RM, Dill CW, Albrecht TB, Alford ES, Garza C, Goldman AS. Rapid high-temperature treatment of human milk. *J Pediatr.* (1984) 104:380–5.
13. Hamprecht K, Maschmann J, Müller D, Dietz K, Besenthal I, Goelz R, et al. Cytomegalovirus (CMV) inactivation in breast milk: reassessment of pasteurization and freeze-thawing. *Pediatr Res.* (2004) 56:529–35. doi: 10.1203/01.PDR.0000139483.35087.BE
14. Schanler RJ, Lau C, Hurst NM, Smith EO. Randomized trial of donor human milk versus preterm formula as substitutes for mothers' own milk in the feeding of extremely premature infants. *Pediatrics* (2005) 116:400–6. doi: 10.1542/peds.2004-1974
15. Cossey V, Vanhole C, Eerdekens A, Rayyan M, Fieuws S, Schuermans A. Pasteurization of mother's own milk for preterm infants does not reduce the incidence of late-onset sepsis. *Neonatology* (2013) 103:170–6. doi: 10.1159/000345419
16. Stock K, Griesmaier E, Brunner B, Neubauer V, Kiechl-Kohlendorfer U, Trawöger R. Pasteurization of breastmilk decreases the rate of postnatally acquired cytomegalovirus infections, but shows a nonsignificant trend to an increased rate of necrotizing enterocolitis in very preterm infants–a preliminary study. *Breastfeed Med.* (2015) 10:113–117. doi: 10.1089/bfm.2014.0108
17. Peila C, Moro GE, Bertino E, Cavallarin L, Giribaldi M, Giuliani F, et al. The effect of holder pasteurization on nutrients and biologically-active components in donor human milk: a review. *Nutrients* (2016) 8:477. doi: 10.3390/nu8080477
18. Le Doare K, Holder B, Bassett A, Pannaraj PS. Mother's Milk: A purposeful contribution to the development of the infant microbiota and immunity. *Front Immunol.* (2018) 9:361. doi: 10.3389/fimmu.2018.00361
19. Baro C, Giribaldi M, Arslanoglu S, Giuffrida MG, Dellavalle G, Conti A, et al. Effect of two pasteurization methods on the protein content of human milk. *Front Biosci.* (2011) 3:818–29. doi: 10.2741/289
20. Goelz R, Hihn E, Hamprecht K, Dietz K, Jahn G, Poets C, Elmlinger M. Effects of different CMV-heat-inactivation-methods on growth factors in human breast milk. *Pediatr Res.* (2009) 65:458–61. doi: 10.1203/PDR.0b013e3181991f18
21. Peila C, Emmerik NE, Giribaldi M, Stahl B, Ruitenberg JE, van Elburg RM, et al. Human milk processing: a systematic review of innovative techniques to ensure the safety and quality of donor milk. *J Pediatr Gastroenterol Nutr.* (2017) 64:353–61. doi: 10.1097/MPG.0000000000001435
22. Giribaldi M, Coscia A, Peila C, Antoniazzi S, Lamberti C, Ortoffi M, et al. Pasteurization of human milk by a benchtop high-temperature short-time device. *Innov Food Sci Emerg Technol.* (2016) 36:228–33. doi: 10.1016/j.ifset.2016.07.004
23. *Commission Regulation (EU) No 605/2010 of 2 July 2010 Laying Down Animal and Public Health and Veterinary Certification Conditions for the Introduction into the European Union of Raw Milk and Dairy Products Intended for Human Consumption.* Available online at: https://eur-lex.europa.eu/LexUriServ/LexUriServ.do?uri=OJ:L:2010:175:0001:0024:EN:PDF (Accessed October 12, 2018)
24. Food and Agriculture Organization of the United Nations ed. *Code of Hygienic Practice for Milk and Milk Products in Milk and Milk Products.* Rome: Food and Agriculture Organization of the United Nations (2004). Available online at: http://www.fao.org/fao-who-codexalimentarius/sh-proxy/en/?lnk=1&url=https%253A%252F%252Fworkspace.fao.org%252Fsites%252Fcodex%252FStandards%252FCAC%2BRCP%2B57-2004%252FCXP_057e.pdf (Accessed October 12, 2018)
25. Lin FJ, Morgan JN, Eitenmiller RR, Barnhart HM, Toledo RT, Maddox F. Thermal destruction of Staphylococcus aureus in human milk. *J Food Prot USA.* (1987) 50:669–72. doi: 10.4315/0362-028X-50.8.669

9

Maternal Supplementation with Krill Oil during Breastfeeding and Long-Chain Polyunsaturated Fatty Acids (LCPUFAs) Composition of Human Milk

Anna Giulia Cimatti[1,2], *Silvia Martini*[1,2*], *Alessandra Munarini*[2,3], *Maximilano Zioutas*[4], *Francesca Vitali*[1,2], *Arianna Aceti*[1,2], *Vilma Mantovani*[2,3], *Giacomo Faldella*[1,2] and *Luigi Corvaglia*[1]

[1] *Neonatal Intensive Care Unit, S. Orsola-Malpighi University Hospital, Bologna, Italy,* [2] *Department of Medical and Surgical Sciences, University of Bologna, Bologna, Italy,* [3] *Department of Clinical Medicine, Center of Applied Biochemical Research, S. Orsola-Malpighi University Hospital, Bologna, Italy,* [4] *Pediatric Endocrinology, Department of Pediatrics, S. Orsola-Malpighi University Hospital, Bologna, Italy*

Correspondence:
Silvia Martini
silvia.martini4@gmail.com

Background: Docosahexaenoic acid (DHA) is a major constituent of neuronal and retinal membranes and plays a crucial role in brain and visual development within the first months of life. Dietary intakes are fundamental to provide neonates with adequate DHA supply; hence, maternal supplementation might represent a useful strategy to implement DHA contents in breast milk (BM), with possible benefits on neonatal neurodevelopment. *Antarctic krill* is a small crustacean rich in highly available phospholipid-bound DHA. This pilot study aimed to evaluate whether maternal supplementation with krill oil during breastfeeding increases long-chain polyunsaturated fatty acids (LCPUFAs) BM contents.

Methods: Mothers of infants admitted to the Neonatal Intensive Care Unit were enrolled in this open, randomized-controlled study between 4 and 6 weeks after delivery and randomly allocated in 2 groups. Group 1 received an oral krill oil-based supplement providing 250 mg/day of DHA and 70 mg/day of eicosapentaenoic acid (EPA) for 30 days; group 2 served as control. BM samples from both groups were collected at baseline (T0) and day 30 (T1) and underwent a qualitative analysis of LCPUFAs composition by gas chromatography/mass spectrometry.

Results: Sixteen breastfeeding women were included. Of these, 8 received krill-oil supplementation and 8 were randomized to the control group. Baseline percentage values of DHA (%DHA), arachidonic acid (%AA), and EPA (%EPA) did not differ between groups. A significant increase in %DHA (T0: median 0.23% [IQR 0.19;0.38], T1:0.42% [0.32;0.49], *p* 0.012) and %EPA (T0: median 0.10% [IQR 0.04;0.11], T1:0.11% [0.04;0.15], *p* 0.036) and a significant reduction in %AA (T0: median 0.48% [IQR 0.42;0.75], T1:0.43% [0.38;0.61], *p* 0.017) between T0 and T1 occurred in Group 1, whereas no difference was seen in Group 2. Consistently, a significant between-group difference was observed in percentage changes from baseline of DHA (Δ%DHA, group 1: median 64.2% [IQR 27.5;134.6], group 2: −7.8% [−12.1;−3.13], *p* 0.025) and

EPA (Δ%EPA, group 1: median 39% [IQR 15.7;73.4]; group 2: −25.62% [−32.7;−3.4], *p* 0.035).

Conclusions: Oral krill oil supplementation effectively increases DHA and EPA contents in BM. Potential benefits of this strategy on brain and visual development in breastfed preterm neonates deserve further evaluation in targeted studies.

Keywords: LCPUFA, DHA, AA, EPA, breast milk, supplementation, krill oil, lactation

INTRODUCTION

Long-chain polyunsaturated fatty acids (LCPUFAs), such as docosahexaenoic (DHA, 22:6 n−3) and arachidonic acid (AA, 20:4 n−6), are major building blocks for the lipid bilayer of neurons and retina. Brain maturation and visual development start during pregnancy and continue throughout the first year of life; consistently, LCPUFAs and, in particular, DHA, exert their greatest effect during this period (1, 2), and benefits on visual acuity and cognitive development have been largely established in term (3, 4) and preterm (5, 6) infants fed LCPUFAs-supplemented formula.

Like all mammals, humans lack enzymes for the synthesis of n−3 and n−6 precursors of DHA and AA, which are therefore essential fatty acids and need to be provided by dietary sources (7). Furthermore, consistently with the growth spurt of human brain occurring during the third trimester of pregnancy, placental transfer of AA and DHA is highest during this period (8); however, premature birth may preclude this LCPUFAs accretion, therefore dietary intakes are even more crucial in preterm neonates, who are at increased risk of neurodevelopmental impairment (9). In this delicate population, moreover, low blood DHA levels have been associated with a higher incidence of prematurity-related complications, such as intraventricular hemorrhage (IVH), bronchopulmonary dysplasia (BPD), and infections (10, 11).

Due to its several nutritional and non-nutritional benefits, breast milk (BM) is the optimal feeding choice for both term and preterm neonates (12, 13), and is generally regarded as providing adequate intakes of essential fatty acids. LCPUFAs contents of BM, however, are significantly influenced by maternal dietary intakes: as an example, fish-rich diets have been associated with high DHA levels in BM, whereas vegan dietary habits may lead to low concentrations of these compounds (14–16).

Antarctic krill, a small crustacean belonging to the order Euphausiacea, is by far the most dominant member of the Antarctic zooplankton community, and also represents a rich source of n-3 LCPUFAs (i.e., DHA and eicosapentaenoic acid [EPA]). Differently from other LCPUFAs sources, krill oil DHA and EPA are mainly bound to phosphatidylcholine, resulting in a significantly improved bioavailability (17). Hence, maternal krill oil supplementation might represent an effective strategy to enhance LCPUFAs contents in human milk, with possible beneficial effects on visual and brain development of breastfed neonates, especially if born preterm. To date, however, whether oral maternal supplementation with krill oil during breastfeeding increases BM concentration of LCPUFAs has not been investigated yet.

The aim of this pilot study was to evaluate the effect of a combined krill and fish oil oral supplementation, administered in breastfeeding women, on LCPUFAs composition of BM.

Abbreviations: AA, arachidonic acid; ALA, alpha-linolenic acid; BM, breast milk; BPD, bronchopulmonary dysplasia; DHA, docosahexaenoic acid; EPA, eicosapentaenoic acid; FAMEs, fatty acid methyl esters; FFQ, food frequency questionnaire; IQR, interquartile range; IVH, intraventricular hemorrhage; LA, linoleic acid; LCPUFAs, long-chain polyunsaturated fatty acids; MSD, mass spectrometric detector; PTV, programmed temperature vaporizing; RDA, recommended daily allowance.

METHODS

Study Population and Ethics

Breastfeeding mothers of infants admitted at the Neonatal Intensive Care Unit of Sant'Orsola-Malpighi University Hospital, Bologna, Italy, were consecutively enrolled between 4 and 6 weeks after delivery, when peak lactation was already established and breast milk can be considered fully mature (18), if a written informed consent to participate in the present study was obtained. Ongoing LCPUFAs supplementation at the time of enrollment was considered an exclusion criterion.

The study protocol was approved by the Ethics Committee of Sant'Orsola-Malpighi University Hospital, Bologna, Italy (Study ID: 114/2015/U/Sper) and is registered in the Protocol Registration System ClinicalTrials.gov (NCT03583502).

Study Design

The lactating women enrolled in this open, randomized, controlled trial were randomly allocated to 2 groups. Group 1 received 2 gelatin soft capsules per day of a combined krill and fish oil supplement (Krilling D®, Italchimici S.P.A., Milan, Italy), providing 250 mg/day of DHA and 70 mg/day of EPA, for overall 30 days, whereas group 2 served as control. Approximately 10 ml of fresh mid-BM samples were collected from both groups at baseline (T0) and at day 30 (T1). In order to minimize the effect of dynamic changes in LCPUFAs excretion within the day (18, 19), the study samples were collected at early morning. After collection, the samples were stored at −80°C until ready for extraction to minimize lipid oxidation and degradation.

At T0, the enrolled women were also asked to fill out a food frequency questionnaire (FFQ, **Supplementary Table 1**), aimed at calculating individual dietary intakes of LCPUFAs based on their food habits over the last month. This FFQ investigated the consumption of 20 food types containing polyunsaturated fatty acids, including supplements. For each one, average portions (never consumed, less than once a week, 1/week, 2/week, 3/week, or more than 3/week) were reported. If the average portion consumption was >3 times a week, the patient was instructed to provide the exact number of portions actually consumed per week. Once the FFQ was completed, the average consumption of linoleic acid (LA), alpha-linolenic acid (ALA), AA, EPA, DHA, n-6, and n-3, expressed in grams per week, was calculated for each study subject. Based on population reference intakes in pregnancy and breastfeeding, according to the Italian recommended daily allowance (RDA) (20), the proportion of breastfeeding women who did not reach the recommended EPA and DHA intakes (EPA+DHA: 2.8 g/week) was calculated.

An intermediate evaluation (by visit or phone call) of group 1 compliance and adherence to the ongoing supplementation was performed at day 15.

Gas Chromatography/Mass Spectrometry (GC-MS) Analysis

Qualitative analysis of BM LCPUFAs composition was performed at the laboratory of the Center for Applied Biomedical Research (CRBA) of Sant'Orsola-Malpighi University Hospital, Bologna, Italy, by means of GC-MS.

After bringing BM samples at room temperature under continuous mixing, 0.5 ml from each sample were transferred to Sovirel extraction tubes and extracted twice with chloroform/methanol (2:1 vol/vol, 3+2 ml) containing butylated hydroxytoluene 0.01% as anti-oxidant[10].

After centrifugation (400xG, 10 min 25°C), the organic phases were combined, re-extracted with chloroform/H_2O (1:1, vol/vol, 2+2 ml) and separated by centrifugation; the lowest organic phase was then transferred to a new tube and dried under nitrogen stream at 30°C.

The phospholipid fraction was saponified into free fatty acids via a base-catalyzed reaction (KOH 0.5 M, 2 ml in methanol) and esterified to fatty acid methyl esters (FAMEs) by acid reaction with boron trifluoride (14% in methanol), 1 ml for 10 min at 80°C.

After cooling, FAMEs were extracted twice into hexane (3+2 ml), dried under nitrogen stream and dissolved in cyclohexane for direct injection into a gas chromatograph (Agilent HP5890), equipped with a programmed temperature vaporizing (PTV) injector.

FAMEs were then separated and identified by a mass spectrometric detector (MSD, Agilent 5973, Agilent Technologies Cheadle, UK) in electron impact ionization mode (70 eV) using a Supelco SP™ 2330 column (30 mt × 0.25 mm × 0.2 µm film thickness) with helium as carrier gas (initial flow 0.5 ml/min, constant pressure mode, 10.8 psi).

PTV injections were carried out in solvent vent mode; the initial temperature was set at 60°C, with a purge flow of 50 mL/min for 0.30 sec; the temperature was then ramped at 720°C/min to 220°C, and held for the whole analysis period.

The oven temperature was initially held at 100°C (cold-trapping technique) for 1.25 min, then ramped at rate of 30°C/min to 185°C, held 10 min, further increased at 5°C/min to 205°C and held 10 min (total run time: 28.08 min). The MSD ion source, quadrupole and transfer line temperatures were 150, 230, and 280°C, respectively. Total ion chromatography (40–550 m/z, 100 dwell time) was used for spectral percentage quantitation.

The analytes were identified by comparison with standards retention time (Supelco 37 Component FAME Mix, Sigma Aldrich), whereas mass spectral identity was confirmed by comparison with WileyN and NIST mass spectral databases. Peak areas calculations were performed using the Agilent G1701 BA software.

Within-batch and day-to-day reproducibility were calculated splitting a basal sample into 3 aliquots, which were independently analyzed on the same day; the obtained values are reported in **Supplementary Table 2**. Accuracy was tested vs. FAMEs certified standard material (Supelco, CRM 47885).

Percentage quantitation of each FA was expressed as its percentage over total fatty acid contents (i.e., palmitic, stearic, oleic, docosapentaenoic acid, LA, ALA, AA, EPA, DHA), calculated according to the following formula:

$$Analyte\ percentage(\%) = \frac{Analyte\ Peak\ area * 100}{(\sum peak\ areas\ of\ the\ identified\ analytes)}$$

Statistical Analysis

IBM SPSS Statistics (Statistical Package for the Social Sciences, SPSS Inc., Chicago, IL, USA) version 25 was used for statistical analysis. Intra-group differences in median percentage values of DHA, EPA and AA between T0 and T1 were evaluated by Wilcoxon signed-rank test. Mann-Whitney *U*-test was used to compare clinical characteristics, LCPUFAs dietary intakes and percentage changes from baseline of DHA, EPA, and AA between the two study groups. Fisher's exact test was used to compare the prevalence of inadequate DHA+EPA dietary intakes between the two groups. Eventually, a linear regression model was built to adjust the results for possible influencing factors. Significance level was set at $p < 0.05$.

RESULTS

In total, twenty breastfeeding women were enrolled and randomly allocated in the two study groups. Of these, 4 (2 in group 1 and 2 in group 2) had a significant decrease in breast milk supply between T0 and T1, and were excluded from the study due to the unavailability of T1 sample; therefore, 8 women in group 1 and 8 in group 2 were included in the study. The flowchart summarizing the progress of women enrolled through the trial is provided in **Figure 1**. Baseline BM samples were collected at a median of 34 (interquartile range [IQR]: 31–38) days after delivery. No difference between the two groups was observed in LCPUFAs dietary intakes, estimated by FFQ and summarized in **Table 1**. The infants' characteristics are provided in **Supplementary Table 3**; no between-group

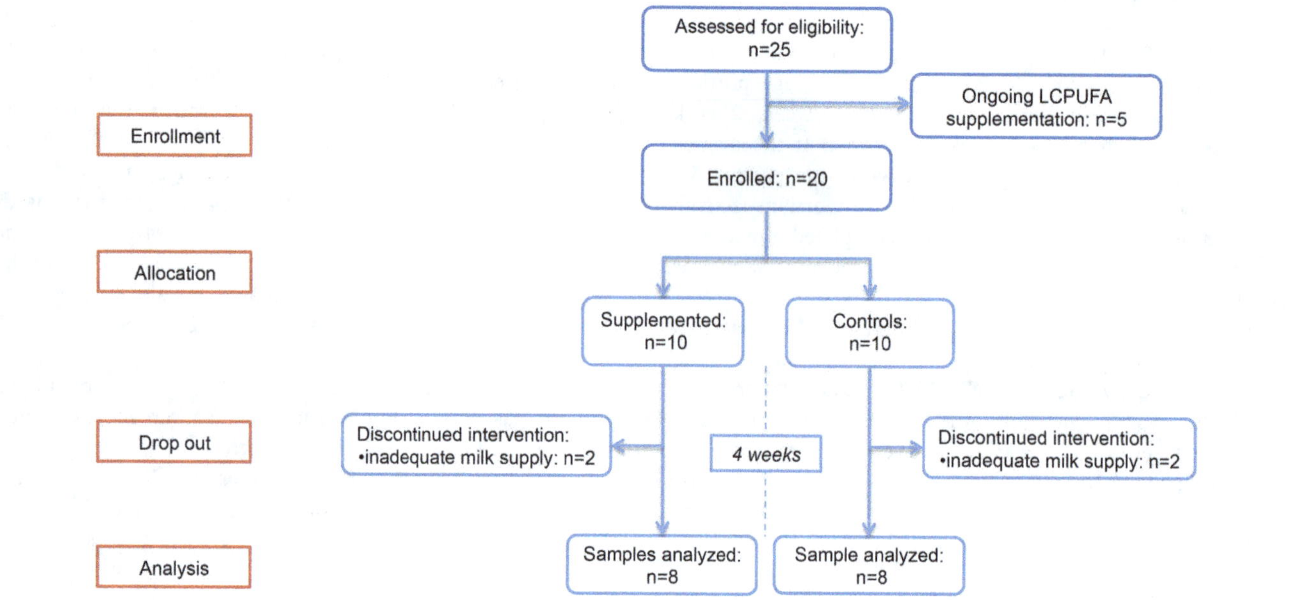

FIGURE 1 | Flow diagram of the main study phases.

TABLE 1 | Weekly dietary intakes of linoleic acid (LA), alpha-linolenic acid (ALA), arachidonic acid (AA), eicosapentaenoic acid (EPA), docosahexaenoic acid (DHA), ω-6 and ω-3 in the study groups, estimated by food-frequency questionnaire.

Dietary intakes, median (interquartile range [IQR])	Group 1 ($n = 8$)	Group 2 ($n = 8$)	Group 1 vs. 2, *p*-value
LA, g/sett	33.70 (24.82–48.25)	36.41 (32.20–44.41)	0.606
ALA, g/sett	3.15 (2.64–4.65)	3.39 (2.92–4.31)	0.797
AA, g/sett	0.94 (0.53–1.24)	1.04 (0.72–2.41)	0.298
EPA, g/sett	0.77 (0.65–1.55)	0.76 (0.50–2.28)	0.898
DHA, g/sett	1.42 (1.03–2.65)	1.12 (0.67–3.95)	1.000
ω-6, g/sett	34.78 (25.79–49.24)	37.30 (32.99–46.83)	0.606
ω-3, g/sett	5.67 (4.64–8.12)	5.53 (4.12–10.39)	1.000

difference in postconceptional age was observed at the time of sample collection ($p = 0.798$).

Based on FFQ reports, 5 women in group 1 and 3 in group 2 (between-group difference $p = 0.399$) had lower DHA intakes than the recommended dietary reference. Of interest, DHA and EPA supplementation (250 and 75 mg/die, respectively) normalized DHA and EPA intakes in the 5 women, randomized to group 1, with inadequate dietary intakes.

Median percentage values of DHA (%DHA), AA (%AA), and EPA (%EPA) for the two study groups are detailed in **Table 2**. Baseline %DHA, %AA, and %EPA did not differ between groups. Group 1 showed a significant increase in %DHA and %EPA and a significant reduction of %AA between T0 and T1. Group 2 showed a decrease in %DHA, %EPA, and %AA between T0 and T1; statistical significance was observed for %AA reduction.

Consistently, a significant between-group difference was observed in percentage changes from baseline of DHA (Δ%DHA, group 1: median 64.2% [interquartile range, IQR: 27.5;134.6], group 2: −7.8% [−12.1; −3.13], p 0.025) and EPA (Δ%EPA, group 1: median 39% [IQR 15.7;73.4]; group 2: median −25.62% [−32.7;−3.4], *p* 0.035).

The ratio between AA and DHA (AA:DHA), which provides an estimation for n−6/n−3 fatty acid ratio, was also calculated for each study group at T0 and T1. As shown in **Figure 2**, a significant decrease ($p = 0.012$) in AA:DHA was observed in the supplemented group between T0 an T1, resulting in significantly lower AA:DHA values at T1 compared to the control group ($p = 0.010$).

Given the well-known influence of maternal dietary intakes on BM LCPUFA composition, a multivariate linear regression model was built to adjust Δ%DHA and Δ%EPA (dependent variables) for the respective dietary intakes calculated by the FFQ and baseline %DHA and %EPA concentrations (independent variables). The regression analysis, whose results are summarized

TABLE 2 | Median percentage values of docosahexaenoic acid (DHA), arachidonic acid (AA) and eicosapentaenoic acid (EPA) for the two study groups and results of intra-group comparison between T0 and T1.

Percentage values, median (interquartile range [IQR])	Group 1 (n = 8)			Group 2 (n = 8)		
	T0	T1	T0 vs. T1, p-value	T0	T1	T0 vs. T1, p-value
DHA, %	0.23 (0.19–0.38)	0.42 (0.32–0.49)	0.012	0.38 (0.21–0.57)	0.28 (0.20–0.50)	0.208
EPA, %	0.10 (0.04–0.11)	0.11 (0.04–0.15)	0.036	0.14 (0.08–0.20)	0.10 (0.08–0.13)	0.093
AA, %	0.48 (0.42–0.75)	0.43 (0.38–0.61)	0.017	0.65 (0.52–0.95)	0.60 (0.44–0.74)	0.036

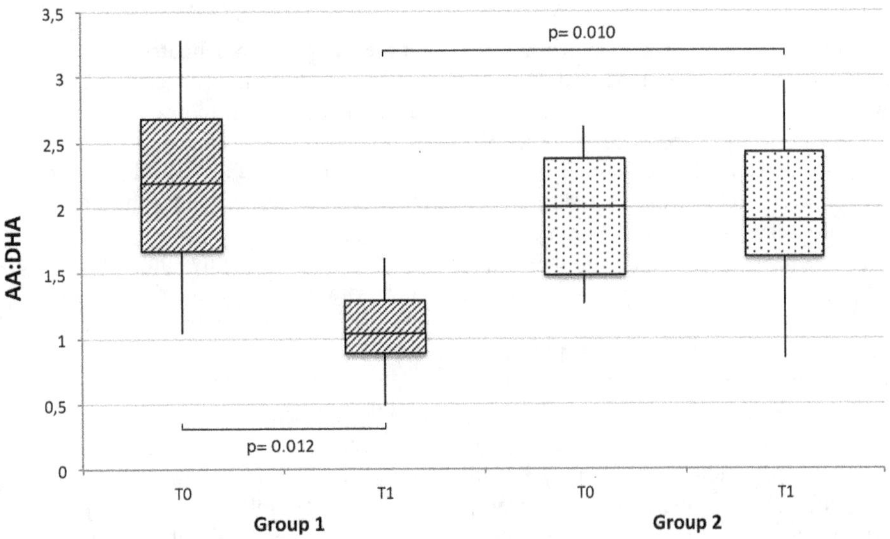

FIGURE 2 | Arachidonic (AA) to docosahexaenoic acid (DHA) ratio (AA:DHA), expressed as median, interquartile range and range, at baseline and T1 in breast milk of supplemented (group 1) vs. non-supplemented (group 2) lactating women.

in **Table 3**, confirmed a significant effect of DHA and EPA supplementation on the percentage observed.

DISCUSSION

According to the present results, a 30-day combined supplementation with fish and krill oil in breastfeeding women significantly increases BM DHA and EPA levels.

The supportive effects of n−3 fatty acids and, in particular, of DHA, on visual and cognitive development in early life have long been known. On the other hand, poor dietary intakes of DHA have been shown to decrease DHA contents in cerebral cortex and retinal membranes, with possible consequences on visual and cognitive functions (21), and low blood levels in preterm infants have been associated with increased rates of IVH (10), late-onset sepsis and BPD (11).

Human milk is considered the best nutritional choice for both term and preterm infants; BM LCPUFAs composition, however, reflects the nutritional status of the breastfeeding mother. Consistently, either 6 or 12-week maternal DHA supplementation effectively increased plasma DHA levels in breastfed infants compared to the placebo group (22, 23). According to a recent meta-analysis, maternal DHA supplementation during breastfeeding is associated with an improved neurodevelopmental pace up to 3 years of life in BM-fed preterm infants (24); moreover, term neonates whose mothers underwent DHA supplementation for the first 4 month of breastfeeding scored significantly better than controls on sustained attention scales at 5 years of age (25), further contributing to support the beneficial effects of DHA supplementation during breastfeeding.

DHA supplements (22, 26, 27) or fish oil administration (28) during lactation have proved to effectively modify LCPUFAs concentration not only in maternal plasma, but also in BM. However, to the best of our knowledge, this is the first study aimed at investigating the effects of a combined krill and fish oil supplementation on BM LCPUFAs composition. Differently from fish oils, whose EPA and DHA are predominantly bound to triglycerides, *Antarctic Krill* LCPUFAs are incorporated into phospholipids, which seem to be associated with enhanced bioavailability and better absorption (29).

According to our results, a 30-day combined krill and fish oil supplementation has led to a significant increase in BM %DHA and %EPA. On the other hand, a slight decrease in %DHA

TABLE 3 | Linear regression model for percentage changes of docosahexaenoic acid (Δ%DHA) and eicosapentaenoic acid (Δ%EPA) from baseline.

Dependent variable		Model	B	SE B	Beta	*t*	*P*
Δ%DHA	$R^2$0.495	Constant	2.331	55.345		0.042	0.967
		dietary DHA intake	-7.860	14.416	-0.135	-0.545	0.599
		baseline %DHA	-10.435	123.660	-0.022	-0.084	0.935
		supplementation	98.833	36.782	0.666	2.687	0.025
Δ%EPA	$R^2$0.569	Constant	16.614	33.868		0.491	0.635
		dietary EPA intake	-8.108	18.968	-0.112	-0.427	0.679
		baseline %EPA	-246.928	265.832	-0.256	-0.929	0.377
		supplementation	60.321	24.395	0.579	2.473	0.035

(−25%) and %EPA (−29%) was observed in the control group, whereas %AA was significantly reduced in both the study groups.

The latter finding is consistent with the progressive decrease in BM LCPUFAs for increasing lactation phases (30). Moreover, n−3 fatty acids such as DHA and EPA act as competitive substrates for the enzymes and products of arachidonic acid metabolism (31), and this may have further contributed to the significant %AA reduction in the supplemented group.

AA:DHA ratio has been used as a marker for DHA variations in biological samples (22), and its decrease may also reflect the biological effect of n−3 series, due to the above mentioned enzymatic competition between DHA and AA production (32). In neonatal rat models, changes in the dietary n−6/n−3 ratio significantly altered the fatty acid composition of neurons, glial membranes, and developing retinal photoreceptors, which reflected the administered dietary proportion (33, 34). In human preterm neonates, higher DHA and lower LA blood levels in the first few weeks of life, resulting in a decreased AA:DHA ratio, have been associated with improved microstructural brain development, reduced IVH incidence and better developmental scores at follow-up (10).

Placental transfer of DHA is greatest during the third trimester of pregnancy, consistently with the LCPUFAs-dependent growth spurt of human brain occurring during this period (35). In case of premature birth, this transfer is disrupted and inadequate dietary intakes of LCPUFAs may be detrimental. In this phase, particular attention should be paid to achieve and maintain appropriate DHA levels, as suggested by the evidence of improved brain development and better cognitive outcomes in preterm infants with higher DHA levels in red blood cells over the first weeks of life (10).

According to our preliminary results, combined krill and fish oil supplementation might represent an easy and feasible strategy to increase BM DHA levels not only in breastfeeding mothers of preterm neonates, but also in donors of Human Milk Banks, whose milk is often used for preterm infants' enteral nutrition when own mother's milk is lacking, but it is reported to contain significantly lower DHA levels than published values for maternal milk and infant formula and thus may not meet the recommended provision for this delicate population (36).

The following study limitations need to be acknowledged. First, sample size calculation was not performed due to the pilot nature of the study. However, a *post-hoc* calculation based on the observed %DHA values has shown that the actual power of the study is 66.5%, whereas 10 women per group would be adequate to achieve a power of 80%. Moreover, LCPUFAs concentration in maternal plasma, which may have provided additional information on the supplement absorption and excretion rate, was not investigated. Eventually, in this study supplement krill oil was combined to fish oil; hence, it is not possible to determine the exact impact of each of them in determining the observed increase in %DHA and %EPA.

Further studies are needed to confirm these preliminary findings, and to quantify krill oil absorption and excretion in breastfeeding women. Furthermore, potential benefits of krill oil supplementation, such as the increase in LCPUFA blood levels in preterm infants fed either maternal or donor milk, and the improvement of these infants' neurocognitive and visual outcomes, deserve to be assessed in targeted clinical trials.

AUTHOR CONTRIBUTIONS

LC, GF, AM, and VM designed the study. AA, FV, AC, and SM collected the data. AM carried out the laboratory analysis. MZ designed the food-frequency questionnaire and calculated dietary intakes. SM performed statistical analysis. AC and SM wrote the first draft. All the authors critically reviewed the manuscript and approved the final version submitted for publication.

REFERENCES

1. Janssen CIF, Kiliaan AJ. Long-chain polyunsaturated fatty acids (LCPUFA) from genesis to senescence: the influence of LCPUFA on neural development, aging, and neurodegeneration. *Prog Lipid Res.* (2014) 53:1–17. doi: 10.1016/j.plipres.2013.10.002
2. SanGiovanni JP, Chew EY. The role of omega-3 long-chain polyunsaturated fatty acids in health and disease of the retina.

Prog Retin Eye Res. (2005) 24:87–138. doi: 10.1016/j.preteyeres.2004.06.002

3. Agostoni C, Trojan S, Bellù R, Riva E, Giovannini M. Neurodevelopmental quotient of healthy term infants at 4 months and feeding practice: the role of long-chain polyunsaturated fatty acids. Pediatr Res. (1995) 38:262–6.
4. Makrides M, Neumann M, Simmer K, Pater J, Gibson R. Are long-chain polyunsaturated fatty acids essential nutrients in infancy? *Lancet* (1995) 345:1463–8. doi: 10.1016/S0140-6736(95)91035-2
5. O'Connor DL, Hall R, Adamkin D, Auestad N, Castillo M, Connor WE, et al. Growth and development in preterm infants fed long-chain polyunsaturated fatty acids: a prospective, randomized controlled trial. *Pediatrics* (2001) 108:359–71. doi: 10.1542/peds.108.2.359
6. Faldella G, Govoni M, Alessandroni R, Marchiani E, Salvioli GP, Biagi PL, et al. Visual evoked potentials and dietary long chain polyunsaturated fatty acids in preterm infants. *Arch Dis Child Fetal Neonatal Ed.* (1996) 75:F108–2. doi: 10.1136/fn.75.2.F108
7. Uauy R, Hoffman DR, Peirano P, Birch DG, Birch EE. Essential fatty acids in visual and brain development. *Lipids* (2001) 36:885–95. doi: 10.1007/s11745-001-0798-1
8. Hanebutt FL, Demmelmair H, Schiessl B, Larqué E, Koletzko B. Long-chain polyunsaturated fatty acid (LC-PUFA) transfer across the placenta. *Clin Nutr.* (2008) 27:685–93. doi: 10.1016/j.clnu.2008.05.010
9. Salas AA, Carlo WA, Ambalavanan N, Nolen TL, Stoll BJ, Das A, et al. Gestational age and birthweight for risk assessment of neurodevelopmental impairment or death in extremely preterm infants. *Arch Dis Child Fetal Neonatal Ed.* (2016) 2016:fetalneonatal-2015-309670. doi: 10.1136/archdischild-2015-309670
10. Tam EWY, Chau V, Barkovich AJ, Ferriero DM, Miller SP, Rogers EE, et al. Early postnatal docosahexaenoic acid levels and improved preterm brain development. *Pediatr Res.* (2016) 79:723–30. doi: 10.1038/pr.2016.11
11. Martin CR, Dasilva DA, Cluette-Brown JE, Dimonda C, Hamill A, Bhutta AQ, et al. Decreased postnatal docosahexaenoic and arachidonic acid blood levels in premature infants are associated with neonatal morbidities. *J Pediatr.* (2011) 159:743–9.e1–2. doi: 10.1016/j.jpeds.2011.04.039
12. Agostoni C, Buonocore G, Carnielli VP, De Curtis M, Darmaun D, Decsi T, et al. Enteral nutrient supply for preterm infants: commentary from the European Society of Paediatric Gastroenterology, Hepatology and Nutrition Committee on Nutrition. *J Pediatr Gastroenterol Nutr.* (2010) 50:85–91. doi: 10.1097/MPG.0b013e3181adaee0
13. Gartner LM, Morton J, Lawrence RA, Naylor AJ, O'Hare D, Schanler RJ, et al. Breastfeeding and the use of human milk. Pediatrics (2012) 129:e827-41. doi: 10.1542/peds.2004-2491
14. Koletzko B, Thiel I, Abiodun PO. The fatty acid composition of human milk in Europe and Africa. *J Pediatr.* (1992) 120:S62–70. doi: 10.1016/S0022-3476(05)81238-7
15. Kumar H, du Toit E, Kulkarni A, Aakko J, Linderborg KM, Zhang Y, et al. Distinct patterns in human milk microbiota and fatty acid profiles across specific geographic locations. *Front Microbiol.* (2016) 7:1619. doi: 10.3389/fmicb.2016.01619
16. Meneses F, Torres AG, Trugo NMF. Essential and long-chain polyunsaturated fatty acid status and fatty acid composition of breast milk of lactating adolescents. *Br J Nutr.* (2008) 100:1029–37. doi: 10.1017/S0007114508945177
17. Kidd PM. Omega-3 DHA and EPA for cognition, behavior, and mood: clinical findings and structural-functional synergies with cell membrane phospholipids. *Altern Med Rev.* (2007) 12:207–27.
18. Ballard O, Morrow AL. Human milk composition. *Pediatr Clin North Am.* (2013) 60:49–74. doi: 10.1016/j.pcl.2012.10.002
19. Kent JC, Mitoulas LR, Cregan MD, Ramsay DT, Doherty DA, Hartmann PE. Volume and frequency of breastfeedings and fat content of breast milk throughout the day. *Pediatrics* (2006) 117:e387–95. doi: 10.1542/peds.2005-1417
20. Marangoni F, Cetin I, Verduci E, Canzone G, Giovannini M, Scollo P, et al. Maternal diet and nutrient requirements in pregnancy and breastfeeding. an italian consensus document. *Nutrients* (2016) 8:629. doi: 10.3390/nu8100629
21. Molloy C, Doyle LW, Makrides M, Anderson PJ. Docosahexaenoic acid and visual functioning in preterm infants: a review. *Neuropsychol Rev.* (2012) 22:425–37. doi: 10.1007/s11065-012-9216-z
22. Sherry CL, Oliver JS, Marriage BJ. Docosahexaenoic acid supplementation in lactating women increases breast milk and plasma docosahexaenoic acid concentrations and alters infant omega 6:3 fatty acid ratio. *Prostaglandins Leukot Essent Fatty Acids* (2015) 95:63–9. doi: 10.1016/j.plefa.2015.01.005
23. Gibson RA, Neumann MA, Makrides M. Effect of increasing breast milk docosahexaenoic acid on plasma and erythrocyte phospholipid fatty acids and neural indices of exclusively breast fed infants. *Eur J Clin Nutr.* (1997) 51:578–84. doi: 10.1038/sj.ejcn.1600446
24. Wang Q, Cui Q, Yan C. The effect of supplementation of long-chain polyunsaturated fatty acids during lactation on neurodevelopmental outcomes of preterm infant from infancy to school age: a systematic review and meta-analysis. *Pediatr Neurol.* (2016) 59:54–61.e1. doi: 10.1016/j.pediatrneurol.2016.02.017
25. Jensen CL, Voigt RG, Llorente AM, Peters SU, Prager TC, Zou YL, et al. Effects of early maternal docosahexaenoic acid intake on neuropsychological status and visual acuity at five years of age of breast-fed term infants. *J Pediatr.* (2010) 157:900–5. doi: 10.1016/j.jpeds.2010.06.006
26. Fidler N, Sauerwald T, Pohl A, Demmelmair H, Koletzko B. Docosahexaenoic acid transfer into human milk after dietary supplementation: a randomized clinical trial. *J Lipid Res.* (2000) 41:1376–83.
27. Valentine CJ, Morrow G, Pennell M, Morrow AL, Hodge A, Haban-Bartz A, et al. Randomized controlled trial of docosahexaenoic acid supplementation in midwestern U.S. human milk donors. *Breastfeed Med.* (2013) 8:86–91. doi: 10.1089/bfm.2011.0126
28. Dunstan JA, Mitoulas LR, Dixon G, Doherty DA, Hartmann PE, Simmer K, et al. The effects of fish oil supplementation in pregnancy on breast milk fatty acid composition over the course of lactation: a randomized controlled trial. *Pediatr Res.* (2007) 62:689–94. doi: 10.1203/PDR.0b013e318159a93a
29. Ulven SM, Holven KB. Comparison of bioavailability of krill oil versus fish oil and health effect. *Vasc Health Risk Manag.* (2015) 11:511–24. doi: 10.2147/VHRM.S85165
30. Moltó-Puigmartí C, Castellote AI, Carbonell-Estrany X, López-Sabater MC. Differences in fat content and fatty acid proportions among colostrum, transitional, and mature milk from women delivering very preterm, preterm, and term infants. *Clin Nutr.* (2011) 30:116–23. doi: 10.1016/j.clnu.2010.07.013
31. Schmitz G, Ecker J. The opposing effects of n−3 and n−6 fatty acids. *Prog Lipid Res.* (2008) 47:147–55. doi: 10.1016/j.plipres.2007.12.004
32. Simopoulos AP. Evolutionary aspects of diet: the omega-6/omega-3 ratio and the brain. *Mol Neurobiol.* (2011) 44:203–15. doi: 10.1007/s12035-010-8162-0
33. Bowen RAR, Clandinin MT. Maternal dietary 22 : 6n-3 is more effective than 18 : 3n-3 in increasing the 22 : 6n-3 content in phospholipids of glial cells from neonatal rat brain. *Br J Nutr.* (2005) 93:601–11. doi: 10.1079/BJN20041390
34. Suh M, Wierzbicki AA, Lien EL, Clandinin MT. Dietary 20:4n-6 and 22:6n-3 modulates the profile of long- and very-long-chain fatty acids, rhodopsin content, and kinetics in developing photoreceptor cells. *Pediatr Res.* (2000) 48:524–30. doi: 10.1203/00006450-200010000-00017
35. Robinson DT, Martin CR. Fatty acid requirements for the preterm infant. *Semin Fetal Neonatal Med.* (2017) 22:8–14. doi: 10.1016/j.siny.2016.08.009
36. Baack ML, Norris AW, Yao J, Colaizy T. Long-chain polyunsaturated fatty acid levels in US donor human milk: meeting the needs of premature infants? *J Perinatol.* (2012) 32:598–603. doi: 10.1038/jp.2011.152

Analytical Study of Donor's Milk Bank Macronutrients by Infrared Spectroscopy Correlations with Clinic-Metabolic Profile of 100 Donors

Stefania Sbrizzi, Pasqua Anna Quitadamo, Domenico Ravidà, Giuseppina Palumbo, Pier Paolo Cristalli and Massimo Pettoello-Mantovani*

NICU, Casa Sollievo della Sofferenza Hospital, San Giovanni Rotondo, Italy

***Correspondence:**
Stefania Sbrizzi
stefaniasbrizzi@gmail.com

For its specific qualitative characteristics human donor milk (DM) is the main alternative to preterm infants nutrition and growing. How several studies suggest child's physical and mental development is influenced by breastfeeding that prevents the necrotizing enterocolitis (NEC), retinopathy of prematurity (ROP), and sepsis common in preterm newborns. Our research was conducted in NICU's Human Milk Bank (HMB) "Allattiamolavita." Our study was based on macronutrients analysis (MA) of 100 DM samples taken until 10 days since childbirth and analyzed by spectroscopic infrared innovative method (MIRIS). This is a specific method to analyse fat (F), crude proteins (CP), true proteins (TP), carbohydrate (CHO), and total solids (TS). We also analyzed the 100 donors' clinic-metabolic profile by blood tests (PMT). Both data was collected between September 2015 and February 2018. The research was structured in two parts. In the first part we compared PMT with qualitative and quantitative characteristics of MA while in the second one we studied every DM macronutrient finding furthermore possible relations between them. Statistical Package for Social Sciences (SPSS-IBM 24) was used to compare data and reporting coefficient of determination using Spearman's Rho and Kendall's Tau. We also analyzed samples using Kolmogorov–Smirnov test, Student *T*-test, ANOVA, Whitney *U*-test, and chi-square test. Statistically significant correlations were noted between maternal serum proteins and CP—TP of DM. The research showed also significant correlations between azotaemia and TP and an inverse correlation between serum creatinine and CP. No statistically significant correlation was observed between donors' glycaemia and CHO. Mineral concentrations of DM emerged independent of blood minerals (P, Ca, Fe, Na). We also calculated a normal range for individual macronutrient of human transitional milk (TM) that was not established in literature yet. Our experience allowed us to underline that human milk is a privileged site compared to donors' clinical and metabolic disorders. Our analysis showed the major role of the HMB to provide DM to improve clinical status, growing, and neurocognitive short and long term outcome of preterm infants.

Keywords: donor human milk, human milk bank, breast milk, macronutrients human milk, clinic-metabolic profile of donors, preterm newborns, infrared spectroscopy

INTRODUCTION

Breast milk (BM) is the first-choice food for the preterm newborn: it brings important benefits at gastrointestinal, immunological, nutritional, and cognitive levels (1). When this food is not available or not sufficient, such as in cases of very critical maternal conditions or transient separation by transfer of the newborn, DHM is the most suitable alternative. The main advantages of using BM in the diet of preterm infants are: low incidence of necrotizing enterocolitis (2, 3), reduced incidence of sepsis and other infections (4–7), reduced incidence of bronchopulmonary dysplasia (8), high food tolerance (9), prevention of arterial hypertension and insulin resistance (10, 11). The national guideline on the protection, promotion, and support of breastfeeding states that "breast milk is, where not contraindicated, the most appropriate food for the nutritional needs of premature and hospitalized infants" (12). Breast milk is currently being researched—several new bioactive components have been identified and described, thanks to the advancement of biotechnology (13). It is important to focus on the aspects of its composition in order to optimize the use, especially for the VLBW for whom it is considered a life-saving drug (14, 15).

PURPOSE

This study aims to:

- establish ranges of normal values for human transitional milk;
- research possible correlations between the clinical-metabolic situation of mothers and the nutritional values of their milk;
- analyze individual macronutrients of donor human milk (DHM);
- search for possible correlations between the above nutrients;
- study how to positively deal with the caloric-energetic contribution of BM.

METHODS

The Human Milk bank (HMB) "AllattiamolaVita" of the Hospital "Casa Sollievo della Sofferenza" (CSS) in San Giovanni Rotondo is part of NICU. It provides the donated human milk for the feeding of preterm newborns on medical prescription. A database containing all the data useful for the objectives of the research has been created at the beginning of our study, namely:

- identification code referred to units;
- personal data of mothers: date of birth, age at the delivery, date of donation to HMB;
- clinical situation of the pregnant woman;
- date of hospitalization for delivery;
- fill personal forms "Donors' Form": free donation of milk, explain exclusion criteria;
- infection of HBV, CMV, HIV, HCV, Syphilis, smoke, drugs and tattoos, piercing and surgical operations on last 6 months; **(Image 1)**
- blood tests of mothers;
- macronutrients of DHM.

Abbreviations: BM, Breast Milk; CSS, Casa Sollievo della Sofferenza; DHM, Donor Human Milk; HMB, Human Milk Bank; VLBW, birth weight < 1,500 g.

The status of the blood tests has been defined according to the reference parameters of the CSS Analysis Laboratory.

Laboratory examinations on undiluted human milk were carried out without additives at the HMB of the same hospital, via Miris-HMA, an infrared spectroscopic analyzer. This method permitted to detect, specifically: fat (F), crude-proteins (CP), carbohydrates (CHO), total solids (TS), true-proteins (TP), and energy (E).

PARTICIPANTS AND PROCEDURES

The analysis of the blood tests of 100 women who have given birth at the CSS Gynecology and obstetrics department are related to glucose, azotemia, creatininemia, total proteins, sodium, phosphorus, calcium, and iron. The macronutrients of 100 samples taken within the 17th post-partum day, were subsequently analyzed by the methodical MIRIS. The study included samples of fresh donated milk and stored refrigerated milk at −20°C. Both analyses were carried out between September 2015 and February 2018. In detail, correlations have been sought between:

- levels of maternal blood glucose and CHO concentration in DHM;
- levels of maternal azotemia and TP in DHM;
- levels of maternal creatininemia and CP in DHM;
- maternal serum proteins and CP-TP proteins of DHM;
- maternal blood trace elements and mineral concentration of DHM;
- maternal iron and macronutrients of DHM.

STATISTICAL ANALYSIS

The group comparison was made using the statistical software Package for Social Sciences version 24 (SPSS-IBM). The results were expressed as mean ± standard deviation with confidence interval to 95% for continuous variables and as percentages for categorical and discrete variables. The computation of the Spearman Rho coefficients and the Kendall Tau β were performed to assess the degree of correlations between the variables. The Kolmogorov–Smirnov test was used to sample the normality of the data. Finally, the data were analyzed by Student *T*-tests, ANOVA, Whitney *U*-test, and Chi-Quadro test. Statistically significant values were considered with $p < 0.05$.

RESULTS

Analysis of the Blood Tests

The data obtained in our study are presented in **Tables 1–5**. The tested blood glucose is 77.29 ± 14.80 mg/dl, range 53.00–151.00 mg/dl, and median 76.00 mg/dl. In the sample analyzed, 30 subjects report a condition of hypoglycemia (30% of the general population), 6 subjects (6%) hyperglycemia, and the remaining 64 (64%) average blood glucose. Serum nitrogen is 18.75 ± 5.14 mg/dl, range 6.00–34.00 mg/dl, and median 18.00 mg/dl. In the general population 18 donors (18% of the sample) report azotemia values below the lower limit and the remaining 82% (82 subjects) report the standard serum values. The creatininemia

TABLE 1 | Descriptive statistics of blood glucose, azotemia, creatitinemia, and total maternal serum proteins and concentrations of carbohydrates, true proteins, crude proteins, and energy of DHM.

	N	Minimum	Maximum	Middle	Standard deviation
CHO in hypoglycemic	30	1.40	8.50	5.1733	1.90334
CHO in normoglycemic	64	1.40	8.50	5.3953	1.69719
CHO in hyperglycemic	6	5.00	6.80	6.2500	0.66858
Number of valid cases	100				
TP in ipoazotemic	18	0.40	1.90	1.2056	0.37647
TP in normoazotemic	82	0.08	3.60	1.0654	0.60167
Number of valid cases	100				
CP in ipocreatininemic	50	0.50	5.70	1.6300	1.03967
CP in normocreatininemic	50	0.10	4.20	1.3500	0.95538
Number of valid cases	50				
Total proteins low	34	5.66	6.48	6.1665	0.20084
CP in total proteins low	34	0.10	1.80	0.8906	0.49541
TP in total protein low	34	0.10	4.40	1.1824	0.78450
Total proteins normal	66	6.50	7.52	6.9202	0.27871
CP in total proteins normal	66	0.10	5.70	1.6485	1.07033
TP in total proteins normal	66	0.08	3.60	1.1936	0.57994
Number of valid cases	100				
Energy	100	6.00	110.00	57.3100	17.58598
Number of valid cases	100				

values of people belonging to the population are 0.55 ± 0.11 mg/dl, with range 0.18–0.94 mg/dl, and median 0.93 mg/dl. In the sample, 50% (50 subjects) of the donors report the creatininemia below the normal range, the remaining 50 (50%) have values compatible with the standard. Serum values of total proteins within the entire population are 6.66 ± 0.44 g/dl, with a range of 5.66–7.52 g/dl, and median 6.70 g/dl. In the sample, 30 donors (30%) show blood concentrations of total proteins below the normal range. The sodium blood concentration is equal to 138.11 ± 2.09 mMol/L, with a range of 132.00 ± 143.00 mMol/L, and median of 138.00 mMol/L. Ninety-two patients (92%) have normal sodium blood values while the remaining 8 (8%) show mild hyponatremia conditions (132 mMol/L). The blood values of phosphorus showed the average of 3.23 ± 0.48 mg/dl, range 2.20–4.60 mg/dl with median 3.20 mg/dl. Six percent (3 donors) of the blood phosphorus test has a ipofosforemia condition, while the remaining 94% (47 donors) has blood phosphorus levels compatible with the standard. Serum calcium of 51 blood samples with an average of 8.77 ± 0.37 mg/dl, range 8.10–9.59 mg/dl, and median 8.80 mg/dl was evaluated. The totality of the population in analysis, 51 subjects, has ordinary calcium values. Finally, in a sub-sample of 80 subjects, the iron was found to be equal to 84.10 ± 42.33 mcg/dl, with range 21.00–221.00 mcg/dl, and median 75.00 mcg/dl. A partial deficiency is reported in 21 individuals (26.25% of the entire sub-sample), 3 individuals (3.75%) have an increase of the iron values (>221 mcg/dl) and the remaining 56 (70.00%) show iron blood values in the standard.

Population Overview and Nutrient Analysis

It was observed that:

- lipids of the 100 samples are 3.26 ± 1.77 g/dl, with range 0.20–9.70 g/dl, and median 2.90 g/dl;

TABLE 2 | Statistical analysis by Rho Spearman of the correlations between azotemia and true proteins, creatitinemia, and crude proteins, maternal total blood protein, respectively, with crude proteins and true proteins of BM.

			Azotemia	TP
Rho of Spearman	Azotemia	Correlation coefficient	1.000	−0.259**
		Sign. (two tails)	.	0.009
		N	100	100
	TP	Correlation coefficient	−0.259**	1.000
		Sign. (two tails)	0.009	.
		N	100	100
			Creatininemia	**CP**
Rho of Spearman	Creatininemia	Correlation coefficient	1.000	−0.246*
		Sign. (two tails)	.	0.014
		N	100	100
	CP	Correlation coefficient	−0.246*	1.000
		Sign. (two tails)	0.014	.
		N	100	100
			Total proteins	**CP**
Rho of Spearman	Total proteins	Correlation coefficient	1.000	0.241*
		Sign. (two tails)	.	0.016
		N	100	100
	CP	Correlation coefficient	0.241*	1.000
		Sign. (two tails)	0.016	.
		N	100	100
			Total proteins	**TP**
Rho di Spearman	Total proteins	Correlation coefficient	1	0.232*
		Sign. (two tails)		0.020
		N	100	100
	TP	Correlation coefficient	0.232*	1
		Sign. (two tails)	0.020	
		N	100	100

**The correlation is significant at level 0.05 (two-tailed).*
***The correlation is significant at level 0.01 (two-tailed).*

- the full sample CPs are 1.49 ± 1.00 g/dl, with range 0.10–5.70 g/dl, and median 1.30 g/dl;
- CHO have an average value of 5.36 ± 1.72 g/dl, range 1.40–8.50 g/dl, and a median of 6.10 g/dl;
- the proportion of minerals in the BM tested is 10.10 ± 2.86 g/dl, with range 1.20–17.10 g/dl, and median 10.61 g/dl;
- total sample energy is included in a range of 6.00–110.00 g/dl, with an average value of 57.31 ± 17.59 g/dl, and median 56.21 g/dl;
- TP are 1.09 ± 0.57 g/dl, with range 0.8–3.60 g/dl, and median 1.00 g/dl (**Table 5**).

Blood Glucose Levels and Correlation With CHO Concentration in DHM

The first correlation is between levels of blood glucose and CHO concentration. We analyzed the data of the entire population and the related milk samples, noting that:

TABLE 3 | Student *T*-Test for independent samples between the concentrations of crude and true proteins of DHM in the two levels of total maternal blood proteins.

		Test of Levene		Test *t* for the equality of the averages						
		F	**Sign.**	***t* independent**	**gl**	**Sign. (two tails)**	**Difference middle**	**Difference error standard**	**Range of confidence of the 95% difference**	
									Inferior	**Superior**
Total proteins	Var. equal alleged	7.783	0.006	−12.983	98	0.000	−0.75890	0.05846	−0.87491	−0.64290
	Var. equal not alleged			−15.391	83.087	0.000	−0.75890	0.04931	−0.85698	−0.66083
CP	Var. equal alleged	1.235	0.269	−2.102	98	0.038	−0.45238	0.21525	−0.87954	−0.02522
	Var. equal not alleged			−2.310	68.97	0.024	−0.45238	0.19586	−0.84312	−0.06164
Total proteins	Var. equal alleged	7.783	0.006	−12.983	98	0.000	−0.75890	0.05846	−0.87491	−0.64290
	Var. equal not alleged			−15.391	83.087	0.000	−0.75890	0.04931	−0.85698	−0.66083
TP	Var. equal alleged	0.052	0.820	−2.579	98	0.011	−0.31133	0.12071	−0.55088	−0.07179
	Var. equal not alleged			−2.777	65.525	0.007	−0.31133	0.11211	−0.53521	−0.08746

TABLE 4 | Statistically significant correlations between energy and other nutrients of BM.

			Energy	**Fat**	**CP**	**CHO**	**Total solids**	**TP**
Rho of Spearman	Energy	Correlation coefficient	1.000	0.797**	0.428**	0.229*	0.872**	0.330**
		Sign.	.	0.000	0.000	0.022	0.000	0.001
		N	100	100	100	100	100	100
	Fat	Correlation coefficient	0.797**	1.000	0.235*	−0.099	0.533**	0.088
		Sign.	0.000	.	0.018	0.326	0.000	0.382
		N	100	100	100	100	100	100
	CP	Correlation coefficient	0.428**	0.235*	1.000	0.108	0.531**	0.887**
		Sign.	0.000	0.018	.	0.283	0.000	0.000
		N	100	100	100	100	100	100
	CHO	Correlation coefficient	0.229*	−0.099	0.108	1.000	0.494**	0.234*
		Sign.	0.022	0.326	0.283	.	0.000	0.019
		N	100	100	100	100	100	100
	Total solids	Correlation coefficient	0.872**	0.533**	0.531**	0.494**	1.000	0.489**
		Sign.	0.000	0.000	0.000	0.000	.	0.000
		N	100	100	100	100	100	100
	TP	Correlation coefficient	0.330**	0.088	0.887**	0.234*	0.489**	1.000
		Sign.	0.001	0.382	0.000	0.019	0.000	.
		N	100	100	100	100	100	100

***The correlation is significant at level 0.01 (two-tailed).*
**The correlation is significant at level 0.05 (two-tailed).*

- 30 subjects have blood glucose values below normal values (70–100 mg/dl):
  - carbohydrate levels in milk equal to 5.17 ± 1.90 g/dl with range 1.40–8.50 g/dl;
- 6 subjects have blood glucose values above the normal values:
  - carbohydrate levels in milk equal to 6.10 ± 0.34 g/dl with range 6.10–6.80 g/dl;
- 64 subjects have glucose values in the standard:
  - carbohydrate levels in milk equal to 5.40 ± 1.70 g/dl with range 1.40–8.50 g/dl (**Table 1**).

The correlation between blood glucose and carbohydrate concentration in DHM was statistically insignificant according to the coefficient of Spearman ($p = 0.093$; **Table 2**). We compared, moreover, the averages of carbohydrates between hypoglycemic donors and hyperglycemic ones: they were found to be not statistically different from the Student *T*-Test ($p = 0.131$).

TABLE 5 | Prospectus of normal values of macronutrients of human transitional milk.

Fat	1.49–5.03 g/dl
Crude protein	0.49–2.49 g/dl
Carbohydrate	3.64–7.08 g/dl
Total solids	7.24–12.96 g/dl
Energy	39.72–74.90 g/dl
True protein	0.52–1.66 g/dl

Azotemia and Correlation With TP in DHM

On 100 samples analyzed:

➢ 18 donors have azotemia values below normal range (15–38 mg/dl):

- true protein levels in milk equal to 1.21 ± 0.38 g/dl, with range 0.40–1.90 g/dl;

➢ 72 donors present blood nitrogen values compatible with the normal range:

- true protein levels in milk equal to 1.07 ± 0.60 g/dl, with range 0.80–3.60 g/dl (**Table 1**).

We have demonstrated the presence of an inverse correlation between Azotemia and concentration of True proteins by the coefficient of Spearman ($p = 0.009$; **Table 2**).

Creatininemia and Correlation With the CP of DHM

The subsequent step is represented by the analysis of the blood creatinine levels and the concentrations of crude proteins. We observed that:

➢ 50 donors have values below the normal range of creatininemia (0.55–1.02 mg/dl):

- levels of crude protein are equal to 1.63 ± 1.04, with range 0.5–5.70 g/dl;

➢ 50 remaining donors have normal values of Creatininemia:

- levels of crude protein are equal to 1.35 ± 0.14 g/dl, with range 0.10–4.20 g/dl (**Table 1**).

The correlation coefficient has shown a reverse condition between creatininemia and crude protein concentrations ($p = 0.014$; **Table 2**).

Correlations Between Serum Proteins and Crude-True Proteins

The following step was to look for possible correlations between the total serum proteins and the CP-TP of the BM in analysis. We have therefore observed that:

➢ 30 subjects have total protein values below the standard (6.40–8.20 g/dl):

- the concentrations of crude proteins in DHM are equal to 0.89 ± 0.50 g/dl with range 0.10–1.80 g/dl;
- the concentrations of true proteins are instead of 1.18 ± 0.78 g/dl with range 0.10–4.40 g/dl;

➢ 70 subjects have total protein blood values in the standard, moreover:

- the concentrations of crude proteins are equal to 1.65 ± 0.28 g/dl, with range 0.10–5.70 g/dl;
- the concentrations of true proteins are equal to 1.19 ± 0.58 g/dl with range 0.08–3.60 g/dl (**Table 1**).

We therefore observed that there are statistically significant correlations between the crude protein concentrations and the total blood proteins, and between the latter and the true proteins, both represented by the correlation coefficient (respectively, $p = 0.016$ and $p = 0.020$; **Table 2**). It was thus demonstrated by the Student T-test that the two averages of the crude protein concentrations (with total blood proteins below the standard and in the norm) are statistically different from each other (respectively, with $p = 0.006$ with test of Leneve and $p = 0.024$ with T-Test for the comparator of the averages; **Table 3**). The same statistically significant correlation was, finally, demonstrated with the true proteins by means of the Student T-Test (with respectively, $p = 0.006$ with test of Leneve and $p = 0.007$ with tests of equality of the averages; **Table 3**).

Correlations Between Blood Trace Elements and the Concentration of Minerals

It also sought to demonstrate the possible correlations between calcium, sodium, blood phosphorus, and the concentration of minerals. With regard to blood calcium concentrations we analyzed a sub-sample of 51 subjects and the corresponding samples of BM. It was therefore observed that there are no statistically significant correlations between the blood calcium and the concentrations of the minerals in the milk ($p = 0.116$). The totality of the sample has been analyzed as regards the possible correlations between blood sodium and the concentration of minerals. It has therefore been shown that there are no statistically significant correlations between these two independent variables ($p = 0.327$). Finally, the possible correlation between phosphorus levels and the concentration of minerals in BM samples was sought by analyzing a sub-sample of 50 individuals within the general population with their corresponding milk.

Correlations Between Iron and Nutrients of BM

We also sought the possible correlations of iron with each nutrient of DHM observing iron serum levels of 84.10 ± 4.73 mcg/dl, range 21.00–221.00 mcg/dl, and median 75.00 mcg/dl. No statistically significant correlations between the iron and each nutrient of DHM have been highlighted.

Descriptive Analysis of the Components of Transitional DHM

In this part of the study we focused on the macronutrient composition of DHM samples. We established a range of concentrations for each nutrient and the possible correlations between the variables in question, i.e., fat, carbohydrates, crude proteins, true proteins, total solids, and energy of DHM have been changed. Considering the caloric intake of transitional DHM, it was observed that:

- energy levels are represented by 53.31 ± 17.59 g/dl, with range 6.00–110.00 g/dl, and with median 56.21 g/dl;
- statistically significant correlations between the energy and the other nutrients of the 100 samples can be pointed out (**Table 4**).

DISCUSSION

Breast Milk is a complex and dynamic fluid comprising numerous bioactive factors and different cellular populations making it the natural food par excellence, optimal for the newborn and for the preterm infant (16–19). One of the strengths of our analysis consists in the infrared spectroscopy because it does not foresee neither coloration nor dilution of the sample with a good preservation of the properties of the nutrients promoting the collection and the analysis of more accurate and reliable data (20).

The study is divided into two main phases. In the first phase, the possible influence of the clinical-metabolic structure of the mothers on the qualitative and quantitative characteristics of DHM nutrients was sought. The second phase was based, instead, on the study of the macronutrients of human milk and their possible correlations. The first figure that emerges from our results is the non-correlation between donor blood glucose and the glucose profile of the corresponding milk samples. In fact, there is no statistically significant correlation between the blood glucose itself and the carbohydrates ($p = 0.093$).

Another datum in favor of this thesis is the non-statistically significant difference of the average concentrations of the milk carbohydrates grouped by conditions of hypo/normo/hyperglycemia ($p = 0.131$). At this point we can say that it would be interesting to increase the number of the sample in analysis because, despite being not statistically significant, the increase in blood glucose showed a slight increase in the average concentration of carbohydrates and a gradual reduction in the dispersion of relative values (s.d.).

Our sample presented a close correlation between azotemia and true proteins of DHM ($p = 0.009$). In particular, it was observed that between these two variables there is a reverse relationship represented by the reduction of true proteins in response to the increase of azotemia. As shown in literature, the nitrogen balance, in the assessment of the nutritional status, is calculated as the difference between the intake and the elimination of the nitrogen itself. This balance is positive during pregnancy and breastfeeding but becomes negative in the case of insufficient protein and energy intake and when there is an imbalance between essential and non-essential amino acids (21). It is therefore important not to increase the intake of nitrogen in order to ensure a correct concentration of true proteins in BM.

The data analyzed later were related to creatininemia. A reverse correlation was observed regarding the crude proteins of the corresponding samples of DHM, statistically significant ($p = 0.014$).

We can therefore say that it would be desirable to maintain levels of creatininemia on the lower threshold of the normal limit as this would result in an increase of the concentration of crude proteins within BM. We also remember, as found in the literature, that the latter are responsible for the actual protein content necessary for the correct nourishment of the newborn (21). Another blood test taken into account regarded the total serum proteins. We have researched how these could affect the concentration of macronutrients of human milk. We therefore found a correlation between the total serum proteins (SP) and the protein categories of the milk. Both crude and true proteins are proportional to the value of total blood proteins ($p = 0.016$ and $p= 0.020$, respectively). In this regard, observing that the sample showed 34 values of total proteins lower than the normal range, we divided the general sample into two subsamples relative to the value of the SP calculating the average concentrations of the corresponding rates of BM.

We also found average concentrations between the two statistically different subsamples to confirm the above ($p = 0.006$ and $p = 0.024$). The monitoring of total serum protein values during pregnancy would be useful for a correct protein intake in BM.

We continued our study by analyzing sodium, phosphorus, calcium, and blood iron. We expected to find a close correlation between these and the macronutrients of milk. In particular, a regulation of BM minerals was expected through blood calcium.

These expectations were refuted because all the parameters taken into account, were not statistically correlated with the macronutrients of human milk.

These latest evidences associated with blood glucose results demonstrate that milk is certainly a privileged site because its nutritional characteristics cannot change on the basis of clinical-metabolic alterations.

After the first part of the study, we focused exclusively on milk and its components. Assessed the number of the sample, once the normality of the data has been obtained by means of the Kolmogorov-Smimoy test, we have set ourselves to bring back a range of normal values of the human transitional milk (**Table 5**).

Then we analyzed the possible correlations between the macronutrients of human milk, discussing in particular on the caloric aspect. We can say that all macronutrients play a fundamental role in the caloric-energetic contribution of breast milk, showing statistically significant positive correlation coefficients.

Significant importance in the increase of caloric intake is given by fats and true and crude proteins, according to what is known in the literature ($p < 0.001$, $p = 0.001$, and $p < 0.001$, respectively) (22).

Finally, we found that carbohydrates contribute to caloric intake with a lower significance ($p = 0.020$).

CONCLUSION

This study has given us the opportunity to understand and demonstrate how much BM is a privileged site in relation to certain alterations of maternal biochemical profile. Nitrogen and creatinine are implicated in this process, having observed a reverse proportionality with the increase of true and crude proteins and, respectively, the reduction of the azotemia and the serum creatitinemia ($p = 0.009$ and $p = 0.014$; **Table 2**). Moreover, by observing a directly proportional correlation between the total blood proteins and the overall protein structure of the BM ($p = 0.016$ and $p = 0.020$) during pregnancy and breastfeeding a more careful monitoring of these parameters may be useful (**Table 2**). It would be desirable to continue these studies by increasing the number of the sample and including metabolic growth and clinical parameters of the newborn. Finally, we want to emphasize the role of the HMB which allows preterm infants to benefit from DHM. This proves to be an irreplaceable resource, as widely promoted during the course of this study, for the improvement of the clinical conditions, for the growth and the short and long term outcomes of our newborns (23–29).

AUTHOR CONTRIBUTIONS

SS: introduction, analytical study, results, discussion, and conclusion. PQ: participants and procedures, conclusion. DR: statistical analysis, results, discussion, and conclusion. MP-M: introduction. GP: participants and procedures. PC: introduction.

REFERENCES

1. Koletzko B, Poindexter B, Uauy R. Nutritional care of preterm infants: scientific basis and practical guidelines. *World Rev Nutr Diet.* (2014) 110:1–12. doi: 10.1159/isbn.978-3-318-02641-2
2. McGuire W, Anthony MY. Donor human milk versus formula for preventing necrotising enterocolitis in preterm infants: systematic review. *Arch Dis Child Fetal Neonatal Ed.* (2003) 88:F11–4. doi: 10.1136/fn.88.1.F11
3. Maffei D, Schanler RJ. Human milk is the feeding strategy to prevent necrotizing enterocolitis! *Semin Perinatol.* (2017) 41:36–40. doi: 10.1053/j.semperi.2016.09.016
4. De Silva A, Jones PW, Spencer SA. Does human milk reduce infection rates in preterm infants? A systematic review. *Arch Dis Child Fetal Neonatal Ed.* (2004) 89:F509–13. doi: 10.1136/adc.2003.045682
5. Ronnestad A, Abrahamsen TG, Medbo S, Reigstad H, Lossius K, Kaaresen PI, et al. Late-onset septicemia in a Norwegian national cohort of extremely premature infants receiving very early full human milk feeding. *Pediatrics.* (2005) 115:e269–76. doi: 10.1542/peds.2004-1833
6. Lodge CJ, Tan DJ, Lau MX, Dai X, Tham R, Lowe AJ, et al. Breastfeeding and asthma and allergies: a systematic review and meta-analysis. *Acta Paediatr.* (2015) 104:38–53. doi: 10.1111/apa.13132
7. Schanler RJ, Lau C, Hurst NM, Smith EO. Randomized trial of donor human milk versus preterm formula as substitutes for mothers' own milk in the feeding of extremely premature infants. *Pediatrics.* (2005) 116:400–6. doi: 10.1542/peds.2004-1974
8. Villamor-Martínez E, Pierro M, Cavallaro G, Mosca F, Kramer BW, Villamor E. Donor human milk protects against bronchopulmonary dysplasia: a systematic review and meta-analysis. *Nutrients.* (2018) 10:E238. doi: 10.3390/nu10020238
9. Vieira Borba V, Sharif K, Shoenfeld Y. Breastfeeding and autoimmunity: programing health from the beginning. *Am J Reprod Immunol.* (2018) 79:e12778. doi: 10.1111/aji.12778
10. Singhal A, Cole TJ, Lucas A. Early nutrition in preterm infants and later blood pressure: two cohorts after randomised trials. *Lancet.* (2001) 357:413–9. doi: 10.1016/S0140-6736(00)04004-6
11. Singhal A, Fewtrell M, Cole TJ, Lucas A. Low nutrient intake and early growth for later insulin resistance in adolescents born preterm. *Lancet.* (2003) 361:1089–97. doi: 10.1016/S0140-6736(03)12895-4
12. Linee di indirizzo nazionali sulla protezione, la promozione ed il sostegno dell'allattamento al seno, Conferenza Stato Regioni 20.12.2007 - GU n. 32 del 7-2-2008- Suppl. Ordinario n.32.
13. Kanwar JR, Kanwar RK, Sun X, Punj V, Matta H, Morley SM, et al. Molecular and biotechnological advances in milk proteins in relation to human health. *J Pharm Biomed Anal.* (2017) 146:168–78.
14. Davanzo R,Cannioto Z, Ronfani L, Monasta L, Demarini S. Breastfeeding and neonatal weight loss in healthy term infants. *J Hum Lact.* (2013) 29:45–53. doi: 10.1177/0890334412444005
15. Stefanescu BM, Krakauer MG, Stefanescu AR, Markham M, Kosinski JI. Very low birth weight infant care: adherence to a new nutrition protocol improbe growth outcomes and reduces infectious risk. *Early Hum Dev.* (2016) 94:25–30. doi: 10.1016/j.earlhumdev.2016.01.011
16. Ballard O, Morrow AL. Human milk composition: nutrients and bioactive factors. *Pediatr Clin North Am.* (2013) 60:49–74. doi: 10.1016/j.pcl.2012.10.002
17. Grabarics M, Csernák O, Balogh R, Béni S. Analytical characterization of human milk oligosaccharides - potential applications in pharmaceutical analysis. *J Pharmac Biomed Anal.* (2017) 140:168–78. doi: 10.1016/j.jpba.2017.08.039
18. Hassiotou F, Hartmann PE At the dawn of a new discovery: the potential of breast milk stem cells. *Adv Nutr.* (2014) 5:770–8. doi: 10.3945/an.114.006924
19. Bertino E, Giuliani F, Baricco M, Di Nicola P, Peila C, Vassia C, et al. Benefits of donor milk in the feeding of preterm infants. *Early Hum Dev.* (2013) 89(Suppl. 2):S3–6. doi: 10.1016/j.earlhumdev.2013.07.008
20. Billard H, Simon L, Desnots E, Sochard A, Boscher C, Riaublanc A, et al. Calibration adjustment of the mid-infrared analyzer for an accurate determination of the macronutrient composition of human milk. *J Hum Lact.* (2016) 32:NP19–27. doi: 10.1177/0890334415588513
21. Bedogni G, Cecchetto G. *Manuale di ANDID di Valutazione Della Stato Nutrizionale.* Ed. Universo. Roma (2009).
22. Johnston M, Landers S, Noble L, Szucs K, Viehmann L. American academy of pediatrics. Breastfeeding and the use of human milk. *Pediatrics.* (2012) 129 :827–41. doi: 10.1542/peds.2011-3552
23. Horta BL, Loret de Mola C, Victora CG. Breastfeeding and intelligence: a systematic review and meta-analysis. *Acta Paediatr.* (2015) 104:14–9. doi: 10.1111/apa.13139
24. Victora CG, Horta BL, Loret de Mola C, Quevedo L, Pinheiro RT, Gigante DP, et al. Association between breastfeeding and intelligence, educational attainment, and income at 30 years of age: a prospective birth cohort study from Brazil. *Lancet Glob Health.* (2015) 3:E199–205. doi: 10.1016/S2214-109X(15)70002-1
25. Schanler RJ. Outcomes of human milk-fed premature infants. *Semin Perinatol.* (2011) 35:29–33 doi: 10.1053/j.semperi.2010.10.005
26. Park S, Kim BN, Kim JW, Shin MS, Yoo HJ, Cho SC. Protective effect of breastfeeding with regard to children's behavioral and cognitive problems. *Nutr J.* (2014) 13:111. doi: 10.1186/1475-2891-13-111
27. Madore LS, Bora S, Erdei C, Jumani T, Dengos AR, Sen S. Effects of donor breastmilk feeding on growth and early neurodevelopmental outcomes in preterm infants: an observational study. *Clin Ther.* (2017) 39:1210–20. doi: 10.1016/j.clinthera.2017.05.341

28. Cortez J, Makker K, Kraemer DF, Neu J, Sharma R, Hudak ML. Maternal milk feedings reduce sepsis, necrotizing enterocolitis and improve outcomes of premature infants. *J Perinatol.* (2017) 38:71–4. doi: 10.1038/jp.2017.149

29. Silano M, Vincentini O, Luciani A, Felli C, Caserta S, Esposito S, et al. Early tissue transglutaminase-mediated response underlies K562(S)-cell gliadin-dependent agglutination. *Pediatr Res.* (2012) 71:532–8. doi: 10.1038/pr.2012.4

11

Handling of Breast Milk by Neonatal Units: Large Differences in Current Practices and Beliefs

Daniel Klotz[1]*, *Stefanie Jansen*[1], *Corinna Gebauer*[2] *and Hans Fuchs*[1]

[1] *Department of Neonatology, Center for Pediatrics, Medical Center - University of Freiburg, Faculty of Medicine, University of Freiburg, Freiburg, Germany,* [2] *Department of Neonatology, University Children's Hospital, Leipzig, Germany*

Correspondence:
Daniel Klotz
daniel.klotz@uniklinik-freiburg.de

Background: Breast milk (BM) for premature infants is subjected to multiple steps of processing, storage and distribution. These steps may influence the quality and safety of BM. Guidelines concerning the use of mother's own milk are either not available or limited to specific aspects of BM handling and are based on evidence of variable strength. This may result in diverse BM handling routines by health care professionals.

Objective: We surveyed neonatal units to increase the knowledge about the current practice of BM handling routines of mother's own milk and to identify controversial aspects that could give directions for future research.

Methods: An online-based questionnaire was sent to 307 different neonatal departments providing level III to level I neonatal care within Germany, Austria and Switzerland. Practices concerning screening for cytomegalovirus and BM bacteria, pasteurization, fortification, storage, workforce and the incidence of BM administration errors were surveyed.

Results: A total of 152 units, 56% of contacted level III units and 51% of level II units, participated in the survey (Germany 53%, Switzerland 71%, and Austria 56%). We found differences concerning indication and method of CMV inactivation (performed by 58%), bacterial count screening (48%) and bacterial count reduction (17%) within participating units. Thirty different thresholds for bacterial BM counts were reported by 65 units, resulting in pasteurization or discarding of BM. The use of nutrient analysis (12%) and fortification regimens in addition to standard multicomponent fortifiers (58%) using either individual (93%), targeted (3%), or adjusted (4%) fortification protocols varied profoundly. There is a high variability in staff and available facilities for BM handling. 73% of units report about BM administration errors.

Conclusion: There is a wide variability in most aspects of BM handling in the participating units. Despite limited evidence labor and cost intensive procedures are applied which may have an impact on BM quality.

Keywords: bacterial contamination, cytomegalovirus, breast milk, infant, pasteurization, premature, mothers own milk

INTRODUCTION

Mothers own breast milk (BM) is the preferred source of nutrition for the term and preterm infant (1). However, certain aspects must be considered when feeding BM to premature infants: Viruses, such as cytomegalovirus (CMV), and bacteria are transmitted via BM and may prompt BM treatment (2, 3). BM for the preterm infants needs to be expressed, collected and, depending on the individual organizational structures of the neonatal unit, transported to a designated site for further handling or storage. Upon distribution to the neonatal ward the milk needs to be (re)labeled, fortified to meet the nutritional demand of the preterm infant and reheated before it can finally be fed to premature infant (4).

These BM handling routines may be hazardous to its quality and safety (5). Hence, departmental organizational structures and operational procedures that ensure optimal BM handling and treatment need to be in place (6). However, there is a paucity of evidence-based data concerning optimal BM handling (5). Consequently, existing recommendations are based on evidence of very variable strength and this may result in diverse BM handling practices by health care professionals (7). Few data are available about the current approaches of neonatal departments for handling of mothers own milk (8–10).

The aim of this cross-sectional survey was to describe current practices of BM handling routines of mother's own milk within neonatal units and to identify controversial aspects of BM treatment that may merit further research for guiding daily clinical practice on the neonatal ward.

MATERIALS AND METHODS

A structured and stratified online-based questionnaire was sent to 307 different neonatal units within Germany ($n = 259$), Austria ($n = 34$) and German speaking Switzerland ($n = 14$) between June 8th 2016 and March 1th 2017 using an online survey tool (SurveyMonkey, Portland, OR). We aimed to include all neonatal units within the participating countries, identified via the respective national neonatal and/or pediatric society or internet research. We assessed the level of neonatal care and the number of very low birth weight infants per unit per year. The screening rate for maternal CMV serostatus, the unit specific indications, methods and threshold levels for CMV inactivation and/or bacterial count reduction were surveyed. The feeding regimen for preterm infants according to the maternal CMV serostatus, bacterial BM count and postmenstrual age were inquired. Furthermore, we asked to detail the strategies for BM fortification, the prevalence and applied techniques for BM nutrient analysis as well as the condition of BM storage, departmental organizational structures and allocated staff for BM handling. The questionnaire is available as **Supplementary Material**. Statistical analysis was performed using GraphPad Prism (V5.02, GraphPad, San Diego, CA). Categorical variables are presented in absolute numbers and percentages. Percentages apply to the number of answers for any given question. We reported quantitative data as mean and standard deviation or median and interquartile range (or range) where applicable.

Abbreviations: BM, breast milk; CMV, Cytomegalovirus; HTST, High-temperature short-time.

RESULTS

We received a total of 152 replies. Fifty-six percent of the 189 contacted units that provided level III and 51% of the 75 units that provided level II of neonatal care (definition according to the American Academy of Pediatrics) participated in the survey. Response rate per country was 53% for Germany, 71% for Switzerland and 56% for Austria. Of the 43 contacted well baby units (level I) only eight returned the questionnaire. The median number of very low birth weight infants for level III units was 54 (IQR 36-79).

Cytomegalovirus Screening and Inactivation

Maternal CMV screening was performed by 87 (85%) of level III units and by 25 (63%) of level II units. Untreated raw colostrum of CMV seropositive mothers was fed by 57 units (66%) for a median of 4 days (range 2–10). Thereafter, CMV inactivation using Holder-Pasteurization (heating milk at 62.5 ± 0.5°C for 30 min), high-temperature short-time pasteurization (HTST, in this instance performed at 62°C for 5 s) and/or freeze-thawing of BM was applied by 89 (58%) of participating units (**Table 1**). For the freeze-thawing method milk was frozen with a median freezing time of 1 day (range 0.5–14) at a median temperature of −20°C (range −80 to −8). Discontinuation of BM treatment for CMV inactivation or bacterial count reduction and the initiating of breastfeeding of CMV seropositive mothers were considered based upon the postmenstrual age and the actual body weight of the infant (**Figure 1**).

Bacterial Count Screening and Reduction

Sixty-five units (43%) routinely screened for bacterial BM colonization, either if BM was expressed at home ($n = 7$), expressed at the unit ($n = 2$) or both ($n = 56$). BM was pasteurized by 28 out of 65 units and/or discarded by 48 out of 65 units if bacterial counts exceeded pre-defined thresholds. In general, threshold levels varied considerably between units (**Table 2**). Bacterial count reduction was performed by Holder-pasteurization ($n = 20$) or HTST pasteurization ($n = 3$) (**Table 1**). Again, the duration of BM treatment for bacterial count reduction was depending on the postmenstrual age or the actual body weight of the infant (**Figure 1**).

Nutrient Analysis and Breast Milk Fortification

Only sixteen units (12%) were performing BM nutrient analysis using a bedside infrared analyser. Six of those regularly measured the BM nutrients content as part of a nutritional regime, five units occasionally and five units within clinical trials. Fortification in addition to standard multicomponent fortifier was performed by 75/135 units (58%). Additional protein was added to already

TABLE 1 | Methods applied for CMV inactivation and bacterial count reduction in breast milk.

	Total (*n* = 152) *n* (%)[#]	**Germany (*n* = 126) *n* (%)[#]**	**Level III (*n* = 92) *n* (%)[#]**	**Level II (*n* = 27) *n* (%)[#]**	**Switzerland (*n* = 10) *n* (%)[#]**	**Level III (*n* = 6) *n* (%)[#]**	**Level II (*n* = 4) *n* (%)[#]**	**Austria (*n* = 16) *n* (%)[#]**	**Level III (*n* = 8) *n* (%)[#]**	**Level II (*n* = 7) *n* (%)[#]**
CMV inactivation	89 (58)	74 (58)	61 (66)	13 (48)	3 (30)	3 (50)	0 (0)	12 (75)	6 (75)	6 (86)
Holder-Pasteurization	53 (60)	44 (60)	39 (62)	6 (46)	2 (67)	2 (67)	n.a.	7 (58)	5 (83)	2 (23)
High-temperature short-time pasteurization	11 (12)	10 (14)	9 (15)	1 (8)	1 (23)	1 (13)	n.a.	0 (0)	0 (0)	0 (0)
Freeze-thawing method	25 (28)	20 (27)	13 (21)	6 (46)	0 (0)	0 (0)	n.a.	5 (42)	1 (17)	4 (67)
Bacterial count reduction[¶]	28 (17)	22 (17)	17 (18)[§]	5 (19)	2 (20)	2 (33)	0 (0)	4 (25)	3 (38)	1 (14)
Holder-Pasteurization	23 (82)	18 (86)	14 (82)	4 (80)	1 (50)	1 (50)	n.a.	4 (100)	3 (100)	1 (100)
High-temperature short-time pasteurization	3 (11)	1 (0.5)	1 (6)	1 (20)	1 (50)	1 (50)	n.a.	0 (0)	0 (0)	0 (0)

[#]*Denominator: Units participating in total, in each country and per level of neonatal care within each country.*
[§]*Freeze-thawing method for bacterial count reduction: n = 1.*
[¶]*Missing numbers = answers not given.*
CMV = cytomegalovirus; Holder-Pasteurization = 62.5°C, 30 min; High-temperature short-time pasteurization = 62°C, 5 s.
n.a., not applicable.

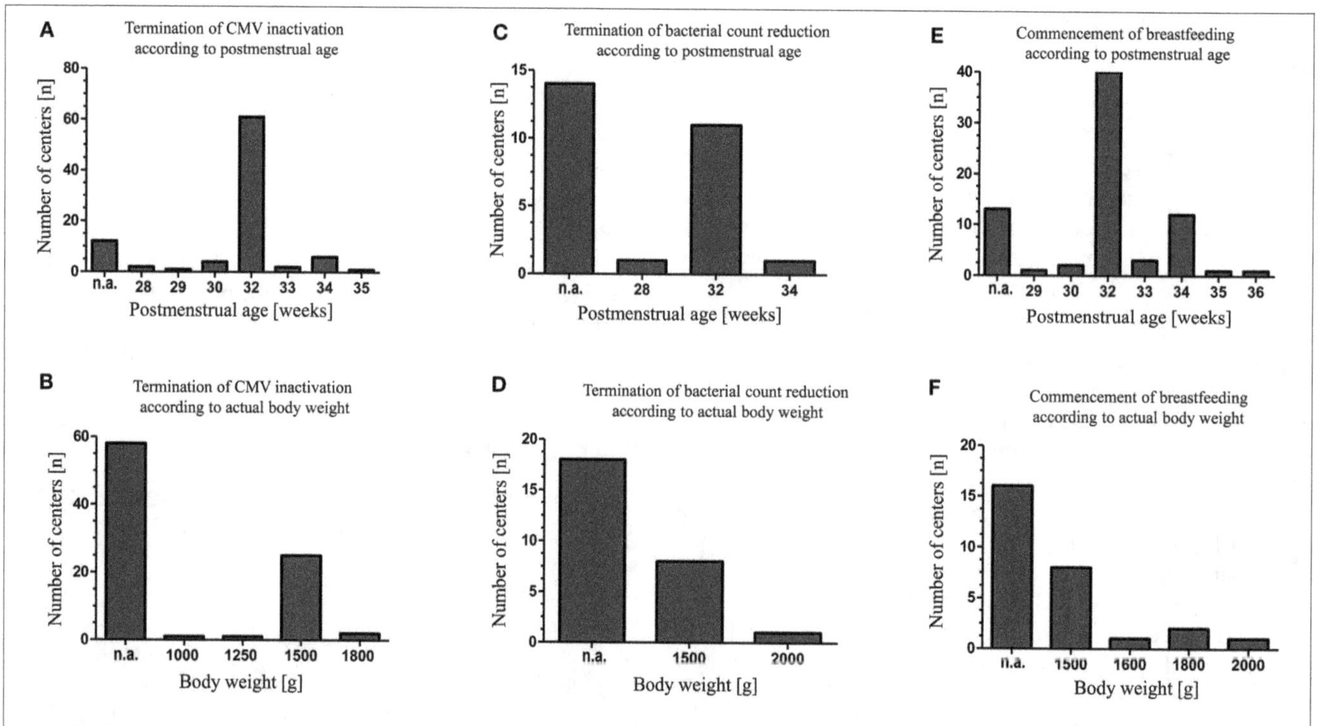

FIGURE 1 | Indications of individual neonatal units for CMV inactivation, reduction of bacterial breast milk count and initiation of breastfeeding in case of maternal CMV seropositivity. The decisions to commence breastfeeding, to terminate CMV inactivation or bacterial count reduction were made either depending on the infants postmenstrual age **(A,C,E)** or depending on the infants' actual body weight **(B,D,F)**. N.a., respective criteria were not applied.

fortified BM by 50%, lipids by 38% and carbohydrates by 15% of units. The decision on which component should be added was not revealed by our survey. In three units, fortification was adapted after nutrient analysis of mothers' own milk (targeted fortification) or according to the periodic determinations of the infant's blood urea nitrogen in four units (adjusted fortification).

Organizational and Departmental Structures

Organizational details for the location of BM handling and storage as well as designated work force and responsibilities for BM handling are given in **Table 3**. BM was stored at a median temperature of −20°C (range −8 to −33) for a median of 6 months (range 0.07–8) before being discarded.

TABLE 2 | Bacterial count thresholds for pasteurization **(A)** and discarding **(B)** of breast milk intended for premature infants <32 weeks postmenstrual age or body weight <1,500 g.

Evidence of	Replies *n* (%)	No pasteurization needed	Bacterial count limits (colony-forming units/mL)				
			>0	$\geq 10^2$	$\geq 10^3$	$\geq 10^4$	$\geq 10^5$
(A) PASTEURIZATION OF BREAST MILK FOR BACTERIAL COUNT REDUCTION ACCORDING TO POSITIVE CULTURE RESULTS							
Skin commensals	27 (100)	12 (44)	0 (0)	0 (0)	0 (0)	5 (19)	10 (37)
Staphylococcus aureus	27 (100)	5 (19)	7 (26)	1 (4)	7 (26)	4 (15)	3 (10)
Gram-negative bacteria	26 (100)	4 (15)	14 (54)	0 (0)	5 (19)	1 (4)	2 (8)
Bacillus cereus	24 (100)	8 (33)	8 (33)	0 (0)	4 (17)	2 (8)	2 (8)
(B) DISCARDING OF BREAST MILK DUE TO BACTERIAL CONTENT ACCORDING TO POSITIVE CULTURE RESULTS							
Skin commensals	48 (100)	30 (63)	0 (0)	3 (6)	4 (8)	2 (4)	9 (19)
Staphylococcus aureus	48 (100)	13 (27)	9 (19)	6 (13)	4 (8)	3 (6)	13 (27)
Gram-negative bacteria	48 (100)	12 (25)	12 (25)	5 (10)	5 (10)	6 (13)	8 (17)
Bacillus cereus	44 (100)	14 (32)	13 (30)	1 (2)	6 (14)	2 (4)	8 (18)

TABLE 3 | Organizational details of breast milk handling.

Location of frozen BM storage	Replies *n* (%)	Neonatal ward	Milk kitchen (separate from neonatal ward)	Milk bank (also preparing donor milk)	Other location (e.g., hospital main kitchen, with parents)
	136 (100)	71 (54)	52 (38)	9 (7)	4 (3)
Location of BM preparation (thawing, pasteurization, portion)	Replies *n* (%) 139 (100)	Neonatal ward 70 (50)	Milk kitchen (separate from neonatal ward) 60 (43)	Milk bank (also preparing donor milk) 9 (6)	Other location (e.g., main hospital kitchen) 4 (0)
BM is prepared by*	Replies *n* (%)	Nursing staff	Designated milk bank personnel	Main hospital kitchen personnel	Other provider (dietician, nutritionist)
	139 (100)	78 (56)	60 (43)	1 (0.7)	4 (3)
BM handling under the direction of	Replies *n* (%)	Nursing staff	Medical team	Other (dietician, nutritionist, IBCLC)	Not explicitly assigned
	138 (100)	92 (67)	21 (15)	2 (1)	23 (17)

**Multiple replies possible.*
BM, breast milk.

Breast Milk Administration Errors

One hundred twenty-five units (82%) replied when queried about the incidence of BM administration errors per year with at least one incident of feeding BM to another than the intended infant in 91/125 units (73%). This relates to 66% of level III, 50% of level II, and 29% of level I units. There were either no cases of BM administration error ($n = 34$), 1–5 errors per year ($n = 78$), 6–10 per year ($n = 9$) or more than 10 per year ($n = 4$) reported.

DISCUSSION

Our survey reveals wide differences concerning many aspects of BM handling within participating units.

CMV inactivation of BM has been promoted to reduce the incidence of BM transmitted CMV infection (11). According to our survey, rates of maternal CMV screening and of CMV inactivation in mothers' own milk are comparable if not increased compared to corresponding data collected nearly a decade ago within the same countries (8) and appear to be more prevalent than in others (9, 10). CMV seropositive mothers' BM treatment for CMV inactivation was on average commenced on day 4 by the participants consistent with the occurrence of CMV in BM after the first week of lactation (12). Interestingly, there appears to be an agreement amongst participant concerning the postmenstrual age and body weight required to terminate BM treatment for CMV inactivation (and/or bacterial count reduction). However, CMV transmission rates, incidence of clinical signs of infection or sepsis and the impact of a postnatal CMV infection on neonatal short- and long-term outcomes remain controversial (13). While some data concerning neurocognitive development or hearing function point toward an unaffected outcome after BM transmitted CMV infection others suggest long-term neuropsychological sequelae (14–19). Therefore, the relevance of BM transmitted CMV infection and thus the role of CMV inactivation remains uncertain and official recommendations are not consistent. The Austrian Society of Pediatrics and Adolescent Medicine recommends freeze-thawing of colostrum and BM of CMV seropositive mothers for all infants <32 weeks gestational age (20). The national German Breastfeeding Committee does not recommend pasteurization for CMV inactivation due to insufficient data (21) and official recommendations for Switzerland are not available.

A substantial number of neonatal units are performing routine BM cultures to assess an apparent need for bacterial count reduction or discarding of BM. Indeed, there are several reports of sepsis and/or death caused by BM transmitted bacteria published (22). However, there was no association between BM pathogens and the subsequent pathogen causing an infant's illness in a single center analysis of 813 BM cultures of 209 infants (3). To the best of our knowledge, no data from observational studies or randomized trials are available to support bacterial count reduction in mother's own BM to reduce neonatal morbidity. In fact, a trend toward an increased rate of necrotizing enterocolitis was observed in an Austrian neonatal unit after its unit policy was changed in favor of pasteurization of BM (23). Furthermore, in their randomized controlled trial Cossey et al. noted a trend toward an increased rate of late onset sepsis in infants fed pasteurized BM compared to those fed raw BM. However, results of this trial need to be interpreted with caution since BM containing any gram-negative organisms, *Staphylococcus aureus* or enterococci, was withheld and replaced by formula (24). The loss of humoral and cellular mediated immunological, antibacterial and enzymatic BM properties due to pasteurization may have an impact on BM mediated neonatal immunocompetence and on above mentioned observations (25). HTST pasteurization may increase protein retention rates compared to Holder-pasteurization but data concerning antibacterial efficacy of HTST pasteurization are controversial (25, 26). Because there is no robust evidence to guide the assessment of a safe bacterial load of BM when feeding premature infants, any distinction between BM colonization and BM contamination remains arbitrary (27). Therefore, interpretation of bacterial BM counts as well as bacterial spectrum differed widely, 30 different cut off values for bacterial content indicating BM treatment or discarding were reported in our survey. A survey of nine neonatal units from Belgium and Luxembourg showed similar inconsistent results (10). The German Breastfeeding Committee does not recommend pasteurization for bacterial count reduction (28). No recommendations for Switzerland and Austria are available. In conclusion, the role of routine BM cultures and bacterial count reduction remains uncertain.

Breast milk services were mostly headed by nursing staff members. In some units however, there was no explicit allocation of responsibility. This may prove unfavorable in terms of organizational management and liability. Only in the minority of units personnel was exclusively tasked with BM handling. In these cases, BM was mostly handled and stored not on the neonatal unit but in separate facilities. However, in most units regular nursing staff was tasked with BM handling next to their obligations as primary caregivers on the neonatal ward. Our survey revealed a high rate of BM administration errors throughout most units. Computerized provider order entry systems and adequate resource allocation may reduce BM administration errors (8).

Bedside BM nutrient analysis is performed in some units. Clinically relevant variations in results obtained from near-infrared compared to wet bench nutrient analysis were demonstrated and despite calibration adjustments concise near-infrared measurement of BM macronutrient content remains challenging (29, 30). Therefore, the Committee on Nutrition of the German Society for Pediatrics issued a statement against the indiscriminate use of human milk analyzers (31).

Standard fortification represents the predominant form of BM fortification. Fortification targeted according to BM nutrients content or adjusted to the infant's metabolic response (i.e., blood urea nitrogen levels) is rarely applied. But most units are adding additional proteins, lipids or carbohydrates to BM that has already been fortified with standard multicomponent fortifier, albeit on what basis remains unclear. Effects of increased osmolality need to be taken into account (32).

There are limitations to our survey. We did not inquire about the preferred feeding regimens if BM of CMV seropositive mothers was not pasteurized. The response rate to our survey was limited and varied between regions and countries, which may have influenced our results. However, comparable studies focused on specific BM handling aspects or included a limited number of units. The strength of our survey lies in the number of participating units within three different countries, providing insight into many different aspects of, to some extent, very diverse BM handling routines.

CONCLUSIONS

There is a wide variability in most aspects of BM handling in the participating units. Despite limited evidence of clinical relevance, labor and cost intensive procedures are applied which may have an impact on BM quality. Evidence based data are needed to formulate reliable guidelines and strong recommendations for handling of human milk for premature infants.

AUTHOR CONTRIBUTIONS

DK conceived and designed the survey, contributed to data collection, analyzed data and wrote the first draft of the manuscript. SJ designed the survey, collected data, contributed to data analysis and reviewed the manuscript. CG designed the survey, contributed to data collection and reviewed the manuscript. HF contributed to data collection and reviewed the manuscript.

ACKNOWLEDGMENTS

The authors are indebted to the participants of this survey: Germany: Klinikum Konstanz: K. Waldecker; Hegau-Bodensee-Klinikum Singen: A. Trotter; St. Elisabethen-Krankenhaus Lörrach: H. Fahnenstich; Ortenau Klinikum Offenburg: M. Rohrbach; Klinikum Villingen-Schwenningen: E. Komini; Klinikum Baden-Baden: M. Kratz; Universitätskinderklinik Tübingen: A. Franz; Klinikum Reutlingen: P. Freisinger; Klinikum Sindelfingen-Böblingen: M. Teufel; Städtisches Klinikum Karlsruhe: A. Krauth; Filderklinik Filderstadt: D. Ecker; Klinikum Stuttgart: M. Vochem; Universitätskinderklinik Ulm: S. Baranowski; Klinikum Schwäbisch Gmünd: B. Schwander; Klinikum Esslingen: C. v. Schnakenburg; Ostalb Klinikum Aalen: J. Freihorst; St. Josefs-Krankenhaus Freiburg: A. Härtling; Universitätskinderklinik Freiburg: U. Grundmann; Klinikum Garmisch-Partenkirchen: C. Stockklausner; Klinikum Starnberg: T. Lang; Klinikum Kempten: H. Müller; Städtisches Klinikum München Harlaching: M. Krüger; Klinikum der Universität München Großhadern: S. Herber-Jonat; Klinikum Augsburg: W. Schenk; Josefinum Kinderkrankenhaus Augsburg: M. Heinrich; Klinikum Deggendorf: M. Welsch; Perinatalzentrum Ingoldstadt/Neuburg: S. Seeliger; Krankenhaus Barmherzige Brüder Regensburg: H. Segerer; Klinikum Nürnberg: C. Fusch; Universitätsklinikum Erlangen: H.-G. Topf, H. Bieberstein; Klinikum St. Marien Amberg: A. Fiedler; Missionsärztliche Klinik Würzburg: C. Kohlhauser-Vollmuth; Universitätskinderklinik Würzburg: E. Frieauff; Sozialstiftung Bamberg: K.-H. Deeg; Vinzentius-Krankenhaus Landau: J. Bensch; St. Marien- und St. Annastiftskrankenhaus Ludwigshafen am Rhein: U. Merz; Universitätskinderklinik Mainz: A. Kidszun; Klinikum Mutterhaus der Borromäerinnen Trier: W. Thomas; Kemperhof Koblenz: T. Hoppen; Klinikum Saarbrücken: J. Möller; Marienhausklinik Kohlhof Neunkirchen: G. Shamdeen; Universitätsklinik des Saarlandes: S. Meyer; Universitätskinderklinik Bonn: A. Müller; GFO Kliniken Bonn: K. Schneider; DRK-Kinderklinik Siegen: M. Hubert; Uniklinik Köln: A. Kribs; Kliniken der Stadt Köln: M. Hoppenz; Klinikum Leverkusen: P.Jahn; Bethlehem- Gesundheitszentrum Stolberg: U. Hannig; Uniklinik RWTH Aachen: T. Orlikowsky; Krankenhaus Mönchengladbach: S. Thushyanthan; Elisabeth-Krankenhaus Rheydt: J. Wintgens; Universitätskinderklinik Düsseldorf: T. Höhn; Florence-Nightingale-Krankenhaus Düsseldorf: M. Berghäuser; Städtisches Klinikum Solingen: J. Adler; Helios Klinikum Krefeld: P. Heister; Helios Klinikum Wuppertal: M. Heldmann; Allgemeines Krankenhaus Hagen: G. Koch; Gemeinschaftskrankenhaus Herdecke: S. Bernitzki; Marien Hospital Witten: B. Gharavi; Klinikum Dortmund: F. Heitmann; St. Elisabeth-Hospital Bochum: N. Teig; Universitätskinderklinik Essen: U. Felderhoff-Müser; Evangelisches Krankenhaus Oberhausen: A. Jenke; Sana Klinikum Duisburg; F. Brevis; Bethanien Moers: M. Wallot; Marienhospital Bottrop: S. Ata; Marien-Hospital Wesel: M. Gappa; Evangelisches Krankenhaus Hamm: G. Selzer; Evangelisches Krankenhaus Lippstadt: T. Hofmann; Klinikum Lippe: U. Wunderle; Klinikum Herford: B. Utsch; Christophorus-Kliniken Coesfeld: H. Gerleve; St. Franziskus Hospital Münster: F. Urlichs; Mathias-Spital Rheine: H.-G. Hoffmann; Darmstädter Kinderkliniken Prinzessin Margaret: G. Frey; Universitätsklinikum Frankfurt: R. Schlößer; Sana Klinikum Offenbach: J. Jochim; Klinikum Hanau: B. Bungert; Perinatalzentrum Gelnhausen: M. Wilhelm; Klinikum Fulda: R. Repp; Universitätsklinikum Marburg: R. Maier; Klinikum Kassel: D. Müller; Universitätsklinikum Jena: M. Vogelsberger; Sophien- und Hufeland-Klinikum Weimar: T. Rusche; St. Georg-Klinikum Eisenach: B. Kretzschmar; Helios Vogtland Klinikum Plauen: S. Pötzsch; Helios Klinikum Aue: K. Prädicow; Heinrich-Braun-Klinikum Zwickau: T. Stuckert; DRK Krankenhaus Chemnitz-Lichtenstein: H. Sirb; DRK Krankenhaus Chemnitz-Rabenstein: A. Huster; Helios Klinikum Pirna: D. Stadthaus; Städtisches Klinikum Dresden Neustadt: S. Schmidt; Helios Klinik Leisnig: H. Issa; Sana Kliniken Leipziger Land: A. Möckel; Kreiskrankenhaus Torgau: H.-U. Thomalla; Städtisches Klinikum Görlitz: H.-C. Gottschalk; Carl-Thiem-Klinikum Cottbus: U. Wetzel; Ernst von Bergmann Klinikum Potsdam: M. Radke; DRK Kliniken Berlin Westend: C. Kluthe; Charité-Universitätsmedizin Berlin: M. Berns; Klinikum im Friedrichshain: K.-U. Schunck; Evangelisches Waldkrankenhaus Spandau: F. Jochum; Klinikum Berlin-Buch: E. Harps; Klinikum Südstadt Rostock: D. Olbertz; Universitätsklinikum Halle/Saale: R. Haase, F. Kaufmann; Städtisches Klinikum Dessau: U. Mathony; Universitätskinderklinik Magdeburg: R. Böttger; St. Bernward Krankenhaus Hildesheim: A. Beider; Helios Klinikum Hildesheim: K. Harms; Helios Klinikum Salzgitter: Y. Roumeih; Auf der Bult Kinderkrankenhaus Hannover: F. Guthmann; Medizinische Hochschule Hannover: B. Bohnhorst; Klinikum Oldenburg: E. Cloppenburg; Helios Klinikum Uelzen: S. Geerken; Städtisches Klinikum Lüneburg: J. Sonntag; Klinikum Links der Weser Bremen: T. Körner; Klinikum Bremen-Nord: M. Heinecke; Klinikum Itzehoe: G. Hillebrand; Krankenhaus Neumünster: I. Yildiz; Universitätsklinikum Schleswig-Holstein: M. Bendiks; Westküstenklinikum Heide: R. Jensen; Diakonissenkrankenhaus Flensburg: M. Dördelmann; Universitätsklinikum Hamburg: D. Singer; Kath. Kinderkrankenhaus Wilhelmstift Hamburg: L. Koch; Klinik Barmbek: S. Schmidtke. Switzerland: Universitäts-Kinderspital beider Basel: R. Glanzmann; Universitätsspital Bern: B. Bubl; Luzerner Kantonspital: M. Stocker; Kantonspital Thurgau/Münsterlingen: B. Erkert; Kantonspital Zollikerberg: M. Mönkhoff; Kantonspital Winterthur: L. Hegi; Stadtspital Triemli: M. Hesse; Kinderspital Zürich: V. Bernet; Kinderzentrum Wildermeth: M. Gebauer; Kantonspital Aurau: P. Meyer. Austria: Gottfried von Preyersches Kinderspital Wien: C. Dau; Semmelweis-Frauenklinik der Krankenanstalt Rudolfstiftung Wien: B. Bechter; Universitätskinderklinik Wien: N. Haiden; Universitätsklinikum St. Pölten: U. Schneider; Universitätsklinikum Tulln: H. Salzer; Landeskrankenhaus

Feldkirch: B. Simma, B. Seidel; Medizinische Universität Insbruck: U. Kiechl-Kohlendorfer; Universitätsklinik Salzburg: M. Wald; Kepler Universitätsklinikum: G. Wiesinger-Eidenberger; Krankenhaus der Barmherzigen Schwestern Ried: A. Wimmer; Krankenhaus Dornbirn: E. Haberlandt; Krankenhaus der Barmherzigen Brüder Eisenstadt: H. P. Wagentristl; Universitätsklinik Graz: B. Urlesberger; Landeskrankenhaus Leoben-Eisenerz: A. Trinkl; Klinikum Klagenfurt am Wörthersee: R. Kraschl; Landeskrankenhaus Villach: R. Birnbacher. One further participant remained.

REFERENCES

1. AAP Section on Breastfeeding. *Breastfeeding and the Use of Human Milk*. The American Academy of Pediatrics. Available online at: http://pediatrics.aappublications.org/content/early/2012/02/22/peds.2011-3552 (Accessed July 13, 2017).
2. Hamprecht K, Maschmann J, Vochem M, Dietz K, Speer CP, Jahn G. Epidemiology of transmission of cytomegalovirus from mother to preterm infant by breastfeeding. *Lancet Lond Engl.* (2001) 357:513–18. doi: 10.1016/S0140-6736(00)04043-5
3. Schanler RJ, Fraley JK, Lau C, Hurst NM, Horvath L, Rossmann SN. Breastmilk cultures and infection in extremely premature infants. *J Perinatol.* (2011) 31:335–8. doi: 10.1038/jp.2011.13
4. Picaud JC, Houeto N, Buffin R, Loys C-M, Godbert I, Haÿs S. Additional protein fortification is necessary in extremely low-birth-weight infants fed human milk. *J Pediatr Gastroenterol Nutr.* (2016) 63:103–5. doi: 10.1097/MPG.0000000000001142
5. Peters MDJ, McArthur A, Munn Z. Safe management of expressed breast milk: a systematic review. *Women Birth J Aust Coll Midwives* (2016) 29:473–81. doi: 10.1016/j.wombi.2016.05.007
6. Steele C, Bixby C. Centralized breastmilk handling and bar code scanning improve safety and reduce breastmilk administration errors. *Breastfeed Med Off J Acad Breastfeed Med.* (2014) 9:426–9. doi: 10.1089/bfm.2014.0077
7. Picaud JC, Buffin R, Gremmo-Feger G, Rigo J, Putet G, Casper C. Working group of the french neonatal society on fresh human milk use in preterm infants. Review concludes that specific recommendations are needed to harmonise the provision of fresh mother's milk to their preterm infants. *Acta Paediatr.* (2018) 107:1145–55. doi: 10.1111/apa.14259
8. Buxmann H, Falk M, Goelz R, Hamprecht K, Poets CF, Schloesser RL. Feeding of very low birth weight infants born to HCMV-seropositive mothers in Germany, Austria and Switzerland. *Acta Paediatr.* (2010) 99:1819–23. doi: 10.1111/j.1651-2227.2010.01954.x
9. Omarsdottir S, Casper C, Akerman A, Polberger S, Vanpée M. Breastmilk handling routines for preterm infants in Sweden: a national cross-sectional study. *Breastfeed Med Off J Acad Breastfeed Med.* (2008) 3:165–70. doi: 10.1089/bfm.2007.0033
10. Cossey V, Johansson A-B, de Halleux V, Vanhole C. The use of human milk in the neonatal intensive care unit: practices in Belgium and Luxembourg. *Breastfeed Med Off J Acad Breastfeed Med.* (2012) 7:302–6. doi: 10.1089/bfm.2011.0112
11. Hamprecht K, Maschmann J, Müller D, Dietz K, Besenthal I, Goelz R, et al. Cytomegalovirus (CMV) inactivation in breast milk: reassessment of pasteurization and freeze-thawing. *Pediatr Res.* (2004) 56:529–35. doi: 10.1203/01.PDR.0000139483.35087.BE
12. Hamprecht K, Vochem M, Baumeister A, Boniek M, Speer CP, Jahn G. Detection of cytomegaloviral DNA in human milk cells and cell free milk whey by nested PCR. *J Virol Methods* (1998) 70:167–76. doi: 10.1016/S1386-6532(03)00074-X
13. Lanzieri TM, Dollard SC, Josephson CD, Schmid DS, Bialek SR. Breast milk-acquired cytomegalovirus infection and disease in VLBW and premature infants. *Pediatrics* (2013) 131:e1937–45. doi: 10.1542/peds.2013-0076
14. Goelz R, Meisner C, Bevot A, Hamprecht K, Kraegeloh-Mann I, Poets CF. Long-term cognitive and neurological outcome of preterm infants with postnatally acquired CMV infection through breast milk. *Arch Dis Child Fetal Neonatal Ed.* (2013) 98:F430–3. doi: 10.1136/archdischild-2012-303384
15. Jim W-T, Chiu N-C, Ho C-S, Shu C-H, Chang J-H, Hung H-Y, et al. Outcome of preterm infants with postnatal cytomegalovirus infection via breast milk: a two-year prospective follow-up study. *Medicine (Baltimore)* (2015) 94:e1835. doi: 10.1097/MD.0000000000001835
16. Kelly MS, Benjamin DK, Puopolo KM, Laughon MM, Clark RH, Mukhopadhyay S, et al. Postnatal Cytomegalovirus infection and the risk for bronchopulmonary dysplasia. *JAMA Pediatr.* (2015) 169:e153785. doi: 10.1001/jamapediatrics.2015.3785
17. Gunkel J, de Vries LS, Jongmans M, Koopman-Esseboom C, van Haastert IC, Eijsermans MCJ, et al. Outcome of preterm infants with postnatal cytomegalovirus infection. *Pediatrics* (2018) 141:e20170635. doi: 10.1542/peds.2017-0635
18. Bevot A, Hamprecht K, Krägeloh-Mann I, Brosch S, Goelz R, Vollmer B. Long-term outcome in preterm children with human cytomegalovirus infection transmitted via breast milk. *Acta Paediatr.* (2012) 101:e167–72. doi: 10.1111/j.1651-2227.2011.02538.x
19. Brecht KF, Goelz R, Bevot A, Krägeloh-Mann I, Wilke M, Lidzba K. Postnatal human cytomegalovirus infection in preterm infants has long-term neuropsychological sequelae. *J Pediatr.* (2015) 166:834–9.e1. doi: 10.1016/j.jpeds.2014.11.002
20. Ernährungskommission der Österreichischen Gesellschaft für Kinder- und Jugendheilkunde, Zwiauer K. Prävention von CMV-Infektionen bei Frühgeborenen durch Muttermilch. *Monatsschr Kinderheilkd* (2009) 157:795–7. doi: 10.1007/s00112-009-2019-5
21. Risiko der Zytomegalievirus-Infektion durch Muttermilchernährung von sehr unreifen Frühgeborenen. Empfehlung der Nationalen Stillkommission. (2006). Available online at: http://www.bfr.bund.de/cm/343/risiko_der_zytomegalievirus_infektion_durch_muttermilchernaehrung_von_sehr_unreifen_fruehgeborenen.pdf (Accessed July 24, 2017).
22. Widger J, O'Connell NH, Stack T. Breast milk causing neonatal sepsis and death. *Clin Microbiol Infect.* (2010) 16:1796–98. doi: 10.1111/j.1469-0691.2009.03071.x
23. Stock K, Griesmaier E, Brunner B, Neubauer V, Kiechl-Kohlendorfer U, Trawöger R. Pasteurization of breastmilk decreases the rate of postnatally acquired cytomegalovirus infections, but shows a nonsignificant trend to an increased rate of necrotizing enterocolitis in very preterm infants–a preliminary study. *Breastfeed Med.* (2015) 10:113–7. doi: 10.1089/bfm.2014.0108
24. Cossey V, Vanhole C, Eerdekens A, Rayyan M, Fieuws S, Schuermans A. Pasteurization of mother's own milk for preterm infants does not reduce the incidence of late-onset sepsis. *Neonatology* (2013) 103:170–6. doi: 10.1159/000345419
25. Klotz D, Joellenbeck M, Winkler K, Kunze M, Huzly D, Hentschel R. High temperature short time pasteurisation of human breast milk is efficient in retaining protein and reducing the bacterial count. *Acta Paediatr.* (2017) 106:763–7. doi: 10.1111/apa.13768
26. Klotz D, Falcone V, Jonas D, Schreiner M, Kunze M, Fuchs H, et al. High-temperature short-time (HTST)-Pasteurisierung zur CMV-Inaktivierung und Keimzahlreduktion in Muttermilch. *Monatsschr Kinderheilkd* (2018) 166:S1–S93. doi: 10.1007/s00112-018-0501-7
27. McGuire MK, McGuire MA. Got bacteria? The astounding, yet not-so-surprising, microbiome of human milk. *Curr Opin Biotechnol.* (2017) 44:63–8. doi: 10.1016/j.copbio.2016.11.013
28. Sammlung, Aufbewahrung und Umgang mit abgepumpter Muttermilch für das eigene Kind im Krankenhaus und zu Hause. Empfehlung der Nationalen Stillkommission vom 2. März (1998). Available online at: https://www.bfr.bund.de/cm/343/sammlung_aufbewahrung_und_umgang_mit_abgepumpter_muttermilch_fuer_das_eigene_kind.pdf (Accessed March 3, 2017).
29. Fusch G, Kwan C, Kotrri G, Fusch C. "Bed side" human milk analysis in the neonatal intensive care unit: a systematic

review. *Clin Perinatol.* (2017) 44:209–67. doi: 10.1016/j.clp.2016.11.001

30. Fusch G, Kwan C, Rochow N, Fusch C. MAMAS study group. milk analysis using milk analyzers in a standardized setting (mamas) study. *Monatsschr Kinderheilkd* (2017) 165(Suppl. 1):S20. doi: 10.1007/s00112-017-0301-5
31. Jochum F, Bührer C, Jochum F, Ganschow R, Kauth T, Körner A, et al. Warning against the indiscriminate use of human milk analyzers. Statement by the committee on nutrition of the German society for pediatrics. *Monatsschr Kinderheilkd* (2016) 164:500–1. doi: 10.1007/s00112-016-0049-3
32. Rosas R, Sanz MP, Fernández-Calle P, Alcaide MJ, Montes MT, Pastrana N, et al. Experimental study showed that adding fortifier and extra-hydrolysed proteins to preterm infant mothers' milk increased osmolality. *Acta Paediatr.* (2016) 105:e555–60. doi: 10.1111/apa.13522

12

Pasteurization Preserves IL-8 in Human Milk

*Marilyn V. Giorgi, Champa N. Codipilly, Debra Potak, Howard S. Heiman and Richard J. Schanler**

Lilling Family Neonatal Research Lab, Division of Neonatal-Perinatal Medicine, Cohen Children's Medical Center, Zucker School of Medicine at Hofstra, Northwell, Feinstein Institute for Medical Research, New York, NY, United States

Correspondence:
Richard J. Schanler
schanler@northwell.edu

Background: Pasteurized donor human milk is an alternative feeding when mothers' own milk is not available for premature infants. The effects of pasteurization on the host defense properties of human milk are unclear. We investigated the effects of Holder pasteurization on concentrations of anti-inflammatory and pro-inflammatory cytokines in human milk.

Objective: To compare concentrations of anti-inflammatory and pro-inflammatory cytokines before and after pasteurization of donor human milk.

Study Design: A single milk sample was obtained from each of 24 mothers of premature infants in the neonatal intensive care unit by electric breast pump and was stored at −80°C. At the time of pasteurization, milk samples were thawed and divided into two aliquots. The first aliquot was re-stored at −80°C and the second aliquot was heat-treated at 62.5°C for 30 min and then re-stored at −80°C. At the time of batch cytokine analyses samples were thawed rapidly.

Results: Most cytokine concentrations declined following pasteurization. The most prevalent cytokine, IL-8, was preserved (89%) following pasteurization. There were no relationships between gestational age, postnatal age of milk collection, duration of milk storage, and the concentrations cytokines.

Conclusion: In contrast to most cytokines after pasteurization, IL-8 is preserved or liberated from another compartment. The maintenance of IL-8 in human milk after pasteurization and the loss of anti-inflammatory cytokines following pasteurization, suggests that the effects of inflammatory activity in pasteurized human milk should be evaluated. These data may account, in part, for the lesser protective effect on the host of pasteurized donor human milk compared with mother's own milk.

Keywords: human milk, premature infants, donor human milk, pasteurized donor human milk, cytokines

INTRODUCTION

There is strong evidence to support feeding premature infants their mother's own milk (1–3). Not all mothers of premature infants, however, are able to supply sufficient milk to meet the needs of their infants throughout the NICU stay. When mother's own milk is not available, most clinicians recommend pasteurized donor human milk (DHM) as the second choice for feeding premature infants (4). There are advantages of using DHM as well as concerns limiting its use. When compared with preterm formula, DHM is associated with lower rates of necrotizing enterocolitis and lower mortality (4 6).

Pasteurized donor milk may not confer the same protective effect as mothers' own milk in the feeding of premature infants (7, 8). Donor milk is dissimilar to mother's own milk because it usually is obtained later in lactation when the contents of certain nutrients (protein, sodium) are lower and nutrient losses may have occurred from the collection and storage processes (lipid). Moreover, specific component concentrations may be affected by the heat-treatment process (7, 8). Holder pasteurization, heating milk to 62.5°C for 30 min, the usual method for processing donor human milk, is associated with substantial losses of immune components, including lactoferrin, secretory IgA, and lysozyme, and these losses are variable (9–11).

The cytokines in human milk (usually IL-1β, IL-2, IL-4, IL-5, IL-6, IL-8, IL-10, IL-12, EGF, TGF-α, TGF-β, TNF-α, and IFN-γ) are believed to provide passive immunity to the neonate (12–15). These cytokines are believed affect the maturation of the developing human intestine (16). As there are scant data on the effect of heat treatment on total cytokine concentrations in donor human milk, the objective of this study was to assess the effect of human milk pasteurization on its cytokine concentrations.

METHODS

A single milk sample of 50 mL from a complete collection of one breast was obtained from 24 mothers of premature infants in the NICU using an electric breast pump. Mothers were free of medical illnesses and not receiving medications, including antibiotics. Milk samples were collected fresh and stored at −80°C in sterile polypropylene containers until studied. Samples were thawed at room temperature and divided into two equal parts. The first part was divided into 2 mL aliquots and re-stored at −80°C until analyzed and the second part was heat-treated in a shaking water bath at 62.5°C for 30 min. A thermometer was placed in a centrally located non-study milk sample to ensure all study samples were maintained at 62.5°C. Subsequently, 2 mL aliquots of the pasteurized milk samples were re-stored at −80°C until analyzed.

Just prior to analyses, milk samples were thawed rapidly and centrifuged at 3000 rpm for 30 min to separate lipid and aqueous layers. Cytokine concentrations in aqueous milk samples were determined by flow cytometry (BD Facscaliber Flow Cytometer, San Diego, CA). Human Inflammation and Human Th1/Th2 cytokine kits (BD Cytometric Bead Array Analysis, San Diego, CA), following manufacturers protocols, were used for individual cytokine analyses. The use of both kits allowed an analysis of 10 cytokines: IL-1β, IL-2, IL-4, IL-5, IL-6, IL-8, IL-10, IL-12p70, TNF-α, IFN-γ. IL-10, and TNF-α measured by both kits were the same suggesting no interassay variation.

Paired samples (before- and after-pasteurization) were evaluated for IL-1β, IL-2, IL-4, IL-5, IL-6, IL-8, IL-10, TNF-α, IL-12p70, and IFN-γ concentrations. The adequacy of pasteurization was confirmed by comparing the concentrations of alkaline phosphatase and lipase in before and after treatment samples.

Sample size was chosen to detect a difference of one standard deviation from the mean. We chose a significance of $p = 0.005$ due to multiple comparisons and a power of 0.80. Pearson correlation coefficients were used to compare relationships between variables. Before- and after-pasteurization results were analyzed by paired t-test. The data were standardized using z-scores, then the changes of IL-8 were compared to the other nine cytokines measured using a RMANOVA model.

The study was approved by the Institutional Review Board of the North Shore Long Island Jewish Health System (now known as Northwell Health). Written informed consent was obtained from all mothers.

RESULTS

Milk samples, collected at 4–54 days postpartum from mothers delivering infants between 27 and 36 weeks gestation, were stored at −80°C for 8–157 days prior to analyses. There were no relationships between gestational age, postnatal age of milk collection, duration of milk storage, and the concentrations of cytokines in milk ($p > 0.05$). The completeness of pasteurization was confirmed by measuring milk alkaline phosphatase (mean 1946 and 9 U/L) and lipase (mean 48.8 and <3 U/L) before and after treatment, respectively, $p < 0.005$.

The concentrations of all cytokines declined following pasteurization (**Figures 1, 2**). There was variable preservation (18–58%) of cytokines following pasteurization. The most abundant cytokine, IL-8, was preserved (89%) after pasteurization compared to other cytokines (**Figure 3**).

DISCUSSION

Mother's milk provides important protection to the premature infant who has a developmentally delayed immune system (17). As not all mothers of premature infants are able to provide 100% of their infants' needs, donor human milk has emerged as an alternative feeding strategy. As a result there is an increased

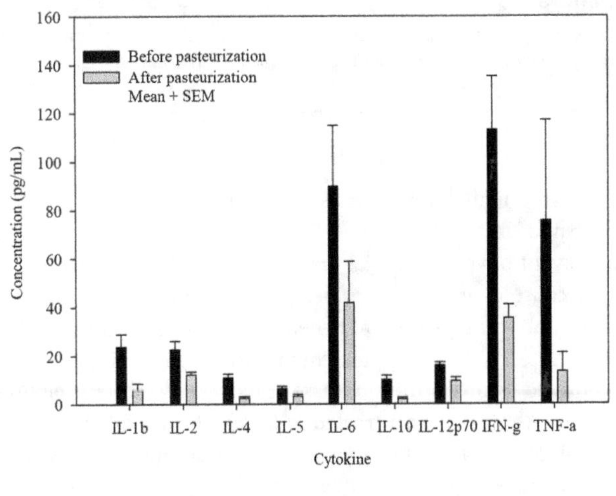

FIGURE 1 | Cytokine concentrations before and after pasteurization. The concentration of cytokines of 24 milk samples measured in duplicates in thawed human milk before and after pasteurization. All cytokine concentrations decreased significantly, $p \leq 0.005$.

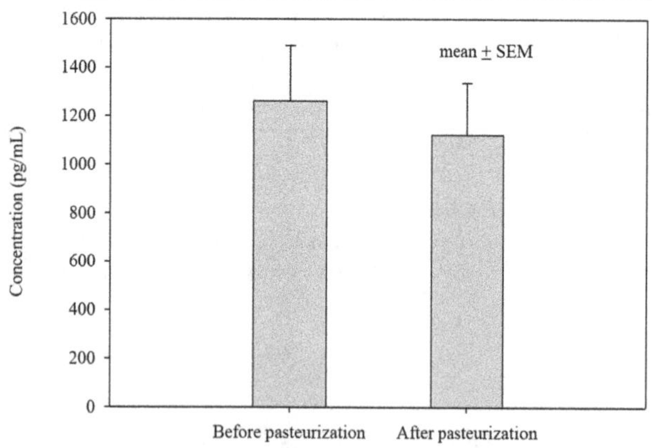

FIGURE 2 | IL-8 concentration before and after pasteurization. The concentration of IL-8 of 24 milk samples measured in duplicates in thawed milk. The concentration after pasteurization was not changed significantly, $p = 0.543$.

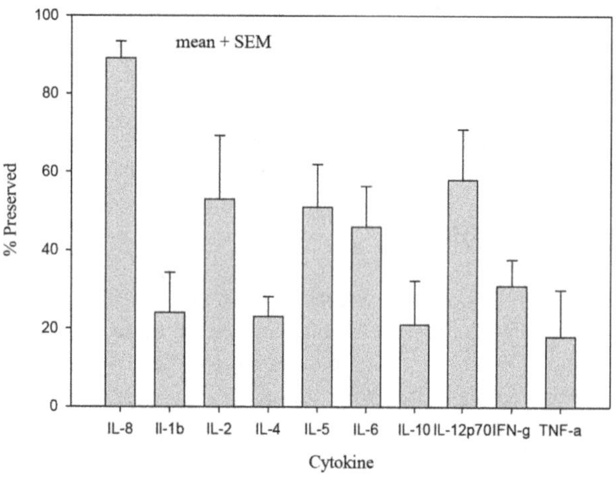

FIGURE 3 | Percentage of cytokine preserved after pasteurization. Only IL-8 concentration in heat treated human milk was preserved (89%) compared with other cytokines which were significantly less preserved after heat treatment, $p < 0.005$.

interest in donated human milk and a marked increase in donor milk banks in the US. Donor human milk is heat treated for the prevention of microbial transmission. There are concerns that because of its heat treatment donor human milk may not provide the same protective benefit as mother's own milk (2, 3, 6, 18). Indeed, when supplemented with bovine milk products, pasteurized human milk is associated with more infectious morbidity than non-heat treated milk, suggesting that there may be some loss of immune properties once human milk is heat-processed (4, 19).

Among the immune components in human milk are a variety of cytokines, whose concentrations vary with lactation stage, from colostrum to mature milk, between foremilk and hindmilk, between mothers delivering at term or prematurely, and with maternal medical conditions (20, 21). We found using a reproducible common laboratory assay that pasteurized human milk contained both pro- and anti- inflammatory cytokines (20, 22–24). We found a generalized reduction in cytokine concentrations after pasteurization. The pro-inflammatory cytokine IL-8 was the most preserved (89%) cytokine after pasteurization. Despite the measured declines in anti-inflammatory cytokines after pasteurization, the retention rates of 18–58% suggest that donor milk still provides potential protection to the recipient infant.

Our data qualitatively reinforce other reports of the preservation of IL-8 after pasteurization (15). We speculate that the preservation of IL-8 in heat-treated milk may be a concern for the premature infant who is susceptible to a variety of inflammatory conditions. IL-8, a major mediator of inflammatory responses and a chemoattractant, is found in leukocytes and endothelial cells. Its preservation may be a result of a strong tertiary structure (25). The other two pro-inflammatory cytokines preserved at a higher levels are IL-2 (53%) and IL-12p70 (58%), probably also due to their protein structure.

The imbalance favoring pro-inflammatory cytokines in pasteurized milk potentially could explain the lack of consistent short-term benefits of this milk when compared with mother's own milk (6, 18, 26). There are inconsistent beneficial outcomes of inflammation-related diseases in premature infants receiving donor human milk: necrotizing enterocolitis, bronchopulmonary dysplasia, and retinopathy of prematurity (6, 26–29). Moreover, long-term studies fail to demonstrate better outcomes of pasteurized donor milk-fed infants (30). Nevertheless, when compared with preterm formula, short-term benefits of pasteurized donor milk are noted (31).

Our data might be used to question the process of pasteurization, classic Holder pasteurization, as short-time high temperature pasteurization methods have been associated with less protein degradation (32). Indeed, the high temperature treatment reported greater retention of bioactive factors in human milk (IgA, alkaline phosphatase, bile salt-stimulated lipase) with similar antibacterial efficacy when compared with Holder pasteurization. The expense and practicality of the high temperature method needs further evaluation to encourage its use.

Thus, we report preservation of pro-inflammatory cytokines after pasteurization of human milk suggesting that heat treatment may have significantly different effects on the premature infant with a developing immune system.

AUTHOR CONTRIBUTIONS

All authors listed have made a substantial, direct and intellectual contribution to the work, and approved it for publication.

REFERENCES

1. Eidelman AI, Schanler RJ. Section on breastfeeding. Breastfeeding and the use of human milk. *Pediatrics* (2012) 129:e827–41. doi: 10.1542/peds.2011-3552
2. Morales Y, Schanler RJ. Human milk and clinical outcomes in VLBW infants: how compelling is the evidence of benefit? *Semin Perinatol.* (2007) 31:83–8. doi: 10.1053/j.semperi.2007.02.002
3. Underwood MA. Human milk for the premature infant. *Pediatr Clin North Am.* (2013) 60:189–207. doi: 10.1016/j.pcl.2012.09.008
4. ESPGHAN Committee on Nutrition, Arslanoglu S, Corpeleijn W, Moro G, Braegger C, Campoy C, et al. Donor human milk for preterm infants: current evidence and research directions. *J Pediatr Gastroenterol Nutr.* (2013) 57:535–42. doi: 10.1097/MPG.0b013e3182a3af0a
5. Abrams SA, Schanler RJ, Lee ML, Rechtman DJ. Greater mortality and morbidity in extremely preterm infants fed a diet containing cow milk protein products. *Breastfeed Med.* (2014) 9:281–5. doi: 10.1089/bfm.2014.0024
6. Schanler RJ, Lau C, Hurst NM, Smith EO. Randomized trial of donor human milk versus preterm formula as substitutes for mothers' own milk in the feeding of extremely premature infants. *Pediatrics* (2005) 116:400–6. doi: 10.1542/peds.2004-1974
7. Akinbi H, Meinzen-Derr J, Auer C, Ma Y, Pallum D, Kusano R, et al. Alterations in the host defense properties of human milk following prolonged storage or pasteurization. *J Pediatr Gastroenterol Nutr.* (2010) 51:347–52. doi: 10.1097/MPG.0b013e3181e07f0a
8. Groer M, Duffy A, Morse S, Kane B, Zaritt J, Roberts S, et al. Cytokines, chemokines, and growth factors in banked human donor milk for preterm infants. *J Hum Lact.* (2014) 30:317–23. doi: 10.1177/0890334414527795
9. Koenig A, de Albuquerque Diniz EM, Barbarosa SF, Vaz FA. Immunologic factors in human milk: the effects of gestational age and pasteurization. *J Hum Lact.* (2005) 21:439–43. doi: 10.1177/0890334405280652
10. Czank C, Prime DK, Hartmann B, Simmer K, Hartmann PE. Retention of the immunological proteins of pasteurized human milk in relation to pasteurizer design and practice. *Pediatr Res.* (2009) 66:374–9. doi: 10.1203/PDR.0b013e3181b4554a
11. Garza C, Hopkinson JM, Schanler RJ. Human milk banking. In: Howell RR, Morriss FH Jr, Pickering LK, editors. *Human Milk in Infant Nutrition and Health*. Springfield, IL: Charles C. Thomas (1986). p. 225–55.
12. Garofalo R. Cytokines in human milk. *J Pediatr.* (2010) 156(Suppl. 2):S36–40. doi: 10.1016/j.jpeds.2009.11.019
13. Goldman AS, Chheda S, Garofalo R, Schmalstieg RC. Cytokines in human milk: properties and potential effects upon the mammary gland and the neonate. *J Mammary Gland Biol Neoplasia* (1996) 1:351–258. doi: 10.1007/BF02018078
14. Chirico G, Gasparoni A. Immunologic components of human milk. *Immunol Infect.* (2006) 2:27–30. doi: 10.4081/hmr.v2i10.448
15. Ewaschuk JB, Unger S, O'Connor DL, Stone D, Harvey S, Clandinin MT, et al. Effect of pasteurization on selected immune components of donated human breast milk. *J Perinatol.* (2011) 31:593–8. doi: 10.1038/jp.2010.209
16. Maheshwari A, Lu W, Lacson A, Barleycorn AA, Nolan S, Christensen RD, et al. Effects of interleukin-8 on the developing human intestine. *Cytokine* (2002) 20:256–67. doi: 10.1006/cyto.2002.1996
17. Polat A, Tunc T, Erdem G, Yerebasmaz N, Tas A, Beken S, et al. Interleukin-8 and its receptors in human milk from mothers of full-term and premature infants. *Breastfeed Med.* (2016) 11:247–51. doi: 10.1089/bfm.2015.0186
18. Corpeleijn WE, de Waard M, Christmann V, van Goudoever JB, Jansen-van der Weide MC, Kooi EM, et al. Effect of donor milk on severe infections and mortality in very low-birth-weight infants: the early nutrition study randomized clinical trial. *JAMA Pediatr.* (2016) 170:654–61. doi: 10.1001/jamapediatrics.2016.0183
19. Narayanan I, Prakash K, Murthy NS, Gujral VV. Randomised controlled trial of effect of raw and Holder pasteurised human milk and of formula supplements on incidence of neonatal infection. *Lancet* (1984) 2:1111–3.
20. Freitas NA, Santiago LTC, Kurokawa CS, Meira Jr JD, Corrente JE, Rugolo LMSS. Effect of preeclampsia on human milk cytokine levels. *J Matern Fetal Neonatal Med.* (2018). doi: 10.1080/14767058.2018.1429395. [Epub ahead of print].
21. Brenmoehl J, Ohde D, Wirthgen E, Hoeflich A. Cytokines in milk and the role of TGF-beta. *Best Pract Res Clin Endocrinol Metab.* (2018) 32:47–56. doi: 10.1016/j.beem.2018.01.006
22. Ernst D, Bolton G, Recktenwald D, Cameron MJ, Danesh A, Persad D, et al. Bead-based flow cytometric assays: a multiplex assay platform with applications in diagnostic microbiology. In: Ernst D, Bolton G, Rectenwald D, Cameron MJ, Danesh A, Persad D, Kelvin DJ, Gaur A, editors. *Advanced Techniques in Diagnostic Microbioilogy*. Boston, MA: Springer (2016). pp. 427–43.
23. Morgan E, Varro R, Sepulveda H, Ember A, Apgar J, Wilson J, et al. Cytometric bead array: a multiplexed assay platform with applications in various areas of biology. *Clin Immunol.* (2004) 110:252–66. doi: 10.1016/j.clim.2003.11.017
24. Holmlund U, Amoudruz P, Johansson MA, Haileselassie Y, Ongoiba A, Kayentao K, et al. Maternal country of origin, breast milk characteristics and potential influences on immunity in offspring. *Clin Exp Immunol.* (2010) 162:500–9. doi: 10.1111/j.1365-2249.2010.04275.x
25. Rajarathnam K, Sykes BD, Dewald B, Baggiolini M, Clark-Lewis I. Disulfide bridges in interleukin-8 probed using non-natural disulfide analogues: dissociation of roles in structure from function. *Biochemistry* (1999) 38:7653–8. doi: 10.1021/bi990033v
26. Sullivan S, Schanler RJ, Kim JH, Patel AL, Trawöger R, Kiechl-Kohlendorfer U, et al. An exclusively human milk-based diet is associated with a lower rate of necrotizing enterocoitis than a diet of human milk and bovine milk-based products. *J Pediatr.* (2010) 156:562–7.e1. doi: 10.1016/j.jpeds.2009.10.040
27. Schanler RJ, Schulman RJ, Lau C. Feeding strategies for premature infants: Beneficial outcomes of feeding fortified human milk vs. preterm formula. *Pediatrics* (1999) 103:1150–7. doi: 10.1542/peds.103.6.1150
28. Kantorowska A, Wei JC, Cohen RS, Lawrence RA, Gould JB, Lee HC. Impact of donor milk availability on breast milk use and necrotizing enterocolitis rates. *Pediatrics* (2016) 137:e20153123. doi: 10.1542/peds.2015-3123.
29. Villamor-Martinez E, Pierro M, Cavallaro G, Mosca F, Kramer BW, Villamor E. Donor human milk protects against bronchopulmonary dysplacia: a systemic review and meta analysis. *Nutrients* (2018) 10:E238. doi: 10.3390/nu10020238
30. O'Connor DL, Gibbins S, Kiss A, Bando N, Brennan-Donnan J, Ng E, et al. Effect of supplemental donor human milk compared with preterm formula on neurodevelopment of very low-birth-weight infants at 18 months: a randomized clinical trial. *JAMA* (2016) 316:1897–905. doi: 10.1001/jama.2016.16144
31. Quigley M, Embleton ND, McGuire W. Formula versus donor breast milk for feeding preterm or low birth weight infants. *Cochrane Database Syst Rev.* (2018) CD002971. doi: 10.1002/14651858.CD002971
32. Klotz D, Jollenbeck M, Winkler K, Kunze M, Huzly D, Hentschel R. High temperature short-time pasteurization of human breastmilk is efficient in retaining protein and reducing the bacterial count. *Acta Pediatr.* (2017) 106:763–7. doi: 10.1111/apa.13768

13

Human Milk Oligosaccharides in the Prevention of Necrotizing Enterocolitis: A Journey from *In Vitro* and *In Vivo* Models to Mother-Infant Cohort Studies

*Lars Bode**

Department of Pediatrics and Larsson-Rosenquist Foundation Mother-Milk-Infant Center of Research Excellence (LRF MOMI CORE), University of California, San Diego, La Jolla, CA, United States

Correspondence:
Lars Bode
lbode@ucsd.edu

Preterm infants who receive human milk instead of formula are 6- to 10-times less likely to develop necrotizing enterocolitis (NEC), one of the most common and devastating intestinal disorders that affects 5–10% of all very-low-birth-weight infants. Combined data from *in vitro* tissue culture models, *in vivo* preclinical studies in animal models, as well human mother-infant cohort studies support the hypothesis that human milk oligosaccharides (HMOs), complex sugars that are highly abundant in human milk but not in infant formula, contribute to the beneficial effects of human milk feeding in reducing NEC. The almost 20-year long journey of testing this hypothesis took an interesting turn during HMO *in vivo* efficacy testing and structure elucidation, suggesting that the original hypothesis may indeed be correct and specific HMO reduce NEC risk, however, the underlying mechanisms are likely different than originally postulated.

Keywords: preterm infant, necrotizing enterocolitis, breast milk, infant nutrition, human milk oligosaccharide

NECROTIZING ENTEROCOLITIS (NEC) IS ONE OF THE MOST COMMON AND DEVASTATING INTESTINAL DISORDERS IN PRETERM INFANTS, BUT THERAPEUTIC OPTIONS ARE LIMITED

Necrotizing enterocolitis (NEC) is one of the most common and devastating intestinal disorders in preterm infants [reviewed in (1)]. In the United States and Canada the mean prevalence of NEC in infants with a birth weight between 500 and 1,500 g is about 7%, but can be much higher in certain neonatal intensive care units (NICUs) (2–5). NEC is one the most common causes of gastrointestinal surgical emergencies among neonates and is also the most common cause of death among neonates requiring gastrointestinal surgery (6–8). The mortality rate for NEC patients ranges from 10 to 50% and approaches 100% for patients with the most severe form of the disease (2). Survivors are often faced with long-term neurological complications (9). The total annual costs to care for infants with NEC in the United States alone are estimated to be between $500 million and $1 billion (1, 10, 11).

Medical interventions to treat NEC are limited and typically include bowel decompression, discontinuation of enteral feeding and broad-spectrum intravenous antibiotics [reviewed in (1, 12, 13)]. Surgical interventions range from drain placement to resection of diseased bowel, but once surgery is required, the outcome is often poor.

The rapid onset, fulminant progression, and limited treatment options make it most desirable to prevent NEC all together before it strikes. Preventative approaches include the use of enteral antibiotics, administering pre-, pro-, or synbiotics, growth factors, cytokines, and glucocorticoids [reviewed in (1, 14, 15)]. Most of these approaches are however controversial (16–18) or have not been validated in preclinical or clinical studies.

Overall, therapeutic options to treat or prevent NEC are highly limited. New safe and effective NEC therapies are urgently needed to meet the clinical needs of preterm infants that suffer from this devastating condition.

NEC ETIOLOGY AND PATHOGENESIS ARE COMPLEX AND IN PART UNDEFINED

Instead of representing one clearly defined disorder, NEC may represent a syndrome, with a variety of etiologies and commonalities in the underlying pathogenetic mechanisms. Although NEC pathogenesis is incompletely understood, it likely involves intestinal immaturity and an excessive inflammatory response to an imbalance in the microbial colonization of the infant's intestine [dysbiosis; reviewed in (1, 19)]. One of the proposed models suggests that perinatal hypoxia or a mild postnatal infection could be the primary insults causing mild mucosal damage and impaired intestinal epithelial barrier function (19). Following (formula) feeding and a proliferation of the intestinal microbiome, an increased uptake of bacteria and bacterial metabolites including lipopolysaccharides (LPS) into the mucosa triggers the endogenous production of inflammatory cytokines such as platelet-activating factor (PAF) and tumor necrosis factor alpha (TNFα), which in turn further enhance intestinal permeability, closing a vicious circle. PAF also synergizes with LPS and TNFα, reaching a threshold necessary to induce an inflammatory cascade, which includes mucosal neutrophil infiltration and activation. Eventually, vasoconstriction occurs and leads to ischemia and subsequent reperfusion. Reactive oxygen species (ROS) produced by activated neutrophils and intestinal epithelial xanthine oxidase may then cause severe tissue necrosis and breakdown of the intestinal barrier. Entry of large amounts of bacteria and LPS leads to sepsis, shock, and death. **Figure 1** shows a flow diagram of the proposed pathogenesis of NEC [modified after Hsueh et al. (19)].

NEC INCIDENCE IS SIGNIFICANTLY LOWER IN HUMAN MILK-FED INFANTS COMPARED TO FORMULA-FED INFANTS

Several studies have shown that NEC incidence is 6- to 10-fold lower in human milk-fed infants compared to formula-fed infants (20–23). It is unclear whether components in infant formula trigger NEC, whether components in human milk protect from NEC, or whether a combination of both is responsible for the gap in NEC incidence between human milk-fed and formula-fed infants. However, a significant number of infants still develop NEC although they exclusively receive human milk and are not exposed to infant formula. These observations speak against the notion that components in infant formula trigger NEC and support the idea that bioactive components in human milk protect from NEC. Interpersonal variation in human milk composition may explain why some infants still develop NEC despite receiving human milk.

HUMAN MILK OLIGOSACCHARIDES (HMOS) ARE THE THIRD MOST ABUNDANT COMPONENT OF HUMAN MILK. HMOS HELP SHAPE THE INFANT GUT MICROBIOME AND MAY PREVENT NEC-ASSOCIATED DYSBIOSIS

Human milk contains a high amount of complex glycans (carbohydrates, sugars) that are not present in infant formula [reviewed in (24–28)], which led us to hypothesize that these human milk oligosaccharides (HMOs) at least in part contribute to the lower incidence of NEC in human milk-fed infants. HMOs are the third most abundant component in human milk (5–20 g/L), surpassed only by the concentrations of lactose (~70 g/L) and lipids (~40 g/L). HMO composition follows a basic blueprint that connects the five building blocks glucose (Glc), galactose (Gal), N-acetylglucosamine (GlcNAc), fucose (Fuc), and the sialic acid derivative N-acetylneuraminic acid (Neu5Ac) in specific linkages. More than 150 different and structurally distinct HMOs have been identified and the composition varies between women as well as over the course of lactation. Once ingested, HMOs withstand the low pH in the infant's stomach (29), resist degradation by pancreatic and brush border membrane enzymes (29, 30), and reach the infant's distal small intestine and colon. Here, HMOs act as prebiotics that serve as metabolic substrates for potentially beneficial bacteria to thrive while supressing other, potentially harmful bacteria. In addition, HMOs are antiadhesives that serve as soluble adhesion receptor decoys and block the attachment of potential viral or bacterial pathogens to the infant's intestinal epithelial cell surface, a process that otherwise allows pathogens to proliferate, and in some cases invade, and cause disease. Moreover, HMOs are antimicrobials that directly kill bacteria (cytotoxic) or at least reduce bacterial proliferation (cytostatic). Altogether, these mechanisms shape the infant gut microbiome early in life (26–28, 31) and may counteract dysbiosis at the early stages of NEC pathogenesis shown in **Figure 1**.

HMOS ARE ABSORBED INTACT, INTERFERE WITH IMMUNE CELL-CELL INTERACTIONS, AND MAY REDUCE NEC-ASSOCIATED INFLAMMATION

HMOs are not only present in the infant's intestinal lumen, they are also absorbed, reach the systemic circulation, and are excreted intact with the infant's urine (32–35). Thus, in addition to effects in the intestinal lumen, HMOs may also interfere with the inflammatory cascade involved in NEC pathogenesis.

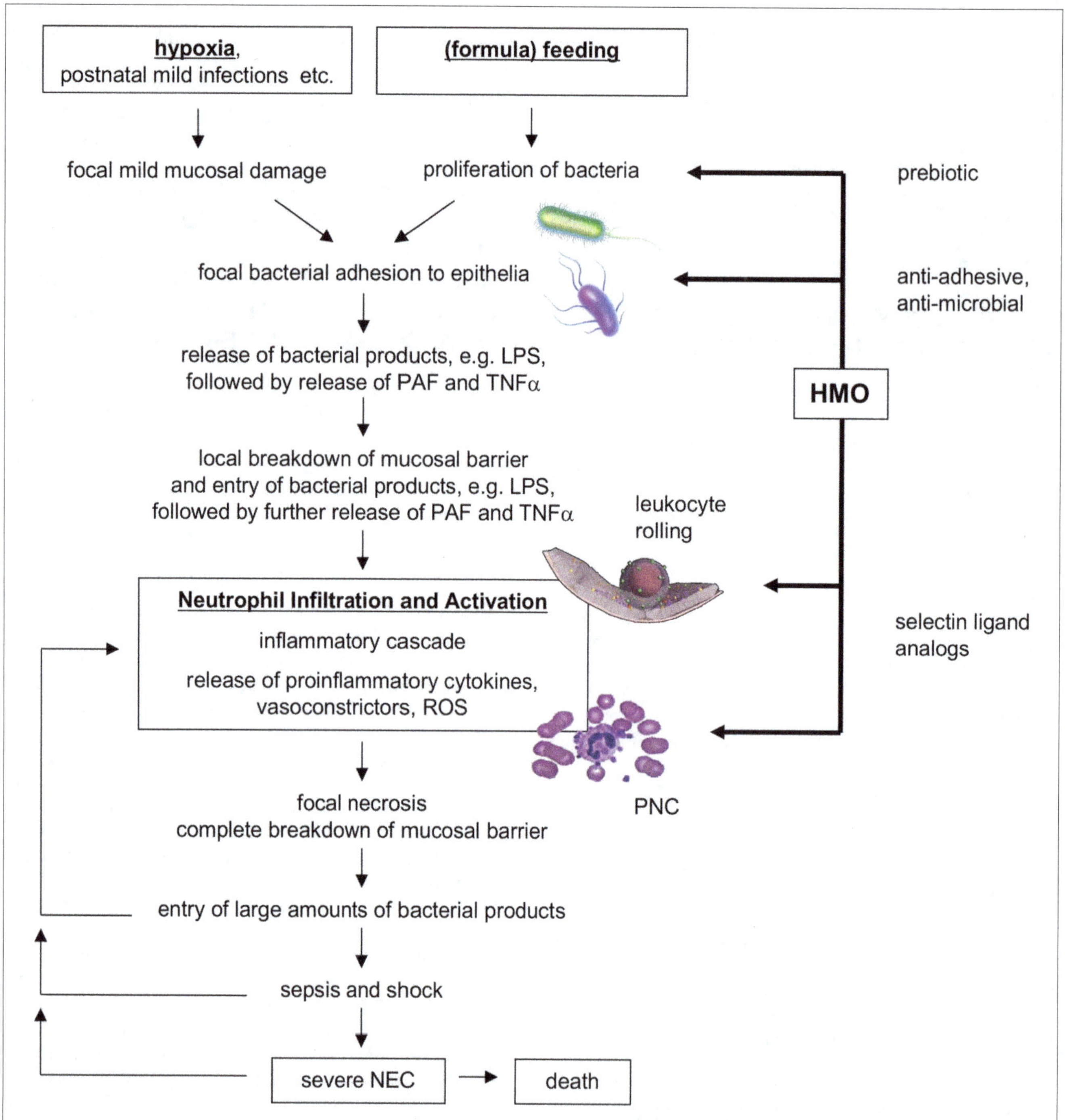

FIGURE 1 | Flow diagram of proposed NEC pathogenesis and potential benefits of HMOs. HMO, human milk oligosaccharides; NEC, necrotizing enterocolitis; PAF, platelet-activating factor; PNC, platelet-neutrophil complexes; ROS, reactive oxygen species [modified after Hsueh et al. (19)].

Mucosal neutrophil infiltration and activation are thought to be early key events in NEC pathogenesis. Neutrophils are first decelerated from the blood stream before they adhere to endothelial cells and transmigrate (**Figure 2A**). Neutrophil deceleration, the "rolling" on activated endothelial cells, is mediated by adhesion molecules of the selectin family (37). Selectins bind to carbohydrate determinants, predominantly Sialyl Lewis x (SLe^x; NeuAcα2-3Galβ1-4(Fucα1-3)GalNAc) (38), on glycoconjugate ligands. While L-selectin (CD62L) is constitutively expressed on leukocytes, P- and E-selectins (CD62P and E) are expressed on platelets and endothelial cells, and their expression is upregulated by inflammatory cytokines such as TNFα. P-selectin expression is increased on intestinal endothelial cells in NEC patients and strongly

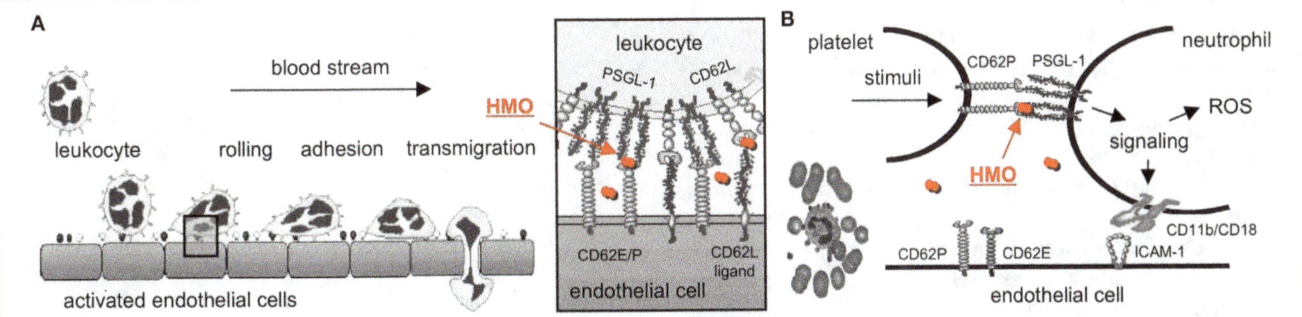

FIGURE 2 | Selectin-mediated cell-cell interactions and potential interference with HMOs. **(A)** Leukocytes decelerate from the blood stream before they adhere and finally transmigrate to the site of inflammation. The initial rolling, the first interaction between leukocytes and activated endothelial cells, is mediated by selectins (box). HMOs (red dots) serve as selectin ligand analogs, reduce selectin ligand binding, and are thought to reduce leukocyte rolling and infiltration (modified after http://ley-leukocyte.liai.org). **(B)** Activated platelets upregulate expression of P-selectin (CD62P), which binds to P-Selectin Glycoprotein Ligand-1 (PSGL-1) on neutrophils, which establishes platelet-neutrophil-complex (PNC) formation and triggers a signaling cascade with an increase in neutrophil adhesion molecules and production of reactive oxygen species (ROS). Once again, HMOs serve as selectin-ligand analogs, reduce P-selectin-PSGL-1 binding, and neutrophil activation [modified after Cerletti et al. (36)]. CD62E/P, E- or P-Selectin; CD62L, L-Selectin; HMO, human milk oligosaccharide; PSGL-1, P-Selectin Glycoprotein Ligand-1.

correlates with neutrophil infiltration (39). P-selectin knockout mice are protected from PAF-induced intestinal necrosis (40), indicating an essential role of P-selectin in NEC pathogenesis.

Neutrophil activation and ROS production lead to progression of NEC pathogenesis. Platelet-neutrophil complexes (PNC) represent a highly activated subpopulation of neutrophils primed for adhesion and increased ROS production. PNC formation is increased after ischemia/reperfusion (41, 42), one of the key events in NEC progression. PNC formation is initiated by the binding of P-selectin on activated platelets to PSGL-1 on neutrophils (**Figure 2B**). PSGL-1 signaling induces ROS production as well as expression of CD11b/CD18 adhesion molecules that facilitate neutrophil binding to platelets and activated endothelial cells (36). Blocking P-selectin with a P-selectin antibody completely inhibits the increase in ROS production and CD11b/CD18 expression (43), documenting the essential role of P-selectin in PNC formation.

While both neutrophil infiltration as well as neutrophil activation and ROS production require selectin-ligand interactions, HMOs have been shown to carry SLex determinants, suggesting they act as soluble selectin ligand analogs (44). Indeed, we were the first to provide evidence that a mixture of sialylated HMOs reduces selectin-mediated neutrophil rolling and adhesion *in vitro* (45) as well as PNC formation and neutrophil activation *ex vivo* (46). However, at this stage it was unclear whether or not these *in vitro*/*ex vivo* results translate to *in vivo*, inhibit key events in NEC pathogenesis, and reduce or prevent NEC.

IN VIVO EFFICACY TESTING IN A NEONATAL RAT MODEL CONFIRMS THAT HMOS REDUCE NEC-LIKE SYMPTOMS AND IMPROVE SURVIVAL

Results from *in vitro* and *ex vivo* studies supported our hypothesis that HMOs contribute to a lower NEC risk in human milk-fed infants, but to confirm this hypothesis, we needed *in vivo* proof—ideally by showing HMO efficacy in preterm infants. However, at this stage, a human intervention study was not feasible for several reasons: (1) We would need to recruit between 800 and 1,000 preterm infants to power the study. (2) We would need several kg of HMOs to administer to the intervention group every 2 to 3 h for at least the first four weeks of life, and HMOs were simply not available in that amount. (3) There was no information which of the more than 150 different HMOs would be effective. It could be that all HMOs are effective, but it could also be that the effects are highly structure-specific and limited to just one or two selective HMOs. (4) The study design itself was (and remains to be) challenging. It is known that formula-fed infants are at a significantly higher NEC risk and it would be unethical to use formula-feeding without HMOs as intervention control. Thus, we selected a rodent NEC model to test our hypothesis first, allowing us to use much smaller amounts of HMOs for initial efficacy testing. Afterwards, the small animal model would also enable us to conduct structure-activity relationship (SAR) studies and elucidate the underlying mechanisms of action.

The NEC model in neonatal rats was originally described by Barlow and Santulli (47) and later modified as follows (48): Pregnant time-dated Sprague-Dawley rats were induced at term. The pups were immediately removed from the dam at birth to ensure they don't receive any rat milk, which also contains some oligosaccharides. The pups were randomized into one of the different study groups. Some pups were returned to the dam to serve as dam-fed control. All other animals remained separated from the dam, housed in a temperature- and humidity-controlled incubator and, twice daily, orally gavaged with a special rodent formula with or without HMOs that were isolated from pooled human donor milk. All animals, dam-fed and gavaged, were exposed to 10 min of hypoxia thrice daily in a modular chamber. All animals were sacrificed 96 h post-partum; their intestines were collected and inspected for the presence of gross necrotic changes or NEC-characteristic *Pneumatosis intestinalis*. A section of the terminal ileum was prepared for H&E staining and scored blindly based on morphological changes that included epithelial sloughing, villus oedema, infiltration of neutrophils, apoptosis of villus enterocytes, crypt hyperplasia, and misaligned nuclei in the epithelium.

The HMO intervention had an immense effect in the neonatal rat NEC model. Pups that received HMOs with their formula had a significantly higher survival rate than their littermates that did not receive HMOs (49). Their intestines were not as dark and bloody with less patchy necrosis and less evidence of haemorrhagic intestine as well as intramural gas cysts (*Pneumatosis intestinalis*). These macroscopic observations were aligned with microscopic evaluation of ileum sections, showing that pups that received HMOs had significantly lower pathology scores than their littermates that did not receive HMOs. From this first set of experiments we concluded that HMOs indeed reduce NEC-like symptoms in the neonatal rat model and even improved survival significantly.

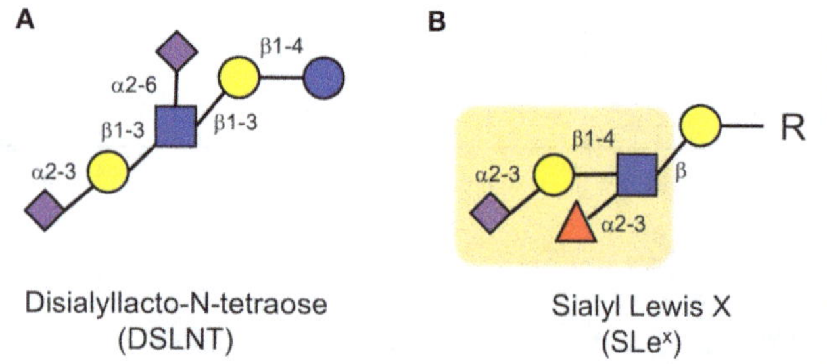

FIGURE 3 | Disialyl-lacto-N-tetraose (DSLNT) **(A)** reduces NEC-like symptoms in neonatal rats, but the HMO does not contain the Sialyl Lewis X (SLe^X) determinant **(B)**. The Sialyl Lewis X is highlighted as an orange background (blue circle, glucose; yellow circle, galactose; blue square, N-acetylglucosamine; red triangle, fucose; purple diamond, sialic acid).

A SPECIFIC HMO, DISIALYLLACTO-N-TETRAOSE (DSLNT) IS MOST EFFECTIVE IN REDUCING NEC IN NEONATAL RATS, BUT THE UNDERLYING MECHANISMS ARE LIKELY DIFFERENT THAN ORIGINALLY POSTULATED

Next, we applied a multidimensional chromatography approach to address the question which of the more than 150 different HMOs was responsible for the beneficial effects we observed in the neonatal rat model (49). In a first dimension, we used anion exchange chromatography to separate the HMOs by charge. Every sialic acid moiety contributes a negative charge to an HMO. HMOs without sialic acid carry no negative charge and are neutral; HMOs with one sialic acid carry one negative charge; HMOs with two sialic acids carry two negative charges, etc. We then tested these charge-fractions in the neonatal rat NEC model and found that HMOs with two sialic acids were most effective. However, there are several HMOs with two sialic acids. Thus, in a second dimension, we used gel filtration chromatography to separate the fraction that contained HMOs with two sialic acids by size. We then tested the generated subfractions for their efficacy in the neonatal rat NEC model and identified one specific subfraction, containing only one HMO, that was most effective. Finally, we used a combination of exoglycosidase enzyme digestion and gas chromatography mass spectrometry (GC-MS) of partially methylated alditol acetate (PMAA) derivatives to structurally characterize the effective HMO as disialyllacto-N-tetraose (DSLNT, **Figure 3A**). We further confirmed that the effect of DSLNT is highly structure-specific. For example, enzymatic removal of sialic acid at the terminal galactose completely abolished the effect.

While these results were very exciting, they were also quite puzzling. The *in vitro* and *ex vivo* data showed that HMOs interfere with selectin-mediated cell-cell interactions, leading to a reduction in neutrophil rolling, adhesion and transmigration as well as a reduction in neutrophil activation, which were considered key elements in NEC pathogenesis. However, we did not observe a reduction in neutrophil infiltration in the neonatal rat NEC model. Moreover, DSLNT, the HMO we identified as being most effective in reducing NEC-like symptoms in rats, did not contain a SLe^x determinant that is part of selectin ligands (**Figure 3**). While there is some structural ambiguity around the glycan determinant for selectin ligands (50), fucose is an essential component for a glycan to serve as a selectin ligand as demonstrated in patients with congenital disorder of glycosylation (CDG) type IIc, also known as leukocyte adhesion deficiency (LAD) type 2 (51). The genetic defect in CDG IIc patients leads to impaired intracellular fucose metabolism, which results in decreased fucosylation of cell surface proteins (52), including selectin ligands. Consequently, CDG IIc patients present with impaired neutrophil motility and extravasation and recurrent infections (51). Although DSLNT is effective in reducing NEC-like symptoms in the neonatal rat model, it is not fucosylated. Thus, it appears unlikely that DSLNT interferes with selectin-mediated neutrophil infiltration and activation. Therefore, while the hypothesis that HMOs contribute to a lower NEC risk in human milk-fed infants may indeed be correct, the underlying protective mechanisms are likely different than originally anticipated.

While it is known that HMOs shape microbial communities (26–28, 31), it remains challenging to establish direct cause-and-effect relationships. There are at least two different scenarios to connect DSLNT, the microbiome, and NEC-like symptom improvement: (1) DSLNT affects the microbiome which then affects the host and improves NEC-like symptoms, and (2) DSLNT affects the host, and the host response leads to an improvement in NEC-like symptoms and also, and independently, to a change in microbiome.

In addition to influencing the microbiome and targeting a NEC-associated dysbiosis, HMOs can also alter host epithelial cell or host immune cell responses. These interactions are often receptor-mediated and highly structure-dependent, which would explain why DSLNT is effective, but the removal of just one sialic acid moiety from DSLNT renders the HMO ineffective. While selectins require their glycan binding partners to be fucosylated and DSLNT is not fucosylated, other glycan-binding receptors like galectins or siglecs play major roles in facilitating and modulating immune responses and represent potential DSLNT targets (53).

We have since explored the chemical space around DSLNT and tested *in vivo* efficacy of chemoenzymatically synthesized derivatives in the neonatal rat NEC model (54–56). Interestingly, the HMO 2′-fucosyllactose (2′FL), which is structurally unrelated to DSLNT, available at commercial scale, and now added to some term infant formula, had a moderate effect in the neonatal rat and mouse NEC models (55, 57), but failed to improve NEC in a piglet model (58). So far, DSLNT remains to be the most effective HMO or derivative we have studied in the context of NEC to date.

HUMAN MOTHER-INFANT COHORT STUDIES CONFIRM THAT DSLNT IS ASSOCIATED WITH LOWER NEC RISK

While the data obtained from HMO efficacy testing in the neonatal rat NEC model are encouraging, the use of preclinical NEC models in rodents or piglets is challenging (59). Animals are exposed to rather artificial insults like external hypoxia and/or hypothermia. In general, the use of animals itself is considered a major limitation due to interspecies differences in anatomy, physiology, and pathophysiology. Therefore, advancing a potential therapeutic like DSLNT from preclinical models, that are controversial, to clinical treatment trials, that are challenging and expensive, comes with a tremendous risk of failure. To narrow this wide gap between preclinical models and clinical intervention studies, we applied an intermediate approach and conducted a prospective cohort study with mothers and their very low-birth-weight (VLBW) infants fed predominantly human milk (60). The study is based on the observation that some of the infants who receive predominately human milk still develop NEC. However, not all human milk is equal. In fact, there is strong interindividual variation in HMO composition, which led us to hypothesize that human milk fed to infants who develop NEC contains less DSLNT than human milk fed to infants who do not develop NEC.

The study was conducted in five different neonatal intensive care units across North America (US and Canada), recruited 200 mothers, and analyzed HMO composition in human milk fed to their VLBW infants over the first 28 days post partum (60). We then matched each of the eight identified NEC cases with five controls, and used logistic regression and generalized estimating equation to show that DSLNT concentrations were significantly lower in almost all milk samples in all eight NEC cases when compared to controls. The association between low DSLNT concentrations in human milk and NEC was highly significant ($p < 0.001$), corroborating the results that DSLNT reduces NEC-like symptoms and improves survival in neonatal rats (49).

In parallel, we analyzed the HMO composition in human milk samples from a mother-infant cohort in South Africa,

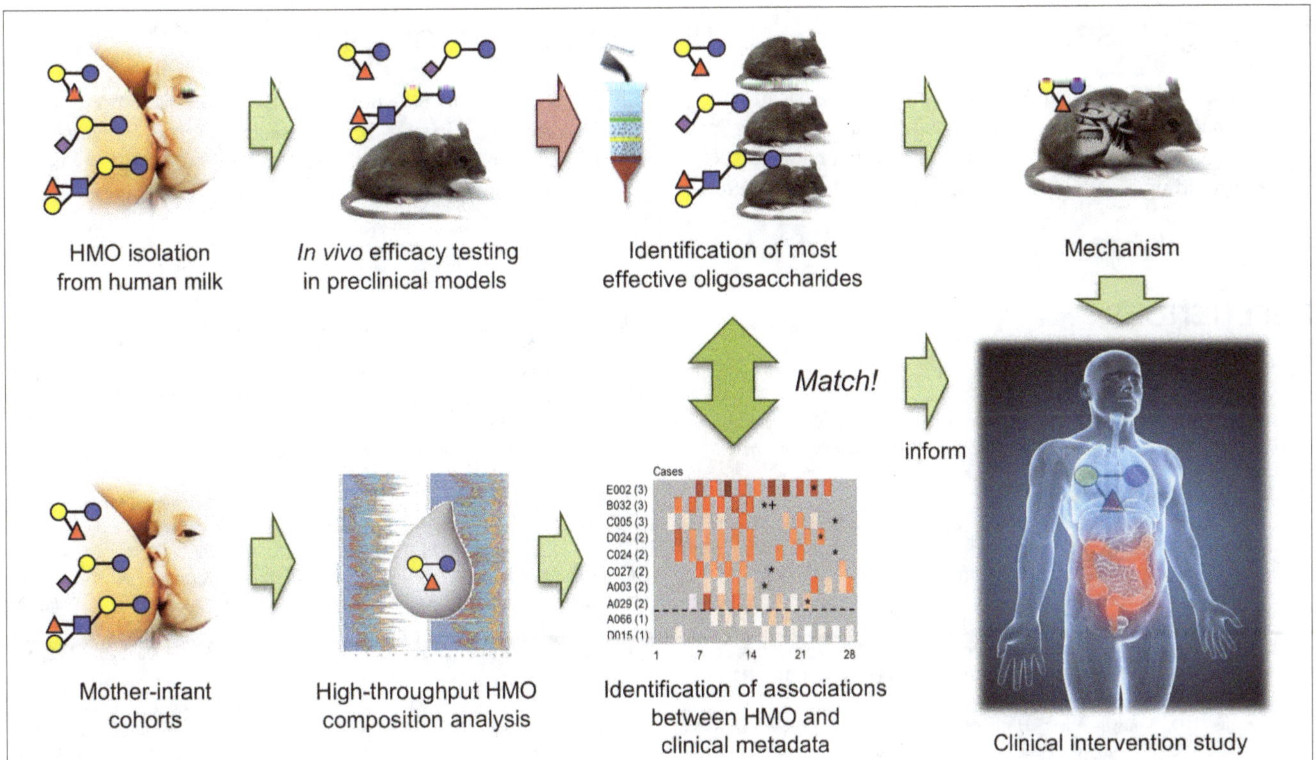

FIGURE 4 | The combination of *in vivo* HMO efficacy and structure-function testing in neonatal rats with association studies in human mother-infant cohorts led to the identification of DSLNT as the protective HMO in NEC and informs future invention studies.

and found overlapping results (61). Although the original and primary objective of the South Africa study was to investigate the role of HMOs in reducing HIV-transmission in preterm infants, the cohort included several VLBW infants who developed NEC. Independent of the HIV-status, DSLNT concentrations in the milk that these infants with NEC received were significantly lower than those in the milk given to infants who did not develop NEC. Thus, data from two independent cohort studies, one in North America and one in South Africa, strongly support our hypothesis that a specific HMO, DSLNT, contributes to the lower NEC risk in human milk-fed infants.

As the two cohort studies have shown, DSLNT concentrations vary greatly between women with preterm infants, but seem to be fairly constant within the same woman over the first four weeks of lactation (60, 61). The variability in DSLNT concentrations between different donors may be one justification for donor milk to be pooled or synthetic DSLNT to be added. Like other HMOs, DSLNT concentrations are not affected by pasteurization (62–64). However, when comparing HMO composition in donor milk batches from the San Jose Milk Bank with that in milk from moms with preterm infants in the neonatal intensive care unit at the University of California, San Diego, we discovered that DSLNT is slightly lower in donor milk batches, potentially reflecting the fact that donor milk is often from women with healthy term infants, which might be different from milk of women with preterm infants (63).

FUTURE PERSPECTIVE

The results from the North American and South African cohort studies match the results from *in vivo* efficacy testing and structure-activity relationship studies in the neonatal rat NEC model, providing a strong foundation to further explore DSLNT as a therapeutic for NEC and setting a powerful example of how the combination of *in vitro/ex vivo*, *in vivo*, and cohort studies can advance a field (**Figure 4**).

Even though some of the control milk samples in the North American cohort occasionally had low levels of DSLNT concentrations, the aggregate assessment of DSLNT in milk fed to the same infant over multiple days greatly increased the ability to discriminate between NEC cases and controls (60). Therefore, in addition to exploring DSLNT as a new NEC therapeutic, measuring DSLNT content in mother's own milk has the potential to serve as a non-invasive marker to identify infants at risk of developing NEC. Furthermore, DSLNT could become a quality control parameter for donor milk and products like human milk-based human milk fortifiers to avoid feeding low DSLNT products to infants at risk to develop NEC. Although other HMOs like 2′FL or lacto-N-(neo)tetraose have been successfully synthesized at large scale and are currently added to some formula for healthy term infants, the synthesis of DSLNT remains to be challenging and is not yet available for preterm infants at risk of NEC.

AUTHOR CONTRIBUTIONS

The author confirms being the sole contributor of this work and has approved it for publication.

ACKNOWLEDGMENTS

LB is the Larsson-Rosenquist Foundation Endowed Chair of Collaborative Human Milk Research at the University of California, San Diego, and the support of the Family Larsson-Rosenquist Foundation is gratefully acknowledged.

REFERENCES

1. Neu J, Walker WA. Necrotizing enterocolitis. *N Engl J Med.* (2011) 364:255–64. doi: 10.1056/NEJMra1005408
2. Holman RC, Stoll BJ, Curns AT, Yorita KL, Steiner CA, Schonberger LB. Necrotising enterocolitis hospitalisations among neonates in the United States. *Paediatr Perinat Epidemiol.* (2006) 20:498–506. doi: 10.1111/j.1365-3016.2006.00756.x
3. Guillet R, Stoll BJ, Cotten CM, Gantz M, McDonald S, Poole WK, et al. Association of H2-blocker therapy and higher incidence of necrotizing enterocolitis in very low birth weight infants. *Pediatrics* (2006) 117:e137–42. doi: 10.1542/peds.2005-1543
4. Horbar JD, Badger GJ, Carpenter JH, Fanaroff AA, Kilpatrick S, LaCorte M, et al. Trends in mortality and morbidity for very low birth weight infants, 1991-1999. *Pediatrics* (2002) 110:143–51. doi: 10.1542/peds.110.1.143
5. Erasmus HD, Ludwig-Auser HM, Paterson PG, Sun D, Sankaran K. Enhanced weight gain in preterm infants receiving lactase-treated feeds: a randomized, double-blind, controlled trial. *J Pediatr.* (2002) 141:532–7. doi: 10.1067/mpd.2002.127499
6. Stoll BJ. Epidemiology of necrotizing enterocolitis. *Clin Perinatol.* (1994) 21:205–18.
7. Holman RC, Stoll BJ, Clarke MJ, Glass RI. The epidemiology of necrotizing enterocolitis infant mortality in the United States. *Am J Public Health* (1997) 87:2026–31. doi: 10.2105/AJPH.87.12.2026
8. Hall N, Pierro A. Necrotizing enterocolitis review. *Hospital Med.* (2004) 65:220–5.
9. Rees CM, Pierro A, Eaton S. Neurodevelopmental outcomes of neonates with medically and surgically treated necrotizing enterocolitis. *Arch Dis Child Fetal Neonatal Ed.* (2007) 92:F193–8. doi: 10.1136/adc.2006.099929
10. Bisquera JA, Cooper TR, Berseth CL. Impact of necrotizing enterocolitis on length of stay and hospital charges in very low birth weight infants. *Pediatrics* (2002) 109:423–8. doi: 10.1542/peds.109.3.423
11. Spencer AU, Kovacevich D, McKinney-Barnett M, Hair D, Canham J, Maksym C, et al. Pediatric short-bowel syndrome: the cost of comprehensive care. *Am J Clin Nutr.* (2008) 88:1552–9. doi: 10.3945/ajcn.2008.26007
12. Bell MJ, Ternberg JL, Feigin RD, Keating JP, Marshall R, Barton L, et al. Neonatal necrotizing enterocolitis: therapeutic decisions based upon clinical staging. *Ann Surg.* (1978) 187:1–7. doi: 10.1097/00000658-197801000-00001

13. Walsh MC, Kliegman RM. Necrotizing enterocolitis: treatment based on staging criteria. *Pediatr Clin North Am.* (1986) 33:179–201.
14. Grave GD, Nelson SA, Walker WA, Moss RL, Dvorak B, Hamilton FA, et al. New therapies and preventive approaches for necrotizing enterocolitis: report of a research planning workshop. *Pediatr Res.* (2007) 62:510–4. doi: 10.1203/PDR.0b013e318142580a
15. Neu J. Neonatal necrotizing enterocolitis: an update. *Acta Paediatr.* (2005) 94:100–5. doi: 10.1080/08035320510043637
16. Anderson DM, Kliegman RM. The relationship of neonatal alimentation practices to the occurrence of endemic necrotizing enterocolitis. *Am J Perinatol.* (1991) 8:62–7.
17. Moss RL, Kalish LA, Duggan C, et al. Clinical parameters do not adequately predict outcome in necrotizing enterocolitis: a multi-institutional study. *J Perinatol.* (2008) 28:665–74. doi: 10.1038/jp.2008.119
18. Cotton CM, Taylor S, Stoll B, Goldberg RN, Hansen NI, Sánchez PJ, et al. Prolonged duration of initial empirical antibiotic treatment is associated with increased rates of necrotizing enterocolitis and death for extremely low birth weight infants. *Pediatrics* (2009) 123:58–66. doi: 10.1542/peds.2007-3423
19. Hsueh W, Caplan MS, Qu XW, Tan XD, De Plaen IG, Gonzalez-Crussi F. Neonatal necrotizing enterocolitis: clinical considerations and pathogenetic concepts. *Pediatr Dev Pathol.* (2003) 6:6–23. doi: 10.1007/s10024-002-0602-z
20. Lucas A, Cole TJ. Breast milk and neonatal necrotising enterocolitis. *Lancet* (1990) 336:1519–23. doi: 10.1016/0140-6736(90)93304-8
21. Meinzen-Derr J, Poindexter B, Wrage L, Morrow AL, Stoll B, Donovan EF. Role of human milk in extremely low birth weight infants' risk of necrotizing enterocolitis or death. *J Perinatol.* (2009) 29:57–62. doi: 10.1038/jp.2008.117
22. Quigley MA, Henderson G, Anthony MY, McGuire W. Formula milk versus donor breast milk for feeding preterm or low birth weight infants. *Cochrane Database Syst Rev.* (2007) 4:CD002971. doi: 10.1002/14651858.CD002971.pub2
23. Sullivan S, Schanler RJ, Kim JH, Patel AL, Trawöger R, Kiechl-Kohlendorfer U, et al. An exclusively human milk-based diet is associated with a lower rate of necrotizing enterocolitis than a diet of human milk and bovine milk-based products. *J Pediatr.* (2010) 156:562–7.e1. doi: 10.1016/j.jpeds.2009.10.040
24. Kunz C, Rudloff S, Baier W, Klein N, Strobel S. Oligosaccharides in human milk: structural, functional, and metabolic aspects. *Annu Rev Nutr.* (2000) 20:699–722. doi: 10.1146/annurev.nutr.20.1.699
25. Newburg DS, Ruiz-Palacios GM, Morrow AL. Human milk glycans protect infants against enteric pathogens. *Annu Rev Nutr.* (2005) 25:37–58. doi: 10.1146/annurev.nutr.25.050304.092553
26. Bode L. Recent advances on structure, metabolism, and function of human milk oligosaccharides. *J Nutr.* (2006) 136:2127–30. doi: 10.1093/jn/136.8.2127
27. Bode L. Human milk oligosaccharides: every baby needs a sugar mama. *Glycobiology* (2012) 22:1147–62. doi: 10.1093/glycob/cws074
28. Moukarzel S, Bode L. Human milk oligosaccharides and the preterm infant. *Clin Perinatol.* (2017) 44:193–207. doi: 10.1016/j.clp.2016.11.014
29. Gnoth MJ, Kunz C, Kinne-Saffran E, Rudloff S. Human milk oligosaccharides are minimally digested *in vitro*. *J Nutr.* (2000) 130:3014–20. doi: 10.1093/jn/130.12.3014
30. Engfer MB, Stahl B, Finke B, Sawatzki G, Daniel H. Human milk oligosaccharides are resistant to enzymatic hydrolysis in the upper gastrointestinal tract. *Am J Clin Nutr.* (2000) 71:1589–96. doi: 10.1093/ajcn/71.6.1589
31. Chichlowski M, German JB, Lebrilla CB, Mills DA. The influence of milk oligosaccharides on microbiota of infants: opportunities for formulas. *Annu Rev Food Sci Technol.* (2011) 2:331–51. doi: 10.1146/annurev-food-022510-133743
32. Ruhaak LR, Stroble C, Underwood MA, Lebrilla CB. Detection of milk oligosaccharides in plasma of infants. *Anal Bioanal Chem.* (2014) 406:5775–84. doi: 10.1007/s00216-014-8025-z
33. Goehring KC, Kennedy AD, Prieto PA, Buck RH. Direct evidence for the presence of human milk oligosaccharides in the circulation of breastfed infants. *PLoS ONE* (2014) 9:e101692. doi: 10.1371/journal.pone.0101692
34. Rudloff S, Obermeier S, Borsch C, Pohlentz G, Hartmann R, Brosicke H, et al. Incorporation of orally applied (13)C-galactose into milk lactose and oligosaccharides. *Glycobiology* (2006) 16:477–87. doi: 10.1093/glycob/cwj092
35. Dotz V, Rudloff S, Blank D, Lochnit G, Geyer R, Kunz C. 13C-labeled oligosaccharides in breastfed infants' urine: individual-, structure- and time-dependent differences in the excretion. *Glycobiology* (2014) 24:185–94. doi: 10.1093/glycob/cwt099
36. Cerletti C, Evangelista V, de Gaetano G. P-selectin-beta 2-integrin cross-talk: a molecular mechanism for polymorphonuclear leukocyte recruitment at the site of vascular damage. *Thrombosis Haemostasis* (1999) 82:787–93. doi: 10.1055/s-0037-1615912
37. Springer TA. Traffic signals for lymphocyte recirculation and leukocyte emigration: the multistep paradigm. *Cell* (1994) 76:301–14. doi: 10.1016/0092-8674(94)90337-9
38. Varki A. Selectin ligands: will the real ones please stand up? *J ClinInvest.* (1997) 99:158–62.
39. Stefanutti G, Lister P, Smith VV, Peters MJ, Klein NJ, Pierro A, et al. P-selectin expression, neutrophil infiltration, and histologic injury in neonates with necrotizing enterocolitis. *J Pediatr Surg.* (2005) 40:942–7. doi: 10.1016/j.jpedsurg.2005.03.027
40. Sun X, Rozenfeld RA, Qu X, Huang W, Gonzalez-Crussi F, Hsueh W. P-selectin-deficient mice are protected from PAF-induced shock, intestinal injury, and lethality. *Am J Physiol.* (1997) 273:G56–61. doi: 10.1152/ajpgi.1997.273.1.G56
41. Fitzgerald DJ, Roy L, Catella F, FitzGerald GA. Platelet activation in unstable coronary disease. *N Eng J Med.* (1986) 315:983–9. doi: 10.1056/NEJM198610163151602
42. Grande P, Grauholt AM, Madsen JK. Unstable angina pectoris. platelet behavior and prognosis in progressive angina and intermediate coronary syndrome. *Circulation* (1990) 81:I16–9.
43. Peters MJ, Dixon G, Kotowicz KT, Hatch DJ, Heyderman RS, Klein NJ. Circulating platelet-neutrophil complexes represent a subpopulation of activated neutrophils primed for adhesion, phagocytosis and intracellular killing. *Br J Haematol.* (1999) 106:391–9. doi: 10.1046/j.1365-2141.1999.01553.x
44. Rudloff S, Stefan C, Pohlentz G, Kunz C. Detection of ligands for selectins in the oligosaccharide fraction of human milk. *Eur J Nutr.* (2002) 41:85–92. doi: 10.1007/s003940200012
45. Bode L, Kunz C, Muhly-Reinholz M, Mayer K, Seeger W, Rudloff S. Inhibition of monocyte, lymphocyte, and neutrophil adhesion to endothelial cells by human milk oligosaccharides. *Thrombosis Haemostasis* (2004) 92:1402–10. doi: 10.1160/TH04-01-0055
46. Bode L, Rudloff S, Kunz C, Strobel S, Klein N. Human milk oligosaccharides reduce platelet-neutrophil complex formation leading to a decrease in neutrophil beta 2 integrin expression. *J Leukocyte Biol.* (2004) 76:820–6. doi: 10.1189/jlb.0304198
47. Barlow B, Santulli TV. Importance of multiple episodes of hypoxia or cold stress on the development of enterocolitis in an animal model. *Surgery* (1975) 77:687e90.
48. Nadler EP, Dickinson E, Knisely A, Zhang XR, Boyle P, Beer-Stolz D, et al. Expression of inducible nitric oxide synthase and interleukin-12 in experimental necrotizing enterocolitis. *J Surg Res.* (2000) 92:71e7 doi: 10.1006/jsre.2000.5877
49. Jantscher-Krenn E, Zherebtsov M, Nissan C, Goth K, Guner YS, Naidu N, et al. The Human milk oligosaccharide disialyllacto-N-tetraose prevents Necrotizing Enterocolitis in neonatal rats. *GUT* (2011) 61:1417–25. doi: 10.1136/gutjnl-2011-301404
50. Varki A. Selectin ligands: will the real ones please stand up? *J Clin Invest.* (1997) 99:158–62.
51. Becker DJ, Lowe JB. Leukocyte adhesion deficiency type II. *Biochim Biophys Acta* (1999) 1455:193e204.
52. Lühn K, Wild MK, Eckhardt M, Gerardy-Schahn R, Vestweber D. The gene defective in leukocyte adhesion deficiency II encodes a putative GDP-fucose transporter. *Nat Genet.* (2001) 28:9e72. doi: 10.1038/88289
53. Triantis V, Bode L, van Neerven RJJ. Immunological effects of human milk oligosaccharides. *Front Pediatr.* (2018) 6:190. doi: 10.3389/fped.2018.00190
54. Yu H, Lau K, Thon V, Autran CA, Jantscher-Krenn E, Xue M, et al. Synthetic disialyl hexasaccharides protect neonatal rats from necrotizing enterocolitis. *Angew Chem Int Ed Engl.* (2014) 53:6687–91. doi: 10.1002/anie.201403588

55. Autran CA, Schoterman MHC, Jantscher-Krenn E, Kamerling JP, Bode L. Sialylated galacto-oligosaccharides and 2'-fucosyllactose reduce necrotizing enterocolitis in neonatal rats. *Br J Nutr.* (2016) 116:294–9. doi: 10.1017/S0007114516002038
56. Yu H, Yan X, Autran C, Li Y, Etzold S, Latasiewicz J, et al. Enzymatic and chemoenzymatic syntheses of disialyl glycans and their necrotizing enterocolitis preventing effects. *J Org Chem.* (2017) 82:13152–60. doi: 10.1021/acs.joc.7b02167
57. Good M, Sodhi CP, Yamaguchi, Y. The human milk oligosaccharide 2'-fucosyllactose attenuates the severity of experimental necrotising enterocolitis by enhancing mesenteric perfusion in the neonatal intestine. *Br J Nutr.* (2016) 116:1175–87. doi: 10.1017/S0007114516002944
58. Rasmussen SO, Martin L, Østergaard MV, Rudloff S, Roggenbuck M, Nguyen DN, et al. Human milk oligosaccharide effects on intestinal function and inflammation after preterm birth in pigs. *J Nutr Biochem.* (2017) 40:141–54. doi: 10.1016/j.jnutbio.2016.10.011
59. Tanner SM, Berryhill TF, Ellenburg JL, Jilling T, Cleveland DS, Lorenz RG, et al. Pathogenesis of necrotizing enterocolitis: modeling the innate immune response. *Am J Pathol.* (2015) 185:4–16. doi: 10.1016/j.ajpath.2014.08.028
60. Autran CA, Kellman BP, Kim JH, Asztalos E, Blood AB, Hamilton Spence EC, et al. Human milk oligosaccharide composition predicts risk of necrotizing enterocolitis in preterm infants. *Gut* (2018) 67:1064–70. doi: 10.1136/gutjnl-2016-312819
61. Van Niekerk E, Autran CA, Nel DG, Kirsten GF, Blaauw R, Bode L. Human milk oligosaccharides differ between HIV-infected and HIV-uninfected mothers and are related to necrotizing enterocolitis incidence in their preterm very-low-birth-weight infants. *J Nutr.* (2014) 144:1227–33. doi: 10.3945/jn.113.187799
62. Bertino E, Coppa GV, Giuliani F. Effects of Holder pasteurization on human milk oligosaccharides. *Int J Immunopathol Pharmacol.* (2008) 21:381–5. doi: 10.1177/039463200802100216
63. Marx C, Bridge R, Wolf AK, Rich W, Kim JH, Bode L. Human milk oligosaccharide composition differs between donor milk and mother's own milk in the NICU. *J Hum Lact.* (2014) 30:54–61. doi: 10.1177/0890334413513923
64. Daniels B, Coutsoudis A, Autran C, Amundson Mansen K, Israel-Ballard K, Bode L. The effect of simulated flash heating pasteurisation and Holder pasteurisation on human milk oligosaccharides. *Paediatr Int Child Health* (2017) 37:204–9. doi: 10.1080/20469047.2017.1293869

14

Mother's Own Milk and Bronchopulmonary Dysplasia: A Systematic Review and Meta-Analysis

*Eduardo Villamor-Martínez [1], Maria Pierro [2], Giacomo Cavallaro [3], Fabio Mosca [3] and Eduardo Villamor [1]**

[1] Department of Pediatrics, School for Oncology and Developmental Biology (GROW), Maastricht University Medical Center (MUMC+), Maastricht, Netherlands, [2] UOC TIN e Neonatologia, Dipartimento Salute Mamma e Bambino, Fondazione Poliambulanza, Brescia, Italy, [3] Neonatal Intensive Care Unit, Department of Clinical Sciences and Community Health, Fondazione IRCCS Cà Granda Ospedale Maggiore Policlinico, Università degli Studi di Milano, Milan, Italy

***Correspondence:**
Eduardo Villamor
e.villamor@mumc.nl

Background: Bronchopulmonary dysplasia (BPD) is the most common complication of very preterm birth and can lead to lifelong health consequences. Optimal nutrition is a cornerstone in the prevention and treatment of BPD. In very preterm infants, mother's own milk (MOM) feeding is associated with lower risks of necrotizing enterocolitis, retinopathy of prematurity, and sepsis. Although several studies have shown that MOM may protect against BPD, a systematic analysis of the evidence has not been performed to date.

Methods: A comprehensive literature search was conducted using PubMed/MEDLINE and EMBASE, from their inception to 1 December 2017. Longitudinal studies comparing the incidence of BPD in preterm infants fed with exclusive MOM, MOM supplemented with preterm formula (PF), and/or exclusively fed with PF were selected. A random-effects model was used to calculate the Mantel Haenszel risk ratio (RR) and 95% confidence interval (CI).

Results: Fifteen studies met the inclusion criteria (4,984 infants, 1,416 BPD cases). Use of exclusive MOM feedings was associated with a significant reduction in the risk of BPD (RR 0.74, 95% CI 0.57–0.96, 5 studies). In contrast, meta-analysis could not demonstrate a significant effect on BPD risk when infants fed with more than 50% MOM were compared with infants fed with <50% MOM (RR 0.98, 95% CI 0.77–1.23, 10 studies) or when infants fed with MOM supplemented with PF were compared with infants fed with exclusive PF (RR 1.00, 95% CI 0.78–1.27, 6 studies). Meta-regression showed that differences in gestational age were a significant confounder of the effect of MOM.

Conclusion: To our knowledge, this is the first systematic review and meta-analysis that specifically evaluates the role of MOM on BPD. Our data indicate that MOM may reduce the incidence of BPD when used as an exclusive diet, but this result needs to be interpreted with caution. We did not find the same difference in analyses with other dosages of MOM. Further studies adequately powered to detect changes in BPD rates and that adjust for confounders are needed to confirm the beneficial effects of MOM on BPD.

Keywords: mother's own milk, human milk, bronchopulmonary dysplasia, preterm formula, meta-analysis, systematic review, meta-regression

INTRODUCTION

Mother's own milk (MOM), fresh or frozen, is the normative standard for preterm infant feeding and nutrition (1–4). If MOM is unavailable despite significant lactation support, pasteurized donor human milk (DHM) is the recommended alternative over the use of bovine milk-based preterm formula (PF) (1–4). However, it is increasingly recognized that numerous MOM components which could contribute to its protective effects against adverse outcomes of prematurity are reduced or absent in DHM (5).

Bronchopulmonary dysplasia (BPD) is one of the most common complications of prematurity, and it predicts multiple adverse outcomes including chronic respiratory impairment and neurodevelopmental delay (6, 7). Optimal nutritional support is considered a cornerstone in the treatment/prevention of BPD (8). Recently, we performed a systematic review and meta-analysis on the effects of DHM on BPD (9). Meta-analysis of randomized controlled trials (RCTs) could not demonstrate that supplementation of MOM with DHM had a significant effect on BPD risk when compared to supplementation with PF. However, meta-analysis of observational studies showed a protective effect of DHM supplementation on BPD (9). Two very recent systematic reviews confirmed that the protective effects of human milk (i.e., MOM and/or DHM) on BPD are only observed in meta-analysis of observational studies (10, 11). Using the GRADE-system (12), the authors of these meta-analyses consider the evidence to be inconclusive.

Despite the important differences between DHM and MOM, the umbrella term "human milk" is frequently used to encompass both MOM and DHM, implying that the beneficial effects of MOM can be directly extrapolated to DHM (5, 13). Moreover, many of the studies and meta-analyses have compared PF feedings with various combinations of PF, MOM, and DHM. A recent meta-analysis evaluated the effects of MOM on retinopathy of prematurity (ROP) (14). This analysis excluded data on DHM and showed that the overall incidence of ROP was reduced among infants fed MOM compared with those fed PF. To the best of our knowledge, no systematic review has focused on the role of MOM in the development of BPD. The analysis of exclusive MOM vs. PF was beyond the scope of our previous study (9), and Miller et al. and Huang et al. did not study the effect of MOM separately from that of DHM (10, 11). Therefore, we aimed to conduct a systematic review and meta-analysis on the association between MOM/PF feeding and BPD development. The present meta-analysis does not include data on DHM.

METHODS

This study is a continuation of our previous review on DHM and BPD (9), and shares much of the same methodology. We expanded on the protocol of our earlier study, and specified the objectives, criteria for study inclusion, method for evaluating study quality, outcomes and statistical methodology. We report this study according to the guidelines of the Preferred Reporting Items for Systematic Reviews and Meta-Analysis (PRISMA) (15). The PRISMA checklist for this report can be found in the **Supplementary Material.**

Data Sources and Search Strategy

We modified and expanded on the search strategy of our earlier review (9). We carried out a comprehensive literature search using PubMed/Medline and EMBASE, from their inception to March 1, 2018. The search strategy for PubMed used the following terms, including Mesh terms: (breast milk OR infant feeding OR mother's own milk) AND (preterm infant OR very low birth weight infant) AND (outcome OR bronchopulmonary dysplasia OR BPD) AND (observational study OR cohort study OR case-control). We used a similar strategy in EMBASE. We applied no language restrictions. We translated articles when needed. We included cohort and case-control studies in this review, as well as RCTs with an observational arm. Other types of studies were excluded, but when considered relevant, they were read to identify additional studies to include. We also used the "cited by" tool in Google Scholar and Web of Science to identify studies for inclusion. Moreover, we included articles which we came across in the elaboration of our earlier review (9).

Eligibility Criteria and Study Selection

We included studies if they were original cohort or case-control studies, which examined very preterm (gestational age, GA <32 weeks) or very low birth weight (VLBW, BW <1,500 g) infants receiving either MOM or PF, and which included at least two groups divided according to feeding policy. Only full-length published studies were considered for inclusion. Studies were included if they reported results on the incidence of BPD. We defined BPD as oxygen dependence at 28 days of life (BPD28) or as oxygen dependence at 36 weeks adjusted gestational age (BPD36). Studies were excluded if the group receiving MOM or PF also received DHM. Two reviewers (EV-M, EV) independently screened the results of the searches, and included studies according to the inclusion criteria using EndNote (RRID:SCR_014001), using the methodology of Bramer et al. (16). Studies on which reviewers disagreed for inclusion were identified, and discrepancies were resolved through discussion or by consulting the other authors.

Data Extraction

We collected the following information per study: citation information, study design, number of patients, number of centers, location of study, inclusion and exclusion criteria, patient characteristics (GA, BW), type of feeding received (MOM, PF, combination of MOM and PF, and type of fortifier), and incidence of BPD per group. Two researchers (EV-M, EV) extracted the data using an Excel sheet designed for this review. We resolved discrepancies in data extraction through discussion, or by consulting the other authors. Another researcher (MP) independently validated the accuracy of the data extracted.

Assessment Risk of Bias

Two researchers (EV-M, MP) assessed the risk of bias in included studies. We used the Newcastle-Ottawa Scale (NOS) for quality assessment of cohort and case-control studies. The NOS is used to assign a score to studies on selection (0–4 points), comparability (0–2 points), and outcome/exposure (0–3 points), for a total score of up to 9 points. Discrepancies were resolved through discussion.

Statistical Analysis

We used Comprehensive Meta-Analysis V3.0 software (RRID:SCR_012779) to combine and analyze studies. The Mantel Haenszel (MH) risk ratio (RR) for BPD with 95% confidence interval (CI) was calculated in each study. Due to anticipated heterogeneity, we used a random-effects model to combine studies. This model accounts for heterogeneity between and within studies and it does not assume that "true" effect sizes are identical across studies. Subgroup analyses were conducted according to the mixed-effects model (17). In this model a random-effects analysis is used to combine studies within each subgroup, and a fixed-effect model is used to combine subgroups and yield the overall effect. The model does not assume study-to-study variance (tau-squared) to be the same for all subgroups. We assessed statistical heterogeneity using the Cochran's Q statistic, and the I^2 statistic which is derived from it. We planned to evaluate the risk of publication bias through visual inspection of the funnel plot and with Egger's regression test (18). We decided *a priori* to analyze the effect of GA as a confounding factor, by analyzing the mean difference in this covariate between groups, and through subgroup analysis, by removing studies with large differences in GA from analysis. We decided to use the group with the higher MOM intake as the reference group in all our analyses. We carried out sensitivity analyses by removing one study from analyses at a time. We used an $\alpha = 0.05$ for statistical significance ($\alpha = 0.10$ for statistical heterogeneity).

RESULTS

After removing duplicates, our comprehensive search found 965 articles, of which we identified 84 as potentially relevant, and 15 met our inclusion criteria (19–33) after full-text review. The PRISMA search diagram is shown in **Figure 1**. The characteristics of the included studies are shown in **Supplementary Table 1**. Fourteen included studies were observational cohorts, of which seven were prospective (20, 21, 23, 25, 30, 31, 33) and seven were retrospective (19, 22, 24, 26, 28, 29, 32), and one study was a retrospective case-control (27). One study was excluded from meta-analysis because it did not group by type of feeding (22). We divided studies according to the proportion of feeding that was MOM or PF in each group, and we made three comparisons for analysis: (1) Exclusive MOM vs. Any PF; (2) Mainly MOM vs. Mainly PF; (3) Any MOM vs. Exclusive PF.

Quality Assessment

Three studies scored six points on the NOS, 10 studies scored seven points, and two studies scored the maximum of 9 points. We downgraded studies in quality for not adjusting for confounders ($k = 13$), for excluding infants who were lost to follow-up ($k = 2$) and for not defining BPD clearly ($k = 1$).

Exclusive MOM vs. Any PF

Five studies (19–21, 27, 30) compared infants who received a diet of exclusive MOM to infants who received MOM and any supplementation with PF. Meta-analysis of these studies found that the exclusive MOM group had a reduced risk of BPD (RR 0.74, 95% CI 0.57–0.96, $p = 0.021$, **Figure 2**). When we excluded the study of Fewtrell et al. which used a different definition of BPD (BPD28), the effect of MOM on BPD remained significant (RR 0.71, 95% CI 0.54–0.93 $p = 0.014$). Sensitivity analysis showed that removing the study of Madore et al. (27) or the study of Schanler et al. (30) made the overall association no longer significant (**Supplementary Figure 1**).

When we analyzed the difference in GA between groups, meta-analysis did not find a significant difference (MD GA −0.06 weeks, 95% CI −0.38–0.25, $p = 0.689$, **Supplementary Figure 2**). None of the included studies had a mean difference in GA between groups which was larger than 0.3 weeks.

Out of the five studies which had an exclusive MOM group, three studies (19–21) also provided data on a group of infants receiving exclusive PF. We carried out a subgroup analysis of these studies. When pooled, meta-analysis could not find a significant difference in BPD risk between groups (RR 1.08, 95% CI 0.63–1.87, $p = 0.770$ **Figure 3**). When we excluded the study of Fewtrell et al., which defined BPD as BPD28 instead of BPD36, the effect of MOM did not change in significance (RR 1.10, 95% CI 0.58–2.09, $p = 0.777$). When we removed the study of Assad et al. for having a MD in GA (of 1.5 weeks) between groups $\geq$0.5 weeks, the results did not change in significance (RR 0.88, 95% CI 0.57–1.37, $p = 0.583$). An analysis on the difference in GA between groups did not find a significant difference overall (MD −0.41 weeks, 95% CI −1.19–0.36, $p = 0.295$, **Supplementary Figure 3**).

Mainly MOM vs. Mainly PF

Ten studies compared infants receiving mainly MOM vs. infants receiving mainly PF. We included studies which had stricter criteria for comparison (i.e., exclusive MOM vs. exclusive PF) in this analysis as well. Meta-analysis could not find a significant difference in risk of BPD between the mainly MOM and the

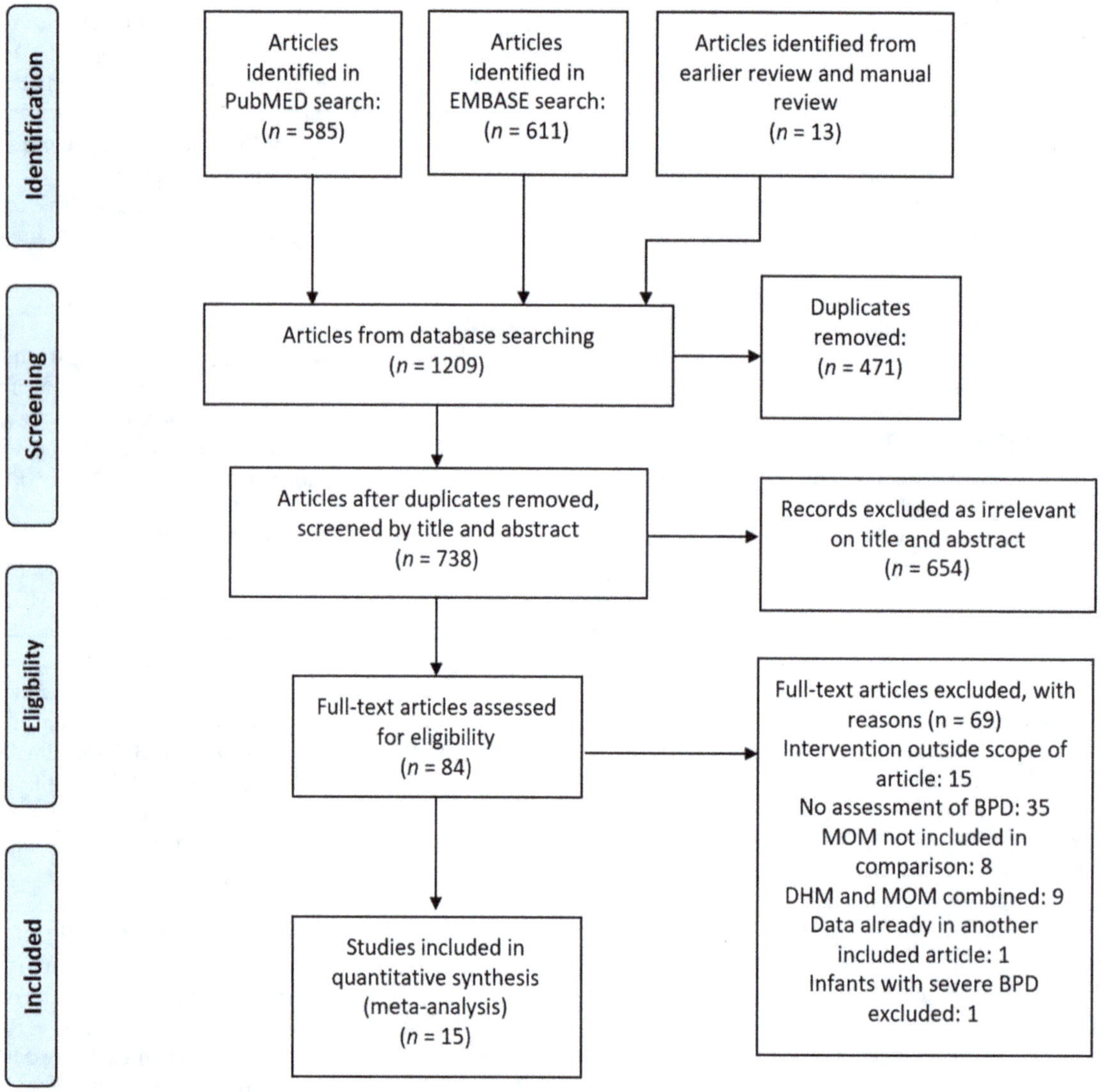

FIGURE 1 | PRISMA diagram of the search.

mainly PF group (RR 0.98, 95% CI 0.77–1.23, $p = 0.833$, **Figure 4**). When we excluded the study of O'Connor et al. for using a definition of BPD at 28 days of life instead of at 36 weeks PMA, the effect of MOM on BPD development remained non-significant (RR 0.99, 95% CI 0.75–1.31, $p = 0.938$). Excluding any study one at a time did not change the significance of the effect of MOM on BPD (**Supplementary Figure 4**).

We used meta-analysis to study the differences in GA between the MOM and PF groups in each study. Meta-analysis found no significant MD in GA when pooling all studies together (MD −0.31 weeks, 95% CI −0.78–0.17, $p = 0.204$, **Supplementary Figure 5**). However, individual studies showed significant differences in GA between groups, and the heterogeneity was very high ($p < 0.001$, $I^2 = 92.1\%$), which indicated that GA could be a significant confounder. When we used subgroup analysis to exclude studies where the difference in GA between groups was larger than 0.5 weeks, we were left with 6 studies, but the effect of MOM on BPD did not change significantly (RR 0.99, 95% CI 0.82–1.18, $p = 0.890$).

We used meta-regression to explore the role of GA in potentially modifying the effect of MOM on BPD development. Meta-regression found a significant association between MD in GA and the risk of BPD in the MOM group (Coefficient: −0.59, 95% CI −0.95 to −0.23, $p = 0.001$, $R^2 = 1.00$, **Figure 5**). This indicates that in studies where the MOM group had a higher risk of BPD, this group was also more premature than the PF group, and in studies where the MOM group had a lower risk of BPD, this group was also more mature than the PF group.

Any MOM vs. Exclusive PF

Six studies (19, 20, 23–25, 33) compared infants who received any MOM to infants who received exclusive PF. We also included

Study name	BPD-Yes / Total MOM	BPD-Yes / Total PF	MH risk ratio	Lower limit	Upper limit	p-Value	Relative weight
Schanler 2005	9 / 70	25 / 92	0.47	0.24	0.95	0.035	13.8
Madore 2017	11 / 29	14 / 25	0.68	0.38	1.21	0.189	19.8
Assad 2016	30 / 127	24 / 79	0.78	0.49	1.23	0.281	31.9
Cortez 2017	19 / 63	20 / 55	0.83	0.50	1.39	0.475	25.3
Fewtrell 2002	7 / 81	16 / 195	1.05	0.45	2.46	0.905	9.2
OVERALL			**0.74**	**0.57**	**0.96**	**0.021**	

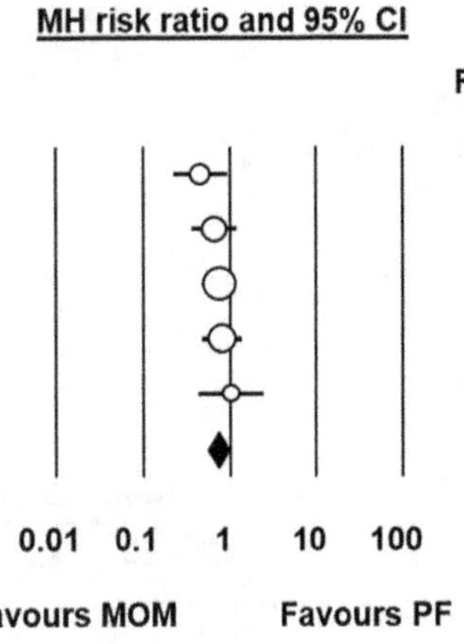

Heterogeneity: Q= 3; $p = 0.631$; $I^2 = 0.0\%$

FIGURE 2 | Meta-analysis of exclusive MOM vs. any PF and risk of BPD. MOM, mother's own milk; PF, preterm formula; BPD, bronchopulmonary dysplasia; CI, confidence interval; MH, Mantel-Haenszel.

Study name	BPD-Yes / Total MOM	BPD-Yes / Total PF	MH risk ratio	Lower limit	Upper limit	p-Value	Relative Weight (%)
Cortez 2017	19 / 63	20 / 55	0.83	0.50	1.39	0.475	52.1
Fewtrell 2002	7 / 81	16 / 195	1.05	0.45	2.46	0.905	28.8
Assad 2016	30 / 127	3 / 30	2.36	0.77	7.23	0.132	19.0
OVERALL			**1.08**	**0.63**	**1.87**	**0.770**	

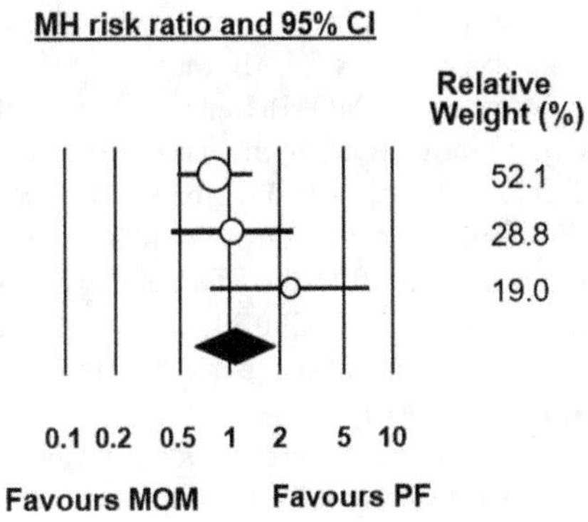

Heterogeniety: Q= 3; $p = 0.224$; $I^2 = 33.2\%$

FIGURE 3 | Meta-analysis of exclusive MOM vs. exclusive PF and risk of BPD. MOM, mother's own milk; PF, preterm formula; BPD, bronchopulmonary dysplasia; CI, confidence interval; MH, Mantel-Haenszel.

Study name	BPD-Yes / Total Mainly MOM	BPD-Yes / Total Mainly PF	MH risk ratio	Lower limit	Upper limit	p-Value	Relative weight
Patra 2017	26 / 99	47 / 101	0.56	0.38	0.83	0.004	14.6
Madore 2017	11 / 29	14 / 25	0.68	0.38	1.21	0.189	9.7
Cortez 2017	19 / 63	20 / 55	0.83	0.50	1.39	0.475	11.2
O' Connor 2003	34 / 141	79 / 322	0.97	0.68	1.38	0.871	15.8
Jacobi-Polishook 2016	61 / 283	68 / 329	1.04	0.77	1.42	0.789	17.3
Fewtrell 2002	7 / 81	16 / 195	1.05	0.45	2.46	0.905	5.7
Sisk 2007	19 / 156	5 / 46	1.12	0.44	2.84	0.810	5.0
Sisk 2017	53 / 299	14 / 113	1.43	0.83	2.47	0.200	10.4
Maayan-Metzger 2012	17 / 50	7 / 36	1.75	0.81	3.77	0.154	6.6
Assad 2016	30 / 127	3 / 30	2.36	0.77	7.23	0.132	3.7
OVERALL			**0.98**	**0.77**	**1.23**	**0.833**	

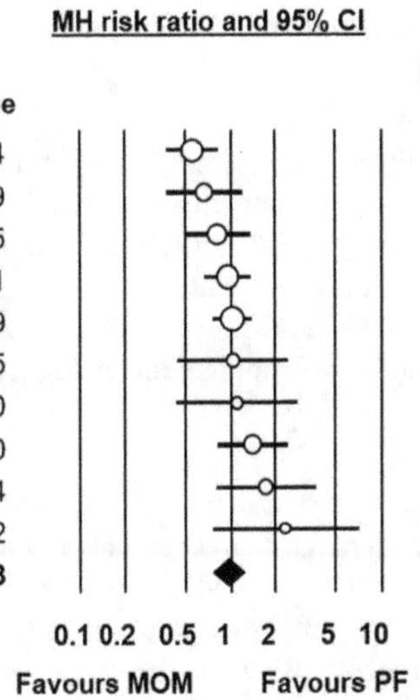

Heterogeneity: Q= 16; $p = 0.061$; $I^2 = 44.8\%$

FIGURE 4 | Meta-analysis of mainly MOM vs. mainly PF and risk of BPD. MOM, mother's own milk; PF, preterm formula; BPD, bronchopulmonary dysplasia; CI, confidence interval; MH, Mantel-Haenszel.

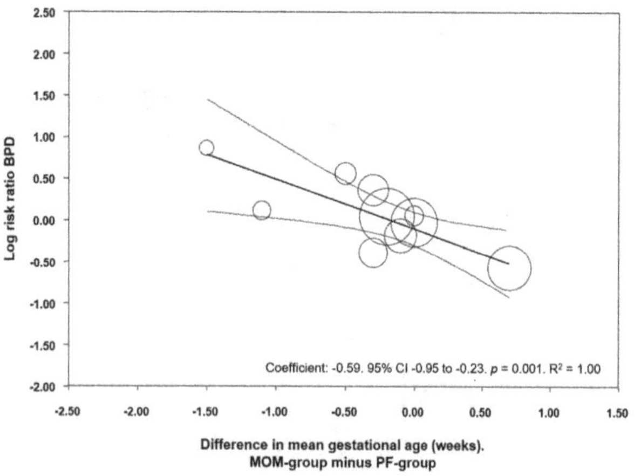

FIGURE 5 | Meta-regression of MD in GA between the MOM and PF group, and risk of BPD. CI, confidence interval; BPD, bronchopulmonary dysplasia.

studies in this comparison where the infants of the MOM group received larger proportions of MOM (e.g., infants receiving mainly MOM or exclusive MOM). Meta-analysis could not find a significant effect of any MOM on the risk of developing BPD (RR 1.00, 95% CI 0.78–1.27, $p = 0.975$, **Figure 6**). When we removed the study of Hylander et al. from the analysis, which did not clarify their definition of BPD, the effect of any MOM remained non-significant (RR 1.07, 95% CI 0.80–1.42, $p = 0.665$). Removal of any one study did not affect the significance of the results (**Supplementary Figure 6**).

Meta-analysis found that there was a significant difference in mean GA between the any MOM group and the exclusive PF group, with the infants receiving any MOM being born earlier (MD −0.50 weeks, 95% CI −0.99 to −0.01, $p = 0.045$, **Figure 7**). Removing studies where the groups differed by more than 0.5 weeks in GA left us with three studies (20, 24, 33), but the effect of MOM on BPD remained non-significant (RR 0.93, 95% CI 0.82–1.05, $p = 0.236$, **Supplementary Figure 7**).

Publication Bias

We tested the three comparisons for publication bias (**Supplementary Figure 8**), but neither visual inspection of the funnel plot nor Egger's regression test could find significant evidence of publication bias. A small number of studies made the analyses on "Exclusive MOM vs. Any PF" and "Any MOM vs. Exclusive PF" inconclusive (**Supplementary Figure 8**).

Adjusted Data

Two studies (23, 26) reported data on BPD incidence that was adjusted for confounders. Furman et al. (23) reported incidence of BPD by amount of maternal milk received, and they adjusted for several confounders (BW, sex, and ethnicity). They found no significant difference in BPD risk for varying levels of MOM intake, compared to receiving exclusive PF. Maayan-Metzger et al. (26) used logistic regression to adjust for confounders including GA, BW and sex. They found that receiving only or mainly MOM, compared to receiving only or mainly PF, did not significantly affect the risk of developing BPD. They found the same result in the subgroup of infants with GA 24–28 weeks.

Other Studies

One study (22) did not group according to MOM or PF intake. Instead they compared infants with BPD to infants without BPD and studied median intake of MOM in the first 6 weeks of life. In their study infants were given MOM, supplemented by PF when necessary. They found infants with BPD had a significantly lower median daily MOM intake compared to infants without BPD (2.3 mL/kg/d vs. 10.8). The protective effect on BPD of a higher MOM intake at 42 days remained after adjustment for confounding factors (RR 0.98, 95% CI 0.96–0.99, $p = 0.030$).

DISCUSSION

RCTs are widely regarded to provide the highest degree of evidence (34). However, the random allocation of infants to a group receiving PF instead of MOM is not ethical and, therefore, evidence must be based on observational studies (14, 35). To our knowledge, this is the first systematic review and meta-analysis that specifically evaluated the role of MOM on BPD. We found that MOM reduced the risk of developing BPD but only when used as an exclusive diet. In contrast, meta-analysis could not find significant changes in BPD risk when comparing infants fed mainly with MOM with those fed mainly with PF, or when comparing any MOM vs. exclusive PF.

The reduction of BPD rates when MOM is used as an exclusive diet may have various explanations. The major pathogenetic clue of BPD is the arrest in the alveologenesis and vasculogenesis of the lung due to very preterm birth (36). Superimposed inflammatory events complete this detrimental picture (37, 38). Prenatally, in the setting of chorioamnionitis, the overwhelming inflammatory cascade may interfere with lung development (37). Postnatally, the intensive care support needed by very preterm infants, including resuscitation, mechanical ventilation, and oxygen administration, carries a high grade of inflammation to the immature lung, leading to the establishment of BPD (38). When postnatal infections occur, the incidence of BPD sharply increases (39–41). Finally, inadequate nutrition can further worsen BPD (42). MOM may reduce the incidence of BPD thanks to nutritional and bioactive components, counteracting oxidative stress (43), inflammation (44, 45), and nutritional flaws involved in the BPD pathogenesis (46, 47). In addition, MOM may also impact the risk of BPD indirectly by reducing the incidence of necrotizing enterocolitis (NEC) and late-onset sepsis (LOS).

Due to the observational character of the studies included in the meta-analysis, the MOM and PF groups may differ in a number of maternal and infant characteristics which may affect the development of BPD. Previous studies have shown associations between characteristics such as ethnicity, socioeconomic status, maternal education, pregnancy hypertensive disorders, smoking during pregnancy, GA, BW, infant sex, Apgar score, or respiratory distress syndrome, and rate of MOM feeding in preterm infants (32, 48–54). We evaluated one possible major confounder: difference in GA between groups. GA played a role in modifying the association

Study name	BPD-Yes / Total MOM	BPD-Yes / Total PF	MH risk ratio	Lower limit	Upper limit	p-Value	Relative weight
Jacobi Polishook 2016	7 / 46	122 / 565	0.70	0.35	1.42	0.327	9.2
Cortez 2017	19 / 63	20 / 55	0.83	0.50	1.39	0.475	14.2
Hylander 1998	64 / 123	55 / 89	0.84	0.67	1.07	0.152	28.6
Vohr 2006	349 / 775	120 / 260	0.98	0.84	1.14	0.752	33.9
Furman 2005	32 / 79	8 / 40	2.03	1.03	3.98	0.040	9.7
Assad 2016	51 / 186	3 / 30	2.74	0.91	8.23	0.072	4.3
OVERALL			**1.00**	**0.78**	**1.27**	**0.975**	

Heterogeneity: Q= 11; $p = 0.056$; $I^2 = 53.7\%$

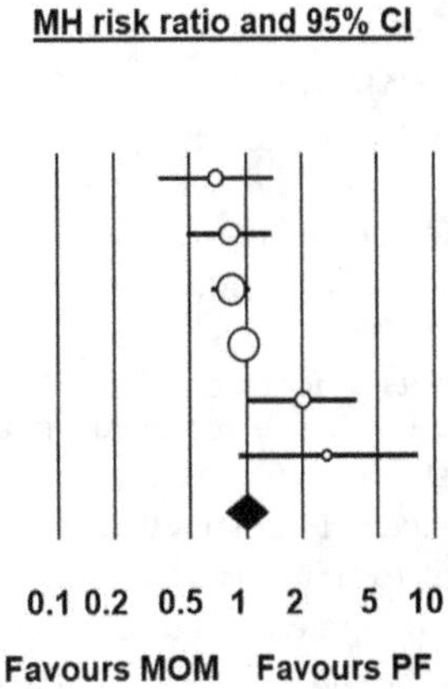

FIGURE 6 | Meta-analysis of Any MOM vs. Exclusive PF and risk of BPD. MOM, mother's own milk; PF, preterm formula; BPD, bronchopulmonary dysplasia; CI, confidence interval; MH, Mantel-Haenszel.

Study name	MOM	PF	Difference in means	Lower limit	Upper limit	p-Value	Relative weight
Assad 2016	176	30	-1.70	-2.77	-0.63	0.002	11.28
Furman 2005	79	40	-1.00	-1.79	-0.21	0.013	14.94
Jacobi Polishook 2016	565	46	-0.90	-1.44	-0.36	0.001	18.79
Vohr 2006	775	260	-0.20	-0.48	0.08	0.163	22.46
Cortez 2017	63	55	-0.10	-0.86	0.66	0.796	15.36
Hylander 1998	123	89	0.40	-0.24	1.04	0.220	17.18
Mean difference in GA			**-0.50**	**-0.99**	**-0.01**	**0.045**	

Heterogeneity: Q= 20; $p = 0.001$; $I^2 = 74.5\%$

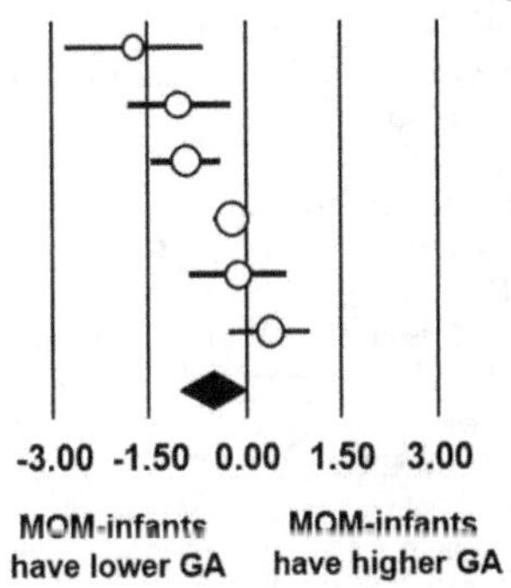

FIGURE 7 | Meta-analysis of Any MOM vs. Exclusive PF, mean difference (MD) in gestational age (GA) between groups. MOM, mother's own milk; PF, preterm formula.

between MOM and BPD, as we have shown through meta-regression and sub-group analyses. This is relevant since the incidence of all the complications of prematurity, including NEC, LOS, and BPD, is inversely related to GA. In studies which compared mainly MOM vs. mainly PF, the comparison that included the highest number of studies, meta-regression showed a significant correlation between difference in GA and the protective effect of MOM on BPD (**Figure 5**). In other words, in the studies where the mainly MOM group had a higher BPD risk, this group was also more premature than the mainly PF group. Interestingly, in the comparison where we found a significant positive result (exclusive MOM vs. any PF), the differences in GA between groups were small. This suggests that the protective effects of exclusive MOM are not affected by GA as confounder in this analysis.

Several studies have reported that the effects of human milk in reducing the incidence of adverse outcomes of prematurity are dose-dependent (14, 23, 31, 55–58). It has been suggested that at least 50% of the infant's total enteral intake should be MOM in order to achieve a decreased incidence of NEC (13). With regards to BPD, Patel et al. have shown a 9.5% reduction in the risk of BPD for each 10% increase in MOM received from birth to 36 weeks PMA. This may generate a reduction in BPD risk up to 63% when an exclusive MOM diet is compared with an exclusive PF diet (55). Surprisingly, the present meta-analysis could not demonstrate a different rate of BPD in infants fed exclusive MOM when compared with infants fed exclusive PF. However, this analysis was based on only three studies (**Figure 3**). Moreover, in one of the studies the infants in the PF group had a markedly higher GA (1.5 weeks) than the infants of the MOM group. To date, there are no exact limits set in the amount of MOM that would produce benefits in terms of BPD reduction (59). The studies that we analyzed documented a high variability of MOM amount in their study groups. Since the relation between MOM and BPD, may not be as direct as for NEC and LOS, it is possible that higher minimum amounts of MOM may be needed to detect significant differences. In addition, the conditions of storage and the use of fresh, refrigerated, frozen, or deep-frozen MOM may affect the antioxidant as well as other biological properties of MOM (60).

CONCLUSION

Our data indicate that MOM may reduce the incidence of BPD when used as an exclusive diet, but this result needs to be interpreted with caution. We did not find the same difference in analyses with other dosages of MOM, which may be related to the high variability in the available studies and the dose-dependent beneficial effects of MOM. It may also be due to differences in GA between infants who receive MOM and infants who receive PF, which we found had modified the protective effects of MOM against BPD. Moreover, there may be other differences in infant and maternal characteristics that play a role and which we could not account for. Further studies, adequately powered to detect changes in BPD rates, and that adjust for the different characteristics of infants who receive MOM and PF are needed to confirm the beneficial effects of MOM on BPD.

AUTHOR CONTRIBUTIONS

EV-M designed the study, performed the search, selected studies for inclusion, collected data, performed the statistical analyses, contributed to the interpretation of the results, and drafted the initial manuscript. MP revised collected data, contributed to statistical analysis and interpretation of the results, and reviewed and revised the manuscript. GC contributed to interpretation of results and reviewed and revised the manuscript. FM contributed to interpretation of results and reviewed and revised the manuscript. EV conceptualized and designed the study, performed the search, selected the studies for inclusion, supervised data collection, contributed to the statistical analyses and interpretation of the results, and reviewed and revised the manuscript. All authors approved the final manuscript as submitted.

ACKNOWLEDGMENTS

We thank Paula M. Sisk for kindly providing additional clarification on their study.

REFERENCES

1. Eidelman AI, Schanler RJ, Johnston M, Landers S, Noble L, Szucs K, et al. Breastfeeding and the use of human milk. *Pediatrics.* (2012) 129:e827–41. doi: 10.1542/peds.2011-3552
2. World Health Organization. *Guidelines on Optimal Feeding of Low Birth-Weight Infants in Low-and Middle-Income Countries.* Geneva: World Health Organization (2011). p. 55.
3. Arslanoglu S, Corpeleijn W, Moro G, Braegger C, Campoy C, Colomb V, et al. Donor human milk for preterm infants: current evidence and research directions. *J Pediatr Gastr Nutr.* (2013) 57:535–42. doi: 10.1097/MPG.0b013e3182a3af0a
4. McNelis K, Fu TT, Poindexter B. Nutrition for the extremely preterm infant. *Clin Perinatol.* (2017) 44:395–406. doi: 10.1016/j.clp.2017.01.012
5. Meier P, Patel A, Esquerra-Zwiers A. Donor human milk update: evidence, mechanisms, and priorities for research and practice. *J Pediatr.* (2017) 180:15–21. doi: 10.1016/j.jpeds.2016.09.027
6. McEvoy CT, Jain L, Schmidt B, Abman S, Bancalari E, Aschner JL. Bronchopulmonary dysplasia: NHLBI Workshop on the primary prevention of Chronic Lung Diseases. *Ann Am Thorac Soc.* (2014) 11(Suppl 3):S146–53. doi: 10.1513/AnnalsATS.201312-424LD
7. Jensen EA, Barbara S. Epidemiology of bronchopulmonary dysplasia. *Birth Defects Res A.* (2014) 100:145–57. doi: 10.1002/bdra.23235
8. Wemhoner A, Ortner D, Tschirch E, Strasak A, Rudiger M. Nutrition of preterm infants in relation to bronchopulmonary dysplasia. *BMC Pulm Med.* (2011) 11:7. doi: 10.1186/1471-2466-11-7
9. Villamor-Martínez E, Pierro M, Cavallaro G, Mosca F, Kramer B, Villamor E. Donor human milk protects against bronchopulmonary dysplasia: a systematic review and meta-analysis. *Nutrients.* (2018) 10:238. doi: 10.3390/nu10020238
10. Huang J, Zhang L, Tang J, Shi J, Qu Y, Xiong T, et al. Human milk as a protective factor for bronchopulmonary dysplasia: a systematic review and meta-analysis. *Arch Dis Child Fetal.* (2019) 104:F128–36. doi: 10.1136/archdischild-2017-314205
11. Miller J, Tonkin E, Damarell RA, McPhee AJ, Suganuma M, Suganuma H, et al. A systematic review and meta-analysis of human milk feeding and morbidity in very low birth weight infants. *Nutrients.* (2018) 10:E707. doi: 10.3390/nu10060707
12. Guyatt GH, Oxman AD, Vist GE, Kunz R, Falck-Ytter Y, Alonso-Coello P, et al. GRADE: an emerging consensus on rating quality of evidence and strength of recommendations. *BMJ.* (2008) 336:924–6. doi: 10.1136/bmj.39489.470347.AD
13. Cacho NT, Parker LA, Neu J. Necrotizing enterocolitis and human milk feeding: a systematic review. *Clin Perinatol.* (2017) 44:49–67. doi: 10.1016/j.clp.2016.11.009
14. Zhou J, Shukla VV, John D, Chen C. Human milk feeding as a protective factor for retinopathy of prematurity: a meta-analysis. *Pediatrics.* (2015) 136:e1576–86. doi: 10.1542/peds.2015-2372
15. Moher D, Liberati A, Tetzlaff J, Altman DG, Group P. Preferred reporting items for systematic reviews and meta-analyses: the PRISMA statement. *BMJ.* (2009) 339:b2535. doi: 10.1136/bmj.b2535
16. Bramer WM, Milic J, Mast F. Reviewing retrieved references for inclusion in systematic reviews using endnote. *J Med Libr Assoc.* (2017) 105:84–7. doi: 10.5195/JMLA.2017.111
17. Borenstein M, Hedges LV, Higgins J, Rothstein HR, editors. Subgroup analyses. In: *Introduction to Meta-Analysis.* Hoboken, NJ: John Wiley and Sons Ltd (2009). p. 149–86.
18. Egger M, Smith GD, Schneider M, Minder C. Bias in meta-analysis detected by a simple, graphical test. *BMJ.* (1997) 315:629–34. doi: 10.1136/bmj.315.7109.629
19. Assad M, Elliott M, Abraham J. Decreased cost and improved feeding tolerance in VLBW infants fed an exclusive human milk diet. *J Perinatol.* (2016) 36:216–20. doi: 10.1038/jp.2015.168
20. Cortez J, Makker K, Kraemer D, Neu J, Sharma R, Hudak M. Maternal milk feedings reduce sepsis, necrotizing enterocolitis and improve outcomes of premature infants. *J Perinatol.* (2018) 38:71–4. doi: 10.1038/jp.2017.149
21. Fewtrell MS, Morley R, Abbott RA, Singhal A, Isaacs EB, Stephenson T, et al. Double-blind, randomized trial of long-chain polyunsaturated fatty acid supplementation in formula fed to preterm infants. *Pediatrics.* (2002) 110(1 Pt 1):73–82. doi: 10.1542/peds.110.1.73
22. Fonseca LT, Senna DC, Silveira RC, Procianoy RS. Association between breast milk and bronchopulmonary dysplasia: a single center observational study. *Am J Perinatol.* (2017) 7:264–9. doi: 10.1055/s-0036-1586503
23. Furman L, Taylor G, Minich N, Hack M. THe effect of maternal milk on neonatal morbidity of very low-birth-weight infants. *Arch Pediat Adol Med.* (2003) 157:66–71. doi: 10.1001/archpedi.157.1.66
24. Hylander MA, Strobino DM, Dhanireddy R. Human milk feedings and infection among very low birth weight infants. *Pediatrics.* (1998) 102:e38. doi: 10.1542/peds.102.3.e38
25. Jacobi-Polishook T, Collins CT, Sullivan TR, Simmer K, Gillman MW, Gibson RA, et al. Human milk intake in preterm infants and neurodevelopment at 18 months corrected age. *Pediatr Res.* (2016) 80:486–92. doi: 10.1038/pr.2016.114
26. Maayan-Metzger A, Avivi S, Schushan-Eisen I, Kuint J. Human milk versus formula feeding among preterm infants: short-term outcomes. *Am J Perinatol.* (2012) 29:121–6. doi: 10.1055/s-0031-1295652

27. Madore LS, Bora S, Erdei C, Jumani T, Dengos AR, Sen S. Effects of donor breastmilk feeding on growth and early neurodevelopmental outcomes in preterm infants: an observational study. *Clin Ther.* (2017) 39:1210–20. doi: 10.1016/j.clinthera.2017.05.341
28. O'Connor DL, Jacobs J, Hall R, Adamkin D, Auestad N, Castillo M, et al. Growth and development of premature infants fed predominantly human milk, predominantly premature infant formula, or a combination of human milk and premature formula. *J Pediatr Gastroenterol Nutr.* (2003) 37:437–46. doi: 10.1097/00005176-200310000-00008
29. Patra K, Hamilton M, Johnson TJ, Greene M, Dabrowski E, Meier PP, et al. NICU human milk dose and 20-month neurodevelopmental outcome in very low birth weight infants. *Neonatology.* (2017) 112:330–6. doi: 10.1159/000475834
30. Schanler RJ, Lau C, Hurst NM, Smith EOB. Randomized trial of donor human milk versus preterm formula as substitutes for mothers' own milk in the feeding of extremely premature infants. *Pediatrics.* (2005) 116:400–6. doi: 10.1542/peds.2004-1974
31. Sisk P, Lovelady C, Dillard R, Gruber K, O'shea T. Early human milk feeding is associated with a lower risk of necrotizing enterocolitis in very low birth weight infants. *J Perinatol.* (2007) 27:428–33. doi: 10.1038/sj.jp.7211758
32. Sisk PM, Lambeth TM, Rojas MA, Lightbourne T, Barahona M, Anthony E, et al. Necrotizing enterocolitis and growth in preterm infants fed predominantly maternal milk, pasteurized donor milk, or preterm formula: a retrospective study. *Am J Perinatol.* (2017) 34:676–83. doi: 10.1055/s-0036-1597326
33. Vohr BR, Poindexter BB, Dusick AM, McKinley LT, Wright LL, Langer JC, et al. Beneficial effects of breast milk in the neonatal intensive care unit on the developmental outcome of extremely low birth weight infants at 18 months of age. *Pediatrics.* (2006) 118:e115–23. doi: 10.1542/peds.2005-2382
34. Djulbegovic B, Guyatt GH. Progress in evidence-based medicine: a quarter century on. *Lancet.* (2017) 390:415–23. doi: 10.1016/S0140-6736(16)31592-6
35. Binns C, Lee MK, Kagawa M. Ethical challenges in infant feeding research. *Nutrients.* (2017) 9:59. doi: 10.3390/nu9010059
36. Jobe AH, Bancalari E. Bronchopulmonary dysplasia. *Am J Respir Crit Care Med.* (2001) 163:1723–9. doi: 10.1164/ajrccm.163.7.2011060
37. Kramer BW. Antenatal inflammation and lung injury: prenatal origin of neonatal disease. *J Perinatol.* (2008) 28(Suppl 1):S21–7. doi: 10.1038/jp.2008.46
38. Shahzad T, Radajewski S, Chao CM, Bellusci S, Ehrhardt H. Pathogenesis of bronchopulmonary dysplasia: when inflammation meets organ development. *Mol Cell Pediatr.* (2016) 3:23. doi: 10.1186/s40348-016-0051-9
39. Shah J, Jefferies AL, Yoon EW, Lee SK, Shah PS. Risk factors and outcomes of late-onset bacterial sepsis in preterm neonates born at <32 weeks' gestation. *Am J Perinatol.* (2015) 32:675–82. doi: 10.1055/s-0034-1393936
40. Hintz SR, Kendrick DE, Stoll BJ, Vohr BR, Fanaroff AA, Donovan EF, et al. Neurodevelopmental and growth outcomes of extremely low birth weight infants after necrotizing enterocolitis. *Pediatrics.* (2005) 115:696–703. doi: 10.1542/peds.2004-0569
41. Brener Dik PH, Nino Gualdron YM, Galletti MF, Cribioli CM, Mariani GL. Bronchopulmonary dysplasia: incidence and risk factors. *Arch Argent Pediatr.* (2017) 115:476–82. doi: 10.5546/aap.2017.eng.476
42. Biniwale MA, Ehrenkranz RA. The role of nutrition in the prevention and management of bronchopulmonary dysplasia. *Semin Perinatol.* (2006) 30:200–8. doi: 10.1053/j.semperi.2006.05.007
43. Friel JK, Martin SM, Langdon M, Herzberg GR, Buettner GR. Milk from mothers of both premature and full-term infants provides better antioxidant protection than does infant formula. *Pediatr Res.* (2002) 51:612–8. doi: 10.1203/00006450-200205000-00012
44. Collado MC, Santaella M, Mira-Pascual L, Martinez-Arias E, Khodayar-Pardo P, Ros G, et al. Longitudinal study of cytokine expression, lipid profile and neuronal growth factors in human breast milk from term and preterm deliveries. *Nutrients.* (2015) 7:8577–91. doi: 10.3390/nu7105415
45. Underwood MA, Gaerlan S, De Leoz ML, Dimapasoc L, Kalanetra KM, Lemay DG, et al. Human milk oligosaccharides in premature infants: absorption, excretion, and influence on the intestinal microbiota. *Pediatr Res.* (2015) 78:670–7. doi: 10.1038/pr.2015.162
46. Dvorak B, Fituch CC, Williams CS, Hurst NM, Schanler RJ. Concentrations of epidermal growth factor and transforming growth factor-alpha in preterm milk. *Adv Exp Med Biol.* (2004) 554:407–9. doi: 10.1007/978-1-4757-4242-8_52
47. Hassiotou F, Hartmann PE. At the dawn of a new discovery: the potential of breast milk stem cells. *Adv Nutr.* (2014) 5:770–8. doi: 10.3945/an.114.006924
48. Sisk PM, Lovelady CA, Dillard RG, Gruber KJ, O'Shea TM. Maternal and infant characteristics associated with human milk feeding in very low birth weight infants. *J Hum Lact.* (2009) 25:412–9. doi: 10.1177/0890334409340776
49. Jones JR, Kogan MD, Singh GK, Dee DL, Grummer-Strawn LM. factors associated with exclusive breastfeeding in the United States. *Pediatrics.* (2011) 128:1117–25. doi: 10.1542/peds.2011-0841
50. Sisk PM, Lovelady CA, Dillard RG, Gruber KJ. Lactation counseling for mothers of very low birth weight infants: effect on maternal anxiety and infant intake of human milk. *Pediatrics.* (2006) 117:e67–75. doi: 10.1542/peds.2005-0267
51. Furman L, Minich N, Hack M. Correlates of lactation in mothers of very low birth weight infants. *Pediatrics.* (2002) 109:e57. doi: 10.1542/peds.109.4.e57
52. Meier PP, Engstrom JL, Mingolelli SS, Miracle DJ, Kiesling S. The rush mothers' milk club: breastfeeding interventions for mothers with very-low-birth-weight infants. *J Obstet Gynecol Neonatal Nurs.* (2004) 33:164–74. doi: 10.1177/0884217504263280
53. Jones JR, Kogan MD, Singh GK, Dee DL, Grummer-Strawn LM. Factors associated with exclusive breastfeeding in the United States. *Pediatrics.* (2011) 128:1117–25. doi: 10.1542/peds.2011-0841d
54. Lessen R, Crivelli-Kovach A. Prediction of initiation and duration of breast-feeding for neonates admitted to the neonatal intensive care unit. *J Perinat Neonatal Nurs.* (2007) 21:256–66. doi: 10.1097/01.JPN.0000285817.51645.73
55. Patel AL, Johnson TJ, Robin B, Bigger HR, Buchanan A, Christian E, et al. Influence of own mother's milk on bronchopulmonary dysplasia and costs. *Arch Dis Child Fetal Neonatal Ed.* (2017) 102:F256–61. doi: 10.1136/archdischild-2016-310898
56. Schanler RJ, Shulman RJ, Lau C. Feeding strategies for premature infants: beneficial outcomes of feeding fortified human milk versus preterm formula. *Pediatrics.* (1999) 103(6 Pt 1):1150–7. doi: 10.1542/peds.103.6.1150
57. Abrams SA, Schanler RJ, Lee ML, Rechtman DJ. Greater mortality and morbidity in extremely preterm infants fed a diet containing cow milk protein products. *Breastfeed Med.* (2014) 9:281–5. doi: 10.1089/bfm.2014.0024
58. Meinzen-Derr J, Poindexter B, Wrage L, Morrow AL, Stoll B, Donovan EF. Role of human milk in extremely low birth weight infants' risk of necrotizing enterocolitis or death. *J Perinatol.* (2009) 29:57–62. doi: 10.1038/jp.2008.117
59. Spiegler J, Preuss M, Gebauer C, Bendiks M, Herting E, Gopel W. Does breastmilk influence the development of bronchopulmonary dysplasia? *J Pediatr.* (2016) 169:76–80 e4. doi: 10.1016/j.jpeds.2015.10.080
60. Hanna N, Ahmed K, Anwar M, Petrova A, Hiatt M, Hegyi T. Effect of storage on breast milk antioxidant activity. *Arch Dis Child Fetal Neonatal Ed.* (2004) 89:F518–20. doi: 10.1136/adc.2004.049247

15

Strategies of Increased Protein Intake in ELBW Infants Fed by Human Milk Lead to Long Term Benefits

Elisa Mariani[1], Augusto Biasini[2], Lucia Marvulli[1], Silvia Martini[3], Arianna Aceti[3], Giacomo Faldella[3], Luigi Corvaglia[3], Alessandra Sansavini[4], Silvia Savini[3], Francesca Agostini[4], Marcello Stella[1] and Erica Neri[4]*

[1] Pediatric and Neonatal Intensive Care Unit, M. Bufalini Hospital, Cesena, Italy, [2] Donor Human Milk Bank Italian Association (AIBLUD), Milan, Italy, [3] Neonatology and Neonatal Intensive Care Unit—S. Orsola-Malpighi Hospital, Bologna, Italy, [4] Department of Psychology, University of Bologna, Bologna, Italy

***Correspondence:**
Elisa Mariani
elisa.mariani@auslromagna.it

Objective: The aim of this observational study was to evaluate the effects of two different protein intake regimes on feeding tolerance, in-hospital growth, anthropometric data and psychomotor outcome up to 24 months corrected age (CA) in extremely low birth-weight (ELBW; birth weight <1000 g) infants.

Methods: During the period 2008–2013, 52 ELBW infants admitted at birth to two Neonatal Intensive Care Units of Emilia Romagna (Italy) were fed according to different protocols of protein fortification of human milk: an estimated protein intakes at maximum fortification levels of 3.5 gr/kg/day in the Standard Nutrition Population-SNP group ($n = 26$) and 4.8 g/kg/day in the Aggressive Nutrition Population-ANP group ($n = 26$). During hospitalization, infants' growth, biochemical indices of nutritional status, enteral intake, feeding tolerance, clinical history and morbidity were evaluated. After discharge, anthropometric data and psychomotor outcome, evaluated by Revised Griffiths Mental Development Scales (GMDS-R) 0–2 years, were assessed up to 24 months CA.

Results: During hospitalization, the ANP group showed significantly higher weight (18.87 vs. 15.20 g/kg/day) and head circumference (0.70 vs. 0.52 cm/week) growth rates compared to SNP, less days of parenteral nutrition (7.36 ± 2.7 vs. 37.75 ± 29.6) and of hospitalization (60.0 ± 13.3 vs. 78.08 ± 21.32). After discharge, ANP infants had a greater head circumference compared to SNP (45.64 ± 0.29; 46.80 ± 0.31). Furthermore, the General Quotient of GMDS-R mean scores in the SNP group significantly decreased from 12 to 24 months CA, while no difference was seen in the ANP group.

Conclusions: Increased protein intake may provide short and long term benefits in terms of growth and neurodevelopment in human milk-fed ELBW infants.

Keywords: nutrition ELBW, protein intake, long term neurologic advantages, full feeding achievement, speed of growth

INTRODUCTION

The main goals of preterm infants' nutrition are the achievement of postnatal growth rates similar to those of normal fetuses of the same gestational age, a mimic fetal body composition and neurodevelopmental outcomes comparable to term-born infants (1).

In-hospital weight, length, and head circumference (HC) growth rates are positively correlated with neurodevelopment and, possibly, with an improved brain growth and neurological maturation in the preterm population (2, 3). Conversely, extra-uterine growth restriction (EUGR), defined as weight, length, or HC ≤10th percentile of intra-uterine growth expectation for correspondent postmenstrual age at hospital discharge (4), is a negative prognostic factor for long-term neurodevelopment (2). Adequate nutrition during hospitalization is fundamental in order to prevent EUGR and to optimize long-term growth and neurodevelopment in the preterm population. However, due to their gastro-intestinal immaturity, very preterm infants often experience poor feeding tolerance during their stay in Neonatal Intensive Care Unit (NICU), and this contributes to hinder the achievement of optimal nutritional intakes over the first weeks of life (5). As a consequence, significant energy and nutrients deficits are frequently established during NICU stay, and inadequate protein and energy intakes may account for up to 45% of postnatal weight restriction in very-low-birth-weight preterm infants at hospital discharge (6, 7).

The beneficial effects of human milk feeding have been currently acknowledged to overcome the delayed weight gain associated to the lower protein and energy contents of human milk compared to formula (8, 9). However, it has been previously shown that actual protein intakes after standard protein fortification of human milk are substantially lower than those recommended over the first weeks of life (10, 11). Furthermore, data on the possible influence of protein intakes on neonatal growth and neurodevelopment in extremely low birth weight (ELBW) infants are still limited (12).

This study aimed to evaluate the effect of two nutritional approaches, providing different protein regimens, on in-hospital and post-discharge growth and psychomotor outcomes in ELBW preterm infants followed up to 24 months of corrected age (CA).

MATERIALS AND METHODS

During the period 2008–2013, all preterm infants admitted to two level III NICUs of Emilia Romagna region (Italy), Sant'Orsola Malpighi Hospital NICU (Bologna) and Bufalini Hospital NICU (Cesena), were included in the present study if the following inclusion criteria were fulfilled: birth-weight (BW) <1000 g, gestational age (GA) < 32 weeks, exclusive human milk feeding (own mother's milk [OMM] or donor milk [DM] from the local human milk bank) during NICU stay, no presence of sepsis. Conversely, infants developing intraventricular hemorrhage grade 3 or 4 (13), periventricular leukomalacia (14), retinopathy of prematurity ≥grade 3 plus disease (15), or necrotizing enterocolitis (NEC) Bell's stage ≥2 (16) during hospitalization were ruled out from the study, in view of the known negative effects of these conditions on growth and development. Globally, 52 ELBW infants were considered eligible for the study.

This study was conducted in conformity with the principles and regulations of the Helsinki Declaration. A written, informed consent to participate was obtained from the parents/guardians of each infant. The protocol was approved by the local Ethics Committees in both the study centers.

Strategies

The two NICUs had similar protocols for resuscitation, stabilization, ventilation and pharmacological management of ELBW preterm infants, whereas their nutritional approaches were significantly different.

The nutritional protocol of Sant'Orsola Malpighi Hospital's NICU, named Standard Nutrition Protocol (SNP), provided an average protein regimen, administered by combined enteral and parenteral nutrition (PN) according to the European Society of Pediatric Gastroenterology and Nutrition (ESPGHAN) Guidelines (17, 18). This protocol entailed four different phases of enteral nutrition. In phase 1 (minimal enteral feeding [MEF]), minimal milk feeds (10–15 ml/kg/day) were administered to stimulate the anatomical and functional maturation of the gut and to reduce NEC risk (19). During this period, recommended nutrient intakes were guaranteed by PN, started within the first 24 h of life. PN was prescribed according to the ESPGHAN recommendations (17): starting composition consisted of 6 mg/kg/day of glucose and 2–2.5 g/kg/day of aminoacids, which were incremented to 3.5 g/kg/day by day 6. Lipids were introduced from day 3 and gradually increased to 0.5 g/kg/day over the first week of life until the achievement of 3 g/kg/day. Sodium and other electrolytes were added from day 3 onwards and adjusted in relation to serum values and diuresis.

Once feeding tolerance to MEF was obtained, feeds were increased by 15–20 ml/kg/day divided in 8 meals (phase 2) until the achievement of full feeding, defined as enteral volumes of 160 ml/kg/day (phase 3). Human milk fortification was started at volumes of 100 ml/kg/day using Aptamil BMF 4.4% (1,6-1,98 gr proteins/100 ml of milk) at meal administration. If clinical deterioration or symptoms of feeding intolerance (i.e., abdominal distention, absent bowel sounds, persistently bilious or bloody gastric residuals and/or bloody stools) (20), suspected sepsis, NEC or other surgical problems occurred at any phase, enteral feeds were withheld. According to inclusion criteria, 26 ELBW infants were recruited in SNP group.

The nutritional protocol of Bufalini Hospital's NICU was named Aggressive Nutrition Protocol (ANP). According to this protocol, preterm neonates were fed with fresh OMM or DM since their first day of life. Feeds were started at volumes of 10–15 ml/kg/day, divided in 10 meals; when an adequate feeding tolerance was established, feeds were increased by 20–25 ml/kg/die. Protein fortification of HM was started from day 3 (when volume were about 40 ml/kg) onwards at protein intakes of 0.5 g/100 ml of milk with Pro-expert PS (Aptamil) or Protifar (Nutricia), and was incremented to 1% over the next 24 h. When infants tolerated feed volumes of 100 ml/kg/day, BMF (Aptamil) at a concentration of 3 g/100 ml was added to Pro-expert PS, and increased to 5 g/100 ml over the next days. The amount of protein fortification was adjusted according to the newborn's blood urea and acid-base status, monitored twice a week (21): if blood urea was less than 40 mg/dl, protein fortification (Pro-expert PS) was yielded by 1.5%, whereas BMF kept fixed at 5%; no changes were made for levels between 40 and 50 mg/dl and normal acid-base status (pH >7.30 and BE <-4). The maximum level of fortification was obtained with BMF at 5% plus Protifar or Pro-expert PS at 1.5%, depending on the infants' feeding tolerance, blood urea values and acid-base status. According to inclusion criteria, 26 ELBW infants were recruited in ANP group.

Outcome Evaluation

During hospitalization, growth parameters (weight, length and HC), acid-base status, renal function, diuresis, enteral intakes, feeding tolerance, clinical history and the occurrence of clinical complications were regularly assessed and recorded in a clinical report form.

After discharge, as per national recommendations (22), all the enrolled infants were included in the clinical, neurological and neurodevelopmental follow-up of prematurity, which entails a term MRI scan at 40 weeks post-conceptional age and regular evaluations of the infant's growth and neurodevelopmental status up to 24 months CA. At each evaluation, weight, length and HC were measured to assess the infant's growth.

The psychomotor outcome of the enrolled infants was evaluated by two psychologists, with long-standing experience in developmental assessment, blind to the infant's nutrition group, using the Revised Griffiths Mental Development Scales (GMDS-R) 0–2 years (23), which are widely adopted for the evaluation of mental and psychomotor development in the context of the neurodevelopmental follow-up of preterm infants (24–28). These scales investigate five main areas (Locomotor—LOC, Personal-Social - PS, Hearing and Language - HL, Eye-Hand Coordination - EH, Performance—PERF), providing a general quotient (GQ) of the infant's abilities adjusted for corrected age and 5 sub-quotients (SQ) for each functional area.

Data from the 12 and 24-month assessments were included in the present study.

Statistical Analysis

Statistical analysis was performed using Statistical Package for Social Science software for Microsoft Windows (SPSS) version 21.0. Data distribution was checked using Kolmogorov–Smirnov test; all data showed a normal distribution. Clinical characteristics of the study groups were compared by Pearson's chi-squared test and MANOVA.

Possible differences between the study groups in terms of length of NICU stay, growth parameters and in-hospital outcomes were evaluated by MANOVA test. Furthermore, the effects of study group (SNP and ANP), child's age (12 and 24 months CA), and their interaction on anthropometric data and psychomotor scores at post-discharge assessments were tested through Repeated Measure MANOVA. Maternal education and the infant gestational age were included as variables in order to control their possible influence, as emerged in previous literature (9, 24).

Finally, the association among intra-hospital variables and anthropometric data and psychomotor scores at post-discharge assessments was investigated with Pearson correlation coefficients. Fisher test (F) and eta squared (η^2_p) values were reported.

Significance level was set at $p \leq 0.05$.

RESULTS

A total of 52 neonates were included in the present study, 26 in the SNP group and 26 in the ANP group. The infants' characteristics are detailed in **Table 1**; while the two study groups were similar in terms of GA and anthropometric characteristics at birth, a significant difference in the distribution of gender, twinhood and mechanical ventilation [MV] was observed. Subsequent analyses showed that infant gender and twinhood did not significantly influence anthropometric data and GMDS scores. For this reason, these variables were not included in further analyses. On the contrary, MV showed a significant association with the outcome scores and was, therefore, controlled in subsequent analyses.

Globally, 60% of the enrolled infants received OMM and 40% pasteurized DM from the local hospital bank.

Eventually, groups were homogeneous for the following maternal characteristics: education, nationality and age (**Table 1**).

Parenteral and enteral protein intakes for the two groups over the first 4 weeks of life are detailed in **Table 2**. For each week the daily protein intake was significantly higher in the ANP group compared to SNP group. The high-protein nutritional regimen was well tolerated by the ANP group; no difference in the rate of metabolic acidosis and in serum creatinine levels during NICU stay was seen compared to the SNP group.

The rate of infants fed exclusively with OMM at discharge was 62.5% in the ANP group and 65.6% in the SNP group.

In-hospital Outcomes

In-hospital outcomes are detailed in **Table 3**. Infants in the ANP group showed significantly higher growth rates for weight and HC [$F_{(1,47)} = 5.95$; $P = 0.021$; $F_{(1,47)} = 7.60$; $P = 0.010$, respectively], but not for length, when compared to SNP. PN duration and the length of NICU stay were significantly shorter in the ANP group compared to the SNP [$F_{(1,47)} = 15.87$; $P < 0.0005$; $F_{(1,47)} = 21.85$; $P < 0.0005$, respectively] (**Table 3**).

Post-discharge Outcomes

No pathological findings at term MRI were observed in the infants enrolled. At 24 months CA, no child developed cerebral palsy.

Anthropometric measures at 12 and 24 months CA in the two groups are provided in **Table 4**. Repeated measure MANOVA showed no significant effect of the Study Group on weight and length between two groups, whereas head circumference was significant higher in the ANP than in SNP group [SNP mean = 45.64 ± 0.29; ANP mean = 46.80 ± 0.31; $F_{(1,40)} = 7.844$; $P = 0.008$]. A significant interaction between Study Group and Child's Age emerged for the children length [$F_{(1,40)} = 27.170$; $P < 0.0005$]: at 24 months CA SNP

TABLE 1 | Biological, socio-demographic and medical characteristics of the two groups.

	SNP (*n* = 26)	ANP (*n* = 26)	*F/X*²	*P*
Males, *n* (%)	9 (34.6)	16 (61.5)	3.78	0.05
Birth-weight (g), mean (SD), range	773 (165), 445–1000	826 (136), 692–986	0.11	0.74
Head circumference (cm), mean (SD), range	25.3 (2.55), 2 2–31	24.9 (1.59), 22.8–29	0.59	0.44
Gestational age (weeks), mean (SD), range	27.5 (1.68), 23–31	28.0 (1.75), 2 4–31	0.30	0.59
Cesarean section, *n* (%)	23 (88.5)	21 (80.8)	0.60	0.44
Twinhood, *n* (%)	8 (30.8)	2 (7.7)	4.46	0.03
MV, *n* (%)	13 (50.0)	3 (11.5)	9.03	0.003
SGA, *n* (%)	11 (42.3)	12 (46.2)	0.08	0.78
BPD, *n* (%)	9 (34.6)	5 (19.2)	1.56	0.21
PDA, *n* (%)	11 (42.3)	7 (26.9)	1.36	0.24
Maternal education University, *n* (%)	11 (42.3)	10 (39.1)	2.83	0.24
High school, n (%)	11 (42.3)	7 (26.1)		
Primary and secondary school, *n* (%)	4 (15.4)	9 (34.8)		
Maternal foreign nationality, *n* (%)	4 (15.4)	8 (30.8)	1.73	0.18
Maternal age, mean (SD), range	32.54 (4.37), 24–42	34.55 (4.25), 23–41	2.35	0.13

SNP, Standard Nutrition Protocol; ANP, Aggressive Nutrition Protocol; MV, mechanical ventilation, SGA, small for gestational age, BPD, bronchopulmonary dysplasia.

TABLE 2 | Mean values (standard deviation) of parenteral, enteral and total protein intakes in the two groups during the first 4 weeks of life.

		SNP (*n* = 26)	ANP (*n* = 26)	*F*	*P*
Week 1	Enteral	0.05 (0.05)	0.70 (0.65)	9.73	0.003
	Parenteral	1.39 (0.34)	1.20 (0.48)		<0.0005
	Total	1.46 (0.36)	1.99 (0.50)	12.77	0.001
Week 2	Enteral	0.30 (0.37)	3.08 (1.27)	18.31	<0.0005
	Parenteral	1.22 (0.35)	0.10 (0.18)		<0.0005
	Total	1.69 (0.29)	3.65 (0.99)	41.47	<0.0005
Week 3	Enteral	1.03 (0.77)	4.22 (0.87)	51.46	<0.0005
	Parenteral	0.63 (0.52)	0.00 (0.00)		<0.0005
	Total	1.72 (0.52)	4.22 (0.87)	73.68	<0.0005
Week 4	Enteral	1.72 (0.99)	4.36 (0.84)	32.66	<0.0005
	Parenteral	0.64 (0.63)	0.00 (0.00)		<0.0005
	Total	1.96 (0.71)	4.36 (0.84)	55.36	<0.0005

Values describe g/kg/day. SNP, Standard Nutrition Protocol; ANP, Aggressive Nutrition Protocol.

children were taller than ANP ones ($P = 0.04$), whereas no significant difference for weight and head circumference was observed.

Psychomotor data at 12 and 24 months CA in the two groups are provided in **Table 5**. Mean values of GQ and SQ scores fell within normal ranges[22] in both groups at 12 and 24 months except for PERF mean values in the SNP group at 24 months, which fell below the lower normal threshold. Despite no significant differences between SNP and ANP emerged, the interaction between Study Group and Child's Age significantly influenced the GQ [$F_{(1,40)} = 9.062$; $P = 0.005$] and the following SQ: PS [$F_{(1,40)} = 10.743$, $P = 0.002$], and PERF [$F_{(1,40)} = 6.653$, $P = 0.014$] (**Figure 1**). Bonferroni *post hoc* analyses showed that QG, PS and PERF mean scores significantly decreased from 12 to 24 months CA [$P = 0.003$; $P = 0.018$; $P = 0.006$, respectively] but only in SNP group; moreover, PS quotients of ANP children (but non SNP ones) significantly increased from 12 to 24 months CA [$P = 0.047$] (**Figure 1**). Eventually, when compared to SNP, ANP children showed higher PERF scores at 24 months CA [$P = 0.013$] (**Figure 1**).

No significant effect of Child's Age emerged on anthropometric nor psychomotor outcomes.

Protein intakes in the first 2 weeks of life positively correlated with HC at 24 months CA ($P = 0.031$). No significant correlation between protein intakes in the first 2 weeks and GMDS quotients were observed.

TABLE 3 | In-Hospital Outcomes.

	SNP (*n* = 26)	ANP (*n* = 26)	F/X2	*P*
Weight gain (gr/kg/day), mean (SD), range	15.20 (2.8), 9.7–23.9	18.87 (3.0), 13.2–25.0	5.95	0.021
Length growth (cm/week), mean (SD), range	0.95 (0.5), 0.1–2.3	0.88 (0.2), 0.3–1.4	0.62	NS
Head circumference growth (cm/week), mean (SD), range	0.52 (0.2), 0.2–0.9	0.70 (0.2), 0.1–1.1	7.60	0.010
Milk volume, ml/kg, mean (SD), range	150.52 (17.6), 115.6–200.9	160.7 (7.3), 149.3–198.8	0.12	NS
Days of PN, mean (SD), range	38.75 (29.6), 9–106	7.36 (2.7), 2–14	15.86	<0.0005
Days to achieve full feeding, mean(SD), range	28.50 (17.2), 9-78	7.50 (2.0), 4-12	28.40	<0.0005
Weight at full feeding, mean(SD), range	895.42 (294.8), 535–1620	748.8 (112.70),526–940	2.68	NS
Days of hospitalization, mean (SD), range	78.08 (21.32),46–145	60.0 (13.3),31–81	21.85	<0.0005
EUGR, n (%)	22 (84.6%)	16 (61.5%)	3.52	0.06

SNP, Standard Nutrition Protocol; ANP, Aggressive Nutrition Protocol; PN, Parenteral Nutrition; EUGR, Extra-Uterine Growth Restriction.

TABLE 4 | Anthropometric data.

	SNP (*n* = 26)		ANP (*n* = 26)		RM-MANOVA		
	Mean(SD)	**Range**	**Mean(SD)**	**Range**	***F***	***P***	$\eta\, p^2$
Weight (g)					2.509	0.121	0.059
12 mo. ca	8027.7 (1109)	5915–10660	8546.15 (1175.8)	6800–10900			
24 mo. ca	10375.8 (1363)	8110–13700	10572.31 (1280.7)	8530–13200			
Length (cm)					27.170	<0.0005	0.405
12 mo. Ca	72.3 (3.14)	68–81	72.9 (2.79)	67–78			
24 mo. ca	84.7 (3.20)	80–92	82.2 (3.15)	76–89			
HC (cm)					2.985	0.092	0.069
12 mo. ca	44.9 (1.46)	41–47	45.8 (1.57)	43–48			
24 mo.ca	47.15 (1.25)	44.3–49.4	47.8 (1.24)	45.5–50			

The table summarizes mean, SD, range, F, p and eta-squared (?2p) values for MANOVAs on Anthropometric data of SNP (Standard Nutrition Protocol) and ANP (Aggressive Nutrition Protocol) infants at 12 and 24 months (corrected age).

DISCUSSION

According to our results, higher protein intakes over the first 4 weeks of life in ELBW infants are associated with improved growth of HC and psychomotor outcomes at 24 months CA, thus highlighting the importance of in-hospital nutrition. Moreover, the present data confirm that adjustable fortification of HM combining different commercially available concentrated HM fortifiers effectively allows the achievement of protein intakes and protein/energy ratio currently recommended for the ELBW population during the first weeks of life.

While more is known about recommended protein intakes for very-low-birth-weight infants, little data are currently available for ELBW babies. Basing on empirical calculations, an enteral protein intake of 4.0–4.5 g/kg/day is currently recommended for infants up to 1000 g of weight to prevent protein deficit accumulation and to aim at growth patterns similar to intrauterine ones (18). Particular attention should be paid also at protein/energy ratio that, for infants <1000 g, ranges from 3.2 to 4.1 g/100 kcal. In growth-restricted infants, energy intakes can be increased; however, if not accompanied by adequate protein intakes, growth is achieved at the expenses of body composition, ensuing in a high percentage of body fat (19) that could contribute to worsen the increased intraabdominal adiposity observed in ELBW neonates and to heighten their risk of metabolic complications in later life (29).

Assuming HM protein contents between 0.8 and 1.2 g/100 ml (10, 11), the estimated protein intakes at maximum fortification levels and at enteral intakes of 160 ml/kg/day were 3.5 g/kg/ day in the SNP group and 4.8 g/kg/day in the ANP group, whereas the protein/energy ratio (protein g/100 Kcal) ranged between 1.9–2.3 and 3.0–3.3, respectively. Hence, according to the above recommendations, the estimated protein requirements were met in the ANP but not in the SNP group; consistently, the latter showed higher EUGR rates.

In 2013, Cormack et al. (30) investigated the effects of protein intake equal or greater to 4 g/kg/day provided during the first week of life in a predominantly HM fed cohort of ELBW babies, reporting a significant association between protein intake and in-hospital growth: the higher the intake, the smaller the z-score change between birth and discharge.

TABLE 5 | Infant's psychomotor mean scores at post-discharge assessments.

	SNP ($n = 26$)		ANP ($n = 26$)		RM-MANOVA		
	Mean(SD)	**Range**	**Mean(SD)**	**Range**	**F**	**P**	**$\eta\ p^2$**
GQ score, mean (SD), range					9.062	0.005	0.197
12 mo. ca	103.24 (10.66)	72–119	97.03 (11.79)	66–117			
24 mo. ca	97.03 (11.77)	68–113	101.03 (110.76)	81–120			
LOC score, mean (SD), range					3.130	0.085	0.078
12 mo. Ca	95.28 (16.70)	57–117	97.79 (16.38)	57–121			
24 mo. ca	98.94 (19.30)	60–135	113.93 (20.59)	60–135			
PS score, mean (SD), range					10.743	0.002	0.225
12 mo. ca	107.28 (13.60)	64–122	92.36 (13.20)	56-114			
24 mo.ca	99.60 (13.45)	59–119	99.58 (12.87)	66-119			
HL score, mean (SD), range					0.279	0.601	0.007
12 mo. ca	107.28 (17.08)	85–150	102.55 (13.26)	74–129			
24 mo.ca	99.64 (18.43)	50–115	92.53 (14.43)	50–113			
EH score, mean (SD), range					2.825	0.101	0.071
12 mo. ca	102.08 (14.55)	79–128	97.22 (15.93)	68–122			
24 mo.ca	98.89 (14.28)	71–123	103.62 (14.27)	76–123			
PERF score, mean (SD), range					6.653	0.014	0.152
12 mo. ca	102.32 (12.09)	76–122	102.32 (13.12)	63–123			
24 mo.ca	90.99 (18.74)	50–117	105.53 (12.37)	77–121			

The table summarizes mean, SD, range, F, p and eta-squared ($?^2_p$) values for MANOVAs on GQ, General Quotient; LOC, Locomotor; PS, Personal & Social skills; HL, Hearing & Language; EH, Eye & Hand Coordination; and Performance (PERF) standardized scores (GMDS-R) of SNP (Standard Nutrition Protocol) and ANP (Aggressive Nutrition Protocol) infants at 12 and 24 months (corrected age).

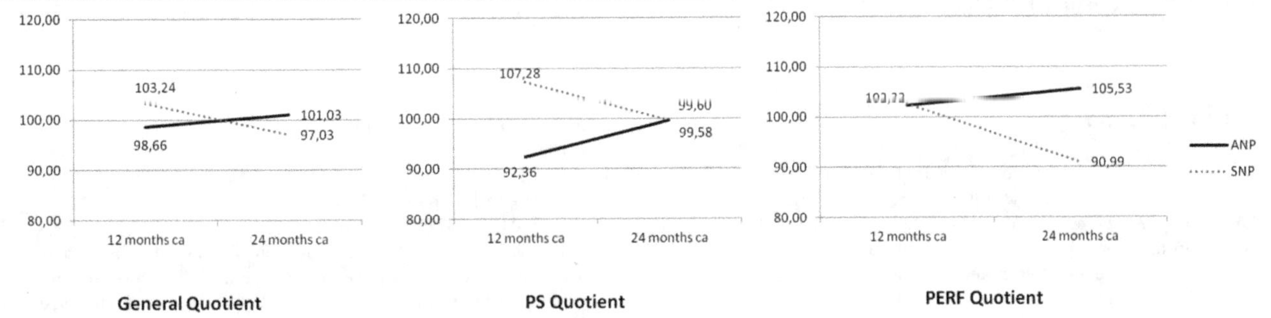

FIGURE 1 | Mean scores on General Quotient (GQ), Personal and Social skills (PS), and Performance (PERF) according to the interaction between Study Group and Child's Age. Continue line denotes ANP (Aggressive Nutrition Protocol) group; dotted line SNP (Standard Nutrition Protocol) group.

In addition to the beneficial effects on in-hospital outcomes and head circumference growth at 12 and 24 months CA, the present study has demonstrated increased length after discharge. However, an unattended result regards the outcome of length, where ANP infants obtained worse scores than those of SNP group. According to previous researches (27, 28), length was measured to the nearest cm using a length board: it could be possible this kind of measure is not adequately sensitive and has a increased risk of measurement bias. Further studies are needed to better explain this result.

Our results are in line with Stephen et al. (12), who had previously described a positive correlation between increased first-week protein and energy intakes and higher Mental Development Index scores at 18 months CA in an ELBW population. Despite ANP and SNP did not differ in the GMDS quotients mean scores, the trajectory of these scores is significantly different in the scales, with a lower decrement and a better psychomotor development at 24 months CA in ELBW infants receiving early and high protein intakes. Specifically, ANP children not only show better personal-social skills outcome at 24 months, but their GQ, PS and PERF mean quotients do not decrease as emerged in SNP group. Despite preliminary, this result is promising: future studies could deepen if this intervention reduce the negative effect of severely preterm birth on long term development. The Hearing and Language quotients is the only where effects did not emerged, confirming as this area is particularly weak for very preterm infants (24, 26, 31).

Taken together, these results suggest a long-lasting beneficial influence of this protein regimen on cerebral maturation.

Recently, a Cochrane review investigating the effect of high protein intake in formula-fed low-birth-weight infants has reported elevated blood urea nitrogen levels and an increased incidence of metabolic acidosis in association with protein intakes ranging between 3 and 4 g/kg/day (32). However, little is known about the incidence of these adverse effects in HM-fed ELBW infants. In the present study, the ANP group did not show increased blood urea or higher rates of metabolic acidosis, suggesting that this high-protein regimen was adequately tolerated by the study ELBW population.

Although a trend toward an earlier introduction of enteral feeds has occurred over the last few years, ELBW infants often do not begin enteral nutrition for several days and do not reach full feeding for weeks. In the ANP population, enteral feeds were introduced since the first day of life and faster rates of feeding advancement were adopted, resulting in earlier full feeding achievement, shortened PN duration -related complications and a significantly briefer length of hospitalization. The combination of these factors may have contributed to the improved psychomotor outcomes of ANP infants at 24 months CA; however, the design of the present study did not allow to define the role of each factor in determining the observed outcome.

A number of limits could be acknowledged for the present study. Firstly, the results need to be confirmed on wider samples. Secondly, a significant difference in the distribution of a clinical complication (mechanical ventilation) emerged. Despite this variables was controlled in analyses, results need replication. Thirdly, the small sample size did not allow to focus on SGA infants, which are known as a high risk population (32). Further studies are therefore recommended which should consider also these factors.

In conclusion, a high-protein regimen, associated with an early introduction and advancement of exclusive HM feeds, can lead to improved in-hospital growth, lower rates of EUGR, shorter length of NICU stay and better psychomotor and growth outcomes at 24 months CA in ELBW preterm infants. Further larger studies are needed to confirm these preliminary data, to assess the contribution of different nutrient components and other clinical or environmental variables on post-discharge growth and neurodevelopment and to investigate possible long-term effects of high-protein regimens in this high-risk population.

AUTHOR CONTRIBUTIONS

EM and AB prepared the study design, organized the sample recruitment, collected data, and contributed to the writing of the manuscript's introduction, discussion, and references sections. LM, SM, AA, and SS contributed to the recruitment of the sample and to data collection. LC, GF, AS, FA, and MS contributed to prepare the study design and supervised data collection and the research team. EN performed statistical analysis, prepared the tables, and contributed to write all sections of the manuscript. All authors reviewed and approved manuscript for publication.

REFERENCES

1. De Curtis M, Rigo J. The nutrition of preterm infants. *Early Hum Dev.* (2012) 88:S5–7. doi: 10.1016/j.earlhumdev.2011.12.020
2. Ehrenkranz RA, Dusick AM, Vohr BR, Wright LL, Wrage LA, Poole WK. Growth in the neonatal intensive care unit influences neurodevelopmental and growth outcomes of extremely low birth weight infants. *Pediatrics* (2006) 117:1253–61. doi: 10.1542/peds.2005-1368
3. Tan MJ, Cooke RW. Improving head growth in very preterm infants - a randomised controlled trial I: neonatal outcomes. *Arch Dis Child.* (2008) 93:F337–41. doi: 10.1136/adc.2007.124230
4. Clark RH, Thomas P, Peabody J. Extrauterine growth restriction remains a serious problem in prematurely born neonates. *Pediatrics* (2003) 111: 986–90. doi: 10.1542/peds.111.5.986
5. Terrin G, De Curtis M. Nutrizione enterale e parenterale nel neonato prematuro. *Prospettive Pediatr.* (2015): 45:41–52.
6. Henriksen C, Westerberg AC, Rønnestad A, Nakstad B, Veierød MB, Drevon CA, et al. Growth and nutrient intake among very-low-birth-weight infants fed fortified human milk during hospitalisation. *Br J Nutr.* (2009) 102:1179–86. doi: 10.1017/S0007114509371755
7. Schneider J, Fischer Fumeaux CJ, Duerden EG, Guo T, Foong J, Graz MB, et al. Nutrient intake in the first two weeks of life and brain growth in preterm neonates. *Pediatrics* (2018) 1414:3. doi: 10.1542/peds.2017-2169
8. Rozé JC, Darmaun D, Boquien CY, Flamant C, Picaud JC, Savagner C, et al. The apparent breastfeeding paradox in very preterm infants: relationship between breast feeding, early weight gain and neurodevelopment based on results from two cohorts, EPIPAGE and LIFT. *BMJ Open* (2012) 2:e000834. doi: 10.1136/bmjopen-2012-000834
9. Gibertoni D, Corvaglia L, Vandini S, Rucci P, Savini S, Alessandroni R, et al. Positive effect of human milk feeding during nicu hospitalization on 24 month neurodevelopment of very low birth weight infants: an italian cohort study. *PLoS ONE* (2015) 10:e0116552. doi: 10.1371/journal.pone.0116552
10. Arslanoglu S, Moro GE, Ziegler EE. Preterm infants fed fortified human milk receive less protein than they need. *J Perinatol.* (2009) 29:489–92. doi: 10.1038/jp.2009.50
11. Corvaglia L, Aceti A, Paoletti V, Mariani E, Patrono D, Ancora G, et al. Standard fortification of preterm human milk fails to meet recommended protein intake: bedside evaluation by Near-Infrared-Reflectance-Analysis. *Early Hum Dev.* (2010) 86:237–40. doi: 10.1016/j.earlhumdev.2010.04.001
12. Stephens BE, Walden RV, Gargus RA, Tucker R, McKinley L, Mance M, et al. First-week protein and energy intakes are associated with 18-month developmental outcomes in extremely low birth weight infants. *Pediatrics* (2009) 123:1337–43. doi: 10.1542/peds.2008-0211
13. McCrea HJ, Ment LR. The diagnosis, management, and postnatal prevention of intraventricular hemorrhage in the preterm neonate. *Clin Perinatol.* (2008) 35:777–92. doi: 10.1016/j.clp.2008.07.014
14. Khwaja O, Volpe JJ. Pathogenesis of cerebral white matter injury of prematurity. *Arch Dis Child - Fetal Neonatal Ed.* (2007) 93: F153–61. doi: 10.1136/adc.2006.108837
15. Hellström A, Smith LEH, Dammann O. Retinopathy of prematurity. *Lancet* (2013) 382:1445–57. doi: 10.1016/S0140-6736(13)60178-6
16. Neu J, Walker WA. Necrotizing enterocolitis. *N Engl J Med.* (2011) 364:255–64. doi: 10.1056/NEJMra1005408
17. Koletzko B, Goulet O, Hunt J, Krohn K, Shamir R. 1. Guidelines on paediatric parenteral nutrition of the european society of paediatric gastroenterology, hepatology and nutrition (ESPGHAN) and the European Society for Clinical Nutrition and Metabolism (ESPEN), Supported by the European Society of Paediatric Research (ESPR). *J Pediatr Gastroenterol Nutr.* (2005) 41:S1–87. doi: 10.1097/01.mpg.0000181841.07090.f4

18. Agostoni C, Buonocore G, Carnielli VP, De Curtis M, Darmaun D, Decsi T, et al. Enteral nutrient supply for preterm infants: commentary from the European Society of Paediatric Gastroenterology, Hepatology and Nutrition Committee on Nutrition. *J Pediatr Gastroenterol Nutr.* (2010) 50:85–91. doi: 10.1097/MPG.0b013e3181adaee0
19. Ramani M, Ambalavanan N. Feeding practices and necrotizing enterocolitis. *Clin Perinatol.* (2013) 40:1–10. doi: 10.1016/j.clp.2012.12.001
20. Schanler RJ. The low-birth-weight infant. In: WA Walker, JB Watkins editors. *Nutrition in Pediatrics: Basic Science and Clinical Applications. 2nd editon.* Hamilton, Ontario: BC Decker Inc., (1996). p. 392–412.
21. Arslanoglu S, Bertino E, Coscia A Tonetto P, Giuliani F, Moro GE. Update of adjustable fortification regimen for preterm infants: a new protocol. *J Biol Regul Homeost Agents* (2012) 26: 65–67.
22. Romagnoli C. *Percorsi Assistenziali Neonatologici.* Milano:Biomedia (2013).
23. Griffiths R. *The Griffiths Mental Development Scales From Birth to Two Years.* Oxford: The 1996 revision Hogrefe (1996).
24. Sansavini A, Savini S, Guarini A, Broccoli S, Alessandroni R, Faldella G. The effect of gestational age on developmental outcomes: a longitudinal study in the first two years of life. *Child Care Health Dev.* (2011) 37:26–36. doi: 10.1111/j.1365-2214.2010.01143.x
25. Giannì ML, Picciolini O, Vegni C, Gardon L, Fumagalli M, Mosca F. Twelve-month neurofunctional assessment and cognitive performance at 36 months of age in extremely low birth weight infants. *Pediatrics* (2007) 120:1012–9. doi: 10.1542/peds.2006-3364
26. Neri E, Agostini F, Baldoni F, Facondini E, Biasini A, Monti F. et al. Preterm infant development, maternal distress and sensitivity: the influence of severity of birth weight. *Early Hum Dev.* (2017) 106–107:19–24. doi: 10.1016/j.earlhumdev.2017.01.011
27. Biasini A, Monti F, Laguardia MC, Stella M, Marvulli L, Neri E. High Protein Intake in human /maternal milk fortification for </=1250 gr infants: intrahospital growth and neurodevelopmental outcome at two years. *Acta Biomed.* (2017) 88:470–6. doi: 10.23750/abm.v88i4.5316
28. Biasini A, Neri E, China M, Monti F, Di Nicola P, Bertino E. Higher protein intake strategy in human milk fortification for preterm infants feeding. Auxological and Neurodevelopmental outcome. *J Biol Regul Homeost Agents* (2012) 26:43–7.
29. Uthaya S, Thomas EL, Hamilton G, Doré CJ, Bell J, Modi N. Altered adiposity after extremely preterm birth. *Pediatr Res.* (2005) 57:211–5. doi: 10.1203/01.PDR.0000148284.58934.1C
30. Cormack BE, Bloomfield FH. Increased protein intake decreases postnatal growth faltering in ELBW babies. *Arch Dis Child Fetal Neonatal Ed.* (2013) 98:F399–404. doi: 10.1136/archdischild-2012-302868
31. Vohr B. Speech and language outcomes of very preterm infants. *Semin Fetal Neonatal Med.* (2014) 19:78–83. doi: 10.1016/j.siny.2013.10.007
32. Fenton TR, Premji SS, Al-Wassia H, Sauve RS. Higher versus lower protein intake in formula-fed low birth weight infants. *Cochrane Database Syst Rev.* (2014) CD003959. doi: 10.1002/14651858.CD003959

16

A Decision Tree for Donor Human Milk: An Example Tool to Protect, Promote, and Support Breastfeeding

Shelley Brandstetter[1,2,3,4*], *Kimberly Mansen*[2,4], *Alessandra DeMarchis*[2], *Nga Nguyen Quyhn*[5], *Cyril Engmann*[2,3,4,6] *and Kiersten Israel-Ballard*[2,3]

[1] School of Nursing, University of Washington, Seattle, WA, United States, [2] Maternal Newborn Health and Nutrition, PATH, Seattle, WA, United States, [3] Department of Global Health, University of Washington, Seattle, WA, United States, [4] Seattle Children's Hospital, Seattle, WA, United States, [5] PATH Vietnam, Hanoi, Vietnam, [6] Department of Pediatrics, University of Washington, Seattle, WA, United States

***Correspondence:**
Shelley Brandstetter
smb59@uw.edu

Despite decades of breastfeeding promotion, exclusive breastfeeding rates for the first 6 months of life remain low: around 40% globally. Infants that are admitted to a neonatal ward are even less likely to be exclusively breastfed. Lactogenesis is frequently delayed in mothers that deliver early, with the added burden of separation of the unstable newborn and mother. For such vulnerable infants, donor human milk is recommended by the World Health Organization, UNICEF, and professional organizations as the next best alternative when mother's own milk is unavailable and can serve as a bridge to full feeding with mother's own milk. Hospital support of optimal breastfeeding practices is essential with thoughtful integration of donor human milk policies for those infants that need it most. We propose a decision tree for neonatal wards that are considering the use of donor human milk to ensure donor human milk is used to replace formula, not to replace mothers' own milk. By first evaluating barriers to full feeding with mother's own milk, healthcare workers are encouraged to systematically consider the appropriateness of donor human milk. This tool also seeks to prevent overuse of donor human milk, which has the potential to undermine successful lactation development. In settings where donor human milk supplies are limited, prioritization of infants by medical status is also needed. Readily available and easy-to-use tools are needed to support healthcare staff and mothers in order to improve lactation development and neonatal nutrition.

Keywords: breastfeeding, decision tree, donor human milk, pre-term, NICU

INTRODUCTION

Breastfeeding is well known as the optimal source of nutrition for infants, and is recommended as the sole food until 6 months of age (1–3). Although this public health message has been widely disseminated, exclusive breastfeeding rates for the first 6 months are not optimal, and are estimated to be <40% globally (4). Premature, low-birth-weight, and small-for-gestational-age babies are at increased risk for feeding issues. Concurrently, mothers of premature infants are also at risk of delayed lactogenesis, impacting short-term ability to express or pump sufficient volumes to meet the infant's immediate needs and increases the potential for insufficient long-term breast milk supply (5–7). Prematurity of the infant is associated with an underdeveloped suck, swallow, and breathe reflex: necessary for safe and effective oral feeding (8). The combination of these factors demands increased attention for this vulnerable mother-infant dyad to receive additional support for lactation and neonatal nutrition.

Being born too soon or too small is a nutritional emergency, requiring close monitoring to ensure adequate growth (9). The increased nutritional needs of the small baby require thoughtful, evidence-based facility policies to ensure all infants have access to human milk to reach their growth goals. Compared to infants that receive exclusive human milk diets, infants that receive formula are at increased risk for complications such as necrotizing enterocolitis, bronchopulmonary dysplasia, and sepsis (10–13). For mothers who experience delayed lactogenesis, optimal alternatives are needed to ensure optimal infant health and to protect the mother's ability to build her milk supply.

BACKGROUND FOR THE DEVELOPMENT OF THIS DECISION TREE

The World Health Organization, UNICEF, and other policy leaders recommend donor human milk (DHM) as the preferred alternative if mother's own milk is not available (2, 14–17). Preterm formula is preferred to term formula for premature infants where DHM is unavailable (18). Donor human milk is expressed breast milk donated by one mother, then processed by a human milk bank to be given to another mother's infant. Guidelines for the prioritization of donor human milk vary by setting, with no global unified guidance for the use or prioritization of donor human milk. Although the minutiae of prioritization criteria must be decided at the national or local level based on a number of factors including supply, broad prioritization guidance is needed to prevent the misuse, including overuse, of DHM, at the expense of providing the optimal nutrition of mother's own milk.

One benefit of DHM is its ability to serve as a bridge to full feeding with mother's own milk (19, 20). In addition to the stresses of premature birth, the mother may also experience challenges with lactogenesis (5, 21). DHM can provide the neonate with a more optimal source of nutrition than formula, while the mother builds up her breast milk supply through alternative methods of expression. Lactation support is vital in the first few days after birth, especially for mothers of premature infants (5). The volume of feeds required by premature infants are minimal, Even a small amount of DHM per infant could provide enough volume to allow the mother the time to come-to-volume, resulting in her own milk being available for her infant (22).

Evidence suggests there may be potential overuse of DHM, as it may be seen as a more convenient source of nutrition than expressed mother's milk for the hospitalized infant (21). Settings may face a variety of barriers to optimal feeding with mother's own milk, including transportation challenges, harried health care workers, and fractured health care systems. In areas that are not set up to support mothers, routinely separate mothers and infants, and are not baby-friendly, DHM may truly be more easily *available* than mother's own milk, but should not be considered an equal replacement. Systems are needed that support mothers to develop their own milk supply and prioritize their milk for their infants. Research has shown that mothers who reach full volume by 14 days post-delivery, estimated as 500 mL of breast milk per day, are more likely to be able to continue breastfeeding at discharge (22). Robust hospital policies and guidelines are needed to ensure all efforts have been made to prioritize mother's own milk and support maternal lactation, not only prior to the allocation of DHM, but routinely during the infant's hospitalization.

In order to support breastfeeding, ensure optimal nutrition for all infants, and prevent misuse, a decision tree was requested by clinicians and experts in human milk banking and neonatal care. This decision tree was intended to help guide prioritization and allocation of DHM, as well as evaluate barriers to feeding with mother's own milk.

OVERVIEW OF THE DECISION TREE

The overarching goal of the decision tree is to first protect, promote, and support breastfeeding, by encouraging thoughtful use of DHM, taking into account neonatal needs and maternal lactation considerations. This decision tree (**Figure 1**), when utilized with early and essential newborn care as an integrated package of interventions, including kangaroo mother care, will help ensure optimal neonatal nutrition and maternal lactation support.

A decision tree model was chosen to provide clinicians with a visual guide that evaluates and promotes maternal lactation support. This should occur at neonatal admission and whenever nutrition orders are being reevaluated throughout the hospital stay. The staff member should first evaluate if the mother intends to provide breast milk to her infant. If the mother does not plan to provide breast milk, staff are encouraged to explore barriers to breastfeeding or expressing breast milk, and ensure that her decision is informed. In cases where the mother is physiologically unable to provide any breast milk (a rare event), or deceased, additional counseling, or education is not appropriate or feasible. For all other mothers, education and assistance should be provided; if the mother is still unwilling to provide breast milk to her infant, staff must respect her autonomy to feed her infant how she chooses. Regardless of the mother's ability or willingness to breastfeed, the source of nutrition should be determined based on the needs of the infant; in some cases, DHM may still be appropriate.

In situations where the mother is willing and able to provide her breast milk to her infant, but sufficient volumes are not available for her infant's feed, the decision tree will assist the health care worker in evaluating next steps. In settings without a mechanism for the mother's expressed breast milk to be available in the neonatal ward, the decision tree will prompt clinicians to evaluate these barriers. For example, a mother delivers prematurely due to her poor health. She is remains hospitalized in the maternity ward while the infant is hospitalized in the neonatal ward. In health systems without strong communication structures between different units or hospitals, the ill mother may be pumping and freezing her breast milk, while her infant is receiving DHM or formula due to lack of maternity-neonatal staff communication and ability to efficiently transfer milk across

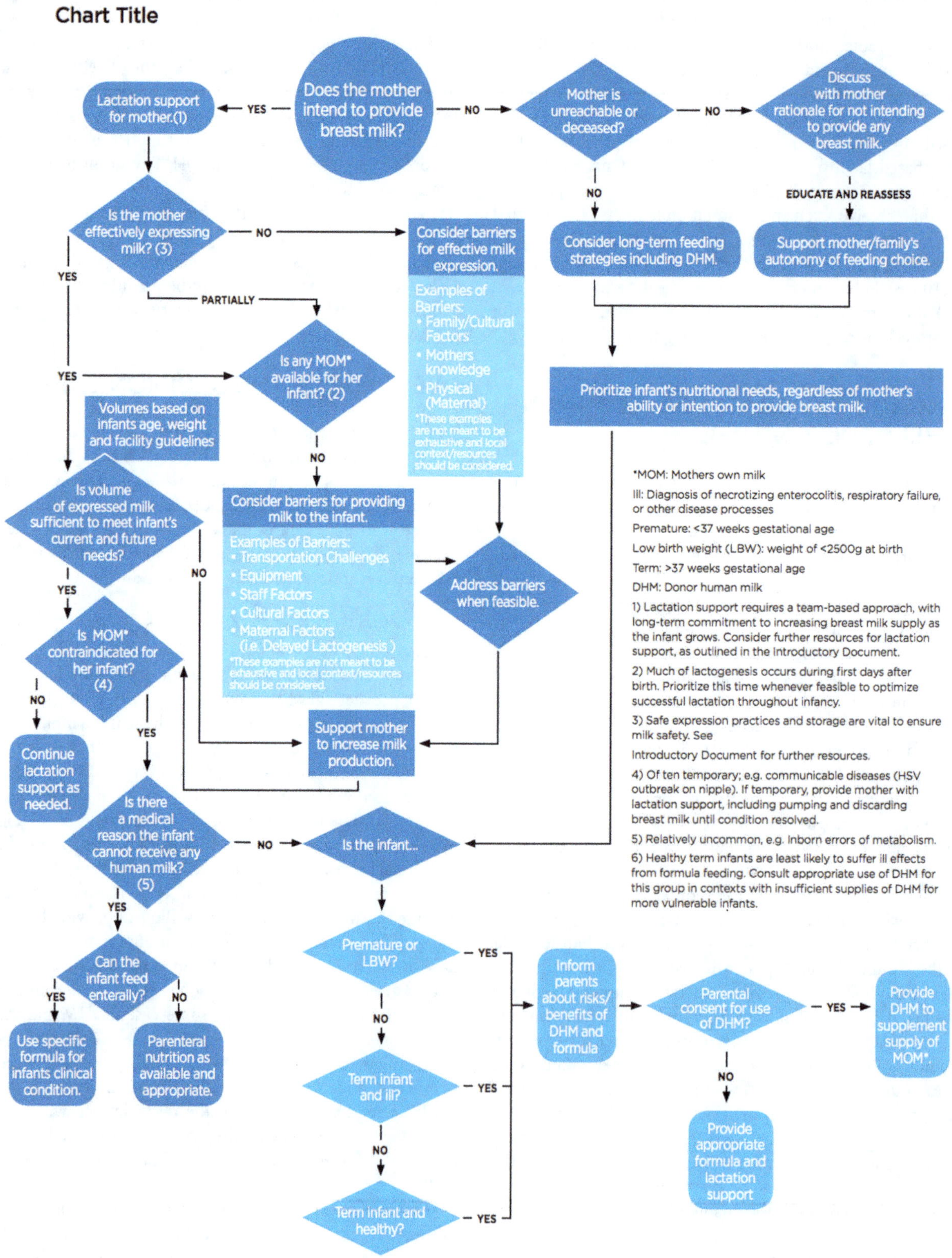

FIGURE 1 | Decision Tree.

units. Using this decision tree will prompt staff in these scenarios to discover and address these barriers.

When infant needs are unmet despite best-efforts to feed with mother's own milk, only then are staffs encouraged to use DHM. In settings where supply of DHM is limited, these small babies are prioritized by medical conditions: those that are at highest risk for morbidity and mortality should receive DHM first. This determination was made based on available evidence for use of DHM for efficacy and cost-effectiveness (23–26). Need for DHM should be reassessed routinely by clinicians to ensure ongoing need. Ideally, infants will transition to full feeding with mother's own milk during hospitalization. Early, and ongoing lactation support and encouragement to build up a mother's milk supply is vital if mothers are to successfully breastfeeding their infants post-discharge.

PRELIMINARY USAGE AND FUTURE STEPS

A preliminary version of the tool was pre-tested in neonatal wards in India and Vietnam. Clinical staff in India recommended simplification of language used, and target use by new nursing staff and resident physicians. As the foundational elements of this tool are already integrated into current practice, the decision tree was considering most applicable for staff education and training. Also identified was the opportunity to modify facets of this into breastfeeding promotion education adverts for parents. Assessment of the decision tree in Vietnam provided feedback that the tool can be adapted into other formats, such as a decision checklist used by staff on admission to the NICU. This provides further evidence that the decision tree may have uses beyond its original intent.

Future steps for the decision tree include rigorous pre-testing and trialing the preliminary tool in additional settings to assess applicability, appropriateness, usability, and possible impact on increased use of mother's own milk, while also preventing overuse of DHM. This feedback will be integrated into the final decision tree, which will be globally accessible as part of a comprehensive package of resources for strengthening newborn nutrition. As differing settings will have specific policies and procedures that may not be covered by this decision tree, we will encourage adaptation of the tool to local settings.

CONCLUSION

This decision tree fills a gap for systematically identifying and addressing barriers for vulnerable neonates to receive human milk. Although many hospitals have policies and protocols for the utilization and prioritization of DHM, these are not always readily available, nor do they address barriers to breastfeeding, provision of mother's own expressed milk, or neonatal nutritional needs. The intent for publishing this decision tree is to reframe the use of DHM to focus on provision of mother's own milk whenever possible. Hospitals and other settings that use DHM should evaluate their current systems and consider strategies for optimizing mechanisms to document and track current infant feeding practices. Better monitoring of actual infant feeding practices will facilitate improved accountability for prioritization of mothers' own milk.

Further research is needed to understand barriers and facilitators for optimal provision of human milk in the NICU in different settings globally. Current research supports the use of donor human milk for preterm and low-birth-weight infants, however evidence is limited in infants with other health conditions or beyond the first weeks of life. Future research may support the use in broader disease states, such as those infants with congenital heart defects, or those who are several months old. Additionally, enhanced indicators should be established to track global progress toward supporting mothers and use of human milk in NICU settings, beyond the traditional early initiation of breastfeeding indicators. Improved and rigorous data collection will help improve quality within the unit to ensure that all infants have the best start in life through equitable access to human milk.

AUTHOR CONTRIBUTIONS

SB, KI-B, KM, AD, NN, and CE conceptualized and developed the decision tree. SB wrote the first draft of the manuscript. SB, KI-B, KM, and CE reviewed and finalized manuscript. All authors approved the final manuscript.

ACKNOWLEDGMENTS

The authors would like to thank Gillian Weaver for thought leadership of this activity and Ruchika Chugh Sachdeva (PATH India), Debbie Barnett (Greater Glasgow and Clyde Donor Milk Bank, Scotland) and staff at the Lokmanya Tilak Municipal Medical College Hospital, Mumbai, India for preliminary pre-testing of the decision tree. Thanks also to the workshop attendees of the 2017 European Milk Banking Association Conference and the 2018 Human Milk Banking Association of North America Conference that provided technical review and feedback.

REFERENCES

1. Kramer MS, Kakuma R. Optimal duration of exclusive breastfeeding. *Cochrane Database Syst Rev.* (2012) 2012:CD003517. doi: 10.1002/14651858.CD003517.pub2
2. World Health Organization, UNICEF. *Global Strategy for Infant and Young Child Feeding.* Geneva: WHO (2003).
3. Hagan JF, Shaw, SJ, Duncan PM, editors. *Bright Futures Guidelines for Health Supervision of Infants, Children, and Adolescents.* 4th Edn. Elk Grove Village, IL: American Academy of Pediatrics (2017).

4. UNICEF, WHO. *Global Breastfeeding Scorecard, 2017: Tracking Progress for Breastfeeding Policies and Programmes.* New York, NY: UNICEF (2017).
5. Cregan MD, De Mello TR, Kershaw D, McDougall K, Hartmann PE. Initiation of lactation in women after preterm delivery. *Acta Obstet Gynecol Scand.* (2002) 81:870–7. doi: 10.1034/j.1600-0412.2002.810913.x
6. Hill PD, Ledbetter RJ, Kavanaugh KL. Breastfeeding patterns of low-birth-weight infants after hospital discharge. *J Obstet Gynecol Neonatal Nurs.* (1997) 26:189–97. doi: 10.1111/j.1552-6909.1997.tb02132.x
7. Ryan AS, Wenjun Z, Acosta A. Breastfeeding continues to increase into the new millennium. *Pediatrics* (2002) 110:1103–9. doi: 10.1542/peds.110.6.1103
8. Browne JV, Ross ES. Eating as a neurodevelopmental process for high-risk newborns. *Clin Perinatol.* (2011) 38:731–43. doi: 10.1016/j.clp.2011.08.004
9. Kumar RK, Singhal A, Vaidya U, Banerjee S, Anwar F, Rao S. Optimizing nutrition in preterm low birth weight infants: consensus summary. *Front Nutr.* (2017) 4:20. doi: 10.3389/fnut.2017.00020
10. Quigley M, Embleton ND, McGuire W. Formula versus donor breast milk for feeding preterm or low birth weight infants. *Cochrane Database Syst Rev.* (2018) 6:CD002971. doi: 10.1002/14651858.CD002971.pub4
11. Sisk PM, Lambeth TM, Rojas MA, Lightbourne T, Barahona M, Anthony E, et al. Necrotizing enterocolitis and growth in preterm infants fed predominantly maternal milk, pasteurized donor milk, or preterm formula: a retrospective study. *Am J Perinatol.* (2017) 34:676–83. doi: 10.1055/s-0036-1597326
12. Villamor-Martínez E, Pierro M, Cavallaro G, Mosca F, Kramer BW, Villamor E. Donor human milk protects against bronchopulmonary dysplasia: a systematic review and meta-analysis. *Nutrients* (2018) 10:2. doi: 10.3390/nu10020238
13. Hair AB, Peluso AM, Hawthorne KM, Perez J, Smith DP, Khan JY, et al. Beyond necrotizing enterocolitis prevention: Improving outcomes with an exclusive human milk-based diet. *Breastfeed Med.* (2016) 11:70–4. doi: 10.1089/bfm.2015.0134
14. Lawn JE, Blencowe H, Oza S, You D, Lee AC, Waiswa P, et al. Every Newborn: progress, priorities, and potential beyond survival. *Lancet* (2014) 384:189–205. doi: 10.1016/S0140-6736(14)60496-7
15. Abrams SA, Landers S, Noble LM, Poindexter BB. Donor human milk for the high-risk infant: preparation, safety, and usage options in the United States. *Pediatrics* (2017) 139:1. doi: 10.1542/peds.2016-3440
16. Arslanoglu S, Corpeleijn W, Moro G, Braegger C, Campoy C, Colomb V, et al. Donor human milk for preterm infants: current evidence and research directions. *J Pediatr Gastroenterol Nutr.* (2013) 57:535–42. doi: 10.1097/MPG.0b013e3182a3af0a
17. WHO. *Guidelines on Optimal Feeding of Low Birth-Weight Infants in Low- and Middle-Income Countries.* Geneva: WHO (2011).
18. Arnold LD. Global health policies that support the use of banked donor human milk: a human rights issue. *Int Breastfeed J.* (2006) 1:26. doi: 10.1186/1746-4358-1-26
19. Williams T, Nair H, Simpson J, Embleton N. Use of donor human milk and maternal breastfeeding rates: a systematic review. *J Hum Lact.* (2016) 32:212–20. doi: 10.1177/0890334416632203
20. Rabinowitz MR, Kair LR, Sipsma HL, Phillipi CA, Larson IA. Human donor milk or formula: a qualitative study of maternal perspectives on supplementation. *Breastfeed Med.* (2018) 13:195–203. doi: 10.1089/bfm.2017.0114
21. Meier PP, Johnson TJ, Patel AL, Rossman B. Evidence-based methods that promote human milk feeding of preterm infants: an expert review. *Clin Perinatol.* (2017) 44:1–22. doi: 10.1016/j.clp.2016.11.005
22. Hoban R, Bigger H, Schoeny M, Engstrom J, Meier P, Patel AL. Milk volume at 2 weeks predicts mother's own milk feeding at neonatal intensive care unite discharge for very low birthweight infants. *Breastfeed Med.* (2018) 13:135–41. doi: 10.1089/bfm.2017.0159
23. Trang S, Zupancic JAF, Unger S, Kiss A, Bando N, Wong S, et al. Cost-effectiveness of supplemental donor milk versus formula for very low birth weight infants. *Pediatrics* (2018) 141:e20170737. doi: 10.1542/peds.2017-0737
24. Buckle A, Taylor C. Cost and cost-effectiveness of donor human milk to prevent necrotizing enterocolitis: systematic review. *Breastfeed Med.* (2017) 12:528–36. doi: 10.1089/bfm.2017.0057
25. Spatz DL, Robinson AC, Froh EB. Cost and use of pasteurized donor human milk at a children's hospital. *J Obstet Gynecol Neonatal Nurs.* (2017) 47:583–8. doi: 10.1016/j.jogn.2017.11.004
26. Assad M, Elliott MJ, Abraham JH. Decreased cost and improved feeding tolerance in VLBW infants fed an exclusive human milk diet. *J Perinatol.* (2016) 36:216–20. doi: 10.1038/jp.2015.168

17

Processing of Donor Human Milk: Update and Recommendations from the European Milk Bank Association (EMBA)

Guido E. Moro [1]*, Claude Billeaud [2], Buffin Rachel [3], Javier Calvo [4], Laura Cavallarin [5], Lukas Christen [6], Diana Escuder-Vieco [7], Antoni Gaya [4], David Lembo [8], Aleksandra Wesolowska [9], Sertac Arslanoglu [10], Debbie Barnett [11], Enrico Bertino [12], Clair-Yves Boquien [13], Corinna Gebauer [14], Anne Grovslien [15], Gillian A. Weaver [16] and Jean-Charles Picaud [3,17]

[1] Associazione Italiana delle Banche del Latte Umano Donato, Milan, Italy, [2] Neonatology Nutrition, Lactarium Bordeaux-Marmande, CIC Pédiatrique 1401 Children's Hospital, Bordeaux, France, [3] Lactarium Auvergne Rhone Alpes, Hospices Civils de Lyon, Lyon, France, [4] Fundació Banc Sang i Teixits de les Illes Balears, Palma de Mallorca, Spain, [5] Institute of Sciences of Food Production, National Research Council, Turin, Italy, [6] CARAG AG, Baar, Switzerland, [7] Banco Regional de Leche Materna, Hospital Universitario 12 de Octubre, Madrid, Spain, [8] Laboratory of Molecular Virology, Department of Clinical and Biological Sciences, University of Turin, Turin, Italy, [9] Department of Neonatology, Faculty of Health Science, Medical University of Warsaw, Warsaw, Poland, [10] Division of Neonatology, Department of Pediatrics, Istanbul Medeniyet University, Istanbul, Turkey, [11] Greater Glasgow and Cycle Donor Milk Bank, Royal Hospital for Sick Children, Glasgow, United Kingdom, [12] Neonatal Unit of Turin University, City of Health and Science, Turin, Italy, [13] PhAN, Institut National de la Recherche Agronomique, Université de Nantes, CRNH-Ouest, Nantes, France, [14] Abteilung Neonatologie Klinik und Poliklinik für Kinder und Jugendliche, Leipzig, Germany, [15] Breast Milk Bank, Oslo University Hospital, Oslo, Norway, [16] The Milk Bank, Imperial College Healthcare NHS Trust, London, United Kingdom, [17] CarMeN Unit, INSERM U1397, Claude Bernard University Lyon 1, Lyon, France

***Correspondence:**
Guido E. Moro
guidoemoro@tiscali.it

Background: A mother's own milk (MOM) is the gold standard for the feeding and nutrition of preterm and full term infants. When MOM is not available or there is not enough, donor human milk (DHM) should be used. Milk delivered to Human Milk Banks (HMBs) should be pasteurized to inactivate viral and bacterial agents. Currently, a pasteurization process at 62.5°C for 30 min (Holder pasteurization, HoP) is recommended in all international HMBs guidelines.

State of the art: It is known that HoP affects some of the nutritional and biological components of human milk. Studies have demonstrated that temperature cycle in HoP is not always controlled or calibrated. A better check of these parameters in the pasteurizers on the market today may contribute to an improvement of the quality of HM, still maintaining some of the negative effects of the heat treatment of human milk. So, food industry, and dairy industry in particular, are evaluating innovative methodologies alternative to HoP to better preserve the nutritional and biological properties of fresh human milk, while assuring at least the same microbiological safety of HoP. The most studied processing techniques include High-Temperature Short Time (HTST) pasteurization, High Pressure Processing (HPP), and Ultraviolet-C (UV-C) irradiation. HTST is a thermal process in which milk is forced between plates or pipes that are heated on the outside by hot water at a temperature of 72°C for 5–15 s. HPP is a non-thermal processing method that can be applied to solid and liquid foods. This technology inactivates pathogenic microorganisms by applying a high hydrostatic pressure (usually 300–800 MPa) during short-term treatments (<5–10 min). UV irradiation utilizes short-wavelength ultraviolet radiation in the UV-C region (200–280 nm), which is harmful to microorganisms. It is effective in destroying the nucleic acids in these organisms, so that their DNA is disrupted by UV radiation.

Aim: The aim of this paper is to present the EMBA recommendations on processing of HM, based on the most recent results obtained with these new technologies.

Conclusions: Although research on the most promising technologies that will represent an alternative to HoP (HTST, HPP, UV-C) in the future is progressing, it is now important to recognize that the consistency and quality assurance of the pasteurizers on the market today represent a fundamental component that was previously lacking in the Holder approach.

Keywords: processing of human milk, donor human milk, human milk, human milk bank, preterm infants, infant nutrition

BACKGROUND

The increasing number of infants who are born extremely preterm and survive at birth and beyond, with a gestational age as low as 22 weeks, represents a new challenge for neonatal nutrition. In the last few decades, human milk (HM) has been identified as the normative standard for premature infant feeding and nutrition by health organizations and scientific societies (1–3). HM confers to these infants protection against necrotizing enterocolitis, sepsis and other infections, and severe retinopathy, decreases the risk of death, and improves their long-term neurocognitive development and cardiovascular health. In addition, the benefits of breast-feeding to promote psychological health and mother-infant bonding are well-known. A mother's own milk (MOM) is the first choice for premature infant feeding. When there is not sufficient MOM (a common occurrence in Neonatal Intensive care Units), donor human milk (DHM) obtained from well-established human milk banks (HMBs) is the best alternative. The WHO/UNICEF Joint Statement clearly indicates: "HMBs should be made available in appropriate situations" (4).

DHM delivered to HMBs should be pasteurized to inactivate viral and bacteriological agents (5). The ideal pasteurization process should consist of a rapid heating phase, followed by a phase in which the temperature is maintained constant, and a final rapid cooling phase. Currently, a pasteurization process performed at a temperature of 62.5°C for 30 min, which is known as the Holder pasteurization (HoP) method, is recommended in all international guidelines for the establishment and management of HMBs (5, 6). Pasteurized HM is known to retain many beneficial and protective components of fresh HM (5). However, it also affects some of the nutritional and biological properties of HM and eliminates the beneficial microbiota of fresh HM, thus resulting in the reduction of some bacteriostatic mechanisms that render milk more susceptible to postheating bacterial contamination, and decreases in its nutritional value (5).

Due to the present limitations of HoP in processing of HM, there is the need to evaluate alternative processing methods able to preserve better the bioactivity of a higher number of HM components in order to improve the nutritional and immunological quality of DHM.

New technologies are under study and the purpose of this manuscript is to evaluate the results obtained from the most promising ones.

STATE OF THE ART AND FUTURE TRENDS

HM is a functional and dynamic biologic system: it provides nutrients, bioactive components and immune factors, and it promotes an adequate and healthy growth of newborn infants. Milk delivered to HMBs should be pasteurized to inactivate viral and bacterial agents, as well as a mother's own milk in specific clinical situations.

Currently, HoP is the most frequently studied and recommended method for the heat treatment of donor HM (5–8). A recent review has shown a significant variability in the data reported in scientific literature concerning the effects of HoP on the biological components of HM (9). Possible explanations for this variability could be the heterogeneity of the test protocols applied in the studies, the fact that HoP is often simulated in laboratories on small aliquots of milk rather than being performed with commercial instruments on the larger volumes of milk utilized inside the HMBs, and, last but not least, modern pasteurizers require significantly less time for heating and cooling than older ones, thus changing the kinetics of the thermal response for heat-sensitive compounds (9–12).

The loss of some biologically active components as a result of HoP, including immunological components, is the main limit to the spread of donor HM utilization in the feeding of preterm infants (10, 11).

The optimization of the biological and nutritional quality of DHM is considered, by the European Association of Human Milk Banks (EMBA), as a scientific and social priority. In order to investigate this aspect, the EMBA Board of Directors set up a Working Group (WG), that is, a dynamic network of scientists who perform research in the field of HMBs and HM treatment, and who operate in different European countries. This WG is aimed to evaluate old and new methodologies in order to determine their effects on the final quality of DHM delivered from HMBs. The objective is to obtain optimum levels of quality and safety of DHM from milk banks in Europe and to decrease the variability of HM, at least as far as the aspects related to the effects of heat treatment are concerned. Quality has been discerned as a powerful tool for the improvement of the well-being of premature infants. A better management of DHM in HMBs will improve the services for donor women (those who donate milk) and for the recipients (the newborn infants who receive it).

The main technologies taken into considerations by this WG are the following: low-temperature long-time pasteurization (LTLT), which has been evaluated by a French group in Lyon (RB and JCP); high-temperature short-time pasteurization (HTST), evaluated by two Italian groups located in Turin and Milan (EB, LC, DL, and GEM); high pressure processing (HPP), evaluated by a French group located in Bordeaux (CB and GD) and a Polish group located in Warsaw (AW); and ultraviolet (UV) irradiation, performed by the Spanish group located in Palma de Mallorca (JC and AG).

Low-Temperature Long Time Pasteurization

At present, the most common practice utilized for the treatment of DHM is a low-temperature (62.5°C) long-time (30 min) pasteurization (LTLT), which is known as Holder pasteurization (HoP). HoP is recommended in all the international guidelines. Milk pasteurization with HoP is known to retain many of the beneficial and protective effects of HM, such as a reduction in NEC and sepsis, protection against bronchopulmonary dysplasia, and a lower rate of long-term complications, such as cardiovascular diseases and neurodevelopmental disabilities (3).

However, some significant concerns have arisen, related to the possible alterations of the nutritional and biological properties of DHM, as a result of the heat treatment. HoP produces a loss in the quantity and/or activity of some biologically functional milk components to varying degrees (9). Other nutritional and biological components, such as oligosaccharides, lactose, glucose, LCPUFAs, gangliosides, vitamins A, D, E, and B12, folic acid, some cytokines, and some growth factors are instead preserved (9).

Different devices have been produced to perform LTLT pasteurization. The most common heat source for pasteurization is hot water, but moving hot air has also been used in some other devices. In 2017, Buffin et al. showed that air pasteurizers have a very different pasteurization pattern from water pasteurizers (12). When the temperature recorded in the different bottles inside at pasteurizer's bath was measured, it was not homogenous, with a difference of 21.7 min between the first probe and the last probe reaching 62.5°C. Moreover, the plateau duration was on average 10 min longer in air pasteurizers than in water pasteurizers. Therefore, the exposure to temperature seems to be more prolonged in the former devices (12). In fact, air is a less effective thermal conductor than water. Its propulsion is uneven and leads to temperature inhomogeneity in pasteurizer. This phenomenon leads to the bottles undergoing a different treatment from each other, and it is difficult to provide adjustments to improve the process.

Water is the most homogeneous environment heat conducting source, and it is therefore the most widely used medium for HoP. Different devices exist on the market today, but not all of them are provided with a temperature control system. The duration of the heat treatment and the maximum temperature of milk exposure have been shown to be essential for the preservation of human milk. Evans et al. already showed, back in 1978, that the alteration of the immunological components of human milk began at a temperature of 60°C and became more significant at 65°C (13). This was later confirmed by Czank et al. who demonstrated a significant impact of the temperature and an early alteration starting at 58°C (14). The study also demonstrated the influence of the duration of pasteurization, with a loss of 1.6, 1.7, and 2.4%, respectively, for IgA, lysozyme and lactoferrin per each minute spent at a temperature of 62.5°C (14).

The recording of the temperature of milk in several bottles, by means of external probes, during the pasteurization cycle showed significant differences, in terms of temperature or the duration of exposure of HM, depending on the device. The increase in the temperature of milk is in fact fast up to 58°C, but the inertia of heating is then responsible for a slowing down of the rise in temperature up to 62.5°C. It has been demonstrated that HM immune components start to be damaged significantly from 58°C (14). The regulation of each pasteurizer is therefore crucial to minimize the exposure time responsible for the damage to HM. Buffin et al. reported that the difference in exposure above 58°C could be as much as 10 min longer, depending on the device. In addition, the average temperature of the plateau can vary by nearly 0.8°C. These effects are only visible when several calibrated probes are used (12, 15). It is important to note that the milk was shaken during the heat treatment in both types of tested pasteurizers (12).

A single recording probe in just one of the bottles does not allow either the whole pasteurizing process to be understood or deviances in the system to be detected. Since HoP is currently conducted at a relatively high temperature (62.5°C), it is important to control this temperature and the duration of exposure (12, 15). Furthermore, most of the studies that have evaluated or compared HoP with other techniques have not described the pasteurizer cycle precisely. The differences that exist between pasteurizers can be important and can have an important impact on the assessed components. This could explain the discrepancies that have been found between the different results in literature. These inconsistencies make it difficult to make a definitive statement on the effects of HoP. For these reasons, any future study on HoP should adopt a standardized approach to ensure consistency. However, it is important to recognize that where research on HoP is being carried out, consistency, and quality assurance adds a necessary component that was previously lacking in the approach.

Therefore, a routine recording of the milk temperature in one bottle located in the middle of a bath is important to control each pasteurization cycle. This probe is not present in all the pasteurizers available on the market today, and is present even less in a simple water bath. Each pasteurizer should be made to undergo regular quality controls, performed by each HMB using several external probes. Some criteria have recently been proposed (**Table 1**) (12, 15). Since 2016, such quality controls have been performed regularly, at least once a year, in the 36 French HMBs. Manufacturers should provide these criteria when they propose qualified pasteurizers to HMBs.

This qualification has two purposes:

- The first is to highlight a dysregulation of the pasteurizer;
- The second, which is based on the results, is to require the manufacturer to adjust and optimize the regulation of the pasteurizer in order to minimize the temperature plateau range, the duration of the pasteurization plateau, and to ensure cycle accuracy and repeatability.

Moreover, since HoP is the most frequently used technique, it should be considered, as part of the optimization, whether a value of 62.5°C is the best temperature for the treatment of human milk. Czank et al. have shown the effectiveness of pasteurization on bacteria at temperatures above 57°C. However, it is known that Cytomegalovirus persists at this temperature, but it could be useful to test intermediate temperatures, such as 60°C and / or shorter exposure times (14).

Finally, it should be kept in mind that the heating phase should be followed immediately by a rapid chilling phase to 4°C to minimize the additional time during which the milk is exposed to the high water bath temperatures and to reduce the further destruction of heat labile components. This thermic shock could also prevent aerobic spore-forming bacteria from multiplying.

As long as HoP remains the main technique utilized in HMBs, it should be made as optimal as possible, with quality assurance being obtained through checks and calibration. When comparing HoP with new techniques, it should be ascertained that HoP is performed correctly, and the comparison should be made in conditions as close as possible to the routine daily practices in the HMBs.

TABLE 1 | Criteria for qualification of human milk pasteurizers (12, 14, 15).

- Measurement by calibrated temperature probes Independent of the pasteurizer
- Regular distribution of the probes inside the pasteurizer
- One probe for 8–10 bottles
- Qualification repeated once a year and after major intervention, and performed on three pasteurization cycles
- Temperature of the plateau as close as possible to 62.5°C and below 64°C
- Duration of the plateau as close as possible to 30 min and <35 min (time calculated when all probes have reached 62.5°C)
- Exposition time over 58°C <50 min for each probe
- Exposition time from 62.5 to 6°C ≤ 1 h

High-Temperature Short-Time (HTST) Pasteurization

HTST was the first non-HoP technique tested to improve the nutritional and immunological quality of milk, and it was first established in the dairy industry in the 1930s (16). HTST is usually performed by heating thin layers of milk in continuous flow systems at 72°C for 15 s. This technology has been applied to the treatment of DHM with promising results (9). Immunological components, and in particular immunoglobulins (Igs), are known to be affected by HoP (17–19), and have often been targeted as qualitative/functional parameters in studies on alternative HM pasteurization technologies. Goldsmith et al. were the first to test HTST pasteurization on HM using a stainless steel laboratory capillary heat exchanger (20). They reported comparable degradation after HTST and HoP for Igs and lactoferrin. The retention of HM Igs was found to decrease as the temperature and holding time increased. Therefore, the search for an optimal compromise between microbiological safety and biological quality should be made considering the pasteurization equipment and the working conditions. Data regarding the effect of HTST pasteurization on lactoferrin and lysozyme concentrations and activities are sometimes divergent, due to the fact that different methods were used to apply the HTST technology in the different studies.

Overall, it has emerged that HTST performed at a laboratory scale or pilot scale is at least equivalent to HoP in ensuring HM microbiological safety, but is better at preserving the HM antioxidant potential, lactoferrin content and structure, B and C vitamins, and some cytokines.

Two HTST pasteurizers have recently been specifically designed and validated for human milk processing (21, 22).

In the first study, a new small-scale, continuous-flow, HTST pasteurizer was designed to treat HM. The efficacy of the new HTST device was assessed on inoculated *Listeria monocytogenes, Staphylococcus aurous, and Chronobacter sakazakii*, as well as on raw human milk bacteria. The biological quality of the milk was assessed after HTST pasteurization and compared with a standard HoP, by determining the secretory IgA (sIgA) content, the protein profile, lysozyme and the Bile Salt Stimulated Lipase (BSSL) activities. No pathogen or bacterial growth was detected after HTST pasteurization with the new instrument. Changes in the protein profile were observed in the milk pasteurized with both processes. The sIgA content and BSSL activity were significantly higher in the milk pasteurized with the new device than in the same milk treated with the standard HoP. In conclusion, the new HTST apparatus was able to effectively pasteurize HM and showed a better retention of the sIgA content and a better BSSL activity (21). However, these results still have to be confirmed in HMB conditions.

Escuder-Vieco et al. described HTST equipment designed specifically for the continuous and adaptable (time-temperature combination) processing of DHM, considering the specific needs of a human milk bank (22). Microbiological quality, the activity of the indicator enzymes and indices for thermal damage to HM were evaluated before and after HTST treatment using different temperature and time combinations and the results were compared with the results obtained after HoP (22). The HTST system had an accurate and simple operation mechanism, which allowed the pasteurization of variable amounts of DHM and reduced both the processing time and the labor force. HTST processing at 72°, for at least 10 s, effectively destroyed all the vegetative forms of the microorganisms that were initially present in the raw DHM. Alkaline phosphatase was completely destroyed after HTST processing at 72 and 75°, but γ-glutamil transpeptidase showed higher thermoresistance, thus indicating that this could be used as a quick, simple, and inexpensive test. The furosine concentrations in HTST-treated donor HM were lower than those obtained after HoP, and the lactulose content for HTST-treated DHM was below the detection limit of the analytical method (10 mg/L). The absence of lactulose and the small amount of furosine found in HTST-treated DHM indicated that a heat treatment with this new HTST equipment did not induce any significant heat damage to DHM. In addition, a higher retention of immunoglobulins, some hormones, BSSL activity and antioxidant capacity were found in HTST-treated DHM samples than in the samples treated by means of HoP (22).

High Pressure Processing (HPP)

HPP is a well-known technique in the food industry, and it is considered a promising alternative to the thermal pasteurization of HM. HPP is a non-thermal processing method that can be applied to solid and liquid foods to provide microbiologically safe, nutritionally intact, and sensory high-quality products (23). This technique inactivates pathogenic microorganisms by applying high hydrostatic pressure (usually 400–800 MPa) through short term treatments (<5–10 min) (24).

Viazis et al. were the first to point out the retention of nutrients and the bioactivity and microbial safety of pascalized HM (25, 26).

Other researchers have shown that HM activity after processed over a 300 to 650 MPa HPP range is similar to heat-treated milk. IgA, IgM, IgG, lysozyme, lactoferrin, cytokines (EGF, TGF-β1 and TGF-β2, IL-6, IL-8, TNF-α, IL-12, IL-17, and IFN-γ) α- and δ-tocopherol, and free nucleotide monophosphates are partly preserved (27–32).

The destruction *of Listeria monocytogenes, Escherícha coli, Staphylococcus aurous, and Salmonella spp,* within the 300–400 MPa pressure range, is comparable with the microbiological purity obtained after thermal pasteurization (25, 28, 33).

Moreover, recently obtained results suggest that anHPP treatment, at pressures below 600 MPa for 15 min, allows the antirotaviral activity to be retained (34).

This technique respects the sensorial and nutritional properties of food better than HoP, because of the absence of a heat treatment (35, 36). As far as the safety and taste satisfaction of donor milk recipients are concerned, the profile of the volatile milk components has been examined after processing. Generally, the change in the sensory quality of human milk after a high-pressure treatment has been found to be less than that caused by HoP (35, 36).

It should be taken into consideration that a change in the lipid fraction may take place as a result of HPP. Milk fat is distributed as globules in colloidal fluid produced by the mammary gland. Any physical factor that is able to influence the stabilization of this component, either pressurization or a warm temperature, causes a decreased fat globule size, which is defined as a homogenization (37).

Exposure to pressures below 600 MPa has not been found to influence the content or composition of the lipid fraction of HM. However, increasing pressure above this limit might result in undesirable changes in the content of selected fatty acids in human milk. A risk of lipid oxidation products in HM after processing has been reported (38, 39).

The HPP technique seems to offer clear advantages over HoP: it results in an improved nutritional quality product; it is faster and perhaps more convenient than HoP; it can be applied to frozen milk samples and it can be used on samples of variable size.

A French team from Bordeaux and a Polish team from Warsaw, with representatives from the EMBA Working Group (CB and AW), have evaluated this technology with positive results. HPP seems to be able to better maintain some milk proteins (HGF, lactoferrin, IgG), and to preserve active hormones (leptine, adiponectine, insulin, erythropoietin) and enzymes (lipase) (EMBA International Conference on Donor Human Milk, Glasgow, October 5-6th, 2017). Until recently, it was considered that vegetative cells are more effectively destroyed by HPP than endosporic forms. Billaud and Demazeau have recently optimized the operational parameters (pressure, rate, decompression, and application mode) and this has allowed the inactivation of *B. cereus* spores. Under these conditions, the activity of certain important human milk biological components, such as lipase activity and immune proteins, is maintained. These results were obtained with a pressure of 350 MPa (40).

The main obstacle to the use of HPP in human milk treatment, is the scaling down of the equipment and the investment and operating costs. It has been calculated on the basis of a cost consequence analysis conducted with a regional model of human milk banking operating in Poland, that the cost of pascalized donor milk will be 130% higher than milk treated by means of Holder (unpublished data). However, there are some small and medium-size enterprises in Poland that are interested in investing in the human milk bank market. The prototype equipment for human milk pascalization has already been described, and the next step will be to obtain the money to construct and validate the device (**Figure 1**).

At present, only prototypes of these HPP devices exist, and this technique still has to be tested under HMB conditions.

Ultraviolet-C Irradiation

Ultraviolet (UV) irradiation utilizes short-wavelength ultraviolet radiation in the UV-C region (200–280 nm), which is harmful to microorganisms. It is effective in destroying the nucleic acids in these organisms, so that their DNA is disrupted by the UV radiation, leaving them unable to perform vital cellular functions. The greater the exposure to UV rays, the better the result, and this ensures a complete destruction of all the microorganisms (1, 3).

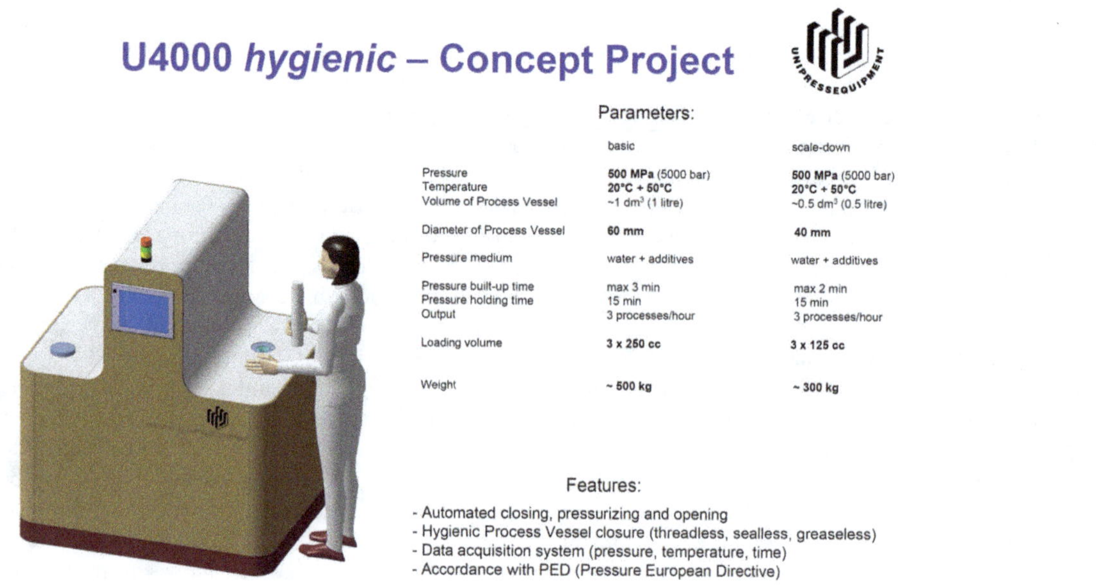

FIGURE 1 | Prototype and parameters utilized for high pressure processing of human milk.

UV light only penetrates food materials by several millimeters, depending on the optical properties of the product. Ultraviolet light penetrates the cells, but does not alter the food that is being treated. The color and/or turbidity of the liquid influences its optical absorption coefficient. UV light cannot penetrate milk or other cloudy foods, like other opaque foods. As a consequence, these substances must be presented to the system as a thin layer, and this constitutes a concern when large volumes of donor HM in HMBs are being treated daily (41, 42).

Some preliminary reports have shown that UV irradiation is able to produce a reduction of 5 log 10 in the exogenously-added bacteria in HM, without affecting the lipase activity (43). The concentrations of lactoferrin, lysozyme and immunoglobulin A (IgA) have been described as basically being unaltered (44), and it has also recently been reported that ultraviolet -C radiation is able to inactivate cytomegalovirus in HM under the correct conditions (45).

The main challenge to testing this methodology is the lack of appropriate equipment in the human milk bank context. In order to further analyze the potential application of UV-C irradiation in this context, a Spanish group from Palma de Mallorca (JC and AG), has designed an instrument in which milk is kept in motion, through the use of a magnetic stirrer bar, which creates a low velocity, laminar flow vortex, thus transporting and overcoming the low penetrance of UV irradiation. **Figure 2** demonstrates the instrument, which allows 500 ml of milk to be processed: it consists of a graduated cylinder glass tube in which a 26 cm long UV-C lamp with 8 w power has been introduced, so that 10 min of treatment equals 9,600 Joules/Liter (LIT-06; Instrumentación Científico Técnica S.L., La Rioja, Spain). In this treatment, the milk is kept at room temperature and agitated with a magnetic bar and a stirrer at 200 rpm.

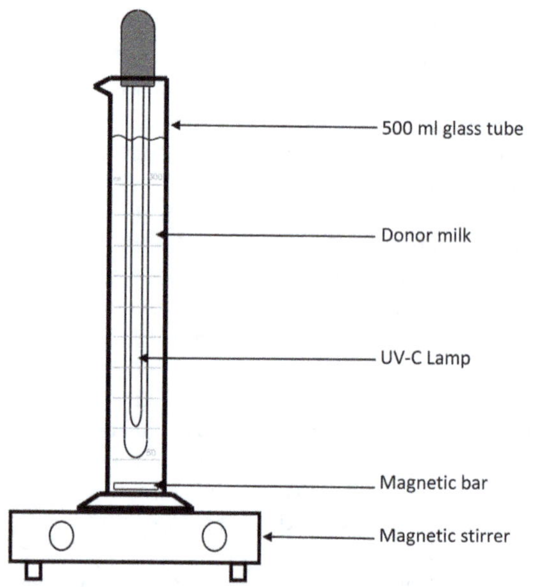

FIGURE 2 | Schematic representation of the device used to treat donor human milk with UV-irradiation.

With this device, Calvo and Gaya tested five different 500 ml batches of DHM that had been discarded during routine processing in their HMB due to the presence of high levels of contamination. Of the five analyzed samples, two presented $>10^5$ CFU/ml and three $>10^6$ CFU/ml. In all cases, the contamination was due to a mixed flora, including gram-negative bacteria. A sample was taken at different times after the treatment was started (0, 15, 30, 45, and 60 min) and the number of CFU was quantified by means of conventional microbiological techniques. These experiments showed that, after 30 min of treatment, the amount of CFU/ml was reduced by five orders of magnitude (log10) in all cases. The fact that the used samples were representative of the DHM samples usually treated in a HMB is of particular relevance.

Bacillus is a bacteria genus that is frequently found in DHM, and it represents a special concern for HMBs, as these bacteria are capable of producing heat-resistant toxins and forming spores that are resistant to pasteurization (46, 47). In the HMB of Palma de Mallorca, about 10% of the milk is generally discarded due to the presence of *Bacillus sp.* In order to test the susceptibility of *Bacillus sp* to the UV treatment, the researchers used two different batches of donor milk that had been discarded as a result of contamination with *Bacillus* sp., 3,000 CFU/ml in both cases. The results showed that after 45 min of treatment, the *Bacillus sp.* were eliminated.

The Spanish group then evaluated the effect on the biological components of HM. One of the main biological components is IgA, which constitutes 90% of all the immunoglobulins present in colostrum and HM. Its importance lies not only in its concentration, but also in its biological activity (48). It has been pointed out that pasteurization affects IgA levels to different extents, depending on the pasteurization temperature (14). In the case of HoP, a clear decrease in IgA concentration was observed, although there were large discrepancies in the range of reduction, from 20 to 60% (9). The results of this group have shown that, after testing seven different batches of DHM, the IgA levels measured by conventional nephelometry techniques, were 96% of the pre-treatment levels, and in five samples, a 100% activity was preserved.

From these results, it can be concluded that the treatment with UV-C light has a number of features that make it a good candidate as an alternative to HoP. In addition to providing a better protection of the biological components than other methods, it is also capable of producing an at least 5-log10 decrease in the number of bacteria (including *Bacillus* sp) present in DHM. Furthermore, the ability of UV-C radiation to eliminate active forms of Cytomegalovirus in HM has also been demonstrated (45). Unfortunately, until now, there is neither a device nor even a prototype that would enable the use of this technology in an HMB setting.

EMBA Working Group Recommendations

One important aspect that should be considered when evaluating the processing of human milk is the viral inactivation effect of the new methodologies.

The ability of LTLT pasteurization to inactivate viral pathogens is well-known. The list of human viruses inactivated by HoP includes pathogens for which transmission through breastfeeding has been conclusively demonstrated (i.e., the human immunodeficiency virus, human T-cell lymphotrofic virus, cytomegalovirus), and viruses that can be transmitted via breast milk, such as human papillomavirus, Zikavirus, Ebola and the Marbourg virus (49–55).

On the other hand, virus inactivation still has to be carefully evaluated for each alternative technique and device designed to treat breast milk. This is an important issue for future research.

We can state that fundamental knowledge of new technologies of HM processing is still lacking. Their effects on safety and bioactive components of HM need further evaluation. **Table 2** presents the "state of the art" at the moment, explaining advantages, and disadvantages of the processing techniques described in this paper.

On the basis of evidence taken from the literature and on the personal experience of its members, the Working Group on the Processing of Human Milk makes the following recommendations:

When testing new technologies, the following requirements should be fulfilled:

- The equipment should be described precisely
- The control of the equipment and repeatability of the process should be demonstrated
- The process parameters should be recorded
- Tests should not be performed only at a lab scale, but also in an HMB environment

The final aim of HM processing performed with new technologies should be:

- To improve the preservation of the nutritional and bioactive components of raw HM (in order to at least ensure the same microbiological safety as HoP)
- To improve the microbiological safety of treated DHM, taking into account the inactivation of spores, even though this aspect is not at present considered in all the guidelines that regulate the activity of HMBs
- To inactivate the viral effect on human viruses for which transmission through breastfeeding has been demonstrated

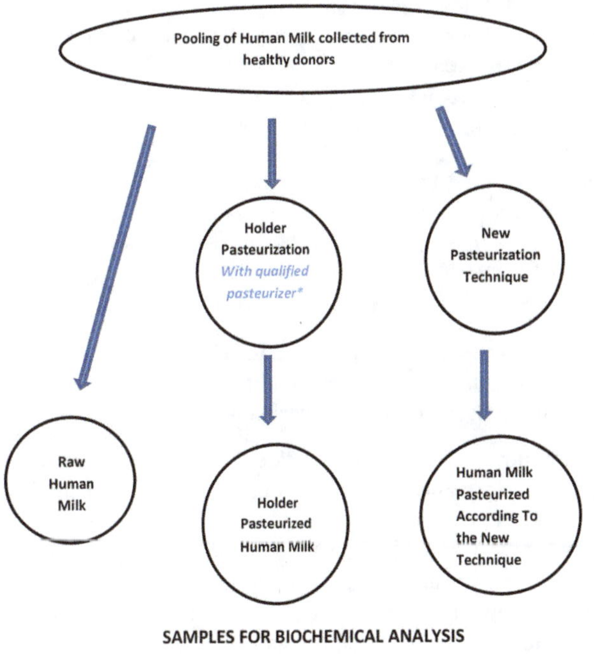

FIGURE 3 | Workflow for assessing the performance of new pasteurization technologies for human milk. *For the qualification of the Holder pasteurizer, see Buffin et al. (12).

TABLE 2 | Advantages and disadvantages of the processing techniques described in this paper.

Processing Technique	Advantages	Disadvantages
Low-Temperature Long-Time Pasteurization (LTLT), known as Holder Pasteurization (HoP)	- Best known methodology - Recommended in all international guidelines for the constitution of Human Milk Banks - Well-established antimicrobial and antiviral activity - Retention of many beneficial and protective effects of human milk	- Reduction/disruption of important nutritional and immunological factors of human milk - Ineffective against bacterial spores (*Bacillus cereus*) - Need of regular requalification of the pasteurizer
High-Temperature Short-Time Pasteurization (HTST Pasteurization)	- Utilized in dairy industry since 1930s - Less thermal stress (processing time in seconds and not in minutes) - Better retention of sIgA and lipase activity in comparison to HoP - Smaller loss in antioxidant potential than HoP	- Prototypes have been used for comparative studies - No device available on the market today - Ineffective against bacterial spores (*Bacillus cereus)*
High Pressure Processing (HPP)	- No thermal stress (processing at low temperature) - Better retention of some important biological components (lipase, lysozyme, lactoferrin, IgA) in comparison to HoP - Inactivation of bacterial spores - Higher microbial safety	- Antiviral activity needs a more deep evaluation - Investment and operating costs are significantly higher than a conventional pasteurizer - Scaling down of the equipment represents a practical problem - Dimensions and weight of the apparatus make difficult the placing in human milk banks
Ultraviolet-C irradiation (UV irradiation)	- Emerging food preservation technique that retains higher quantities of bioactive components - Better retention of IgA in comparison to HoP - Effective on elimination of *Bacillus cereus* spores	- Application of UV-C technology is difficult in human milk - Only few preliminary reports are available - Antiviral activity has to be evaluated - Lack of appropriate equipment in a human milk bank setting

TABLE 3 | Parameters to evaluate for validation of new pasteurization technologies.

BIOCHEMICAL QUALITY			
Parameter	**Unit**		**Method**
sIgA	ng/ml		Giribaldi et al. (21)
BSSL activity	μmol/min/ml		Giribaldi et al. (21)
Lysozyme activity	U/μl		Giribaldi et al. (21)
MICROBIOLOGICAL QUALITY§			
Inoculated bacteria	**Initial loads in raw milk (CFU/mL)**	**Final loads in pasteurized milk (CFU/ml)**	**Method**
Listeria monocytogenes	1.2×10^6	Absent in 25 ml	EN/ISO 11290, 1996 (21)°
Staphylococcus aureus	3.0×10^6	<100	EN/ISO 6888, 1999 (21)°
Chronobacter sakazakii	1.6×10^6	Absent in 10 ml	AFNOR V08-054, 2009 (21)°
CMV		Absent	Hamprecht et al. (51)°
HIV		Absent	Giribaldi et al. (21)°

§ For the design of the microbiological challenge test, see Giribaldi et al. (21).
° Or equivalent methods.

- Easy placement of the new plant in HMBs
- Low cost, in order to overcome the problem of the limited financial resources of the majority of HMBs.

A workflow that can be considered suitable to assess the basic performance of new pasteurization technologies for HM is shown in **Figure 3** and **Table 3**. Since Holder pasteurization is not efficient in eradicating spore-forming bacteria, this parameter has not been included in the validation targets. However, any new pasteurization system that could prove to be efficient against spore-forming bacteria (while maintaining all the other aforementioned characteristics) would represent a great advantage for the improvement of HM safety.

CONCLUSIONS

This paper presents the recommendations of the EMBA Working Group on the "Processing of HM." Although research on the most promising technologies, which will represent a reasonable alternative to HoP in the future (HTST, HPP, UV-C) is progressing, at the moment it is important to recognize that the consistency and quality assurance of the pasteurizers currently available on the market today represent a fundamental approach that was previously lacking in HoP practice.

EMBA recognizes that HoP is at present the safest compromise for the treatment of DHM; however, further studies are needed to improve this technology in order to minimize its effects on the biological components of HM. The new technologies evaluated and studied by the Working Group are being developed rapidly, and EMBA recommends that the final aim of these technologies should be an improved preservation of the nutritional and bioactive components of raw human milk, while assuring microbiological safety of the product, at least at the same level as optimized HoP.

AUTHOR CONTRIBUTIONS

GEM wrote the manuscript. CB, BR, JC, LaC, LuC, DE-V, AGa, DL, and AW are components of the EMBA Working Group on Processing of Donor Human Milk and contributed to the content of this manuscript. SA, EB, AGr, DB, C-YB, CG, GW, and J-CP are components of the Board of Directors of EMBA and made comments and gave suggestions for the final preparation of the manuscript.

ACKNOWLEDGMENTS

The authors are grateful to the Italian Association of Human Milk Banks (Associazione Italiana Banche del Latte Umano Donato = AIBLUD) for its continuous efforts to promote research in the field of donor human milk and Human Milk Banks, and for the financial support for the publication of this manuscript.

REFERENCES

1. World Health Organization (WHO). *Guidelines on Optimal Feeding of Low Birth-Weight Infants in Low- and Middle-Income Countries*. Geneva: WHO. (2011).
2. American Academy of Pediatrics (AAP). Breastfeeding and use of human milk. *Pediatrics*. (2012) 129:e827–41. doi: 10.1542/peds.2011-3552
3. Arslanoglu S, Corpeleijn W, Moro G, Braegger C, Campoy C, Colomb V, et al. Donor human milk for preterm infants: current evidence and research directions. *J Pediatr Gastroenterol Nutr.* (2013) 57:535–42 doi: 10.1097/MPG.0b013e3182a3af0a
4. World Health Organization (WHO)/United Nations Children's Fund (UNICEF). Meeting on infant and young child feeding. *J Nurs Midw.* (1980) 25:31–8.
5. Arslanoglu S, Bertino E, Tonetto P, e Nisi G, Ambruzzi AM, Biasini A, et al. Guidelines for the establishment and operation of a donor human milk bank. *J Matern Fetal Neonatal Med.* (2010) 23:1–20 doi: 10.3109/14767058.2010.512414
6. Human Milk Bank Association of North America (HMBANA). *Guidelines for the Establishment and Operation of a Donor Human Milk Bank.* 10th ed. Raleigh, NC: Human Milk Bank Association of North America (2018).
7. Hartmann BT, Pang WW, Keil AD, Hartmann PE, Simmer K. Best practice guidelines for the operation of a donor human milk bank in an Australian NICU. *Early Hum Dev.* (2007) 83:667–73 doi: 10.1016/j.earlhumdev.2007.07.012
8. Hartmann BT, Pang WW, Keil AD, Hartmann PE, Simmer K. *National Guidelines on Lactation Management Centres in Public Health Facilities.* Child Health Division, Ministry of Health and family Welfare, Government of India. (2017).
9. Peila C, Moro GE, Bertino E, Cavallarin L, Giribaldi M, Giuliani F, et al. The effect of holder pasteurization on nutrients and biologically-active components in donor human milk: a review. *Nutrients.* (2016) 8:477–95. doi: 10.3390/nu8080477
10. Moro GE, Arslanoglu S. Heat treatment of human milk. *J Pediatr Gastroenterol Nutr.* (2012) 54:165–6 doi: 10.1097/MPG.0b013e318235d629
11. Tully DB, Jones F, Tully MR. Donor milk: what's in it and what's not. *J Hum Lact.* (2001) 17:152–5 doi: 10.1177/089033440101700212
12. Buffin R, Pradat P, Trompette J, Ndiaye I, Basson E, Jordan I, et al. Air and water processes do not produce the same high-quality pasteurization of donor human milk. *J Hum Lact.* (2017) 33:717-24. doi: 10.1177/0890334417707962
13. Evans TJ, Ryley HC, Neale LM, Dodge JA, Lewarne VM. Effect of storage and heat on antimicrobial proteins in human milk. *Arch Dis Childhood.* (1978) 53:239–41. doi: 10.1136/adc.53.3.239
14. Czank C, Prime DK, Hartmann B, Simmer K, Hartmann PE. Retention of the immunological proteins of pasteurized human milk in relation to pasteurizer design and practice. *Pediatr R Search.* (2009) 66:374–79. doi: 10.1203/PDR.0b013e3181b4554a
15. Picaud JC, Buffin R. Human milk-treatment and quality of banked human milk. *Clin Perinatol.* (2017) 44:95–119 doi: 10.1016/j.clp.2016.11.003
16. Holsinger VH, Rajkowski KT, Stabel JR. Milk pasteurisation and safety: a brief history and update. *Rev Sci Tech.* (1997) 16:441–51 doi: 10.20506/rst.16.2.1037
17. Silvestre D, Ferrer E, Gayá J, Jareño E, Miranda M, Muriach M, et al. Available lysine content in human milk: stability during manipulation prior to ingestion. *Biofactors.* (2006) 26:71–9. doi: 10.1002/biof.5520260107
18. Góes HC, Torres AG, Donangelo CM, Trugo NM. Nutrient composition of banked human milk in Brazil and influence of processing on zinc distribution in milk fractions. *Nutrition.* (2002) 18:590–4. doi: 10.1016/S0899-9007(02)00813-4
19. Ford JE, Law BA, Marshall VME, Reiter B. Influence of the heat treatment of human milk on some of its protective constituents. *J Pediatric.* (1977) 90:29–35. doi: 10.1016/S0022-3476(77)80759-2
20. Goldsmith SJ, Dickson JS, Barnhart HM, Toledo TR, Eiten-Miller RR. IgA, IgG, IgM and lactoferrin contents of human milk during early lactation and the effect of processing and storage. *J Food Protec.* (1983) 1:4–7 doi: 10.4315/0362-028X-46.1.4
21. Giribaldi M, Coscia A, Peila C, Antoniazzi S, Lamberti C, Ortoffi M, et al. Pasteurization of human milk by a benchtop High-temperature Short-Time device. *Innov Food Sci Emerg Tech.* (2016) 36:228–33. doi: 10.1016/j.ifset.2016.07.004
22. Escuder-Vieco D, Espinosa-Martos I, Rodríguez JM, Corzo N, Montilla A, Siegfried P, et al. High-temperature short-time pasteurization system for donor milk in a human milk bank setting. *Front Microbiol.* (2018) 9:1-16. doi: 10.3389/fmicb.2018.00926
23. Considine KM, Kelly AL, Fitzgerald GF, Hill C, Sleator RD. High-pressure processing-effects on microbial food safety and food quality. *FEMS Microbiol Lett.* (2008) 281:1–9. doi: 10.1111/j.1574-6968.2008.01084.x
24. Huppertz T, Fox PF, de Kruif KG, Kelly AL. High-pressure-induced changes in bovine milk: a review. *Int J Dairy Tech.* (2006) 59:58–66. doi: 10.1111/j.1471-0307.2006.00246.x
25. Viazis S, Farkas BE, Jaykus LA. Inactivation of bacterial pathogens in human milk by high-pressure processing. *J Food Protec.* (2008) 71:109–18. doi: 10.4315/0362-028X-71.1.109
26. Sousa SG, Delgadillo I, Saraiva JA. Effects of high-pressure processing on immunoglobulin and lysozyme activity in human milk. *J Hum Lact.* (2007) 23:253–61. doi: 10.1177/0890334407303945
27. Sousa SG, Delgadillo I, Saraiva JA. Effect of thermal pasteurisation and high-pressure processing on immunoglobulin content and lysozyme and lactoperoxidase activity in human colostrum. *Food Chem.* (2014)151:79–85. doi: 10.1016/j.foodchem.2013.11.024
28. Permanyer M, Castellote C, Ramírez-Santana C, Audí C, Pérez-Cano FJ, Castell M, et al. Maintenance of breast milk immunoglobulin A after high-pressure processing. *J Dairy Sci.* (2010) 93:877–83. doi: 10.3168/jds.2009-2643
29. Mayayo C, Montserrat M, Ramos SJ, Martínez-Lor nzo MJ, Calvo M, Sánchez L, et al. Effect of high pressure and at treatments on IgA immunoreactivity and lysozyme activity in human milk. *Eur Food Res Technol.* (2016) 242:891–8. doi: 10.1007/s00217-015-2595-7

30. Franch A, Audi C, Ramírez-Santana C, Permanyer M, Pérez-Cano FJ, Moltó-Puigmartí C, et al. Banked human milk treatment and immunoactive factors content. *Eur Food Res Tech.* (2009) 242:891–8. doi: 10.1017/S0029665110000777
31. Mayayo C, Montserrat M, Ramos SJ, Martínez-Lorenzo MJ, Pérez MD. Kinetic parameters for high-pressure-induced denaturation of lactoferrin in human milk. *Int Dairy J.* (2014) 39:246–52. doi: 10.1016/j.idairyj.2014.07.001
32. Delgado FJ, Cava R, Delgado J, Ramirez R. Tocopherols, fatty acids and cytokines content of holder pasteurized and high pressure processed human milk. *Dairy Sci Technol.* (2014) 94:145–56. doi: 10.1007/s13594-013-0149-y
33. Windyga B, Rutkowska M, Sokołowska B, Skapska S, Wesołowska A, Wilinska M, et al. Inactivation of *Staphylococcus aureus* and native microflora in human milk by high pressure processing. *High Pressure Res.* (2015) 35:181–8. doi: 10.1080/08957959.2015.1007972
34. Parrón JA, Ripollés D, Ramos SJ, Pérez MD, Semen Z, Rubio P, et al. Effect of thermal and high-pressure treatments on the antirotaviral activity of human milk fractions. *Innov Food Sci Emerg Tech.* (2018) 47:262–70. doi: 10.1016/j.ifset.2018.03.008
35. Garrido M, Contador R, García-Parra J, Delgado FJ, Delgado-Adámez J, Ramírez R. Volatile profile of human milk subjected to high-pressure thermal processing. *Food Res Int.* (2015) 78:186–94. doi: 10.1016/j.foodres.2015.10.016
36. Contador R, Delgado FJ, García-Parra J, Garrido M, Ramírez R. Volatile profile of breast milk subjected to high-pressure processing or thermal treatment. *Food Chem.* (2015) 180:17–24. doi: 10.1016/j.foodchem.2015.02.019
37. Huppertz T, Zobrist MR, Uniacke T, Upadhyay V, Fox PF, Kelly AL. Effects of high pressure on constituents and properties of milk. *Int Dairy J.* (2002) 12:561–72. doi: 10.1016/S0958-6946(02)00045-6
38. Huppertz T, Zobrist MR, Uniacke T, Upadhyay V, Fox PF, Kelly AL. Effect of high pressure and sub-zero temperature on total antioxidant capacity and the content of Vitamin C, fatty acids and secondary products of lipid oxidation in human milk. *Pol J Food Nutr Sci.* (2017) 67:117–22. doi: 10.1515/pjfns-2016-0011
39. Moltó-Puigmartí C, Permanyer M, Castellote AI, López-Sabate MC. Effects of pasteurization and high-pressure processing on vitamin C, tocopherols and fatty acids in mature human milk. *Food Chem.* (2011) 124:697–702. doi: 10.1016/j.foodchem.2010.05.079
40. Demazeau G, Plumecocq A, Lehours P, Martin P, Couëdelo L, Billeaud C. A new high hydrostatic pressure process to assure the microbial safety of human milk while preserving the biological activity of its main components. *Front Public Health.* (2018) 6:306. doi: 10.3389/fpubh.2018.00306
41. Tran MTT, Farid M. Ultraviolet treatment of orange juice. *Innov Food Sci Emerg Technol.* (2004) 5:495–502. doi: 10.1016/j.ifset.2004.08.002
42. Bintsis T, Litopoulou-Tzanetaki E, Robinson RK. Existing and potential applications of ultraviolet light in the food industry – a critical revision. *J Sci Food Agric.* (2000) 80:637–45. doi: 10.1002/(SICI)1097-0010(20000501)80:6%3C637::AID-JSFA603%3E3.0.CO;2-1
43. Christen L, Lai CT, Hartmann B, Hartmann PE, Geddes DT. The effect of UV-C pasteurization on bacte iostatic properties and immunological proteins of donor human milk. *PLoS ONE.* (2013) 8:e85867. doi: 10.1371/journal.pone.0085867
44. Christen L, Lai CT, Hartmann B, Hartmann PE, Geddes DT. Ultraviolet-C irradiatio: a novel pasteurization method for donor human milk. *PLoS ONE.* (2013) 8:e68120. doi: 10.1371/journal.pone.0068120
45. Lloyd ML, Hod N, Jayaraman J, Marchant EA, Christen L, Chiang P, et al. Inactivation of cytomegalovirus in breast milk using ultraviolet-C irradiation: opportunities for a new treatment option in breast milk banking. *PLoS ONE.* (2016) 11:1–12. doi: 10.1371/journal.pone.0161116
46. Walker-York-Moore L, Moore SC, Fox EM. Characterization of enterotoxigenic bacillus cereus sensu lato and *Staphylococcus aureus* isolates and associated enterotoxin production dynamics in milk or meat-based broth. *Toxins.* (2017) 9:1–15. doi: 10.3390/toxins9070225
47. Rigourd V, Barnier JP, Ferroni A, Nicloux M, Hachem T, Magny JF, et al. Recent actuality about Bacillus cereus and human milk bank: a new sensitive method for microbiological analysis of pasteurized milk. *Eur J Clin Microbiol Infect Dis.* (2018) 37:1297–303. doi: 10.1007/s10096-018-3249-z
48. Palmeira P, Carneiro-Sampaio M. Immunology of breast milk. *Rev Assoc Med Bras.* (2016) 62:584–93. doi: 10.1590/1806-9282.62.06.584
49. Eglin RP, Wilkinson AR. HIV infection and pasteurization of breast milk. *Lancet.* (1987) 1:1093. doi: 10.1016/S0140-6736(87)90521-6
50. Orloff SL, Wallingford JC, McDougal JS. Inactivation of human immunodeficiency virus type I in human milk: effects of intrinsic factors in human milk and of pasteurization. *J Hum Lact.* (1993) 9:13–7. doi: 10.1177/089033449300900125
51. Hamprecht K, Maschamann J, Muller D, Dietz K, Besenthal I, Goelz R, et al. Cytomegalovirus (CMV) inactivation in breastmilk: reassessment of pasteurization and freeze-thawing. *Pediatr Res.* (2004) 56:529–35. doi: 10.1203/01.PDR.0000139483.35087.BE
52. Friis H, Andersen HK. Rate of inactivation of cytomegalovirus in raw banked milk during storage at−20°C and pasteurisation. *Br Med J.* (1982) 285:1604–5. doi: 10.1136/bmj.285.6355.1604
53. Donalisio M, Cagno V, Vallino M, Moro GE, Arslanoglu S, Tonetto P, et al. Inactivation of high-risk human papillomaviruses by Holder pasteurization: implications for donor human milk banking. *J Perinat Med.* (2014) 42:1–8. doi: 10.1515/jpm-2013-0200
54. Pfaender S, Vielle NJ, Ebert N, Steinmann E, Alves MP, Thiel V. Inactivation of Zika virus in human breast milk by prolonged storage or pasteurization. *Virus Res.* (2017) 228:58–60. doi: 10.1016/j.virusres.2016.11.025
55. Hamilton Spence E, Huff M, Shattuck K, Vickers A, Yun N, Paessler S. EbolaVirus and marburg virus in human milk are inactivated by holder pasteurization. *J Hum Lact.* (2017) 33:351–4. doi: 10.1177/0890334416685564

18

Human Milk–A Valuable Tool in the Early Days of Life of Premature Infants

Ekhard E. Ziegler[1,2*]

[1] The University of Iowa, Iowa City, IA, United States, [2] Department of Pediatrics, University of Iowa, Iowa City, IA, United States

***Correspondence:**
Ekhard E. Ziegler
ekhard-ziegler@uiowa.edu

The objective of early premature infant nutrition is to maintain, during the turbulent early days of life, a flow of nutrients that differs only minimally from that which would have prevailed had the infant remained *in utero*. Out of necessity, nutrients have at first to be provided mainly via the parenteral route. While that is going on, the feeding of small amounts of human milk (gut priming) is initiated as soon as practical. As mother's own milk is not available in sufficient quantity at this time, donor milk needs to be used temporarily. If not available, formula should be used. Gastric residuals are physiologic at this stage and are monitored to guide the increase of the size of feedings. As the volume of milk is gradually increased, nutrient fortification is initiated when the milk volume reaches around 20 ml/kg/day. There is no need to start with less than full-strength fortification. Fortification should employ one of the liquid fortifiers. Adjustable fortification may be employed but is labor-intensive and is not a necessity as long as full feeding volumes of around 170 ml/kg/day are maintained. As the infant grows beyond 1,500 g the level of fortification can be reduced gradually by omitting fortification first from one, and then from more feedings. After discharge there is still a need for fortification, which requires the mother to express some of her milk so it can be fortified. Nutrient supplementation directly to the infant would obviate the need for milk expression.

Keywords: human milk, early, premature infant, parenteral nutrition, avoidance of nutrient deficit

INTRODUCTION

There is no time in the premature infant's life that is more important than the first few days. It is a time when the provision of nutrients meets with technical difficulties and nutrient intakes frequently fall short of needs. It is a time when the rich flow of nutrients that has been supporting rapid growth and development *in utero* has just been cut off abruptly. The trauma of this disruption is intense and has severe consequences unless the flow of nutrients is restored promptly. Restoring the flow of nutrients is challenging, technically, and otherwise, and that is the reason why prompt restoration is so often not occurring. But this is a time of exquisite vulnerability to the lack of adequate nutrients and prompt restoration is mandatory. Failure to provide adequate amounts of protein and energy during this early period has serious consequences (1). Whether and to what extent nutrient deficits can be made up later is not known exactly, but the widespread occurrence of impaired cognitive development among former preterm infants suggests that the ability to make up is limited (2).

Fortunately, we have the techniques for promptly restoring the flow of key nutrients. If nevertheless the restoration of nutrient intakes does not always occur in a timely fashion, it is because of misperceptions and misinterpretation of physiologic signs, such as gastric residuals. While restoration of the nutrient flow has absolute primacy, it is closely followed in urgency by the need to establish enteral feedings. This is where human milk with its unique properties plays a crucial role, a role that is not always fully utilized.

The benefits of human milk for the premature infant are well-established. They are of particular importance during the early days and weeks of life. The property of human milk that makes it so valuable at this time is its strong trophic effect on the immature gut. This maturational effect not only enables earlier establishment of full feedings, it also provides protection against necrotizing enterocolitis (NEC) and against late-onset sepsis. But for these effects to come to bear, human milk must be fed, and not be withheld, as is too often the case, for various reasons. That is why sound feeding practices are of such crucial importance during the early days of life. One essential condition is the acceptance of gastric residuals as what they are, namely mere manifestations of gut immaturity rather than as signs of "feeding intolerance" or, worse, "impending NEC." Gastric residuals eventually subside, the faster so if the necessary stimulation by feeding of human milk is provided. The only disadvantage of human milk is its low nutrient content relative to the high needs of the premature infant that must be overcome by nutrient fortification.

The objective of the present essay is to foster feeding practices that maximize the utilization of the beneficial effects of human milk. Good feeding practices are part of the overall effort to minimize the hazards that premature birth presents to the baby. The present discussion makes the assumption that parenteral nutrition is being provided starting within hours of birth, that it is providing adequate amounts of amino acids and energy, and that it is not terminated until enteral nutrition has reached near-full levels.

The opinions offered are derived largely from personal experience and anecdotal reports, but are overall consistent with the current literature.

To begin with, it is useful to review some basic facts about the preterm infant and to agree on some of the principles that govern nutrition of the premature infant:

1. The amounts of nutrients the fetus is receiving are known and serve as a model of the nutrient needs of the preterm infant.
2. The flow of nutrients to the recently born preterm infant should not be interrupted for more than a few hours.
3. The gastrointestinal (GI) tract of the preterm infant is at birth in an immature state and incapable of handling a full load of nutrients.
4. If properly stimulated (primed), the GI tract acquires, in a matter of days, the functional maturity for accepting and absorbing full nutrients.
5. While the GI tract is immature, maintaining an adequate supply of nutrients requires the use of parenteral nutrition.
6. The GI tract is susceptible to necrotizing enterocolitis (NEC) and is presumed to remain so for a while even after acquiring adequate motility.
7. The risk of NEC is not modified by the volume and timing of feedings.
8. The risk of NEC increases if formula instead of human milk is fed.
9. The infant should incur no weight loss except that which is explained by the birth-related shrinking of the extracellular fluid space.
10. If weight loss is greater, every effort must be made to recover lost ground as quickly as possible.

PARENTERAL NUTRITION

As the gut is at the outset unable to absorb nutrients, the provision of nutrients must of necessity be via the parenteral route, which has been shown to be effective and safe (3). Parenteral nutrition administered through an umbilical vessel is initiated within a few (preferably <2) hours of birth. It should provide protein/amino acids of at least 2.0 g/kg/day but preferably 3.0 g/kg/day. Blood glucose concentration must be monitored at regular intervals, and hyperglycemia and hypoglycemia, if present, must be treated appropriately. Monitoring of blood urea is not necessary, but monitoring of acid-base status is. After a few days, the administration of parenteral nutrition is shifted to a peripherally placed central venous catheter. As the volume of enteral feedings increases, parenteral nutrition is tapered while maintaining at all times an adequate total nutrient intake. Parenteral nutrition should not be discontinued prematurely as that practice leads to a temporary slowdown or cessation of growth. Parenteral nutrition should be continued until enteral feeds have reached at least 90% of full feedings.

THE INITIATION OF FEEDINGS (GUT PRIMING)

The main reason for the common hesitation to provide enteral feedings during the early days of life is the frequent occurrence of gastric residuals. It is therefore, important to recognize that residuals are merely a manifestation of immaturity of the GI tract and have nothing to do with NEC. Immature motility needs to be overcome by GI priming, which is done better by human milk than by anything else. Until immaturity is overcome, full feedings are not possible. The manifestations of gut immaturity are physiologic and subside in time with proper management. The risk of NEC, while ever present, is not eliminated by withholding of feedings.

The sole purpose of providing enteral feedings early on, also known as trophic feedings or gut priming, is to facilitate maturation of the immature gastrointestinal tract. The progress of gut maturation is, for lack of a better parameter, judged by the decrease of the size of gastric residuals. The goal of gut priming is to reach a rate of gastric emptying that permits the administration of full or near-full feedings. Until that goal

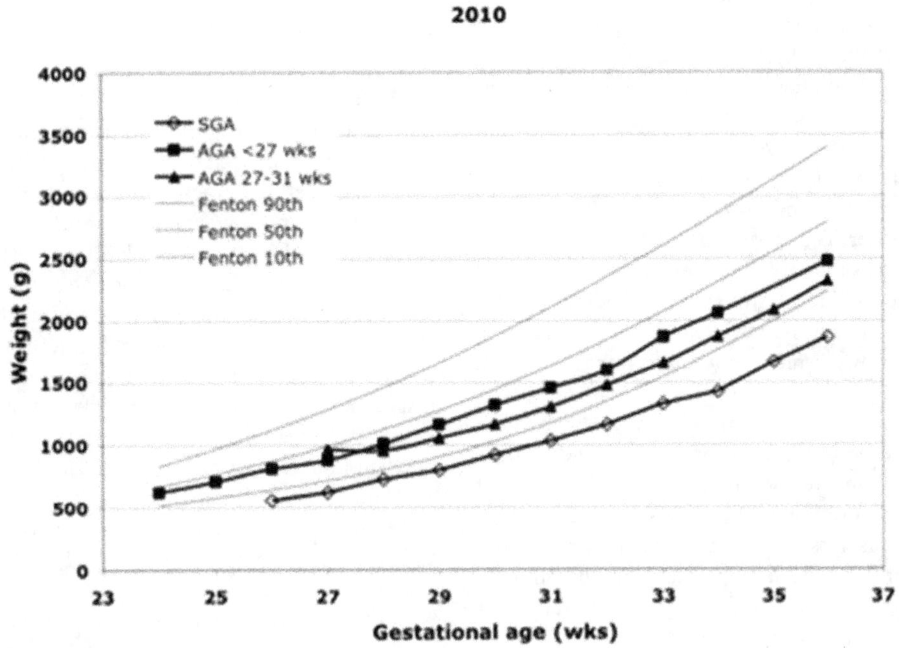

FIGURE 1 | Growth of premature infants.

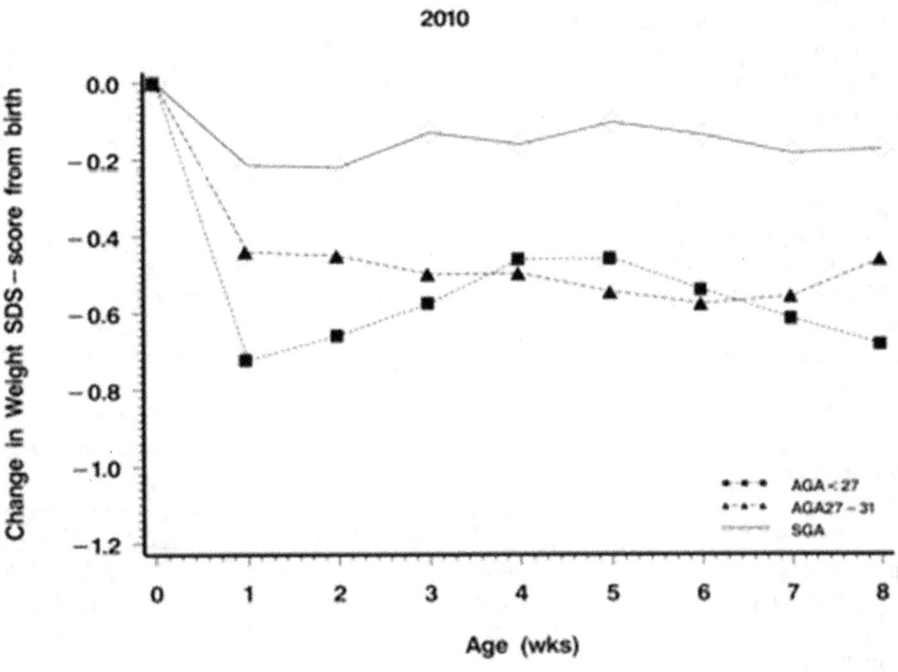

FIGURE 2 | Growth of premature infants.

is reached, parenteral nutrition must be continued to ensure an adequate supply of nutrients at all times. In practice, the initiation of feedings is often delayed by one or more days after birth due to the belief that the risk of NEC is thereby reduced. Practice for many years has shown that such a delay does not reduce the risk of NEC and only causes a delay in reaching full feeds. Thus, gut priming should always be initiated within a few hours of birth, at the latest within the first 24 h of life, and should not be interrupted due to the occurrence of gastric residuals.

There is no evidence that the frequency of early feedings or the strength of feedings are of importance. What is important is that gastric residuals are monitored because the rate of advancement of feeds needs to be based on the occurrence and size of gastric residuals. Historically, before the phenomenon of gut immaturity was fully appreciated, feedings were often advanced too rapidly, and the ensuing gastric residuals were interpreted as constituting NEC grade I (incipient NEC) and prompted the withholding of feedings for 24 h or longer. Today we know that gastric residuals are physiologic, as long as they are of modest size and of normal color, and may require a reduction in the size of feedings but not a cessation of feedings. There is no evidence that the volume of feedings or the rate of advancement of feedings impacts the risk of NEC.

The choice of feeding for GI priming is important because human milk offers several strong advantages, including that it enhances the maturation of the GI tract. Every effort must therefore be made to secure the mother's milk for gut priming. Freezing of milk entails loss of all cellular components and diminution of some of the valuable components of human milk. But the logistics of providing fresh milk are such that much milk is provided after a shorter or longer period of freezing.

Since the availability of mother's own milk is typically limited in the first few days after birth, the temporary (until mother's milk comes in) use of donor milk is necessary. Donor milk is pooled milk from multiple donors who are typically in advanced stages of lactation with its decreases of some components of breast milk. It is always frozen and heat treated, which causes a decrease of the content of nutrients and other components, and the complete elimination of components such as lipase. Despite these decreases, donor milk is the preferred feeding during the first few days after birth when mother's own milk is not available in sufficient quantity. It is also the preferred feeding whenever a mother experiences diminishing milk supply in spite of efforts to maintain her milk supply, which, unfortunately, is a rather common occurrence. If donor milk is not available, formula is a second choice for gut priming. NEC is extremely uncommon in the first few days of life and the feeding of formula temporarily is preferred over not giving any feedings at all.

FORTIFICATION OF HUMAN MILK

Growth and nutrient needs of premature infants are shown in **Table 1**. Infants weighing <1,200 g require an intake of protein of around 4.0 g/kg/day in order to grow like the fetus. If human milk is fed at 150 ml/kg/day, it provides only about 2 g/kg/day of protein (except during the first 2 weeks of lactation when the protein content of human milk tends to be higher). The need for extra protein is thus evident. Although their requirements are not shown in **Table 1**, the intakes of electrolytes, minerals, and vitamins from human milk are similarly not adequate to cover the needs of the small premature infant. Most of the nutrients in short supply are provided by fortifiers. Powder fortifiers have been available for some time but were woefully inadequate mainly in the amount of protein they provide. If used, the addition of extra protein is mandatory (4). The newer liquid fortifiers provide more protein so that the total intake from fortified human milk approaches the required 4.0 g/kg/day.

Initiation of Fortification

Fortification with a liquid multicomponent fortifier should be initiated when the feeding volume reaches around 25 ml/day, which has been the practice at the author's institution for many years. There is nothing gained by waiting any longer, nor is there any advantage from starting at less than full strength fortification. Concerns about an increase in osmolality of feedings caused by the fortifier are unfounded. It has been the practice in many NICU's to initiate fortification when feedings reach a volume of around 100 ml/kg/day. The origin of this practice is murky as is its rationale. The disadvantage from delaying fortification is a deficit in nutrient intakes and a delay in the achievement of a full nutrient intake. Whether the early addition of fortifier delays the attainment of full feedings is a matter of debate. Individualized fortification, if used, is usually initiated only after the first week of life. Fortification with one of the liquid fortifiers in standard fashion is recommended as individualized methods have not been shown to yield superior nutrient intakes.

MONITORING OF GROWTH

As growth provides the ultimate proof of nutritional adequacy (or inadequacy), the monitoring of growth assumes central importance. It is complicated by the fact that all infants undergo a physiologic weight loss, which is not caused by nutritional inadequacy but which is due to constriction of the infant's body water after birth. The decrease of body water is somewhat variable but usually is equivalent to about −0.6 weight z-scores. A loss of 0.6 weight z-scores is therefore physiologic, but any greater weight loss is abnormal and is associated with a risk of neurocognitive impairment.

Daily weight is routinely monitored in every unit, and length and head circumference are measured periodically in most units. The problem lies in the interpretation of measurements. The calculation of average weight gain over some period of time is not an appropriate method because normative values decrease with increasing body weight and are generally not known. An acceptable way of interpreting growth measurements is to display them on charts of fetal growth, where growth in parallel to percentile lines is the expected norm (**Figure 1**). A fall-off from percentile lines indicates growth failure. The preferred way to interpret growth measurements is to transform them into z-scores derived from current references of fetal growth (5) and to express them as deviations from the birth z-score (**Figure 2**). The weight z-score should not drop by more than 0.6, and if it does, every effort should be made to make up the deficit as soon as possible. The z-scores for length and head circumference should not drop at all.

The widespread notion that some degree of postnatal weight loss is unavoidable is slowly giving way to the notion that loss of more than water is avoidable and loss of water only should be the norm. Examples of avoidance of weight loss are provided by Senterre and Rigo (6).

TABLE 1 | Estimated protein intakes needed for weight gain like the fetus.

Body weight (g)	500–700	700–900	900–1,200	1,200–1,500	1,500–1,800	1,800–2,200
Fetal weight gain (g/d)	13	16	20	24	26	29
(g/kg/d)	21	20	19	18	16	14
Protein (g/kg/d)						
Loss	1.0	1.0	1.0	1.0	1.0	1.0
Growth (accretion)	2.5	2.5	2.5	2.4	2.2	2.0
Required intake						
Parenteral	3.5	3.5	3.5	3.4	3.2	3.0
Enteral	4.0	4.0	4.0	3.9	3.6	3.4
Protein/Energy (g/100 kcal)						
Parenteral	3.9	3.8	3.5	3.1	2.9	2.7
Enteral	3.8	3.7	3.4	3.1	2.8	2.6

TAPERING OF FORTIFICATION

Human milk fortified with a liquid fortifier meets approximately the high nutrient needs of the infant weighing <1,500 g. As the infant grows beyond 1,500 g, this regimen provides a surfeit of nutrients that becomes larger as the infant grows larger. While no adverse consequences of the nutrient surfeit in the short run are known, it is counterintuitive to burden the infant with an excess of nutrients. An excess of a comparable size is not routinely provided to any other group of infants. And, if data in full term infants may be used as guidance, the provision of unduly high intakes of protein in early life has been shown to lead to an increase in adiposity and to a greater risk of obesity later in life (7). It is, of course, not known whether the same mechanism may be at work in premature infants, but prudence would suggest that an excess of protein ought to be avoided.

It is suggested that nutrient intakes be reduced as the infant grows. There are no established methods or schedules for the tapering of fortification. A decrease of nutrient intakes could be brought about by diminishing the amount of fortifier added to each feeding. Alternatively, omitting fortification from some feedings and not from others seems to be a simpler way of accomplishing tapering. A suggested schedule would be to omit fortification initially from one feeding per day, then from two feedings per day, and so forth, until at the time of discharge only about 30% of feedings are fortified.

Transition to Breastfeeding

Infants to be discharged from the hospital must be able to feed by mouth. The transition to breastfeeding can be a protracted process. It is sometimes aided by the use breast shields.

FORTIFICATION AFTER DISCHARGE

The usual criteria of discharge readiness include the ability to take all feedings by mouth, whether it is directly from the breast or from a bottle. This readiness is usually reached, in the absence of complications, before the infant's weight reaches 3 kg. Because mother's milk alone does not meet the nutrient needs of infants weighing 3 kg or less, fortification is needed after discharge. Furthermore, infants at discharge are often undergrown and thus have additional nutrient needs for catch-up growth. Post-discharge fortification schemes vary and range from full fortification to token fortification with small amounts of protein. A rational approach would be to fortify two feedings per day in the case of a liquid fortifier, and three feedings per day if a powder fortifier is used. How long fortification should continue is not settled, but a reasonable point at which to discontinue fortification would be the attainment of a weight of 4 kg.

Post-discharge fortification places a large burden on the infant's mother as she needs to express her milk for a portion of the infant's daily consumption. It would be a major advantage if the supplemental nutrients were to be available in the form of a liquid that could be administered in small volume directly to the infant. The infant could then receive all its milk directly from the breast. Unfortunately, such a nutrient solution is not commercially available and would be difficult to prepare in the home.

CONCLUSION

For human milk to exert all its benefits for the premature infant, it has to be fed right from birth when its trophic effects are of crucial importance. As gastric residuals decline and human milk feedings progress, nutrient fortification must be initiated. Weight monitoring must ensure that postnatal weight loss never exceeds −0.6 weight z-scores. As the infant's nutrient needs decline, the level of human milk fortification can be tapered. But at discharge most infants still require nutrient fortification.

AUTHOR CONTRIBUTIONS

The author confirms being the sole contributor of this work and has approved it for publication.

REFERENCES

1. Stephens BE, Walden RV, Gargus RA, Tucker R, McKinley L, Mance M, et al. First-week protein and energy intakes are associated with 18-month developmental outcomes in extremely low birth weight infants. *Pediatrics.* (2009) 123:1337–43. doi: 10.1542/peds.2008-0211
2. Joseph RM, O'Shea TM, Allred EN, Heeren T, Hirtz D, Jara H, et al. Neurocognitive and academic outcomes at age 10 years of extremely preterm newborns. *Pediatrics.* (2016) 137:e20154343. doi: 10.1542/peds.2015-4343
3. Vlaardingerbroek H, Vermeulen MJ, Rook D, van den Akker CHP, Dorst K, Wattimena JL, et al. Safety and efficacy of early parenteral lipid and high-dose amino acid administration to very low birth weight infants. *J Pediatr.* (2013) 163:638–44. doi: 10.1016/j.jpeds.2013.03.059
4. Picaud J-C, Houeto N, Buffin R, Loys C-M, Godbert I, Haÿs S. Additional protein fortification is necessary in extremely low-birth-weight infants fed human milk. *J Ped Gast Nut.* (2016) 63:103–5. doi: 10.1097/MPG.0000000000001142
5. Fenton TR, Kim JH. A systematic review and meta-analysis to revise the Fenton growth chart for preterm infants. *BMC Pediatr.* (2013) 13:59–70. doi: 10.1186/1471-2431-13-59
6. Senterre T, Rigo J. Optimizing early nutritional support based on recent recommendations in VLBW infants and postnatal growth restriction. *J Ped Gast Nutr.* (2011) 53:536–42. doi: 10.1097/MPG.0b013e31822a009d
7. Koletzko B, von Kries R, Closa R, Escribano J, Scaglioni S, Giovannini M, et al. Lower protein in infants formula is associated with lower weight gain up to age 2 years: a randomized clinical trial. *Am J Clin Nutr.* (2009) 89:1837–45. doi: 10.3945/ajcn.2008.27091

19

Improving Pasteurization to Preserve the Biological Components of Donated Human Milk

Antoni Gayà [1,2*] ***and Javier Calvo*** [1,2]

[1] Banc de Llet Materna, Fundació Banc de Sang i Teixits de les Illes Balears, Palma de Mallorca, Spain, [2] Terapia Celular e Ingeniería Tisular, Institut d'Investigació Sanitària Illes Balears, Palma de Mallorca, Spain

***Correspondence:**
Antoni Gayà
agaya@fbstib.org

Donor human milk (DHM) in human milk banks (HMB) is routinely subjected to heat treatment to ensure microbiological security, most guidelines recommending a temperature of 62. 5°C for 30 min. However, this procedure negatively impacts on milk quality, due to the destruction of biological components. Different studies have called for a more respectful treatment of DHM to preserve its properties, and have explored the use of alternative technologies. There is also clear evidence that bacterial and viral contamination in human milk can be effectively destroyed by temperatures lower than that currently recommended (62.5°C). Thus, a simple option would be to optimize the conventional pasteurization technique so the treated milk is free of infectious elements yet retains a maximum amount of biological components. An advantage of this approach is that it would be unnecessary to replace the pasteurization equipment currently available in most HMB. On the basis of a literature review, we here analyze and discuss evidence that pasteurization of human milk at a temperature below 62.5°C results in an improved preservation of its properties without compromising safety regarding the transmission of infectious agents.

Keywords: donated human milk, pasteurization, human milk bank, biological components of milk, temperature

INTRODUCTION

There is general agreement that breastfeeding is the optimal nutritional source for infants (1, 2). Human milk is a synergistic package of essential nutrients and bioactive components that not only covers the nutritional needs of the neonate but also enhances host defenses against infection, actively modulating the immune response. Its consumption facilitates the maturation of various organs and neurological development, modifies the intestinal bacterial flora, and improves the digestion and absorption of nutrients. Beneficial bioactive and immunomodulatory constituents of breast milk include gastrointestinal hormones, immunoglobulins, lactoferrin, lysozyme, oligosaccharides, nucleotides, growth factors, enzymes, antioxidants, and cellular components (3, 4).

When the mother's own milk is not available, the WHO as well as most scientific associations consider DHM, obtained and processed in HMB, as the best alternative, especially in preterm infants (2). As a safety mechanism, HMB usually pasteurize the donated milk to eliminate infectious elements. The technique is named after Pasteur, who first described it in the XIX century as a way of preventing the souring of wine and beer and extending their shelf life. Pasteurization is defined as a process of heating a food, usually a liquid, at a specific temperature for a predefined length of time and then immediately cooling it. The crucial point of the procedure is the selected temperature, which should be high enough to destroy microbial contamination without affecting the properties of the food.

HEAT TREATMENT OF DHM

The use of pasteurization in HMB is based on the experience of the food industry with the treatment of cow's milk (5). Initially, pasteurization of cow's milk was carried out at 61.1°C for 30 min or 71.1°C for 15 s to allow an ample safety margin for the destruction of *Mycobacterium tuberculosis* (6). However, in 1957 these conditions were shown to be inadequate for the inactivation of *Coxiella burnetii*, which causes Q fever in humans if large numbers are present in raw milk (7). New pasteurization conditions of 62.8°C for 30 min for a batch process or 71.7°C for 15 sec for a continuous process were adopted to inactivate *C. burnetii*, and are still in use today (5).

Based on the commercial pasteurization of cow's milk, originally designed to destroy *M. tuberculosis* and *C. burnetii*, Holder pasteurization (HoP) at 62.5°C for 30 min has been recommended as a suitable form of heat treatment for human milk (8). Interestingly, the recommended temperature has evolved over the years. Thus, in 1999 the United Kingdom Association for Milk Banking (UKAMB) guidelines (9) and in 2000 the Human Milk Bank Association of North America (HMBANA) guidelines (10) recommended that milk be heat-treated at a minimum of 57°C or a maximum of 63°C for 30 min. Despite data showing that this degree of heat is more than adequate to eradicate tuberculosis bacilli from cow's milk and that pasteurization at 62.5°C for 30 min may be excessive for rendering human milk bacteriologically safe (11), HoP is widely recommended in most current guidelines.

This point is especially relevant, as several authors have shown that the processing temperature determines the degree of inactivation of the biological components of milk (12, 13). The effect of pasteurization on the composition of human milk has been recently analyzed in two excellent reviews (14, 15). From a nutritional standpoint, the established heat treatment does not significantly affect the macronutrient composition (protein, carbohydrates and lipids, including polyunsaturated fatty acids) of milk. However, there is considerable evidence for a total eradication of lipase activity, as well as a substantial drop in the concentration of various biological components such as IgA, lactoferrin, lysozyme, cytokines, and growth factors.

The discrepancy about the degree of destruction of these biological factors could be explained by the lack of homogeneity in the experimental studies, which generally use small aliquots of milk compared with the volumes usually processed in HMB. In real-life situations, a higher loss of biological properties is expected due to the longer time needed to reach the desired temperature in the center of the milk container (15). Thus, in the process of securing DHM, there is a reduction in quality due to the destruction of biological components.

The literature reflects the enormous importance of biological factors in milk for the development and maturation of the newborn (16). In an interesting study developed in a preclinical model using premature piglets, Li et al. (17) compared two different treatments of the same DHM: HoP and Ultraviolet (UV)-C irradiation. Analysis revealed a markedly higher reduction of several bioactive proteins after HoP compared with UV-C-treated and untreated milk. The authors reported a better weight gain, intestinal health and resistance against bacterial infections in the group receiving the milk with better preserved bioactive factors. They conclude that the differences in the biochemistry of donor milk due to its treatment have potential physiological effects in preterm neonates. Therefore, one of the goals of HMB should be to process human milk with minimum damage to these components.

TABLE 1 | Viral sensitivity to thermal treatment.

Virus	Pasteurization conditions tested	Viral infectivity after treatment	Authors
Parvovirus B19	10′ at 60°C	Completely inactivated	Blümel et al. (33)
Chikungunya virus	30′ at 58 ± 1°C	Completely inactivated	Leydold et al. (35)
Poliovirus	30′ at 55°C	Completely inactivated	Strazynski et al. (34)
West Nile virus	30′ at 58 ± 1°C	Completely inactivated	Leydold et al. (35)
Hepatitis C virus	30′ 56°C	Almost completely inactivated	Song et al. (36)
	40′ at 56°C 10′ at 60°C 4′ at 65°C	Completely inactivated	
Herpes simplex virus	20′ at 50°C	Completely inactivated	Plummer and Lewis (37)
Human Immunodeficiency virus	less than 30′ at 60°C	Completely inactivated	Spire et al. (40) Gregersen et al. (41) Einarsson et al. (42)
Human T lymphotrophic virus	30′ at 56°C	Completely inactivated	Harada et al. (38) Yamato et al. (39)
Zika virus	30′ at 63°C	Completely inactivated	Pfaender et al. (43)
Human papiloma virus	30′ at 62.5°C	Completely inactivated	Donalisio et al. (44)
Ebola virus	30′ at 62.5°C	Completely inactivated	Hamilton Espence et al. (45)
Margburg virus	30′ at 62.5°C	Completely inactivated	Hamilton Espence et al. (45)
Cytomegalovirus	30′ at 62.5°C	Completely inactivated	Hamprecht et al. (47)
	40′ at 50°C	Partially inactivated	Plummer and Lewis (37)
	30′ at 56°C	Partially inactivated	Welsh et al. (46)

ALTERNATIVE TECHNIQUES TO HOP

To optimize the microbiological safety of DHM while maintaining its biological and nutritional quality is an important challenge. In this context, the Committee on Nutrition of the European Society for Pediatric Gastroenterology, Hepatology, and Nutrition (ESPGHAN) has recommended that future research focus on the improvement of milk processing in HMB, including the development and evaluation of different pasteurization techniques to optimize microbiological safety and to preserve the biological and nutritional quality of human milk (18). Thus, to avoid the deleterious effect of HoP on the biological components of human milk, attention has been directed toward the development of new technologies. The most evaluated method is high-temperature short-time (HTST) treatment, which involves the heating of milk at 72°C for 15 s. Several reports confirm that this procedure induces a drastic reduction in bacterial count and CMV infectivity. However, although a better preservation of several components like IgA and lactoferrin has been described, bile salt-stimulated lipase (BSSL) activity is almost completely eliminated (19–21). Two alternative prototypes suitable for use in an HMB have been recently described (22, 23).

Pascalization or high pressure processing (HPP) is a method of preserving and sterilizing food in which a product is processed under very high pressure at low temperatures without the use of additives, leading to the inactivation of certain microorganisms and enzymes. Studies with human milk have shown that in comparison with HoP this kind of treatment may increase the retention of IgA, lisozyme and other cytokines (24, 25). A bactericidal effect of HPP has been reported for different microorganisms with varying degrees of resistance (24, 26). However, these studies do not assure the effectiveness of HPP in banked milk with a high bacterial content, especially because only vegetative bacteria have been analyzed and data is lacking about the effects of high pressure on bacterial spores, viruses or fungi in human milk.

UV irradiation treatment is based on the germicidal properties of light in the UV-C spectrum (200–280 nm). UV light penetrates food materials only up to several millimeters, depending on their optical properties, and cannot be effectively absorbed by milk and other turbid foods unless these are presented to the system as a thin layer.

Preliminary reports indicate that UV irradiation can achieve a reduction of 5 $\log_{10}$ in bacteria exogenously added to human milk without affecting the lipase activity (27), while the concentrations of lactoferrin, lysozyme and immunoglobulin A (IgA) remain essentially unaltered (28). Also, according to a recent report, UV-C irradiation inactivates the cytomegalovirus in human milk under the right conditions (29).

However, although these techniques are commonly used in the food industry, there are no specific devices designed to manage the low volumes of milk usually processed in a milk bank. Thus, until such appropriately scaled and economically affordable equipment is available for HMB use, these methods are unlikely to be put into practice. Meanwhile, since it has been clearly demonstrated that temperatures below 62.5°C have a less negative effect on human milk properties, it is useful to assess temperature modification in the pasteurization process.

A NEED TO IMPROVE THE QUALITY OF HMB PROCESSING

As early as 1982, Wills et al. (13) proposed that "lower temperatures and reduced holding times, if used precisely, will effectively sterilize human milk. At the same time reduced heat treatment results in the preservation of much of the activity of the antimicrobial and other biologically active proteins present in human milk".

Thus, a simpler alternative to the development of new technologies would be to optimize the conventional pasteurization technique used in HMB in a way that guarantees the destruction of infectious elements in human milk with minimum damage to its biological components. This option has the advantage that it would not require the replacement of pasteurization equipment usually available in most HMB. Our hypothesis is that the pasteurization conditions currently used are oversized, and that the same level of elimination of bacterial and viral contamination could be achieved using lower temperatures that are less harmful to the biological factors of milk.

Other improvements could also be made in the pasteurization process. The longer the milk remains above the critical temperature, the greater the detrimental effect on its final quality (30). Hence, the quicker the milk can reach the holding temperature, the lower the overall exposure to damaging heat.

EFFECT OF TEMPERATURE ON BACTERIA

As mentioned above, most of the studies related to the thermosensitivity of bacteria in milk have been conducted with cow's milk for the dairy industry. Among the few that have focused on human milk from a milk bank perspective, the most detailed analysis was published by Czank et al. (12), who reported that the susceptibility of the microbial strains tested was clearly dependent on the pasteurization temperature. There was a reduction of at least 99.9% of all bacterial species when milk samples spiked with 10^5 UFC/ml of *E. coli*, *S. epidermidis*, *E. cloacae*, *B. cereus* or *S. aureus* were treated at 57°C for 30 min or at 62.5°C for 20 min. Also, the data of Lloyd Jones et al (31) suggest that the accepted heating time of 30 min is excessive, since bacterial pathogens commonly contaminating human milk may be eliminated after heating for only 5 min at 62.5°C. This conclusion is in accordance with the results of Wills et al. (13), who showed that over 99% of inoculated organisms are destroyed by heating at 56.0°C for 15 min.

Thus, taking into account that the higher the level of milk contamination, the longer it takes to achieve sterility, reducing the temperature of pasteurization would not constitute a hazard in HMB, where highly contaminated milk is discarded. Moreover, in HMB that pool milk, a high level of contamination is diluted.

EFFECT OF TEMPERATURE ON VIRUSES

In the previous sections, we focused on how the temperature applied in HoP could be considered excessive for the effective removal of bacterial contamination and stability of the main biological components of breast milk. We now turn to viruses and examine if they could also be eliminated at a lower temperature.

In certain maternal viral diseases, there is a substantial risk of maternal-infant transmission by breast milk. This is particularly true for human immunodeficiency virus (HIV)-1, HTLV1/2 and CMV infection. Other viruses are often present in breast milk but transmission is very rare, e.g. other herpes viruses, parvovirus, hepatitis A, B, and C, and rubella (32). It is therefore important that in addition to an accurate anamnesis, including revision of the social, behavioral, and clinical history of the donor, and serological determinations, the donor milk is treated to eliminate possible pathogenic elements.

As mentioned above, pasteurization at 62.5°C may be considered excessive due to its harmful effect on the biological elements in milk. It would therefore be useful to analyse the thermosensitivity of a series of viruses potentially present in donated milk. As it is shown in **Table 1**, evidence in the literature indicates that most such viruses are destroyed at a temperature between 55 and 60°C. Blumel et al. (33) showed that during pasteurization of human serum, albumin parvovirus B19 was immediately inactivated at temperatures above 57.5°C. Moreover, heating at 55°C for 30 min completely inactivated poliovirus in water and milk (34). Also, incubation of Chikungunya- (CHIKV) or West Nile virus- (WNV) spiked albumin solutions at 58±1°C resulted in a rapid and complete inactivation of both viruses to below the limit of detection within 30 min (35). A very small amount of infectious cell culture-derived Hepatitis C virus (HCV) was still detectable after incubation at 56°C for 30 min, and eliminated completely after 40 min; total viral inactivation was also observed after 10 min at 60°C or 4 min at 65°C (36). Although herpes simplex virus (HSV) has been isolated from the breast milk of HSV-infected women, there is no conclusive evidence to support HSV transmission by breastfeeding (32). In any case, HSV is very sensitive to heat treatment, being inactivated after only 20 min at 50°C (37).

HIV and HTLV, potentially the most dangerous viruses, were fully inactivated by treatment at 56°C for 30 min (38–40). Other authors confirmed that at 60°C, HIV in culture supernatants was completely inactivated after only 10 min (41) or after 30 min in stabilized antithrombin III solutions (42).

Another group of viruses are clearly inactivated by conventional HoP conditions but their elimination has not been tested at lower temperatures. Thus, pasteurization of milk spiked with Zika virus (ZIKV) at 63°C for 30 min reduced ZIKV infectivity below the limit of detection, independent of the milk donor or virus strain (43). Also, the infectivity of both high-risk and low-risk human papillomaviruses (HPV) (44) as well as Ebola virus and Marburg virus (45) are completely inactivated after HoP.

Nevertheless, probably the most important virus from the point of view of HMB is CMV. Despite the latency of all herpesviruses, CMV is the only one known to be efficiently transferred to the infant via human milk. There are a few case reports of possible breast milk transmission of HSV and varicella zoster virus (VZV) and strong evidence for the non-transmission of the Epstein-Barr virus (32). Although other members of the herpesvirus group are reported to be destroyed at 50°C, CMV was only partially inactivated at this temperature even after 40 min (37). HoP at 62.5°C for 30 min completely destroyed CMV infectivity in human milk (46, 47), while the treatment of CMV-spiked milk at 56°C for 30 min (46) failed to totally eliminate viral infectivity.

From these data, it could be deduced that a temperature of 62.5°C is required to destroy the CMV, similar to other viruses. Nevertheless, the thermosensitivity of these viruses at temperatures between 56 and 62.5°C has not been reported. Several authors have shown (46, 47) that treatment at 56°C is capable of destroying a significant part of the viral load. Thus, we consider it plausible that the total destruction of the CMV could be achieved at a temperature lower than 62.5°C, and this could be applicable to other viruses not yet tested.

FUTURE RESEARCH DIRECTIONS

According to the previous section, we consider that it is feasible to reduce the pasteurization temperature while maintaining the destruction capacity of the bacteria and viruses potentially present in the DHM. Only the thermal sensitivity of the CMV remains to be confirmed, as there is no data in the range between 56 and 62.5°C.

Therefore, we consider it essential to carry out this analysis, accurately determining the CMV sensitivity to thermal treatment. Once established the temperature at which the CMV is inactivated, and confirmed in exact conditions to those used in a HMB, the effect of this temperature on the essential biological components of the DHM (IgA, lipase, lactoferrin, lysozyme…) should be checked. In both studies, it would be interesting to analyse treatment times of less than 30 min, in order to preserve even more the biological properties of the DHM.

CONCLUSIONS

It is clear that donated human milk must undergo treatment to eliminate potentially transmissible pathogenic elements. Unfortunately, a side effect of such processing, including by the widely accepted HoP, is a reduction in the valuable biological properties of the milk. In accordance with the data presented in this review, we propose the assessment of a lower temperature standard for heat treatment of human milk that would be at least the minimum required to eliminate CMV yet less damaging to the biological components. An added advantage of this proposal is its easy implementation in HMB, since the pasteurizers currently in use would not need to be replaced by new equipment.

AUTHOR CONTRIBUTIONS

AG wrote the initial manuscript. JC edited and finalized the manuscript. All the authors read and approved the final manuscript.

ACKNOWLEDGMENTS

This work was supported in part by funding from Comisión de Docencia e Investigación de la FBSTIB. The Authors also want to acknowledge the financial support of the Associazione Italiana Banche del Latte Umano Donato (AIBLUD) to the publication of this manuscript. We wish to thank Lucy Brzoska for translation support.

REFERENCES

1. World Health Organization. *Global Strategy for Infant and Young Child Feeding*. Report. Geneva: World Health Organization (2003).
2. American Academy of Pediatrics. Breastfeeding and the use of human milk. *Pediatrics* (2012) 129:e827–41. doi: 10.1542/peds.2011-3552
3. Bertino E, Giuliani F, Baricco M, Di Nicola P, Peila C, Vassia C, et al. Benefits of donor milk in the feeding of preterm infants. *Early Hum Dev.* (2013) 89(Suppl. 2):S3–6. doi: 10.1016/j.earlhumdev.2013.07.008
4. Lawrence RM, Pane CA. Human breast milk: current concepts of immunology and infectious diseases. *Curr Probl Pediatr Adolesc Health Care* (2007) 37:7–36. doi: 10.1016/j.cppeds.2006.10.002
5. Holsinger VH, Rajkowski KT, Stabel JR. Milk pasteurisation and safety: a brief history and update. *Rev Sci Tech Off Int Epiz.* (1997) 16:441–51. doi: 10.20506/rst.16.2.1037
6. North CE, Park WH. Standards for milk pasteurization. *Am J Hyg.* (1927) 7:147–73.
7. Enright JB, Sadler WW, Thomas EC. Thermal Inactivation of Coxiella burnetii and its relation to pasteurization of milk. *Public Health Monogr.* (1957) 47:1–30.
8. Evans TJ, Ryley HC, Neale LM, Dodge JA, Lewarne VM. Effect of storage and heat on antimicrobial proteins in human milk. *Arch Dis Child.* (1978) 53:239–41.
9. Royal College of Paediatrics and Child Health. *Guidelines for the Establisment and Operation of Human Milk Banks in the UK*. 2nd ed. London: Royal College of Paediatrics and Child Health (1999).
10. Human Milk Bank Association of North America. *Guidelines for the Establishment and Operation of a Donor Human Milk Bank*. 9th ed. Raleigh, NC: HMBANA (2000).
11. Kells HR, Lear SA. Thermal death time curve of *Mycobacterium tuberculosis* var. bovis in artificially infected milk'. *Appl Microbiol.* (1982) 8:234–6.
12. Czank C, Prime DK, Hartmann B, Simmer K, Hartmann PE. Retention of the immunological proteins of pasteurized human milk in relation to pasteurizer design and practice. *Pediatr Res.* (2009) 66:374–9. doi: 10.1203/PDR.0b013e3181b4554a
13. Wills ME, Han VE, Harris DA, Baum JD. Short-time low-temperature pasteurisation of human milk. *Early Hum Dev* (1982) 7:71–80. doi: 10.1016/0378-3782(82)90009-3
14. Peila C, Emmerik NE, Giribaldi M, Stahl B, Ruitenberg JE, van Elburg RM, et al. Human milk processing: a systematic review of innovative techniques to ensure the safety and quality of donor milk. *J Pediatr Gastroenterol Nutr.* (2016) 64:353–61. doi: 10.1097/MPG.0000000000001435
15. Picaud J-C, Buffin R. Human milk. treatment and quality of banked human milk. *Clin Perinatol.* (2017) 44:95–119. doi: 10.1016/j.clp.2016.11.003
16. AAP Committee on Nutrition; AAP Section on Breastfeeding; AAP Committee on Fetus and Newborn. Donor human milk for the high-risk infant: preparation, safety, and usage options in the United States. *Pediatrics* (2017) 139:e20163440. doi: 10.1542/peds.2016-3440
17. Li Y, Nguyen DN, de Waard M, Christensen L, Zhou P, Jiang P, et al. Pasteurization procedures for donor human milk affect body growth, intestinal structure, and resistance against bacterial infections in preterm pigs. *J Nutr.* (2017) 147:1121–30. doi: 10.3945/jn.116.244822
18. Arslanoglu S, Corpeleijn W, Moro G, Braegger C, Campoy C, Colomb V, et al. Donor human milk for preterm infants: current evidence and research directions. *J Pediatr Gastroenterol Nutr.* (2013) 57:535–42. doi: 10.1097/MPG.0b013e3182a3af0a
19. Baro C, Giribaldi M, Arslanoglu S, Giuffrida MG, Dellavalle G, Tonetto P, et al. Effect of two pasteurization methods on the protein content of human milk. *Front Biosci.* (2011) E3:818–29. doi: 10.2741/289
20. Silvestre D, Miranda M, Muriach M, Almansa I, Jareo E, Romero FJ. Antioxidant capacity of human milk: effect of thermal conditions for the pasteurization. *Acta Paediatr.* (2008) 97:1070–4. doi: 10.1111/j.1651-2227.2008.00870.x
21. Giribaldi M, Antoniazzi S, Gariglio G, Coscia A, Bertino E, Cavallarin L. A preliminary assessment of HTST processing on donkey milk. *Vet Sci.* (2017) 4:50. doi: 10.3390/vetsci4040050
22. Giribaldi M, Coscia A, Peila C, Antoniazzi S, Lamberti C, Ortoffi M, et al. Pasteurization of human milk by a benchtop high-temperature short-time device. *Innov Food Sci Emerg Technol.* (2016) 36:228–33. doi: 10.1016/j.ifset.2016.07.004
23. Escuder-Vieco D, Espinosa-Martos I, Rodríguez JM, Corzo N, Montilla A, Siegfried P, et al. High-temperature short-time pasteurization system for donor milk in a human milk bank setting. *Front Microbiol.* (2018) 9:926. doi: 10.3389/fmicb.2018.00926
24. Permanyer M, Castellote C, Ramírez-Santana C, Audí C, Pérez-Cano FJ, Castell M, et al. Maintenance of breast milk Immunoglobulin A after high-pressure processing. *J Dairy Sci.* (2010) 93:877–83. doi: 10.3168/jds.2009-2643
25. Viazis S, Farkas BE, Allen JC. Effects of high-pressure processing on immunoglobulin a and lysozyme activity in human milk. *J Hum Lact.* (2007) 23:253–61. doi: 10.1177/0890334407303945
26. Viazis S, Farkas BE, Jaykus LA. Inactivation of bacterial pathogens in human milk by high pressure processing. *J Food Prot.* (2008) 71:109–18. doi: 10.4315/0362-028X-71.1.109
27. Christen L, Lai CT, Hartmann B, Hartmann PE, Geddes DT. The effect of UV-C pasteurization on bacteriostatic properties and immunological proteins of donor human milk. *PLoS ONE* (2013) 8:e85867. doi: 10.1371/journal.pone.0085867
28. Christen L, Lai CT, Hartmann B, Hartmann PE, Geddes DT. Ultraviolet-C irradiation: a novel pasteurization method for donor human milk. *PLoS ONE* (2013) 8:e68120. doi: 10.1371/journal.pone.0068120
29. Lloyd ML, Hod N, Jayaraman J, Marchant EA, Christen L, Chiang P, et al. Inactivation of cytomegalovirus in breast milk using ultraviolet-C irradiation: opportunities for a new treatment option in breast milk banking. *PLoS ONE* (2016) 11:e0161116. doi: 10.1371/journal.pone.0161116
30. Weaver G, Sachdeva RC. Treatment methods of donor human milk: recomendations for milk banks in India. *Ann Nutr Metab.* (2016) 69(Suppl. 2):8–15. doi: 10.1159/000452821
31. Lloyd Jones C, Jennison RF, D'Souza SW. Bacterial contamination of expressed breast milk. *Br Med J.* (1979) 2:1320–2.
32. Stiehm ER, Keller MA. Breast milk transmission of viral disease. In: Woodward B, Draper H, editors. *Advances in Nutritional Research.* Boston, MA: Springer (2002). p. 105–22.
33. Blümel J, Schmidt I, Willkommen H, Löwer J. Inactivation of parvovirus B19 during pasteurization of human serum albumin. *Transfusion* (2002) 42:1011–8. doi: 10.1046/j.1537-2995.2002.00158.x
34. Strazynski M, Krämer J, Becker B. Thermal inactivation of poliovirus type 1 in water, milk and yoghurt. *Int J Food Microbiol.* (2002) 74:73–8. doi: 10.1016/S0168-1605(01)00708-5
35. Leydold SM, Farcet MR, Kindermann J, Modrof J, Pölsler G, Berting A, et al. Chikungunya virus and the safety of plasma products. *Transfusion* (2012) 52:2122–30. doi: 10.1111/j.1537-2995.2012.03565.x
36. Song H, Li J, Shi S, Yan L, Zhuang H, Li K. Thermal stability and inactivation of hepatitis C virus grown in cell culture. *Virol J.* (2010) 7:40. doi: 10.1186/1743-422X-7-40
37. Plummer G, Lewis B. Thermoinactivation of herpes simplex virus and cytomegalovirus. *J Bacteriol.* (1965) 89:671–4.
38. Harada S, Yoshiyama H, Yamamoto N. Effect of heat and fresh human serum on the infectivity of human T-cell lymphotropic virus type III evaluated with new bioassay systems. *J Clin Microbiol.* (1985) 22:908–11.
39. Yamato K, Taguchi H, Yoshimoto S, Fujishita M, Yamashita M, Ohtsuki Y, et al. Inactivation of lymphocyte-transforming activity of human T-cell leukemia virus type I by heat. *Jpn J Cancer Res.* (1986) 77:13–5.
40. Spire B, Barré-Sinoussi F, Dormont D, Montagnier L, Chermann JC. Inactivation of lymphadenopathy-associated virus by heat, gamma rays, and ultraviolet light. *Lancet* (1985) 325:188–9.
41. Gregersen JP, Hilfenhaus J, Lemp JF. Heat inactivation of human immunodeficiency virus type 2 (HIV-2). *J Biol Stand.* (1989) 17:377–9. doi: 10.1016/S0092-1157(89)80009-5
42. Einarsson M, Perenius L, McDougal JS, Cort S. Heat inactivation of immunodeficiency virus in solutions of antithrombin III. *Transfusion* (1989) 29:148–52. doi: 10.1046/j.1537-2995.1989.29289146834.x
43. Pfaender S, Vielle NJ, Ebert N, Steinmann E, Alves MP, Thiel V. Inactivation of Zika virus in human breast milk by prolonged storage or pasteurization. *Virus Res.* (2017) 228:58–60. doi: 10.1016/j.virusres.2016.11.025

44. Donalisio M, Cagno V, Vallino M, Moro GE, Arslanoglu S, Tonetto P, et al. Inactivation of high-risk human papillomaviruses by holder pasteurization: implications for donor human milk banking. *J Perinat Med.* (2014) 42:1–8. doi: 10.1515/jpm-2013-0200
45. Hamilton Spence E, Huff M, Shattuck K, Vickers A, Yun N, Paessler S. Ebola virus and marburg virus in human milk are inactivated by holder pasteurization. *J Hum Lact.* (2017) 33:351–4. doi: 10.1177/08903344166 85564
46. Welsh JK, Arsenakis M, Coelen RJ, May JT. Effect of antiviral lipids, heat, and freezing on the activity of viruses in human milk. *J Infect Dis.* (1979) 140:322–8. doi: 10.1093/infdis/140.3.322
47. Hamprecht K, Maschmann J, Müller D, Dietz K, Besenthal I, Goelz R, et al. Cytomegalovirus (CMV) inactivation in breast milk: reassessment of pasteurization and freeze-thawing. *Pediatr Res.* (2004) 56:529–35. doi: 10.1203/01.PDR.0000139483.35087.BE

20

Controversies in Breastfeeding

Riccardo Davanzo [1,2*]

[1] *Division of Pediatrics and Neonatology, Department of Mother and Child Health, Ospedale Madonna delle Grazie, Matera, Italy,* [2] *Task Force on Breastfeeding, Ministry of Health, Rome, Italy*

Correspondence:
Riccardo Davanzo
riccardo.davanzo@gmail.com

When addressing the compatibility of breastfeeding with certain maternal conditions, we need to differentiate between "contraindication" and "obstacle." Failure to distinguish between the two confuses new mothers and their families, and engenders misconceptions about breastfeeding advice by health professionals. Health conditions that may simply impede the initiation and duration of breastfeeding are often wrongly referred to as true contraindications to breastfeed, under the assumption that they might harm the health of the mother and/or that of the nursing infant. Here, we discuss several topics, including breast surgery, prolactinoma, concurrent new pregnancy, hormonal contraception, and use of medications and contrast agents, that continue to raise controversy. While most conditions appear to be compatible with breastfeeding, the major determinants of a woman's final choice of whether to nurse her infant or not are the attitude of health professionals and the state of mind of being an informed mother.

Keywords: breastfeeding, contraindication, maternal health conditions, reproductive health conditions, maternal infections, cytomegalovirus, chemical substances

THE CONCEPT OF CONTRAINDICATION

Breastfeeding, because of its strong health-promoting effect on both the mother (1) and the child (2), affords individual, familial, and social benefits that carry significant economic advantages (3–5). International health authorities (6) and national scientific societies (7) recommend breastfeeding as the nutritional norm, unless an informed choice of the mother or a good medical reason exists for preferring formula feeding (8). There are relatively few evidence-based medical reasons for the use of breastmilk substitutes, yet popular perceptions and beliefs, as well as common attitudes among health professionals, have raised unwarranted concern about breastfeeding. Consequently, many mothers do not start and/or do not continue to breastfeed owing to the confusion between proven and presumed acceptable medical reasons for formula feeding.

When approaching the issue of compatibility of breastfeeding, we need to differentiate between "contraindication" and "obstacle." Failure to distinguish between the two confuses new mothers and their families, and engenders misconceptions among health professionals. All too often, conditions that may simply impede the initiation and the duration of breastfeeding are wrongly taken as true contraindications to breastfeed, under the assumption that they could harm the health of the mother and/or that of the nursing infant. The term contraindication refers to "something (a symptom or condition) that is a medical reason for not doing or using something (a treatment, procedure or activity)"[1]; for example, maternal diabetes is not a contraindication to breastfeeding. In brief, a contraindication is a specific situation in which a drug or a procedure should not be used because it may be harmful for the person. A contraindication can be either relative, when a situation is acceptable and the benefits outweigh the risks, or absolute, when the risks are definitely unacceptable.

[1] https://www.merriam-webster.com/

Quite different from this is the concept of obstacle: an obstacle is "an object that you have to get around or over: something that blocks your path"[1]. For example, a breastfeeding mother may have to cope with mastitis or a tiny baby that is not competent to feed at the breast. These constitute simple obstacles rather than contraindications, although such obstacles might sometimes be very hard to overcome.

The list of true contraindications to breastfeeding is short, clearly stated, and easily available from authoritative scientific sources (7)[2] (**Table 1**); however, health professionals continue to give contradictory advice (9). Here, we review the compatibility of breastfeeding with conditions in which it is often disfavoured or discouraged. The aim is to provide a more balanced perspective on the barriers and challenges to initiating or continuing breastfeeding (**Table 2**).

MATERNAL HEALTH CONDITIONS

Breast Augmentation

Augmentation mammoplasty is a surgical procedure that increases breast size by inserting breast implants under the breast tissue or chest muscles (10). For some women, breast augmentation is a way to enhance self-image and self-confidence. For others, it is part of breast reconstruction after breast cancer surgery or other conditions affecting the breast. Compared to the general population of new mothers, women who had undergone breast augmentation stated they experienced no differences in attempting to breastfeed (11); however, they were noted to have a lower rate of breastfeeding at maternity discharge (79 vs. 89%) (12) and a lower rate of exclusive breastfeeding at 1 month after childbirth (54 vs. 80%) (12).

TABLE 1 | Contraindications to breastfeed.

1. *Mothers should NOT breastfeed*
• Infant galactosemia
• Mother HIV or HTLV positive
• Mother is using an illicit street drug
• Mother has Ebola virus disease
2. *Mothers should temporarily NOT breastfeed*
• Mother with untreated brucellosis
• Mother is taking certain medications
• The mother is undergoing diagnostic imaging with radiopharmaceuticals
• Mother has herpes simplex virus (HSV) lesions present on the breast (Note: Mothers can breastfeed directly from the unaffected breast)
3. *Mothers should temporarily NOT breastfeed, but CAN feed expressed breast milk*
• Mother has untreated, active tuberculosis. The mother may resume breastfeeding when no longer contagious
• Mother has varicella infection at delivery (5 days prior to delivery to the 2 days following delivery).

Modified from the US National Center for Chronic Disease Prevention and Health Promotion (CDC)[2].

[2] https://www.cdc.gov/breastfeeding/breastfeeding-special-circumstances/contraindications-to-breastfeeding.html (Accessed June 30, 2018).

Reduction Mammoplasty

Reduction mammaplasty, commonly known as breast reduction, is a procedure by which excess breast fat, glandular tissue, and skin are removed to achieve a breast size more in proportion with the woman's body and to alleviate the discomfort associated with excessively large breasts (13). Disproportionately large breasts can cause both physical discomfort (due to breast weight) and emotional distress. Most women choose to undergo reduction mammoplasty simply for cosmetic reasons.

Whatever the reason for undergoing mammoplasty, breastfeeding after breast reduction surgery might be challenging, although certain surgical techniques can help preserve the mother's ability to breastfeed. Studies conducted in Brazil (14, 15) suggest that breast reduction surgery is associated with negative breastfeeding performance: compared to controls, women who underwent reduction mammoplasty interrupted exclusive breastfeeding after a median duration of only 5 days and were less disposed to exclusively breastfeed at 4 months (22 vs. 4%) after childbirth.

A systematic review of 51 observational studies found the impact of breast reduction surgery (via 31 different breast reduction techniques) on breastfeeding success to vary widely (4–75%) (16). An important determinant was preservation of the subareolar parenchyma, i.e., the column of parenchyma from the nipple areola complex to the chest wall. When the subareolar parenchyma was not preserved, only 4% of women could be expected to breastfeed successfully (16).

Previous Breast Cancer

Breastfeeding and breast cancer may be linked in two different ways. First, the current literature reports a protective effect of breastfeeding against breast cancer: the relative risk of breast cancer decreases by 4.3% for every 12 months of breastfeeding and by 7.0% for each birth (17). Second, breast cancer survivors may want to become pregnant and possibly to breastfeed. Over the last decade researchers have assessed the risk of stimulation of

TABLE 2 | A selected list of controversial contraindications to breastfeed, discussed in the present paper.

Mother health conditions
• Breast augmentation
• Breast reduction
• Previous breast cancer
• Maternal prolactinoma
Reproductive health conditions
• Pregnancy
• Hormonal contraception
Maternal infections
• CMV infection
• HIV infection
• ZIKV infection
Chemical substances in human milk
• Drugs
• Contrast media agents

the mammary gland following lactation, mainly for reactivation of tumorogenesis, and explored this association (18, 19). In their multicenter case-control study, Lambertini et al. (20) compared 333 patients who became pregnant after surviving breast cancer and 874 nonpregnant patients. They found no difference between disease-free survival and overall survival at a follow-up of 7.2 years after pregnancy. In addition, time to pregnancy following breast cancer treatment and breastfeeding was ascertained to be safe.

Summarizing, cosmetic breast surgery and breast cancer surgery do not constitute a contraindication to breastfeed, although the former may be associated with difficulties in starting to breastfeed and with a shorter duration of breastfeeding because of the altered anatomy of the mammary gland and possible body image concerns (21). Mothers who experience the changes to their body during pregnancy as negative may be less likely to plan or initiate breastfeeding because of the perceived impact of feeding upon their appearance (21).

Prolactinoma

Prolactin (PRL) is a hormone normally released by the anterior pituitary gland after nipple stimulation during a breastfeed (22). Prolactinoma, a pituitary tumor, is one of the most common causes of prolactin excess and results in hypogonadism, infertility, and galactorrhea. As lactation stimulates PRL production, it has been questioned whether breastfeeding might promote the growth of a preexisting prolactinoma.

Opinions on the compatibility of a prolactinoma with breastfeeding differ, as documented by an online survey conducted in the Middle East and North Africa among 468 physicians, 36% of which were endocrinologists (23). Survey results showed that 47% of responders would allow breastfeeding without restrictions, 28% would allow breastfeeding only by patients with microprolactinomas, and 25% would not recommend it at all (23).

Treatment of hyperprolactinemia with dopamine agonists (DAs)(bromocriptine or cabergole) restores fertility in over 90% of cases. Although DAs have a good safety profile during early pregnancy, they are discontinued when a woman becomes pregnant. The risk of prolactinoma enlargement during pregnancy is very low (2–3%) for microprolactinomas but much higher for macroprolactinomas (20–30%) (24). Careful follow-up by magnetic resonance imaging (MRI) and fundoscopic examination of the prolactinoma is advised during pregnancy. If enlargement does occur, reinitiation of DA therapy is advised but it may be delayed as long as breastfeeding is desired. Finally, breastfeeding *per se* has no harmful effect on tumor growth (25).

In their retrospective study on 107 pregnancies of 73 patients with prolactinoma (54 microprolactinoma; 19 macroprolactinoma) (26), Domingue et al. performed MRI prior to pregnancy and at a median follow up of 22 months after delivery or cessation of lactation. MRI at follow-up showed either no tumor (23%) or a decreased adenoma (39%) in the majority of patients. Morevover, the number of pregnancies per woman, breastfeeding and its duration did not influence the remission rate. In conclusion, lactation is compatible with a previous diagnosis of prolactinoma, with no need to limit duration of breastfeeding.

REPRODUCTIVE HEALTH CONDITIONS

Breastfeeding During Pregnancy

Women may be still breastfeeding when they become pregnant again (27). This creates the dilemma of whether to breastfeed or not, as there is millennial cultural and medical pressure to discourage women from breastfeeding during pregnancy. According to Soranus of Ephesus, a famous physician of the Roman Empire, "a woman who nurses the infant either grows prematurely old, having fed one child, or the expenditure for the nourishment of the offspring necessarily makes her own body quite emaciated." (28) This view of the adverse effects of breastfeeding on women's health deeply influenced not only ancient Roman society but has permeated European culture throughout the following centuries until today.

We can understand that breastfeeding during pregnancy may be viewed as a challenge to maternal well-being. The main medical reasons, however, regard maternal nutrition depletion, spontaneous abortion, reduced fetal growth, preterm delivery, impaired quality or quantity of mother's milk, and reduced growth of the nursing infant. Owing to the scarcity of scientific literature on the possible medical effects of breastfeeding during pregnancy, clear medical guidelines on this topic are lacking. To overcome this gap, the Italian Society of Perinatal Medicine (SIMP) Working Group on Breastfeeding and the Task Force on Breastfeeding of the Italian Ministry of Health have reviewed the available literature on breastfeeding during pregnancy and issued a position statement (29). There is no evidence indicating that breastfeeding during pregnancy raises the risk of miscarriage or preterm delivery or intrauterine growth restriction, particularly in women from developed countries. Both the composition of postpartum breast milk and the growth of the newborn might be affected, chiefly in women from developing countries (29). Moreover, we must underline that the impact of breastfeeding during the third trimester of pregnancy has been overemphasized, as it is no longer expected to be exclusive breastfeeding when the nursed infant is older than 6 months of age and possibly already being weaned (30).

In brief, breastfeeding during pregnancy is compatible during the first two trimesters, and it is sustainable in the third trimester unless maternal nutrition is suboptimal or the risk of premature delivery exists (multiple gestation, intrauterine growth retardation, previous preterm delivery) (29).

Hormonal Contraception

Most women who breastfeed exclusively stop having menstrual periods (lactational amenorrhea) and have a lower potential for ovulation; nevertheless, the risk of becoming pregnant cannot be excluded. Some sort of contraceptive method is needed if the mother does not plan to become pregnant again (31). Barrier methods (diaphragms, condoms, etc.) have no effect on milk production and so can be used as a first choice contraceptive method by the breastfeeding mother. Their efficacy is inferior to hormonal contraceptives, however.

Many women incorrectly believe that breastfeeding in itself precludes taking any form of hormonal contraception, although a distinction must be drawn among the many contraceptive methods available. Combined hormonal contraceptives (CHCs) may adversely affect milk supply, making the outcome of breastfeeding unpredictable. As some mothers can completely dry up, women are advised to use the lowest appropriate estrogen dosage and monitor their milk supply. Progesterone only pills (POP) are preferred as they are less likely to reduce milk supply (32), an adverse effect, that is even less welcome in the breastfeeding mother with a basic low milk production or during the first 2 months postpartum when the milk supply is still calibrated.

A contraceptive method's safety should be determined in the context of relevant conditions, including phase of lactation, increased thrombotic risk during the postpartum period, and woman's lifestyle. In other terms, the safety of a contraceptive method should be weighed along with the benefits of preventing unintended pregnancy as indicated by the medical eligibility criteria (MEC) for contraceptive use (33). **Table 3** presents the categories of the United States Medical Eligibility Criteria for Contraceptive Use (US MEC). **Table 4** presents the MEC for hormonal methods in breastfeeding postpartum women. In conclusion, both CHCs and POP, although POP is preferable, can be safely used by breastfeeding women after the first 42 days postpartum.

MATERNAL INFECTIONS

Cytomegalovirus Infection

Between 37 and 93.7% of pregnant women are CMV-IgG seropositive (34) and more than 50% of CMV-IgG positive mothers produce CMV-positive breastmilk (35). CMV can be isolated in milk whey and from milk cells, mainly neutrophils (predominant during the first 30 days of lactation) and macrophages (predominant starting 60 days postpartum onwards) (36). Although human milk contains biological factors (e.g., lactoferrin) that are known to protect against viral infection, inhibition of CMV virulence is only partial and mother-to-child transmission of CMV infection is still possible (37).

Postnatal CMV infection with maternal infected liquids (milk, saliva, urine) rarely causes severe clinical illness in full-term infants (38) and it is usually devoid of relevant late sequelae. Differently, postnatal CMV infection in immunodeficient infants, particularly in moderate-severe preterm infants and/or very low birth weight infants (VLBWIs), was believed until recently to carry significant short- (39) and long-term health consequences (40). In their meta-analysis of studies (41) on mother-to-child transmission of CMV infection among VLBWIs, Lanzieri et al. reported that the risk of transmission is higher with fresh breastmilk (19%; range 11–32%) and lower with frozen (−20°C) breastmilk (13%; range 7–24%). Among the VLBWIs infected with CMV, 4-5% developed a major short-term illness resembling a sepsis like-syndrome (41). Freezing the milk inconsistently reduces CMV infectivity (42, 43), especially when the viral load is high. In contrast, Holder pasteurization (30 min at 62.5°C) completely destroys CMV infectivity in human milk, reducing the transmission rate to almost null (44). Although pasteurized banked human milk from CMV-negative donors may be the least riskiest option of transmission of CMV from the mother to a VLBW infant, the process adversely affects the bioactive properties of human milk. Recently, high-temperature short-time (HTST) pasteurization has been proposed as an alternative method to better preserve some of the biological components of human milk (45, 46).

Regarding the debate over the long-term cognitive consequences of postnatal CMV infection through human milk in preterm infants, a recent large prospective study conducted in the Netherlands involving 356 preterm infants with a gestational age of <32 weeks followed-up until age 6 years reported that neurodevelopmental problems, including hearing loss, are unlikely (47). As pasteurization or freezing reduces the biological and immunological protective value of breastmilk against necrotizing enterocolitis (48), the study concluded that these processes may not be justified (47).

Although options differ (**Table 5**) (49) on how to feed a VLBWI of a CMV-seropositive mother, the value of routine feeding of human milk to preterm infants outweighs the risks of clinical disease (2). Withholding the use of fresh breastmilk in the nutrition of VLBWIs no longer seems justifiable.

Human Immunodeficiency Virus (HIV) Infection

Although breastfeeding is one of the most valuable ways to enhance child survival, until recently HIV-positive mothers in developed countries were discouraged to breastfeed, as mother-to-child transmission of HIV infection can occur not only during pregnancy and delivery but also through breastfeeding (50, 51). Accumulating evidence from countries with a high prevalence of HIV infection in the population of pregnant women has

TABLE 3 | US MEC Categories-2016.

1. No restriction for the use of the contraceptive method for a woman with that condition
2. Advantages of using the method generally outweigh the theoretical or proven risks
3. Theoretical or proven risks of the method usually outweigh the advantages – not usually recommended unless more appropriate methods are not available or acceptable
4. Unacceptable health risk if the contraceptive method is used by a woman with that condition

TABLE 4 | US-MEC (2016) for CHCs and POP in the breastfeeding woman with and without risk factors for venous thromboembolism (VTE).

Time post-partum	CHCs	POP
<21 days postpartum	4	2
21–30 days postpartum		
• With other risk factors for VTE	3	2
• Without other risk factors for VTE	3	2
30–42 days postpartum		
• With other risk factors for VTE	3	1
• Without other risk factors for VTE	2	1
>42 days postpartum	2	1

TABLE 5 | Options when feeding the VLBWI with CMV positive mother's milk.

Option	Comment
1. Pasteurization	• Expensive • Effective • Biological pauperization
2. Freezing before use	• Cheap • Limited effectiveness
3. Application of a MTC transmission protocol, which includes: • Weekly CMV urine test until 32 wks PCA • Informed choice of parents • Weekly CMV urine monitoring by polymerase chain reaction • If the infant becomes positive, fresh milk feeding possibly stopped to reduce viral loads (49)	• Cumbersome • Ambiguous • Causing anxiety
4. Use of fresh mother's milk, in any case	• Priority to the prevention of NEC • Favorable risk/benefit ratio

shown that giving antiretroviral medicines to mothers and baby can significanlty reduce the risk of HIV transmission through breastfeeding (52). In a meta-analysis of the postnatal-mother-to-child transmission (PMTCT) rate of HIV infection, the overall pooled transmission rates for breastfed infants with mothers on antiretroviral treatment (ART) were 3.5 and 4.2% at 6 and 12 months, respectively (53). A substantial reduction in postnatal HIV transmission risk under maternal ART was noted (PMTCT rate 1.1% at 6 months and 2.9% at 12 months) (53). The risk of PMTCT was noted to increase once ART was stopped—usually at 6 months—supporting current recommendations that all women diagnosed as HIV-infected should receive immediate and lifelong ART.

A recent randomized trial involving 14 sites in Sub-Saharan Africa and India compared the efficacy of prolonged infant antiretroviral prophylaxis with nevirapine vs. maternal ART for the prevention of mother-to-child transmission (MTCT) throughout the breastfeeding period (54). Maternal ART or infant nevirapine (iNVP) prophylaxis was safely continued until 18 months after delivery or breastfeeding cessation. The MTCT rate at 24 months was very low in both study arms (ART 0.57%; iNVP 0.58%).

In view of this evidence, in 2016 the World Health Organization (WHO) released updated guidelines on HIV and infant feeding (55). Pregnant women who regularly receive ART before delivery are expected to have a low enough number of HIV copies in their blood that poses a negligible risk of transmission of the virus during labor and delivery, so that they may have a normal vaginal birth and might also eventually breastfeed. According to WHO recommendations, infants born to HIV-positive mothers can be exclusively breastfed for the first 6 months of life, with the introduction of appropriate complementary foods thereafter; they can continue to be breastfed for up to 24 months or longer while the mothers are being fully supported for ART adherence (55).

WHO guidelines refer to limited recourse countries where breastfeeding is the cultural norm and formula feeding is stigmatized in the local community. Though HIV-seropositive status constitutes a potential contraindication to breastfeed, there are good medical as well as social reasons to encourage HIV-positive mothers to breastfeed. Moreover, also in industrialized countries an HIV-positive mother can be supported to breastfeed if she adheres to ART and has a low plasma viral load. When these criteria are met, the postnatal transmission rate at 12 months after delivery for the breastfed infant might be around 3% and even lower if ART is maintained for between 6 and 12 months (52, 54).

Although breastfeeding is still a documented risk factor for MTCT of HIV (56), the British HIV Association (57) and the American Academy of Pediatrics (58) recommend that mothers who choose this option should practice exclusive breastfeeding for no more than 6 months while undergoing regular monitoring of maternal ART compliance, maternal viral load, and infant HIV status. In conclusion, encouraging breastfeeding while the HIV-positive mother is on ART is feasible and may become common practice in the near future also in industrialized countries.

ZIKV Infection

The Zika virus (ZIKV) is a mosquito-borne (*Aedes*) RNA flavivirus that causes a "dengue-like syndrome" as a usual clinical manifestation (59). ZIKV has the potential to spread to areas where the *Aedes* mosquito vector is present, including Southern Europe. ZIKV represents an emerging health threat, particularly due to associated neurological disease in newborns and adults. Consequences of vertical infection include microcephaly with brain and eye abnormalities, and consequences of adult infection include Guillain-Barré syndrome and meningoencephalitis. The route of transmission of ZIKV is multiple (60): sexual, via blood transfusion, intrauterine, perinatal (still unknown spectrum of clinical features), postnatal due to mosquito sting and possibly to breastfeeding.

Following the identification of ZIKV in breastmilk (61, 62), its role as a potential route of transmission has been questioned. Although paucisymptomatic ZIKV infection has been described anecdotally in breastfed infants (63, 64), no proven MTCT of infection via breastmilk has been confirmed. In conclusion, as the benefits of breastfeeding outweigh the risk of possible ZIKV transmission via breastmilk, the WHO (65) and the United States Centers for Disease Control and Prevention (CDC)[3] consider maternal ZIKV infection compatible with breastfeeding.

CHEMICAL SUBSTANCES IN HUMAN MILK

Drugs

Pharmaceutical companies rarely give complete information about the appearance of a drug in breastmilk following assumption by the mother and about the possible side effects for the nursing infant. Drug companies do not provide more detailed information because they choose not to study the problem. Consumers are expected to read the lengthy precautions on the package insert that indicate that the drug should not taken during

[3]https://www.cdc.gov/pregnancy/zika/testing-follow-up/zika-in-infants-children.html

pregnancy and lactation (66). According to the information in the European Summaries of Product Characteristics (SmPCs), the use of 90% of medicines is restricted during both pregnancy and breastfeeding, despite a lack of information to support such indications (67). This defensive position is taken to avoid possible litigation.

It comes as no surprise, therefore, that the use of medications by a nursing mother may be a valid reason for breastfeeding cessation, albeit arguably stemming from an excessively cautious approach. Although almost all drugs pass into breastmilk, the known adverse effects in infants are relatively few. Most adverse effects are reported as being merely associated, without having a certain causal relationship.

Moreover, many side effects are described in the first 2 months of life (68) when breastfeeding is still exclusive or nearly exclusive, limiting the relevance of the passage of a drug into the mother's milk at an older age when semisolids and solids are added to the diet, thus reducing the possible drug burden on the infant.

When documented clinical data on side effects in the infant are unavailable, pharmacokinetic parameters provide the theoretical basis on which the lactation risk is initially assessed (69). From a pharmacological standpoint, we can appreciate that the minimum infant intake of a maternal drug through breastmilk can be expected when its half-life is short, maternal plasma protein binding is high (allowing less unbound drug to pass into the milk), the biochemical characteristics of the drug lead to a low milk-to-plasma ratio, and absorption by the infant gut is slow, resulting in poor bioavailability.

Most drug transfer from the mother's plasma into breastmilk, although rarely exceeding the relative infant dose (RID) of 1 percent of the mother's dose, much less than the upper limit of safety, that is 10% of the maternal dose (69). RID is calculated by dividing the infant dose via milk in mg/kg/day by the maternal dose in mg/kg/day, assuming a mother's body weight of 70 kg.

When giving advice or counseling on the use of medications during breastfeeding, health professionals should use the most authoritative information source that provide pharmacological and toxicological information. LactMed[4] appears to be the most reliable source for quality of citations. After a methodologically appropriate assessment of the safety of a medication in a breastfeeding mother, there is no conflict of interest between the right of the mother to self-treat and the health of her breastfed infant in most cases (70). Nevertheless, assessing the safety profile of a drug in breastfeeding women requires investment by health professional in terms of time, specific scientific knowledge, and empathic approach.

Compared to their older colleagues, few young pediatricians feel that mothers can successfully breastfeed (70% in 1995 vs. 57% in 2014) and that the benefits of breastfeeding outweigh the difficulties (70% in 1995; 50% in 2014) (71). Ultimately, a disfavorable attitude of pediatricians toward the promotion of breastfeeding may hinder the development of well-balanced professional counseling on medication use during breastfeeding. Furthermore, health professionals should also appreciate that some mothers may have a limited willingness to invest in their breastfeeding experience and will ultimately make an informed choice for bottle feeding.

[4]https://toxnet.nlm.nih.gov/newtoxnet/lactmed.htm

Contrast Agents

Contrary to mistaken beliefs that breastmilk is altered by radiation, medical imaging including computed tomography (CT) does not affect the quality of breastmilk or the health of the breastfed infant. Where some uncertainty does, in fact, exist regards the possible health consequences of the passage into breastmilk of contrast agents for imaging studies (CT or MRI). Breastfeeding mothers who require intravascular iodinated or gadolinium-based contrast for an imaging procedure are usually advised to interrupt breastfeeding for 24 to 48 h after exposure to the contrast agent. Because of ethical considerations, no controlled trials have directly examined the safety of breastfeeding after imaging with radiocontrast agents to date.

According to the American College of Radiology (ACR), a negligible dose of contrast agent administered intravenously to the mother is absorbed by the gastrointestinal tract of the breastfed infant: $<0.01\%$ for iodinated X-ray contrast agents and $<0.0004\%$ for gadolinium-based contrast agents (72). Although the final dose of contrast medium absorbed by a breastfeeding infant whose mother receives an intravenous agent is not expected to pose significant toxic or allergic harm to the breastfed infant, the ACR still recommends the option of abstaining from breastfeeding for a period of 12–24 h if this is the preference of an informed mother (72).

An Italian joint working group on the administration of contrast agents to breastfeeding women has come to different conclusions (73), considering the majority of contrast agents safe, except for gadopentetate dimeglumine, gadodiamide, and gadoversetamide. Only these three contrast agents should be precautionally avoided in breastfeeding women due to the high risk of nephrogenic systemic fibrosis (73), although its occurrence has not been reported in infants or young children (74). After MRI or CT examination with a contrast agent: (1) breastfeeding should be temporarily discontinued, the breastmilk expressed and discarded in a limited number of cases; (2) there are no evidence-based reasons for the routine suspension of breastfeeding.

CONCLUSION

The present review provides useful information for developing sound advice for the breastfeeding mother in the context of controversial conditions that are uncritically accepted as true contraindications to breastfeeding. Most conditions appear to be safe and compatible with breastfeeding. The major determinants in the final choice are the attitude of the health professionals consulted and the state of mind of the informed mother.

AUTHOR CONTRIBUTIONS

RD conceived the project and made a substantial, direct and intellectual contribution to the work, and approved it for publication.

REFERENCES

1. Schwarz EB, Nothnagle M. The maternal health benefits of breastfeeding. *Am Fam Physic.* (2015) 91:603–4.
2. Eidelman AI, Schanler RJ. Section on breastfeeding. *Am Acad Pediatr Policy Stat.* (2012) 129:e827–41.
3. Bartick MC, Stuebe AM, Schwarz EB, Luongo C, Reinhold AG, Foster EM. Cost analysis of maternal disease associated with suboptimal breastfeeding. *Obstet Gynecol.* (2013) 122:111–9. doi: 10.1097/AOG.0b013e318297a047
4. Bartick M, Reinhold A. The burden of suboptimal breastfeeding in the United States: a pediatric cost analysis. *Pediatrics* (2010) 125:e1048–56. doi: 10.1542/peds.2009-1616
5. Cattaneo A, Ronfani L, Burmaz T, Quintero-Romero S, Macaluso A, Di Mario S. Infant feeding and cost of health care: a cohort study. *Acta Paediatr.* (2006) 95:540–6. doi: 10.1080/08035250500447936
6. WHO/UNICEF. *Global Strategy for Infant and Young Child Feeding.* Geneva: World Health Organization (2003).
7. DavanzoR, Romagnoli C, Corsello G. Position statement on breastfeeding from the Italian pediatric societies. *Ital J Pediatr.* (2015) 41:80. doi: 10.1186/s13052-015-0191-x
8. World Health Organization/UNICEF. *Acceptable Medical Reasons for Use of Breast-Milk Substitutes.* Geneva: Department of Child and Adolescent Health and Development, World Health Organization (2009).
9. Hauck YL, Graham-Smith C, McInerney J, Kay S. Western Australian women's perceptions of conflicting advicearound breast feeding. *Midwifery* (2011) 27:e156–62. doi: 10.1016/j.midw.2010.02.003
10. Adams WP Jr, Mallucci P. Breast augmentation. *Plast Reconstr Surg.* (2012) 130:597e–611e. 136:531e-44e. doi: 10.1097/PRS.0b013e318262f607
11. Schiff M, Algert CS, Ampt A, Sywak MS, Roberts CL. The impact of cosmetic breast implants on breastfeeding: a systematic review and meta-analysis. *Int Breastfeed J.* (2014) 9:17. doi: 10.1186/1746-4358-9-17
12. Roberts CL, Ampt AJ, Algert CS, Sywak MS, Chen JS. Reduced breast milk feeding subsequent to cosmetic breast augmentation surgery. *Med. J. Aust.* (2015) 202:324–8. doi: 10.5694/mja14.01386
13. Hall-Findlay EJ, Shestak KC. Breast reduction. *Plast Reconstr Surg.* (2015) 136:531e–44e. doi: 10.1097/PRS.0000000000001622
14. Souto GC, Giugliani ER, Giugliani C, Schneider MA. The impact of breast reduction surgery on breastfeeding performance. *J Hum Lact.* (2003) 19:43–9. doi: 10.1177/0890334402239733
15. Andrade RA, Coca KP, Abrão AC. Breastfeeding pattern in the first month of life in women submitted to breast reduction and augmentation. *J Pediatr.* (2010) 86:239–44. doi: 10.2223/JPED.2002
16. Kraut RY, Brown E, Korownyk C, Katz LS, Vandermeer B, Babenko O, et al. The impact of breast reduction surgery on breastfeeding: systematic review of observational studies. *PLoS ONE* (2017) 12:e0186591. doi: 10.1371/journal.pone.0186591
17. Collaborative Group on Hormonal Factors in Breast Cancer. Breast cancer and breastfeeding: collaborative reanalysis of individual data from 47 epidemiological studies in 30 countries, including 50302 women with breast cancer and 96973 women without the disease. *Lancet* (2002) 360:187–95. doi: 10.1016/S0140-6736(02)09454-0
18. Azim HA Jr, Bellettini G, Gelber S, Peccatori FA. Breast-feeding after breast cancer: if you wish, madam. *Breast Cancer Res Treat.* (2009) 114:7–12. doi: 10.1007/s10549-008-9983-7
19. Pagani O, Partridge A, Korde L, Badve S, Bartlett J, Albain K, et al. Breast International Group; North American Breast Cancer Group Endocrine Working Group. Pregnancy after breast cancer: if you wish, ma'am. *Breast Cancer Res Treat.* (2011) 129:309–17. doi: 10.1007/s10549-011-1643-7
20. Lambertini M, Kroman N, Ameye L, Cordoba O, Pinto A, Benedetti G, et al. Long-term safety of pregnancy following breast cancer according to estrogen receptor status. *J Natl Cancer Inst.* (2018) 110:426–9. doi: 10.1093/jnci/djx206
21. Brown A, Rance J, Warren L. Body image concerns during pregnancy are associated with a shorter breast feeding duration. *Midwifery* (2015) 31:80–9. doi: 10.1016/j.midw.2014.06.003
22. Saleem M, Martin H, Coates P. Prolactin biology and laboratory measurement: an update on physiology and current analytical issues. *Clin Biochem Rev.* (2018) 39:3–16.
23. Beshyah SA, Sherif IH, Chentli F, Hamrahian A, Khalil AB, Raef H, et al. Management of prolactinomas: a survey of physicians from the Middle East and North Africa. *Pituitary* (2017) 20:231–40. doi: 10.1007/s11102-016-0767-5
24. Maiter D. Prolactinoma and pregnancy: from the wish of conception to lactation. *Ann Endocrinol* (2016) 77:128–34.
25. Glezer A, Bronstein MD. Prolactinomas: how to handle prior to and during pregnancy? *Minerva Endocrinol.* (2017). doi: 10.23736/S0391-1977.17.02792-4. [Epub ahead of print].
26. Domingue ME, Devuyst F, Alexopoulou O, Corvilain B, Maiter D. Outcome of prolactinoma after pregnancy and lactation: a study on 73 patients. *Clin Endocrinol.* (2014) 80:642–8. doi: 10.1111/cen.12370
27. McNeilly AS, Glasier AF, Howie PW, Houston MJ, Cook A, Boyle H. Fertility after childbirth: pregnancy associated with breast feeding. *Clin Endocrinol.* (1983) 19:167–73. doi: 10.1111/j.1365-2265.1983.tb02978.x
28. Temkin O. *Soranus'Gynecology.* Baltimore, MA: The Johns Hopkins University Press (1991).
29. Cetin I, Assandro P, Massari M, Sagone A, Gennaretti R, Donzelli G, et al. Working group on breastfeeding, Italian Society of Perinatal Medicine and Task Force on Breastfeeding, Ministry of Health, Italy. Breastfeeding during pregnancy: position paper of the Italian Society of Perinatal Medicine and the Task Force on Breastfeeding, Ministry of Health, Italy. *J. Hum. Lact.* (2014) 30:20–7. doi: 10.1177/0890334413514294
30. Butte NF, King JC. Energy requirements during pregnancy and lactation. *Public Health Nutr.* (2005) 8:1010–27. doi: 10.1016/j.mcna.2016.06.004
31. Hughes H. Postpartum contraception. *J Fam Health Care* (2009) 19:9–10.
32. Halderman LD, Nelson AL. Impact of early postpartum administration of progestin-only hormonal contraceptives compared with nonhormonal contraceptives on short-term breast-feeding patterns. *Am J Obstet Gynecol.* (2002) 186:1250–6; discussion 1256-8. doi: 10.1067/mob.2002.123738
33. Curtis KM, Tepper NK, Jatlaoui TC, Berry-Bibee E, Horton LG, Zapata LB, et al. U.S. medical eligibility criteria for contraceptive use, 2016. *MMWR Recomm Rep.* (2016) 65:1–104. doi: 10.15585/mmwr.rr6503a1
34. Antona D, Lepoutre A, Fonteneau L, Baudon C, Halftermeyer-Zhou F, Strat LE Y, et al. Seroprevalence of cytomegalovirus infection in France in 2010. *Epidemiol Infect.* (2017) 145:1471–8. doi: 10.1017/S0950268817000103
35. Vochem M, Hamprecht K, Jahn G, Speer CP. Transmission of cytomegalovirus to preterm infants through breast milk. *Pediatr Infect Dis J.* (1998) 17:53–8. doi: 10.1097/00006454-199801000-00012
36. Maschmann J, Goelz R, Witzel S, Strittmatter U, Steinmassl M, Jahn G, et al. Characterization of human breast milk leukocytes and their potential role in cytomegalovirus transmission to newborns. *Neonatology* (2015) 107:213–9. doi: 10.1159/000371753
37. Harmsen MC, Swart PJ, de Béthune MP, Pauwels R, De Clercq E, The TH, et al. Antiviral effects of plasma and milk proteins: lactoferrin shows potent activity against both human immunodeficiency virus and human cytomegalovirus replication *in vitro*. *J. Infect. Dis.* (1995) 172:380–8.
38. Berardi A, Rossi C, Fiorini V, Rivi C, Vagnarelli F, Guaraldi N, et al. Severe acquired cytomegalovirus infection in a full-term, formula-fed infant: case report. *BMC Pediatr.* (2011) 11:52. doi: 10.1186/1471-2431-11-52
39. Mukhopadhyay S, Meyer SA, Permar SR, Puopolo KM. Symptomatic postnatal cytomegalovirus testing among very low-birth-weight infants: indications and outcomes. *Am J Perinatol.* (2016) 33:894–902. doi: 10.1055/s-0036-1581080
40. Goelz R, Meisner C, Bevot A, Hamprecht K, Kraegeloh-Mann I, Poets CF. Long-term cognitive and neurological outcome of preterm infants with postnatally acquired CMV infection through breast milk. *Arch Dis Child Fetal Neonatal.* (2013) 98:F430–3. doi: 10.1136/archdischild-2012-303384
41. Lanzieri TM, Dollard SC, Josephson CD, Schmid DS, Bialek SR. Breast milk-acquired cytomegalovirus infection and disease in VLBW and premature infants. *Pediatrics* (2013) 131:e1937–45. doi: 10.1542/peds.2013-0076
42. Omarsdottir S, Casper C, Navér L, Legnevall L, Gustafsson F, Grillner L, et al. Cytomegalovirus infection and neonatal outcome in extremely preterm infants after freezing of maternal milk. *Pediatr Infect Dis J.* (2015) 34:482–9. doi: 10.1097/INF.0000000000000619
43. Balcells C, Botet F, Gayete S, Marcos MÁ, Dorronsoro I, de Alba C., et al. Vertically transmitted cytomegalovirus infection in newborn preterm infants. *J Perinat Med.* (2016) 44:485–90. doi: 10.1515/jpm-2015-0325

44. Hamprecht K, Goelz R. Postnatal cytomegalovirus infection through human milk in preterm infants: transmission, clinical presentation, and prevention. *Clin Perinatol.* (2017) 44:121–30. doi: 10.1016/j.clp.2016.11.012
45. Escuder-Vieco D, Espinosa-Martos I, Rodríguez JM, Corzo N, Montilla A, Siegfried P, et al. High-temperature short-time pasteurization system for donor milk in a human milk bank setting. *Front Microbiol.* (2018) 9:926. doi: 10.3389/fmicb.2018.00926
46. Peila C, Emmerik NE, Giribaldi M, Stahl B, Ruitenberg JE, van Elburg RM, et al. Human milk processing: a systematic review of innovative techniques to ensure the safety and quality of donor milk. *J Pediatr Gastroenterol Nutr.* (2017) 64:353–61. doi: 10.1097/MPG.0000000000001435
47. Gunkel J, de Vries LS, Jongmans M, Koopman-Esseboom C, van Haastert IC, Eijsermans MCJ, et al. Outcome of preterm infants with postnatal cytomegalovirus infection. *Pediatrics* (2018) 141:e20170635. doi: 10.1542/peds.2017-0635
48. Stock K, Griesmaier E, Brunner B, Neubauer V, Kiechl-Kohlendorfer U, Trawöger R. Pasteurization of breastmilk decreases the rate of postnatally acquired cytomegalovirus infections, but shows a nonsignificant trend to an increased rate of necrotizing enterocolitis in very preterm infants: a preliminary study. *Breastfeed Med.* (2015) 10:113–7. doi: 10.1089/bfm.2014.0108
49. Kurath S, Resch B. Cytomegalovirus and transmission via breast milk: how to support breast milk to premature infants and prevent severe infection? *Pediatr Infect Dis J.* (2010) 29:680–1. doi: 10.1097/INF.0b013e3181dc4d4a
50. Givens M, Dotters-Katz SK, Stringer E, Rahangdale L, Kuller JA. Minimizing the risk of perinatal human immunodeficiency virus transmission. *Obstet Gynecol Surv.* (2018) 73:423–32. doi: 10.1097/OGX.0000000000000581
51. Fowler MG, Kourtis AP, Aizire J, Onyango-Makumbi C, Bulterys M. Breastfeeding and transmission of HIV1: epidemiology and global magnitude. *Adv Exp Med Biol.* (2012) 743:3–25. doi: 10.1007/978-1-4614-2251-8_1
52. Fowler MG, Flynn P, Aizire J. What is new in perinatal HIV prevention? *Curr Opin Pediatr.* (2018) 30:144–51. doi: 10.1097/MOP.0000000000000579
53. Bispo S, Chikhungu L, Rollins N, Siegfried N, Newell ML. Postnatal HIV transmission in breastfed infants of HIV-infected women on ART: a systematic review and meta-analysis. *J Int AIDS Soc.* (2017) 20:21251. doi: 10.7448/IAS.20.1.21251
54. Flynn PM, Taha TE, Cababasay M, Fowler MG, Mofenson LM, Owor, M. et al. Prevention of HIV-1 transmission through breastfeeding: efficacy and safety of maternal antiretroviral therapy versus infant nevirapine prophylaxis for duration of breastfeeding in HIV-1-infected women with high CD4 cell count (IMPAACT PROMISE): a randomized, open-label, clinical trial. *J Acquir Immune Defic Syndr.* (2018) 77:383–92. doi: 10.1097/QAI.0000000000001612
55. World Health Organization. *Guideline: Updates on HIV and Infant Feeding: The Duration of Breastfeeding, and Support from Health Services to Improve Feeding Practices Among Mothers Living with Geneva.* World Health Organization (2016).
56. Chiappini E, Galli L, Lisi C, Gabiano C, Esposito S, Giacomet V, et al. Strategies for prevention of mother-to-child transmission adopted in the "real world" setting: data from the Italian Register for HIV-1 infection in children. *J Acquir Immune Defic Syndr.* (2018) 79:54–61. doi: 10.1097/QAI.0000000000001774.
57. Taylor GP, Anderson J, Clayden P, Gazzard BF, Fortin J, Kennedy J, et al. British HIV Association and Children's HIV. Association position statement on infant feeding in the UK. HIV Medicine. *HIV Med.* 12:389–93. doi: 10.1111/j.1468-1293.2011.00918.x
58. American Academy of Pediatrics, Committee on Pediatric AIDS. Infant feeding and transmission of human immunodeficiency virus in the United States. *Pediatrics* (2013) 131:391–6. doi: 10.1542/peds.2012-3543
59. Ioos S, Mallet HP, Goffart LI, Gauthier V, Cardoso T, Herida M. Current Zika virus epidemiology and recent epidemics. *Med Mal Infect.* (2014) 44:302–7. doi: 10.1016/j.medmal.2014.04.008
60. Gregory CJ, Oduyebo T, Brault AC, Brooks JT, Chung KW, Hills S, et al. Modes of Transmission of Zika Virus. *J Infect Dis.* (2017) 216 (Suppl_10):S875–83. doi: 10.1093/infdis/jix396
61. Sotelo JR, Sotelo AB, Sotelo FJB, Doi AM, Pinho JRR, Oliveira RC, et al. Persistence of Zika Virus in breast milk after infection in late stage of pregnancy. *Emerg Infect Dis.* (2017) 23:856–7. doi: 10.3201/eid2305.161538
62. Cavalcanti MG, Cabral-Castro MJ, Gonçalves JLS, Santana LS, Pimenta ES, Peralta JM. Zika virus shedding in human milk during lactation: an unlikely source of infection? *Int J Infect Dis.* (2017) 57:70–72. doi: 10.1016/j.ijid.2017.01.042
63. Blohm GM, Lednicky JA, Márquez M, White SK, Loeb JC, Pacheco CA, et al. Evidence for mother-to-child transmission of Zika virus through breast milk. *Clin Infect Dis.* (2018) 66:1120–1. doi: 10.1093/cid/cix968
64. Colt S, Garcia-Casal MN, Peña-Rosas JP, Finkelstein JL, Rayco-Solon P, Weise Prinzo ZC, et al. Transmission of Zika virus through breast milk and other breastfeeding-related bodily-fluids: a systematic review. *PLoS Negl Trop Dis.* (2017) 11:e0005528. doi: 10.1371/journal.pntd.0005528
65. World Health Organization. *Infant Feeding in Areas of Zika Virus Transmission. Summary of Rapid Advice Guideline.* (2016) WHO/ZIKV/MOC/16.6.
66. Brown E, Hotham E, Hotham N. Views of obstetric practitioners and hospital pharmacists on therapeutic goods administration approved product information for pregnancy and lactation. *Aust N Z J Obstet Gynaecol.* (2014) 54:184–8. doi: 10.1111/ajo.12197
67. Arguello B, Salgado TM, Fernandez-Llimos F. Assessing the information in the summaries of product characteristics for the use of medicines in pregnancy and lactation. *Br J Clin Pharmacol.* (2015) 79:537–44. doi: 10.1111/bcp.12515
68. Anderson PO, Manoguerra AS, Valdés V. A review of adverse reactions in infants from medications in breastmilk. *Clin Pediatr.* (2016) 55:236–44. doi: 10.1177/0009922815594586
69. Rowe H, Baker T, Hale TW. Maternal medication, drug use, and breastfeeding. *Child Adolesc Psychiatr Clin N Am.* (2015) 24:1–20. doi: 10.1016/j.chc.2014.09.005
70. Davanzo R, Bua J, De Cunto A, Farina ML, De Ponti F, Clavenna A, et al. Advising mothers on the use of medications during breastfeeding: a need for a positive attitude. *J Hum Lact.* (2016) 32:15–9. doi: 10.1177/0890334415595513
71. Feldman-Winter L, Szucs K, Milano A, Gottschlich E, Sisk B, Schanler RJ. National trends in pediatricians' practices and attitudes about breastfeeding: 1995 to 2014. *Pediatrics* (2017) 140:e20171229. doi: 10.1542/peds.2017-1229
72. American College of Radiology. *Committee on Drugs and Contrast Media. ACR Manual on Contrast Media.* Version 10.3 (2017). American College of Radiology. https://www.acr.org/-/media/ACR/Files/Clinical-Resources/Contrast_Media.pdf
73. Cova MA, Stacul F, Quaranta R, Guastalla P, Salvatori G, Banderali G, et al. Radiological contrast media in the breastfeeding woman: a position paper of the Italian Society of Radiology (SIRM), the Italian Society of Paediatrics (SIP), the Italian Society of Neonatology (SIN) and the Task Force on Breastfeeding, Ministry of Health, Italy. *Eur Radiol.* (2014) 24:2012–22. doi: 10.1007/s00330-014-3198-6
74. Nardone B, Saddleton E, Laumann AE, Edwards BJ, Raisch DW, McKoy JM, et al. Pediatric nephrogenic systemic fibrosis is rarely reported: a RADAR report. *Pediatr Radiol.* (2014) 44:173–80. doi: 10.1007/s00247-013-2795-x

Better Control of Holder Pasteurization Results in Higher Retention of Human Milk Lactoferrin, IgA, and Lysozyme

Rachel Buffin[1,2*], *Stéphane Hays*[2], *Jocelyne Drai*[3], *Marie-Nathalie Sarda*[4] *and Jean-Charles Picaud*[1,2,5]

[1] *Neonatology Department, Croix-Rousse Hospital, Lyon, France,* [2] *Régional Rhône Alpes Auvergne Human Milk Bank, Hôpital de la Croix-Rousse, Lyon, France,* [3] *Biochemistry Laboratory, Lyon-sud Hospital, Pierre-Bénite, France,* [4] *Immunology Laboratory, Lyon-sud Hospital, Pierre-Bénite, France,* [5] *CarMen Unit, INSERM U1060, INRA U197, Claude Bernard University, Pierre-Bénite, France*

***Correspondence:**
Rachel Buffin
rachel.buffin@chu-lyon.fr

Background: Holder pasteurization is commonly used in milk banks. We previously reported that the pattern of temperature and time may be different according to the pasteurizer used.

Aim: The aim of our study was to assess the variances in pasteurization using two different devices: a standard pasteurizer (Past STD) and an optimized pasteurizer (Past OPTI).

Methods: Immunoglobulin A (IgA), lactoferrin (LF), and lysozyme (LZ) content were assessed before and after pasteurization of 24 donor human milk samples. The impact of the pasteurization device was evaluated by testing 50- to 200-mL samples.

Results: Mean temperature and duration of the plateau were 1.5°C lower and 11 min shorter, respectively, with Past OPTI vs. Past STD. The loss of IgA, LF, and LZ was 17.6, 5.6, and 9.8% lower, respectively, with Past OPTI than with Past STD.

Conclusions: Accurate control of temperature enabled better preservation of IgA, LF, and LZ in donor milk. Holder pasteurization should be optimized, and new techniques proposed to treat donor milk should be compared with Holder pasteurization performed with a well-controlled device under realistic conditions.

Keywords: human milk bank, donor human milk, quality control, milk processing, immunity

INTRODUCTION

Human milk (HM) is the gold standard for very-low-birth-weight infant nutrition. Its antimicrobial and immunomodulatory components, such as lactoferrin (LF), immunoglobulin A (IgA), or lysozyme (LZ) compensate for the deficit in neonatal immune system and contribute to the prevention of sepsis in these vulnerable infants (1–5). The mother's milk is the first choice, but when unavailable, donor HM from a milk bank is the best alternative (6). The safety of donor HM is a main concern of HM banks and is achieved by pasteurization. The reference method used worldwide is Holder pasteurization, which consists of heating the milk at a low temperature (62.5°C) for a long duration (30 min). Holder pasteurization partially destroys some

HM components (1). Most relevant studies have been performed *in vitro* with very small samples of HM, with discrepancies in the results (1, 7). These discrepancies could be related to differences in pasteurizer performance, which has not been evaluated and described in most studies, as it is assumed that all pasteurizers have the same performance, which is not the case (8).

Indeed, Czank et al. reported that the impact of heat treatment on HM properties depends on temperature. Between 40 and 57°C, immune components were stable but dramatically decreased above 58°C, lactoferrin being the most affected (9). Moreover, we previously reported that pasteurization temperature was different depending on the type of pasteurizer. Time and temperature during the pasteurization process were inconsistent when using an air-ventilated pasteurizer. Not all bottles were exposed to the same temperature for the same duration, resulting in heterogeneous pasteurization. With a water pasteurizer, pasteurization was more homogenous than with an air-ventilated pasteurizer. Furthermore, we reported that an optimized pasteurizer produced better results than a non-controlled one (8). Optimization was achieved by a precise adjustment of the machine to comply with recommendations (1, 8). It could be helpful to preserve bioactive components of HM (5). The benefits of HM are well-documented (6) and most of them are related to the immune component (2, 3) The aim of the study was to assess LF, IgA, and LZ content of donor HM before and after Holder pasteurization using two water pasteurizers: a standard device (Past STD) and an optimized device (Past OPTI).

MATERIALS AND METHODS

This study was performed at the regional HM bank (Lactarium Auvergne Rhone-Alpes, LARA) at the Croix-Rousse University Hospital in Lyon, France.

Two devices from the same manufacturer (HSC, Décines, France) were used for this study: a standard device (PAS 10000 first version) and an optimized device (PAS 10002). In both devices, bottles were partially immerged and agitated continuously to ensure temperature homogenization. Cooling process differed: Past STD cooled the milk with ambient tap water, while Past OPTI cooled the milk down to 4°C with a tank of refrigerated water. Past STD was an older pasteurizer compliant with standard temperature regulation. Past OPTI was designed with a new regulation system offering a lower temperature and shorter duration of plateau during pasteurization cycle. Prior to study we characterized each pasteurizer by recording the temperature during a pasteurization cycle, using external probes as previously recommended (1, 8). Past STD did not adhere to the following criteria previously proposed (8) (such as the mean temperature between 62.5 and 64°C and plateau duration between 30 and 35 min. By contrast, the temperature pattern of Past OPTI were in agreement with these criteria.

Donors provided written informed consent for the use of their milk for this research purpose. The milk used for the study was frozen donor milk that was collected for research use and could not be used for premature infants because of contraindication according to the French national guidelines (herbal intake, transfusion, >4 months of storage, or smoking) (10).

Study Design

The milk from each donor was thawed, poured into an Erlenmeyer flask and homogenized by manual stirring. The milk was divided into 24 single-use polypropylene bottles (Beldico SA, Marche-en-Famenne, Belgium) (**Figure 1**). A sample of 10 mL was collected from each bottle before pasteurization.

The bottles (50–200 ml) were then similarly distributed within each pasteurizer (Past STD and Past OPTI) and subjected to a routine pasteurization cycle (**Figure 2**). A second 10-mL sample was collected from each bottle after pasteurization.

All samples were anonymously labeled, for blind analysis frozen at −21°C and carried to the laboratory in an icebox. Blinded assessment of LF, IgA, and LZ before and after pasteurization was performed at the biochemistry and immunology laboratories in Lyon-Sud Hospital using enzyme-linked immunosorbent assay.

As the range of LF and IgA values was broad, the coefficients of variation were calculated with a low and high value of each component. The range of values was narrower for LZ, and therefore the coefficient of variation was calculated based on a single value. Because of technical problems, LZ content was not assessed in three samples.

Statistical Analysis

We calculated the mean and standard deviation of the LF, IgA, and LZ content before pasteurization. We evaluated the impact of pasteurization on LF, IgA, and LZ concentrations by expressing the results as the difference between the concentration before and after pasteurization and finally as the percentage of retention after pasteurization. This was calculated for both pasteurizers. Differences in absolute value and percentage of pre-treatment value were compared by a Wilcoxon matched sample test. The threshold of significance was set at 0.05. The software used for analysis was SPSS® version 19 (IBM SPSS Statistics, Boigny-sur-Bionne, France).

RESULTS

The characteristics of the pasteurization cycles of both pasteurizers were different (**Table 1**). The mean plateau temperature and duration were 1.5°C lower and 11 min shorter, respectively, with Past OPTI than with Past STD (**Table 1**).

The coefficient of variation for assessment of LF and IgA was 6.3 and 4.6% for lower values (mean values tested: 106 and 735 mg/L) and 11.4 and 3.6% for higher values (mean values tested: 713 and 1,591 mg/L), respectively. The coefficient of variation for LZ assessment was 7.4% (mean value tested: 143 mg/L).

Median (min, max) values before pasteurization were 631 (465, 915) mg/L for LF, 1,976 (1,103, 2,528) mg/L for IgA, and 195 (135, 357) mg/L for LZ. Reduction in LF, IgA, and LZ was greater when using Past STD compared with Past OPTI, with a median reduction of −559.5 (−813, −410) mg/L vs. −499.5

Abbreviations: HM, Human milk; IgA, Immunoglobulin A; LF, Lactoferrin; LZ, Lysozyme; Past OPTI, Optimized pasteurizer; Past STD, Standard pasteurizer.

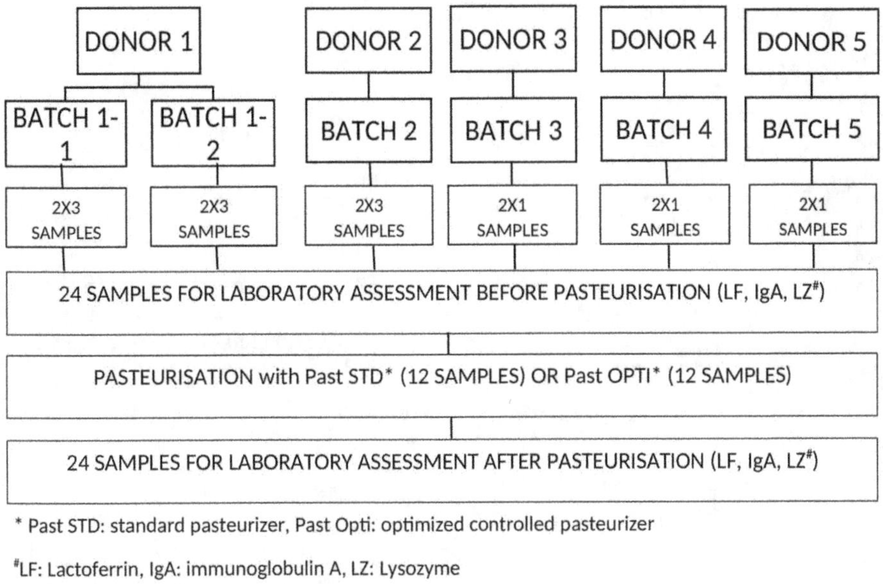

FIGURE 1 | Design of the study and distribution of samples tested with the two pasteurizers: Past STD represents the, standard pasteurizer, while Past OPTI represents the new pasteurizer with better regulation. Each donor's milk was divided in order to be assessed in each device. Each sample was assessed for lactoferrin, IgA, and lysozyme before and after pasteurization.

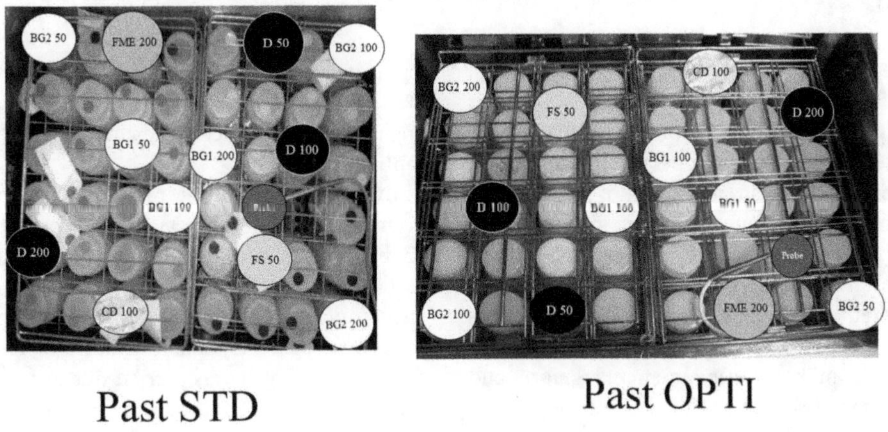

FIGURE 2 | Distribution of the samples in the Past STD and Past OPTI pasteurizers. Capital letters represent the identification of the donor. The volume in each bottle is indicated.

TABLE 1 | Characteristics of pattern of holder pasteurization of Past STD and Past OPTI.

	Past STD	Past OPTI
Mean plateau temperature (°C)	64.4	<62.9
Min plateau temperature (°C)	62.7	62.6
Maximum plateau temperature (°C)	64.8	62.9
Mean plateau duration over 62.5°C (min)	42	31

(−772, −322) mg/L (p = 0.02) for LF, −887.5 (−1,947, −465) mg/L vs. −494.5 (−948, −239) mg/L (p = 0.006) for IgA, and −46.5 (179, −2) mg/L vs. −24 (−109, 13) mg/L (p = 0.037) for LZ, respectively (**Figure 3**). Retention of immune components after pasteurization was ~20% for LF, 60% for IgA, and 80% for LZ (**Figure 3**). Retention was significantly higher with Past OPTI than with Past STD: 21.6 vs. 16% for LF, 71.3 vs. 53.7% for IgA, and 84.2 vs. 74.4% for LZ, which represented a gain of +5.6, +17.8, and +9.8 points for LF, IgA, and LZ, respectively (**Figure 3**).

DISCUSSION

In this study, we observed that an optimized pasteurization better preserved the immune components compared with a standard pasteurization owing to strict control of HM exposure to heat.

The effect of exposure to different temperatures during the Holder pasteurization process is a remaining matter of concern.

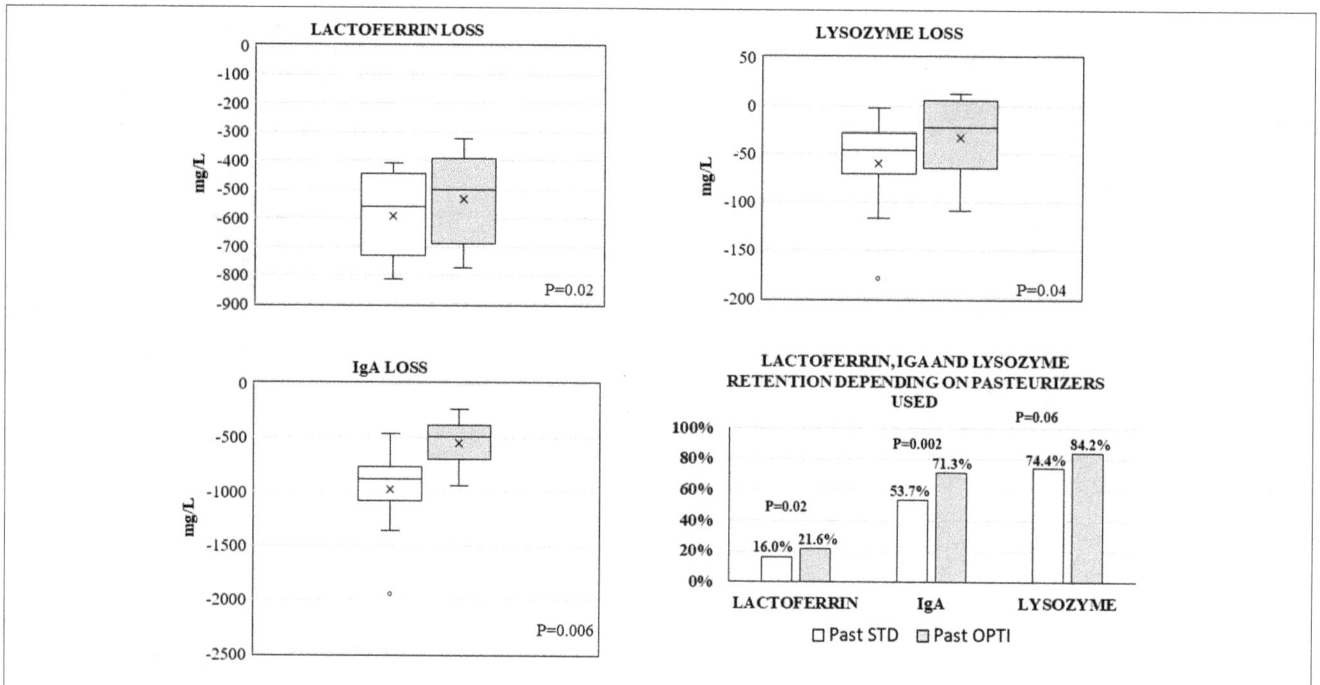

FIGURE 3 | Schematic representation of loss of lactoferrin, IgA, and lysozyme after Past STD (white) and Past OPTI (gray) pasteurization expressed by mean (x) and median (–) in boxplots. The values of preservation are also presented as percentages depending on the pasteurizer used.

Czank et al. described the differences between three types of pasteurizers (bottle immersion (sterifeed), Holding chamber (saurin industries), and an experimental one designed for the study allowing precises' measures of temperature (Carag AC). The impact of the different pasteurizers was not drastic with respect to LF and IgA but was of concern for LZ, in favor of the experimental pasteurizer (9). However, the temperature patterns were not available for these devices, and the composition of treated HM was different. A strength of our study is that we analyzed precisely the temperature pattern of both pasteurizers and we used the same milk for measurements before and after pasteurization to avoid skewing of data due to variations in milk composition (11, 12). Meredith-Dennis et al. also showed differences in LF, IgA, and LZ contents assessed in HM treated with different methods (Holder pasteurization, vat technique or retort sterilization). Indeed, LF, IgA, and LZ— concentrations were greater after Holder pasteurization than after other methods. However, as the samples of HM were different and randomly selected, it was difficult to disentangle effects related to the selection of HM and to the difference in pasteurization methods (11).

In our study, we observed that better temperature control had a statistically significant impact on the retention of three major immune components in HM. We used these components as markers because their effects are well-known, and clinical benefits may be achieved from increasing their concentration in donor HM (13). These markers are commonly used, allowing comparison with levels in other studies (1). In fact, the concentrations of immune components measured in our study were within the range of previously reported values (12, 14–17). Although we did not assess the concentration of other components, we expect that it might also be impacted by the improvement of temperature control.

In recent reviews, the retention after pasteurization ranged from 10 to 65% for LF, 38 to 80% for IgA, and 31 to 80% for LZ, but most articles did not specify the pattern of pasteurization of the devices (1, 7), which could be responsible for these discrepancies (1). Furthermore, nearly all previous studies were performed with very small samples of HM (1). A strength of our study is that it was carried out under conditions closest to routine working conditions of HM banks In such a context we observed that excepted for LF, the retention rates measured in our study were in the upper range of retention reported in the literature (53 and 71% of IgA, 74 and 84% of LZ) (7). It suggests that the impact of Holder pasteurization could be much less than previously published, under the condition that it is a good quality pasteurization (18, 19).

The reduction in immune components following the Holder pasteurization is well-known (1, 7). Therefore, new techniques have been proposed such as high pressure processing, high temperature-short time pasteurization or ultraviolet-C (20–22). The feasibility of their routine use in HM banks is still to be evaluated. Furthermore, the impact on HM bioactive components should be assessed in conditions as close as possible to HM bank, i.e., in large enough milk samples (50–200 mL) and using pasteurizers (not laboratory devices). Finally, it should be compared to the reference method, i.e., Holder pasteurization, performed with devices using a stringent control of temperature during the whole pasteurization cycle (8).

A limitation of our study is that samples were frozen before reaching the laboratory. Indeed, Akinbi et al. reported that freezing induced supplementary loss of immune components (12). However, it is unlikely that the freezing influenced the comparison between pasteurizers, as all HM samples were handled similarly. Furthermore, it suggests that the percentage of immune components preserved after Holder pasteurization was underestimated.

Another limitation is that the only biological parameters measured were the concentrations of three major immune components. Although our study was not designed to investigate the relationship between retention of immune components and clinical evolution, it is well-known that beneficiary effects of HM on health of preterm infants are due in part to its composition (2, 3, 23). HM helps reduce the occurrence of nosocomial bacteremia and the risk of late-onset sepsis in preterm infants (2, 23, 24) It can be assumed that the efficacy of HM is proportional to the quantity of immune components. Therefore, assessing the concentrations of these components may be considered useful until further clinical studies are able to clearly identify benefits related to improvements in pasteurization process.

In conclusion, our results suggest that better control of temperature during Holder pasteurization can improve preservation of LF, IgA, and LZ. Holder pasteurization is used worldwide in HM banks, because it offers the best compromise between efficiency and feasibility. Therefore, it is essential to use only pasteurizers that underwent a stringent control of temperature pattern commercially available. When new techniques are proposed for donor HM treatment, they should be compared under realistic conditions with a well-controlled pasteurizer.

AUTHOR CONTRIBUTIONS

RB and J-CP designed, directed the project wrote the paper with input from all authors. SH, RB, and J-CP analyzed the data. M-NS and JD performed the measurements and analyzed data.

ACKNOWLEDGMENTS

We thank the staff of Auvergne Rhône-Alpes (LARA) regional human milk bank for their help.

REFERENCES

1. Picaud JC, Buffin R. Human milk-treatment and quality of banked human milk. *Clin Perinatol.* (2017) 44:95–119. doi: 10.1016/j.clp.2016.11.003
2. Andreas NJ, Kampmann B, Mehring Le-Doare K. Human breast milk: a review on its composition and bioactivity. *Early Hum Dev.* (2015) 91:629–35. doi: 10.1016/j.earlhumdev.2015.08.013
3. Miller J, Tonkin E, Damarell RA, McPhee AJ, Suganuma M, Suganuma H, et al. A systematic review and meta-analysis of human milk feeding and morbidity in very low birth weight infants. *Nutrients* (2018) 10:E707. doi: 10.3390/nu10060707
4. Ronnestad A. Late-onset septicemia in a Norwegian national cohort of extremely premature infants receiving very early full human milk feeding. *Pediatrics* (2005) 115:e269–76. doi: 10.1542/peds.2004-1833
5. Chen Y. Considerations in donor human milk use in premature infants. *J Pediatr Gastroenterol Nutr.* (2018) 67:550–1. doi: 10.1097/MPG.0000000000002095
6. Arslanoglu S, Corpeleijn W, Moro G, Braegger C, Campoy C, Colomb V, et al. Donor human milk for preterm infants: current evidence and research directions. *J Pediatr Gastroenterol Nutr.* (2013) 57:535–42. doi: 10.1097/MPG.0b013e3182a3af0a
7. Peila C, Moro GE, Bertino E, Cavallarin L, Giribaldi M, Giuliani F, et al. The effect of holder pasteurization on nutrients and biologically-active components in donor human milk: a review. *Nutrients* (2016) 8:E477. doi: 10.3390/nu8080477
8. Buffin R, Pradat P, Trompette J, Ndiaye I, Basson E, Jordan I, et al. Air and water processes do not produce the same high-quality pasteurization of donor human milk. *J Hum Lact.* (2017) 33:717–24. doi: 10.1177/0890334417707962
9. Czank C, Prime DK, Hartmann B, Simmer K, Hartmann PE. Retention of the immunological proteins of pasteurized human milk in relation to pasteurizer design and practice. *Pediatr Res.* (2009) 66:374–9. doi: 10.1203/PDR.0b013e3181b4554a
10. *Règles de Bonnes Pratiques de Collecte, de Préparation, de Qualification, de Traitement, de Conservation, de Distribution et de Délivrance sur Prescription Médicale du lait Humain par les Lactariums* (2008) Available online at: http://sdp.perinat-france.org/ADLF/files/lactarium_guide_bonnes_pratiques_5_janvier_2008_traduction_anglais.pdf (Accessed January 2, 2017)
11. Meredith-Dennis L, Xu G, Goonatilleke E, Lebrilla CB, Underwood MA, Smilowitz JT. Composition and variation of macronutrients, immune proteins, and human milk oligosaccharides in human milk from nonprofit and commercial milk banks. *J Hum Lactation* (2018) 34:120–9. doi: 10.1177/0890334417710635
12. Akinbi H, Meinzen-Derr J, Auer C, Ma Y, Pullum D, Kusano R, et al. Alterations in the host defense properties of human milk following prolonged storage or pasteurization. *J Pediatr Gastroenterol Nutr.* (2010) 51:347–52. doi: 10.1097/MPG.0b013e3181e07f0a
13. Sharma D, Shastri S, Sharma P. Role of lactoferrin in neonatal care: a systematic review. *J Matern Fetal Neonatal Med.* (2017) 30:1920–32. doi: 10.1080/14767058.2016.1232384
14. Rai D, Adelman AS, Zhuang W, Rai GP, Boettcher J, Lönnerdal B. Longitudinal changes in lactoferrin concentrations in human milk: a global systematic review. *Crit Rev Food Sci Nutr.* (2014) 54:1539–47. doi: 10.1080/10408398.2011.642422
15. Trend S, Strunk T, Lloyd ML, Kok CH, Metcalfe J, Geddes DT, et al. Levels of innate immune factors in preterm and term mothers' breast milk during the 1st month postpartum. *Brit J Nutr.* (2016) 115:1178–93. doi: 10.1017/S0007114516000234
16. Hsu YC, Chen CH, Lin MC, Tsai CR, Liang JT, Wang TM. Changes in preterm breast milk nutrient content in the first month. *Pediatr Neonatol.* (2014) 55:449–54. doi: 10.1016/j.pedneo.2014.03.002
17. Mehta R, Petrova A. Biologically active breast milk proteins in association with very preterm delivery and stage of lactation. *J Perinatol.* (2011) 31:58–62. doi: 10.1038/jp.2010.68
18. Viazis S, Farkas BE, Allen JC. Effects of high-pressure processing on immunoglobulin A and lysozyme activity in human milk. *J Hum Lactation* (2007) 23:253–61. doi: 10.1177/0890334407303945
19. Koenig Á, Diniz EM de A, Barbosa SFC, Vaz FAC. Immunologic factors in human milk: the effects of gestational age and pasteurization. *J Hum Lactation* (2005) 21:439–43. doi: 10.1177/0890334405280652
20. Escuder-Vieco D, Espinosa-Martos I, Rodríguez JM, Corzo N, Montilla A, Siegfried P, et al. High-temperature short-time pasteurization system for donor milk in a human milk bank setting. *Front Microbiol.* (2018) 9:926. doi: 10.3389/fmicb.2018.00926
21. Christen L, Lai CT, Hartmann B, Hartmann PE, Geddes DT. Ultraviolet-C irradiation: a novel pasteurization method for donor human milk. *PLoS ONE* (2013) 8:e68120. doi: 10.1371/journal.pone.0068120
22. Sousa SG, Delgadillo I, Saraiva JA. Human milk composition and preservation: evaluation of high-pressure processing as a nonthermal pasteurization technology. *Crit Rev Food Sci Nutr.* (2016) 56:1043–60. doi: 10.1080/10408398.2012.753402

23. Ballard O, Morrow AL. Human milk composition. *Pediatr Clin North Am.* (2013) 60:49–74. doi: 10.1016/j.pcl.2012.10.002

24. Lönnerdal B. Bioactive proteins in human milk-potential benefits for preterm infants. *Clin Perinatol.* (2017) 44:179–91. doi: 10.1016/j.clp.2016.11.013

22

Recommendations for the Establishment and Operation of Human Milk Banks in Europe: A Consensus Statement from the European Milk Bank

Gillian Weaver[1], Enrico Bertino[2], Corinna Gebauer[3], Anne Grovslien[4], Radmila Mileusnic-Milenovic[5], Sertac Arslanoglu[6], Debbie Barnett[7], Clair-Yves Boquien[8], Rachel Buffin[9], Antoni Gaya[10], Guido E. Moro[11], Aleksandra Wesolowska[12,13] and Jean-Charles Picaud[9,14]*

[1] Human Milk Foundation, Harpenden, United Kingdom, [2] Neonatal Unit of Turin University, City of Health and Science of Turin, Turin, Italy, [3] Abteilung Neonatologie Klinik und Poliklinik für Kinder und Jugendliche, Leipzig, Germany, [4] Neonatal Unit, Milk Bank, Oslo University Hospital, Oslo, Norway, [5] First Serbian Milk Bank, Institute of Neonatology, Belgrade, Serbia, [6] Division of Neonatology, Department of Pediatrics, Istanbul Medeniyet University, Istanbul, Turkey, [7] Greater Glasgow and Clyde Donor Milk Bank, Royal Hospital for Sick Children, Glasgow, United Kingdom, [8] PhAN, Institut National de la Recherche Agronomique (INRA), Université de Nantes, CRNH-Ouest, Nantes, France, [9] Neonatal Intensive Care Unit, Hopital de la Croix-Rousse, Hospices Civils de Lyon, Lyon, France, [10] Banc de Teixit, F. Banc de Sang i Teixits de les Illes Balears, Institut d'Investigacio Sanitaria Illes Balears (IdISBa), Barcelona, Spain, [11] Italian Association of Human Milk Banks (AIBLUD), Milan, Italy, [12] Department of Neonatology, Faculty of Health Science, Medical University of Warsaw, Warsaw, Poland, [13] Laboratory of Human Milk and Lactation Research, Holy Family Hospital Regional Human Milk Bank, Warsaw, Poland, [14] CarMeN Unit, INSERM U1060, INRA U1397, Claude Bernard University Lyon 1, Pierre Bénite, France

Correspondence:
Gillian Weaver
gillian.weaver@yahoo.com

Objectives: To develop recommendations from the European Milk Bank Association (EMBA) for the establishment and operation of human milk banks (HMB) in Europe.

Method: A working group comprising members of the EMBA was convened in 2015 to develop Europe-wide recommendations for milk banks. Each member had experience of guideline development and/or milk banking operations. An initial survey was agreed using collated published global recommendations. A total of 108 potential recommendations were included in the survey; responders noted which were included in their national guidelines. The responses were collated, compared, and discussed and the group determined where there was consensus and where substantial or minor differences were identified. Where there was consensus or robust published evidence on which to base recommendations these were included. When there was no consensus and no clear evidence base, a statement of explanation based on collective expert opinion was agreed.

Results: Published, internationally available guidelines with recommendations for human milk banks from France, Italy, and the UK, together with guidelines from Austria, Denmark, Germany, Norway, Slovakia, Spain, Sweden, and Switzerland were included as source materials. These covered: General recommendations; Donor recruitment and screening; Expression, handling, and storage of donor human milk (DHM); Pooling of DHM; Milk screening; Milk treatment (pasteurization); Delivery of DHM to recipients.

Conclusions: Evidence based recommendations and consensus statements from the EMBA will now be published on the EMBA website to assist in the safe establishment and operation of HMBs throughout Europe. These have also been used to inform the chapter on human milk to be included in the 2019 edition of the *Guide to the quality and safety of tissues and cells for human application*, published by the European Directorate for the Quality of Medicines & HealthCare (EDQM).

Keywords: donor human milk (DHM), Human Milk Bank (HMB), breastfeeding, pasteurization, donor screening, bacteriology testing

BACKGROUND

Human milk (HM) is the preferred nutrition for preterm infants (1), but not all mothers are able to provide their child with enough milk. There are specific beneficial effects of breastfeeding in these infants as HM feeding reduces the risk of short term and long term complications related to prematurity. Donor HM (DHM) can supplement the supply of maternal breastmilk when it is insufficient or provide the preferred alternative when the mother is not breastfeeding. DHM is beneficial for the health of preterm infants, first because significant properties are preserved following holder pasteurization (2) and secondly because it prevents feeding these infants with a preterm formula. According to the World Health Organization (1) the American Academy of Pediatrics (3) and the European Society of Pediatric Gastroenterology, Hepatology, and Nutrition (4) the feeding of preterm infants with mother's own milk is recommended as the first choice and if this is not available pasteurized DHM from an established milk bank should be the next alternative.

The main benefits for preterm infants that receive DHM instead of formula are faster gastric emptying, faster attainment of full enteral feedings, improved gut growth and maturation, decreased risk of necrotizing enterocolitis and late onset sepsis, improved neurodevelopmental outcomes, less retinopathy of prematurity and improved visual development (5–9).

HMBs have existed since 1909 in Europe and countries that supported the development of a significant number of HMBs developed national guidelines to harmonize practices. The European Milk Bank Association[1] (EMBA) was officially launched in October 2010. According to the definitions agreed by the EMBA Board of Directors:

- Human milk banks (HMB) collect, screen, store, process, and distribute DHM.
- DHM is breastmilk that has been expressed by a mother and provided freely to a HMB to be fed to another mother's child.

The EMBA constitution is available to view on the EMBA website[1]. The Association welcomes membership from HMBs, milk bank associations and individuals who support the aims of the Association. Membership affords the opportunity to access conference presentations from the past 6 years as well as additional materials of interest to those who bank or use DHM.

The EMBA is a non-profit organization that was established to promote milk banking and to encourage international co-operation between the HMBs of the countries of Europe as well as globally. The association's headquarters are in Milan, Italy but association meetings and conferences are held in different locations within Europe. The primary aim of the EMBA is to support and promote exclusive breastfeeding, which is universally acknowledged to be the optimal method of feeding all infants. The use of DHM from HMBs for preterm and sick infants temporarily without access to their own mother's milk has been widely shown to be linked to increased rates of exclusive breastfeeding on discharge from neonatal units (10, 11).

The EMBA was also established to support human milk banking in Europe by promoting safe practices and fostering sustainable operations. Hence a further aim of the association, as listed in the EMBA Constitution[1] is to "Prepare international and regularly revised guidelines to set standards for the practice of milk banking." The usual methodology for establishing guidelines is to convene appropriate multidisciplinary expertise, consider all of the stages of a process and conduct a review of the evidence before making recommendations linked to the strength of the evidence. In the absence of such a published guideline, aimed at milk banks throughout Europe, it is expected that the development of Europe-wide recommendations by EMBA for HMBs will promote best practice, optimize quality, and safety within the HMBs that are currently operational as well as offer valuable assistance to those who are establishing a new HMB. Evidence and expert opinion based recommendations should be the standard throughout Europe to promote consistent practices both within and between countries.

There are currently 226 HMBs operating in 28 countries in Europe. These include the first milk banks in Estonia, Lithuania, Poland, Portugal, and Russia. A further 16 HMBs are planned. The current status of HMBs in Europe is maintained on the EMBA website[1].

The 226 HMBs in Europe incorporate newly established organizations with a limited history of operational expertise as well as ones that have links to the very early milk banks founded over a century ago. They include national and regionalized services as well as small operations serving a single neonatal unit. The volumes of DHM that are tested and processed and provided mainly to sick and preterm infants vary widely from country to country[1] as well as within a single country (12) as do the criteria for receipt of DHM. An EMBA coordinated survey of all the HMBs in Europe will be carried out in 2019. This will gather up to date information about the extent of milk banking

[1]http://europeanmilkbanking.com

activity including the number of donors recruited, volumes of milk donated and processed, volumes of milk provided to hospitals, and the number of recipients. It will also collate further information about milk banking practices.

There are currently no published Europe-wide guidelines however internationally published guidelines for HMBs are freely available from France[2], Italy (13), and the UK (14). Countries with nationally agreed and recognized guidelines include Austria, Denmark, Germany, Norway, Slovakia, Spain, Sweden, and Switzerland. English translations of recently updated (2017–2018) national guidelines from Sweden and Spain can be downloaded via links from the EMBA website. Differences exist between national guidelines as a result of variations in practices, regulation, and organization of HMBs in each country. Differences in practices are due to the lack of evidence for some points related to the operation of a HMB. DHM status globally is variable; it is either considered a food, a health product food or a tissue; the latter ones being subject to stricter regulation. Organization of HMBs is different when collecting and delivering DHM only for infants hospitalized in the same building, or over a more or less wide area including several health care institutions.

The HMBs of Europe also have very different historical backgrounds[1] and in most cases have operated independently of each other although regular meetings take place between milk banking practitioners in Norway and Sweden and between those of Austria, Germany, and Switzerland.

A major role of the EMBA has, since its inception, been the provision of education, largely via the organization of international congresses. Presentations at these congresses have revealed similarities between the milk banking practices throughout Europe and have also revealed fundamental differences. These have substantiated the results of surveys of HMBs carried out both before and after the establishment of EMBA in 2007 and in 2012. In some cases the official national or local recommendations from various countries lead to significant differences in practice. For example most published guidelines recommend that all DHM should be heat treated [using the standard holder pasteurization method[2] (13, 14)]. However, in Norway mainly raw (non-heat treated) DHM is provided by the country's 12 milk banks. This is considered possible and reasonable because (1) the demand can be met due to very high breastfeeding rates, even with extremely strict donor screening, (2) there is complete traceability of milk from donor to consumer, (3) there is a small population with very low HIV and hepatitis rates, (4) extremely rigorous and regularly repeated testing of donors (every 3 months) is practiced (15, 16). However, in almost half of the 20 official HMBs in Germany both raw and pasteurized DHM is available and used in accordance with local clinical judgment based on the gestation and health of the recipient (17).

OBJECTIVE

One of the clear objectives of the EMBA[1] has been to develop Europe-wide recommendations for HMBs. This is especially needed by countries without experience of human milk banking or the use of DHM. Such recommendations should optimize safety and draw upon the available evidence. The processes and practices within human milk banking do not lend themselves to randomized controlled trials and there are few meta-analyses or systematic reviews available to refer to. In the absence of these, expert opinion is required and where this differs, a consensus and in some cases compromise is sought. The EMBA Guideline Working Group was formed in 2015 to undertake this task. EMBA members from 13 countries contributed to the work of the group. Throughout its 3 year existence, members of the Guideline Working Group have included representatives from Austria, France, Germany, Italy, Norway, Poland, Portugal, Serbia, Slovenia, Slovakia, Spain, Switzerland, and the UK.

METHOD

The three main tasks of the group were:

1) to complete a comprehensive survey of current practices within their national milk banks (See **Appendix** for details of the 108 survey questions)
2) to use the known guidelines to assess where consensus could be achieved
3) identify where research evidence is available to support recommendations.

A useful tool in developing the structure for the survey was the global implementation framework (18) published by the NGO PATH[3]. The framework includes a compilation of practices in HMBs from donor recruitment to delivery of DHM to the recipient.

Each of the group members completed the survey in accordance with their local/regional or national guidelines and, if not included in the guidelines, in accordance with local practice. Once completed, the survey responses were collated and highlighted according to whether international consensus was apparent, whether there was near consensus and where practices and recommendations differed significantly. The next step was to note where no published evidence was available. A list of agreed recommendations that were evidence based and that could form the basis of EMBA recommendations was drawn up and presented to the wider EMBA membership at further meetings. Where there was no consensus and no evidence upon which to determine a recommendation, expert opinion within the group was used to decide whether to include a recommendation or to provide an explanation of why no clear recommendation could be made at that time.

RESULTS

The recommendations that were found to be included in all of the published guidelines or accepted as best practice according to the available evidence or expert opinion and have therefore been agreed by the Working Group are presented below. Many of these are underpinned by principles of good manufacturing

[2]http://ansm.sante.fr/Activites/Elaboration-de-bonnes-pratiques/Bonnes-pratiques-des-lactariums

[3]PATH: http://www.path.org

process (GMP) especially those related to consistency and quality control.

EMBA Recommendations for the Establishment and Operation of Human Milk Banks in Europe

General Recommendations

1. A robust quality assurance plan (e.g., HACCP—Hazard Analysis Quality Control Points) should be in place to ensure the safe operation of the HMB (13, 14).
2. All equipment should be maintained in accordance with manufacturers' instructions and checked and qualified annually to ensure conformity with recommendations (GMP).
3. Containers should be closed or sealed in accordance with manufacturers' recommendations (GMP).
4. Containers should not be overfilled as DHM will expand when frozen (GMP).
5. Containers of human milk should at all times be labeled with the donor's name or unique ID and the date the milk was expressed. In addition, depending on the stage in the process, DHM should also be labeled with the name of the HMB, whether the milk is raw or processed, the milk's expiry date and if the milk is ready (cleared) to use (14).
6. HMBs should at all times minimize exposure of the human milk to sunlight and/or phototherapy lights.
7. HMB staff should have health checks when employed and be immunized in accordance with local hospital or national health service protocols (14).
8. Staff should undertake training by an experienced member of staff (or in accordance with national accredited training programs where available) before undertaking unsupervised work in a HMB (14).
9. DHM should be handled hygienically and HMB staff should wash their hands in accordance with local protocols prior to entering clean areas, handling DHM or equipment used in the collection, storage, testing and processing of DHM (GMP).
10. HMB staff should at all times consider the ethical implications of their work with donors, parents, carers, and infants. For example donors should not be encouraged or coerced to donate more milk than may be optimal for themselves or their infants. The use of DHM should not undermine or interfere with the mother's provision of her own milk or of breastfeeding unless there are concerns about its safety.
11. Records should be kept of all donors and their donations of milk including volumes, dates and any additional relevant information (traceability).
12. Prioritization of recipients should be locally determined (14).
13. Steps should be taken to prevent the temperature of DHM rising during transport e.g., by the use of insulated transport containers (boxes or bags) and thermal (ice) packs or the use of dry ice where necessary (14).
14. The use of tamper evident transport containers is recommended and the temperature of the interior of the container should be monitored during transport using data loggers or checked on arrival. A record of this should be maintained as part of the HMB records (GMP).
15. Transport boxes/bags in which containers of DHM are carried should be insulated and easy to clean.
16. The transport container should be decontaminated between batches of milk. Keep raw milk from different mothers separate. Avoid using the same transport container to transport raw and pasteurized DHM.
17. Containers of DHM should not be placed directly into the transport container—use of clear polythene bags helps the HMB identify the contents and check that they are correctly labeled without the need for unnecessary handling.

Donor Recruitment and Screening

1. Recruit donors using clear, non-technical language in printed and digital media.
2. Screening of donors should include both an oral interview and completion of a health questionnaire.
3. Inform prospective donors that they will be required to undertake serological testing.
4. Exclude prospective donors if they:
    - Smoke cigarettes or use nicotine containing products including "vaping," gums, and other products
    - Use any recreational or "street" drugs.
    - Are known or found to be infected with HIV, hepatitis B or hepatitis C (13, 14)[2]. Additional screening for HTLV (human T-lymphotropic virus), syphilis, and other viral and bacterial infections may be screened for according to local evaluation.
    - Use medications other than those on the EMBA approved medication list[1].
    - Have received a recent blood transfusion, tattoo or piercing, or needle stick injury. The. determination of "recent" should be locally determined in accordance with blood donation/transfusion services and methods used for serology testing.
    - Follow a vegan diet without supplementation with Vitamin B12.
    - Have a sexual partner who has, or is at risk of acquiring, sexually transmitted infections.
5. There is no consensus on safe amounts of alcohol consumption prior to expressing human milk for donation. EMBA recommends therefore that donors avoid alcohol and never donate milk expressed whilst they are under the influence of alcohol or are likely to secrete human milk containing alcohol (within 4 h of moderate drinking). Local guidelines on alcohol consumption by breastfeeding mothers should also be considered.
6. Donors should inform the HMB if there are any changes in their behavior or health status that affects their answers to questions related to any of the above.
7. Before accepting a donor's milk, receive written informed consent for its use in accordance with the HMB's protocols including for approved research if relevant.

8. Train all new donors in hand washing and hygiene requirements for expressing, handling, storing, cooling, freezing, and transporting human milk (GMP).
9. Provide appropriate ongoing support for all donors, including where possible, those rejected by the HMB.
10. Provide additional training and support for donors who repeatedly donate milk that does not meet the microbiological or other testing criteria.
11. Do not exclude bereaved mothers from donating their breastmilk if they meet the donor recruitment and screening requirements (19).
12. Once recruited, exclude donation of HM on a temporary basis in the case of any of the following:

- the presence of mastitis
- temporary use of some pharmacologically active substances[1,4]
- the presence of acute infectious diseases and skin diseases such as herpes simplex or varicella zoster
- fungal infection of the nipple, areola, mammary or thoracic region.

The extent of the temporary deferral of donors will vary according to the duration of the circumstances and medical advice should be sought to exclude the possibility of acceptance of contaminated, unsuitable, or suboptimal milk.

Expression, Handling, and Storage of Human Milk for Donation to the HMB

1. Advise donors to collect expressed milk rather than drip milk (14).
2. Accept hand expressed, manual pump-expressed, and electric pump expressed milk.
3. Advise donors to ensure all breast pump equipment is cleaned and disinfected in accordance with manufacturer's recommendations or local hospital protocols if different (GMP).
4. Emphasize the importance of good hygiene and hand washing at all times when communicating with donors about expressing their milk.
5. Discourage the sharing of breast pumps outside of hospital and the use of second hand or pumps on loan unless by a hospital or health care provider.
6. Request that donors freeze milk for donation as soon as possible but within a maximum of 24 h (48 h if collected and stored in hospital refrigerator/freezer).
7. Only containers provided by or approved by the HMB should be used by donors
8. Ensure donated milk is checked for labeling compliance prior to collection or on arrival at the HMB if delivered by the donor.
9. On its arrival at the milk bank, place donated human milk in a suitable holding freezer (freezer for raw milk only and maintaining −20°C).
10. All refrigeration, freezing, and other chilling equipment should only be used for human milk.
11. Monitor and record refrigeration and freezing equipment continuously or at least every 24 h.
12. Store raw and pasteurized human milk in separate clearly labeled refrigerators and freezers or if not possible in separate clearly labeled fridge and freezer compartments.
13. Thaw frozen raw human milk in a refrigerator to prevent its temperature rising above 8°C or if impractical because of time constraints on a counter where it can be monitored and transferred to a refrigerator immediately once thawed.
14. Pooling of DHM.

    14.1 The pooling of DHM from the same donor is acceptable prior to any heat processing

    14.2 Maintain records of all pooling including the names/ID numbers of the donors, dates the milk was expressed and any medications taken.

Milk Screening; Pre- and Post-pasteurization Testing

Within Europe, as well as globally, there is no consensus for recommendations for the microbiological testing of DHM either before or after pasteurization (see **Table 1**). Throughout Europe, local and national guidelines vary both in the timing and frequency of testing and in the acceptance criteria. There is a lack of published evidence to inform decision making and the working group members concluded that to maximize safety of vulnerable immune-compromised recipients, best practice suggests:

- Before pasteurization
    - All pools of milk be tested prior to pasteurization
    - Each batch of milk be tested after pasteurization
    - Acceptance criteria: 10^5 cfu/ml or less of non-pathogenic organisms and no pathogens for each pool of milk tested prior to pasteurization. Discard all samples of milk from a pool that does not meet this standard.
- After pasteurization
    - Discard the batch if there is any microbial growth detected in a random sample taken after pasteurization.

It is recognized that most published guidelines include less stringent screening criteria (**Table 1**) as part of the overall recommendations. The EMBA therefore recommend that where milk banks follow nationally or locally agreed guidance, alternative microbiological screening criteria may be adopted if done so as part of the overall adherence to the guideline being followed.

Milk Treatment (Pasteurization)

1. Current recommended heat treatment/pasteurization temperature and time is 62.5°C for 30 min followed by rapid cooling to at least 10°C and preferably 4°C prior to transfer to a freezer (2).
2. Monitor the process and record temperatures throughout the treatment (2).
3. Pasteurized milk that has been freeze dried and vacuum packed if performed in a milk bank in accordance with GMP and all relevant safety procedures may be used.

[4]http://ukamb.org/medication-and-breastfeeding

TABLE 1 | Published microbiological screening criteria for acceptance of donor human milk prior to and after pasteurization.

Guideline	Pre-pasteurization: Total confluent bacterial growth	*Pre-pasteurization: Additional criteria*	Post-pasteurization
France: Bonnes pratiques des lactariums[2]	Total (aerobic) flora ≤10^6 CFU/mL	*Staphylococcus aureus* ≤10^4 CFU/mL	Any microbial growth
Italy: Guidelines for the establishment and operation of a donor human milk bank (13)	≤10^5 CFU/mL	*Enterobacteriaceae or Staphylococcus aureus* ≤10^4 CFU/mL	≤10 CFU any organism
Sweden: Guidelines for the use of human milk and milk handling in Sweden[1]	Total aerobic bacteria: No upper limit	• Any pathogenic bacteria from the following': • Betahemolytic Streptococci group A, C, or G, Streptococci group B, Listeria, or Salmonella <10^4 CFU/ml • *Enterobacteriaceae* • *Staphylococcus aureus* • *Pseudomonas aeruginosa* or other Pseudomonas species • *Stenotrophomonas maltophilia* • Acinetobacter species	Total aerobic count ≤10 CFU/ml. No pathogenic bacteria are accepted
United Kingdom: NICE Clinical Guideline 93. Donor milk banks; service operation (14)	≤10^5 CFU/mL	*Enterobacteriaceae or Staphylococcus aureus* ≤10^4 CFU/mL	≤10 CFU any organism
Australia: Best practice guidelines for the operation of a donor human milk bank in an Australian NICU (20)	≤10^5 CFU/mL	Any *Enterobacteriaceae, Enterococci* or potential pathogens capable of producing heat-stable enterotoxins	Any microbial growth
United States of America (HMBANA): Guidelines for the Establishment and Operation of a Donor Human Milk Bank 2018[a]	Pre-pasteurization testing not included in the recommendations	Pre-pasteurization testing not included in the recommendations	"Any bacteriological growth is unacceptable for heat-processed milk"

[a]*Human Milk Bank Association of North America. http://hmbana.org.*

Delivery of DHM to Recipients

1. Never use a microwave oven to defrost or warm milk.
2. All donor milk and containers should be labeled at each stage to ensure traceability and tracking of the milk.
3. The receiving hospital should record/document how donor milk is used including in the infant's hospital notes.
4. Before administration of donor milk, informed consent is required from recipient's mother/parent/carer in accordance with local protocols.
5. It is recognized that some religious beliefs and practices influence the acceptability of anonymized donor human milk and these should be taken into account when discussing donor milk with donors and with parents and carers and when drawing up local protocols.

DISCUSSION

The Working Group was able to arrive at a consensus for recommendations covering most of the major processes involved in recruiting and screening donors, storing, handling, and transporting DHM and in its testing and processing. In these cases, the evidence, as referenced in the relevant national guidelines was checked and noted. Where published evidence was not available, expert opinion was the basis for the recommendation. The group also highlighted several areas for which consensus could not be achieved and where there was no clear evidence to inform a recommendation. In these instances the group provided a statement of explanation and suggested best practice. The group also acknowledged that not all countries that have milk banks were represented within the guideline group. A further consideration was that HMBs are funded in different ways and have varying resources. It was agreed that to make a single recommendation that may undermine a milk bank's ability to continue to operate would not be in the best interests of the overall population of recipients.

The process by which DHM is tested to provide microbiological safety is an example of where no consensus could be found. Very divergent practices are currently in place throughout Europe and there is no agreement within the published guidelines as to the optimal testing regime either before or after pasteurization or both. There is also no clear evidence base on which to determine the recommendations. However, it is possible to make a recommendation as to which practice will offer optimal safety for all recipients, including the most vulnerable neonates, and through which no untested milk reaches the recipients and the strictest published acceptance criteria are used. Recommended testing regimes exist in Europe that include less frequent sampling [e.g., only testing the first donation and randomly testing subsequent donations as in the Italian guidelines (13)]. There are also recommendations in which the acceptance criteria are less strict (e.g., pre-pasteurization criteria of 10^5cfu/ml or less of any organisms and 10^4cfu/ml or less of *Staphylococcus aureus* and *Enterobacteriaceae* and the presence of <10 cfu/ml of any organism post-pasteurization as per the UK's NICE guideline (14). These are acceptable alternatives but do not provide the same assurance of safety. It should be noted however that less strict testing regimes will lead to more processed milk being available. An additional consideration is that if DHM is fed without any heat treatment (as occurs in some parts of Europe), stricter local microbiological testing protocols should be adopted to increase the safety of the recipients.

The tracking of DHM and the traceability of the milk throughout all the HMB processes is an essential component of safety and quality assurance. This is enhanced by the availability of customized and purpose developed barcode tracking systems and the use of the internationally agreed coding system, ISBT128 (21). Regular strict quality control of pasteurization equipment is necessary to maintain optimum safety and quality of DHM (2, 22, 23).

Whilst safety is at the forefront of all recommendations pertaining to HMBs and the use of DHM it is important to ensure that the ethical considerations of banking and sharing human milk and duties of care to the donors as well as the recipients are not overlooked (24).

A limitation of this consensus statement is that no recommendations were made regarding the analysis of HM. HM analysis is a means of assessing protein and energy contents and to facilitate targeted fortification of HM (i.e., to fortify milk according to its individual composition to reach a target composition as a means of helping to cover the theoretical nutritional needs of each infant). Some HMBs include the assessment of HM composition in their practice. This is done either to perform targeted fortification or to select HM with the highest nutrient content for the smallest babies. However, there is no consensus about the best strategy for fortification. Only adjustable fortification, which does not require HM composition assessment, has been shown to improve postnatal growth.

CONCLUSIONS

There are no Europe-wide guidelines covering practices within HMBs. Historically national and/or local guidelines have been developed and although the recommendations include many similarities, clear differences also exist. Developing recommendations for HMBs operating throughout Europe was a challenging task because of the diversity within European countries. However, with the input of leading milk banking experts from a wide range of countries and with additional help from the EMBA Board it was possible to agree a pragmatic approach to where differences could not be resolved through reference to published research. The resultant guidance will now be freely available on the EMBA website to assist in the safe establishment and operation of HMBs throughout Europe. The recommendations have also been used to help inform the chapter on human milk to be included in the 2019 edition of the *Guide to the quality and safety of tissues and cells for human application*, published by the European Directorate for the Quality of Medicines & Health Care (EDQM).

AUTHOR CONTRIBUTIONS

GW, EB, CG, AnnG, RM-M, SA, DB, C-YB, RB, AntG, GM, AW, and J-CP contributed to the working group and/or to the discussions of the findings of the working group and all offered amendments to the previous drafts and/or agreed the manuscript.

ACKNOWLEDGMENTS

We gratefully acknowledge the valuable contribution made to the Guideline Working Group by the following EMBA members and colleagues: Tanya Cassidy (Canada and Ireland), Elena Darol (Poland), Andreja Domjan (Slovenia), Ivana Letenayova (Slovakia), Israel Macedo (Portugal), Daniel Mumblit (Russia), Ingrid Zittera (Austria). We are also extremely grateful to the Italian Association of Human Milk Banks (Associazine Italiana Banche del Latte Umano Donato—AIBLUD) for its continuous efforts to promote research in the field of human milk banking and for the financial support toward the publication of this manuscript.

REFERENCES

1. WHO/UNICEF. *Global Strategy for Infant and Young Child Feeding*. Geneva: WHO (2003). Available online at http://whqlibdoc.who.int/publications/2003/9241562218.pdf
2. Picaud JC, Buffin R. Human milk-treatment and quality of banked human milk. *Clin Perinatol*. (2017) 44:95–119. doi: 10.1016/j.clp.2016.11.003
3. American Academy of Pediatrics. Section on breastfeeding. Breastfeeding and the use of human milk. *Pediatrics*. (2012) 129:e827–41. doi: 10.1542/peds.2011-3552
4. ESPGHAN Committee on Nutrition, Arslanoglu S, Corpeleijn W, Moro G, Braegger C, Campoy C, et al. Donor human milk for preterm infants: current evidence and research directions. *J Pediatr Gastroenterol Nutr*. (2013) 57:535–42. doi: 10.1097/MPG.0b013e3182a3af0a
5. Quigley M, Embleton ND, McGuire W. Formula versus donor breast milk for feeding preterm or low birth weight infants. *Cochrane Database Syst Rev*. (2018) 22:CD002971. doi: 10.1002/14651858.CD002971
6. Maffei D, Schanler RJ. Human milk is the feeding strategy to prevent necrotizing enterocolitis! *Semin Perinatol*. (2017) 41:36–40. doi: 10.1053/j.semperi.2016.09.016
7. Spiegler J, Preuß M, Gebauer C, Bendiks M, Herting E, Göpel W. Does breastmilk influence the development of bronchopulmonary dysplasia? *J Pediatr*. (2016) 169:76–80.e4. doi: 10.1016/j.jpeds.2015.10.080
8. Lucas A, Cole TJ. Breast milk and neonatal necrotising enterocolitis. *Lancet*. (1990) 336:1519–23. doi: 10.1016/0140-6736(90)93304-8
9. Hylander MA, Strobino DM, Pezzullo JC, Dhanireddy R. Association of human milk feedings with a reduction in retinopathy of prematurity among very low birthweight infants. *J Perinatol*. (2001) 21:356–62. doi: 10.1038/sj.jp.7210548
10. Arslanoglu S, Moro GE, Bellù R, Turoli D, De Nisi G, Tonetto P, et al. Presence of human milk bank is associated with elevated rate of exclusive breastfeeding in VLBW infants. *J Perinat Med*. (2013) 41:129–31. doi: 10.1515/jpm-2012-0196
11. Kantorowska A, Wei JC, Cohen RS, Lawrence RA, Gould JB, Lee HC. Impact of donor milk availability on breast milk use and necrotizing enterocolitis rates. *Pediatrics*. (2016) 137:e20153123. doi: 10.1542/peds.2015-3123
12. BAPM. *The Use of Donor Human Expressed Breast Milk in Newborn Infants - A Framework for Practice*. (2016). Available online at: https://www.bapm.org/resources/

13. Italian Association of Human Milk Banks Associazione Italiana Banche del Latte Umano Donato (AIBLUD: https://www.aiblud.com), Arslanoglu S, Bertino E, Tonetto P, De Nisi G, Ambruzzi AM, et al. Guidelines for the establishment and operation of a donor human milk bank. *J Matern Fetal Neonatal Med.* (2010) 23(Suppl. 2):1–20. doi: 10.3109/14767058.2010.512414
14. NICE Clinical Guideline 93. *Donor Milk Banks; Service Operation Published by National Institute for Health and Care Excellence (NICE)* (2010). Available online at: https://www.nice.org.uk/guidance/cg93
15. Lindemann PC1, Foshaugen I, Lindemann R. Characteristics of breast milk and serology of women donating breast milk to a milk bank. *Arch Dis Child Fetal Neonatal Ed.* (2004) 89:F440–1. doi: 10.1136/adc.2003.046656
16. Grøvslien AH, Grønn M. Donor milk banking and breastfeeding in Norway. *J Hum Lact.* (2009) 25:206–10. doi: 10.1177/0890334409333425
17. von Thomas Kühn. *Use of Breast Milk For Feeding Preterm Infants Thomas Kühn, Vivantes Perinatalzentrum Berlin-Neukölln.* 1st ed. UNI-MED Verlag AG (2017).
18. PATH. *Strengthening Human Milk Banking; A Global Implementation Framework.* Version 1.1. Seattle, WA: Bill & Melinda Gates Foundation Grand Challenges Initiative, PATH (2013).
19. Welborn JM. The experience of expressing and donating breast milk following a perinatal loss. *J Hum Lact.* (2012) 28:506–10. doi: 10.1177/0890334412455459
20. Hartmann BT, Pang WW, Keil AD, Hartmann PE, Simmer K. Best practice guidelines for the operation of a donor human milk bank in an Australian NICU. *Early Hum Dev.* (2007) 83:667–73. doi: 10.1016/j.earlhumdev.2007.07.012
21. *ISBT128 Standard: Labelling of Human Milk Banking Products.* ICCBBA (International Council for Commonality in Blood Banking Automation (NGO) (2016). Available online at: https://www.iccbba.org
22. Peila C, Moro GE, Bertino E, Cavallarin L, Giribaldi M, Giuliani F, et al. The effect of Holder pasteurization on nutrients and biologically-active components in donor human milk: a review. *Nutrients.* (2016) 8:E477. doi: 10.3390/nu8080477
23. Buffin R, Pradat P, Trompette J, Ndiaye I, Basson E, Jordan I, et al. Air and water processes do not produce the same high-quality pasteurization of donor human milk. *J Hum Lact.* (2017) 33:717–24. doi: 10.1177/0890334417707962
24. Hartmann BT. Ensuring safety in donor human milk banking in neonatal intensive care. *Clin Perinatol.* (2017) 44:131–49. doi: 10.1016/j.clp.2016.11.006

23

Human Milk: An Ideal Food for Nutrition of Preterm Newborn

Clair-Yves Boquien [1,2*]

[1] *INRA, Université Nantes, Centre de Recherche en Nutrition Humaine-Ouest, IMAD, Physiopathologie des Adaptations Nutritionnelles (UMR PHAN), Nantes, France,* [2] *EMBA (European Milk Bank Association), Milan, Italy*

Correspondence:
Clair-Yves Boquien
clair-yves.boquien@univ-nantes.fr

Human milk is the best food for newborn nutrition. There is no ideal composition of human milk and also no easy way to control the complexity of its nutritional quality and the quantity received by breastfed infants. Pediatricians and nutritionists use charts of infant growth (weight, size, head circumference) and neurodevelopment criteria that reflect the food that these infants receive. These charts reflect first the infant physiology and likely reflect the composition of human milk when infants are breastfed. In a situation of preterm birth, mother physiology impacts partly breast milk composition and this explains how this is more difficult to correlate infant growth or neurodevelopment with milk composition. Some biomarkers (lipids, oligosaccharides) have been identified in breast milk but their function is not always yet known. A better knowledge on how human milk could act on infant development to the mid- and long-term participating thus to nutritional programming is a challenging question for a better management of infants' nutrition, especially for preterm infants who are most fragile.

Keywords: mother milk, breast milk, breastfeeding, preterm, nutritional programming, neonatal growth, infant neurodevelopment

DOHAD (DEVELOPMENTAL ORIGIN OF HEALTH AND ADULT DISEASES) CONTEXT AND NUTRITIONAL PROGRAMMING

The perinatal period is a period of organogenesis in the newborn (at the beginning of pregnancy), and of strong growth of the child during the first 2 years of life, but also in the establishment of the physiological mechanisms that persist throughout life. Since the work of Prof. BARKER (1, 2) and the formalization of the concept of DOHaD (Developmental Origin of Health and adult Diseases), it is recognized that there is a link between the conditions of development during the perinatal period and the health and adult diseases, and nutrition has a key role. It is likely that the growth rate (weight gain during the first few weeks) and the composition of this weight gain (lean body gain and body fat gain) during this key period have major long-term effects. The challenge is that the growth of the child, in this period of life, is achieved by allowing optimal neurodevelopment, without causing increased susceptibility to metabolic diseases (obesity, type-2 diabetes, and cardiovascular disease) at adulthood. And we will see later, that in prematurity of the infant, these objectives are based on nutrition conditions that are sometimes contradictory.

BREASTFEEDING

In this context, the World Health Organization (WHO) recommends exclusive breastfeeding for up to 6 months, starting at the first hour of life. Despite the recommendations of the WHO and pro-breastfeeding messages delivered in hospitals and maternity hospitals, the exclusive breastfeeding rate remains quite low [even in low-income and middle-income countries, only 37% of infants younger than 6 months are exclusively breastfed (3)].

The benefits of breastfeeding, for which there is a broad scientific consensus, provide protection for the health of the infant during the first weeks of life. These are short or medium term effects:

- A highly protective effect on infant mortality, with a 12% decrease in mortality risk compared to non-breastfed (4);
- A decrease in respiratory and gastrointestinal infections during the first weeks of life of the newborn (3), probably related to the composition of colostrum (immature milk for the first 3 days of life) and breast milk that confers immune protection to the child.

Finally, there is also a consensus on the effect of breastfeeding on the improvement of neuro development (5), in children born premature (6), or on term (7). Concerning premature infants, several studies show a positive relationship between the quantity of breast milk received during hospitalization and neuro development (8). Breastfed premature children had better psychomotor development at 2 or 5 years than non-breastfed children (6), but with a slower growth (weight, height) during hospitalization, even if they caught up with non-breastfed children at 3 years of age. This was called "breastfeeding paradox" by Roze et al. (6) as previous studies have shown a positive relationship between growth rate during neonatal hospitalization and neurodevelopment (9).

All these effects are all the more pronounced as breastfeeding lasts a long time, thus highlighting a "dose" effect. However neurodevelopment advantages have been related not only to breastfeeding duration but also to the amount received, reflecting a dose response relationship (10).

Moreover, beside these benefits of breastfeeding for the child, we often forget to mention the benefits for the mother, even in the long term:

- Decreased risk of breast and ovarian cancers (3, 11);
- Decreased risk of type 2 diabetes, with a strong effect of lactation duration (12).

HUMAN MILK COMPOSITION

Breast milk is the best food for the newborn. Human milk consists of 87% water, 1% protein, 4% lipid, and 7% carbohydrate (including 1 to 2.4% oligosaccharides) (**Figure 1**). It also contains many minerals (Calcium, Phosphorus, Magnesium, Potassium, Sodium, etc...) and many vitamins. Compared to cow's milk, human milk contains less protein (3.5% in cow's milk), and especially a proportion of casein (on total protein) lower, max 50% (80% in milk of cow). There is no β-lactoglobulin; some minor proteins are more abundant in human milk (lysozyme, lactoferrin,...) and the same goes for the non-protein nitrogen fraction (urea, free amino acids, including taurine). The protein content of human milk is therefore low (10 g/L), probably the lowest among all mammalian milks, and we can relate this observation with a very low growth rate of the newborn (for comparison, rat milk has a protein content 10 times higher for a growth rate of the pups also higher).

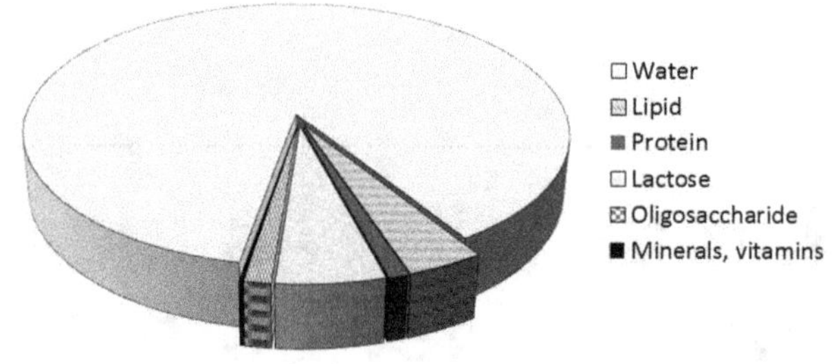

FIGURE 1 | Human milk composition.

Another peculiarity of human milk is the highest proportion of long-chain polyunsaturated fatty acids (APGI-LC), ω6 (such as arachidonic acid) and ω3 (such as eicosapentaenoic and docosahexaenoic acids [DHA]), which are derived from essential fatty acids: linoleic and α-linolenic acid. These fatty acids are important for the brain development of the infant. Compared to cow's milk, breast milk also contains more cholesterol, which is a precursor of hormones and is also involved in brain development.

Finally, oligosaccharides are present in large quantities, from 10 to 20 g/L (only 1 g/L in cow's milk) and with very varied biochemical compositions (more than 100 different compounds) (role mentioned below).

Milk contains compounds that help protect children against infectious diseases (13):

- Either by a direct immune protection, with the many immunoglobulins (including secretory IgA,...);
- Either by modulating this immune protection (by lactoferrin, pro or anti-inflammatory cytokines, or oligosaccharides);
- Either by a non-immune action, by proteins: κ-casein, α-lactalbumin, lactoferrin, haptocorrin, lysozyme (14), and oligosaccharides (see below).

Colostrum, which is produced up to 5 days after birth, also contains many immunity cells (macrophages and lymphocytes).

Milk also contains enzymes including Bile Salt Stimulated Lipase (BSSL), which allows for better lipid digestibility, and better utilization of triglycerides (95% of total lipids), and presumably LC-PUFA, cholesterol, and fat-soluble vitamins.

A certain poverty of vitamins (D and K in particular) is known, whose consequences can be avoided by a supplementation of the children, even of the mothers during the pregnancy (vitamin D). In the same way, the presence in the breast milk of chemical contaminants, highlighted for some years, raises the question of their origin, namely via the nutrition and the environment of the mother (15, 16) and their impact on the breastfed child. These contaminants accumulate in the body of the mother throughout her life because many are fat

Abbreviations: ALA, α-Linolenic Acid; BSSL, Bile Salt Stimulated Lipase; DHA, DocosaHexaenoic Acid; HMO, Human Milk Oligosaccharide; IUGR, Intra-Uterine Growth Restriction; LA, Linoleic acid; LC-PUFA, Long Chain PolyUnsaturated Fatty Acid; MFGM, Milk Fat Globule Membrane.

soluble and are found in adipose tissue. This is all the more pronounced since the first pregnancy of the mother is at an age more and more delayed. Preterm breast milk may also concerned by such contamination. The means to limit their presence in breast milk will be complicated to implement and will require societal, environmental and organizational policies over very long periods.

The richness of breast milk in miRNA is also one of its characteristics (17, 18). MiRNAs are non-coding RNAs that regulate gene expression and control protein synthesis at the post-transcriptional level. They play roles in the regulation of many biological and developmental processes and would be important in the development of the child's immune system. Once the milk is ingested by the child, these maternal miRNAs resist digestion, when they are protected by cellular structures (exosomes). The question of whether they are subsequently absorbed and whether they regulate genes in children is a scientific issue that is still very controversial (19).

Finally, the discovery of a microbiota of breast milk, from the 2000s, has led many teams to question its origin (endogenous entero-mammary or exogenous) and its relative role, compared to other microbiota (particularly maternal), in the colonization of the digestive tract of the newborn (20, 21). There is no complete answer to all these questions, which are complex to solve and require sampling in the most sterile conditions and not to neglect all the necessary methodological controls. Added to this is the additional difficulty of elucidating the potential interactions between all these compounds: the effect of the content of oligosaccharides of breast milk on the microbiota of the newborn is thus well studied (22), and makes it a good example of very current research.

PHYSIOLOGICAL STATE OF THE MOTHER IMPACTS BREAST MILK COMPOSITION

The growth curve of the newborn reflects, in part, the diet (in quality and quantity) that these children receive and whether they are breastfed, presumably the composition of the breast milk they receive. But many other parameters obviously come into play, such as for example, its genetic heritage, and all the events that occur in the first weeks of the child's life (infection, etc.). We will show how it is difficult to distinguish between the effect of nutrition by breast milk and many confounding factors related to the physiological state of the mother and the clinical parameters of the child at birth (prematurity, small weight for gestational age...), knowing that some of these parameters directly influence the composition of breast milk. We can illustrate it in the following situation of prematurity:

Children born prematurely are at risk of experiencing an Extra-Uterine Growth Retardation and, as explained above, their nutritional needs are very important. Except the first days of life where they are fed intravenously (parenteral), because of their intestinal immaturity, they are quickly fed enterally with a nasogastric tube, and most often fed with breast milk (**Figure 2**). It turns out that the prematurity impacts the protein content of mother's milk: protein content in preterm mother's milk is higher than in term mother's milk during the first days of lactation [with maximum mean differences up to 35% (0.7 g/dl)] (23, 24) but it declines afterwards. After postnatal day 3, most of the differences in true protein between preterm and term milk are within 0.2 g/dL or less, and term milk may be the same as preterm milk by the 5th–6th week. Similarly concentration of certain free amino acids, including valine, threonine and arginine is higher in preterm mother's milk (25). Contradictory results have been obtained with lactoferrin (26, 27). Preterm breast milk appears also rich in sIgA (26, 28) and deficient in leptin (26, 29). In one study, the authors observed a decrease in serum albumin (mainly originating from blood flow) in mother's milk of infant born prematurely, which may reflect changes in the oxidative status of breast milk (30). Kunz et al. found no difference in the total amount of HMOs neither in colostrum nor in transitional or in mature milk comparing term and preterm milk samples (31) and authors list all the recent data that are consistent or inconsistent with their.

Finally, the question of whether the total fatty acid composition of mother's milk depends on the gestational age of the child remains still posed. The lower maternal-fetal transfer of fatty acids from mother to child due to a shorter pregnancy would suggest that maternal reserves of LC-PUFA are higher in mothers of premature infants and that milk such mothers would be richer in these fatty acids. However, either there is no difference with the mother's milk full-term, or the studies show quite contradictory results, except possibly for DHA (32).

BREAST MILK IS RECOMMENDED FOR PRETERM INFANT FEEDING

The incidence of prematurity has been steadily increasing for decades: Every year, an estimated 15 million babies are born preterm (before 37 completed weeks of gestation) throughout the world, and this number is rising. Preterm birth complications are the leading cause of death among children under 5 years of age, responsible for ~1 million deaths in 2015 (WHO, http://www.who.int/news-room/fact-sheets/detail/preterm-birth). However, progress in medical technology over the last few decades have allowed for the survival of an ever-increasing proportion of children born with very low birth weight. The challenge is therefore to improve the future of these children, and early nutrition becomes a major player in this objective. All of the expert committees recommend the use of human milk, which reduces, for example, the risk of necrotizing enterocolitis, a serious disease of premature infants in the neonatal period. However, the composition of human milk is extremely variable from one mother to another. Similarly, the long-term prognosis (in particular in terms of psychomotor development, but also in metabolic terms) is very variable among children born premature: thus, recent studies show that the development quotient remains linked to the birth term (33–36), and premature babies are at high risk of insulin resistance and metabolic disorders in adulthood (37). About 40% of premature children have psychomotor disorders at 5 years of age compared to only 12% for full-term children. A very high growth rate during

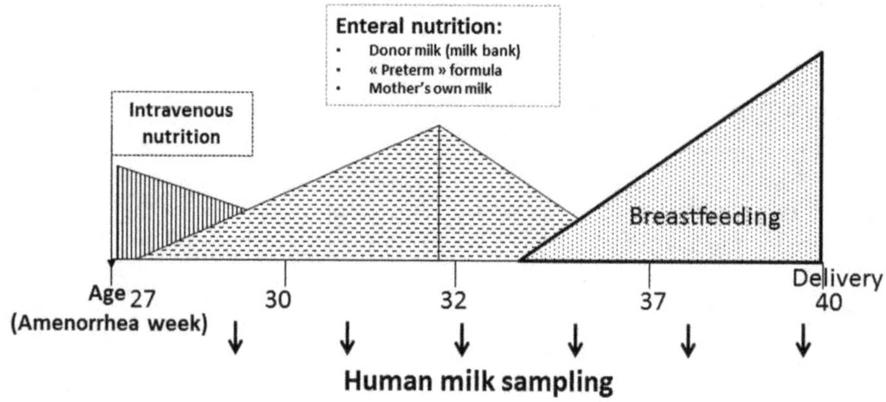

FIGURE 2 | Preterm infant nutrition during early life.

this period can have deleterious effects, in terms of increased susceptibility to metabolic diseases (obesity, type 2 diabetes, cardiovascular diseases) in adulthood (38). It has also been shown that a high growth rate during the first years of life is associated with a better neuro development of the child (9). The nutrition of the child born premature thus raises many questions about the best way to do it and assessing the consequences of neonatal nutrition between susceptibility to metabolic diseases and neuro development is crucial (**Figure 3**).

Although breastfeeding does have a positive effect, particularly on the neuro-development of premature infants, there is great inter-individual variability in the long-term outcome. To date, very little data links the individual growth and development trajectory of a given child to the composition of breast milk received. This analysis is complicated by:

- The many biases related to breastfeeding, the particular psychological relationship between mother and child, the formation and social position of parents, the sociological determinants;
- The fortification of human milk during the hospitalization of premature infants: if breast milk is recommended for children with very low birth weight (8) and for premature infants, it brings, in the first weeks, notoriously insufficient amounts of protein per day compared to the growth needs of these newborns. All the recommendations of the European Society for Pediatric Gastroenterology, Hepatology, and Nutrition (EPSGHAN) are in line with the nutrition of premature infants by breast milk, and a protein enrichment of this milk, as soon as possible, at least until discharge from hospital, in order to increase weight gain and protein accretion (39). Most premature newborns are hospitalized during the first weeks of their postnatal life in Neonatology departments: they need support (*e.g.* respiratory) because of the immaturity of various organs and have important nutritional needs to cover their high energy expenditure in addition to growth during this period. But the debate is lively between neonatologists on the methodology to follow. This topic is debated in an article in the same collection "Human Milk in the Feeding of Preterm Infants: Established and Debated Aspects" (Arslanoglu et al., manuscript under revision). Then, behind this debate between "standardized" vs. "individualized" fortification, there is a low level of knowledge about the variability of the composition of breast milk (micronutrients in particular), from one mother to another, and according to the lactation time, and the consequences on the growth and development of the child, in the short term and even in the medium term.

RELATIONSHIP BETWEEN BREAST MILK COMPOSITION AND GROWTH AND NEURODEVELOPMENT OF INFANT

If breast milk has certain plasticity in its composition, depending on the physiology of the mother, does this affect the physiology of the breastfed child, its growth trajectory, or even its neurological development (**Figure 3**)? The answers to this question are to be found both in experimental researches on animal models and in clinical research, in retrospective studies, which present a longitudinal follow-up of breastfed children.

The breastfed infant receives nutrients from the mother's milk, which, once hydrolyzed or not, passes the intestinal barrier and ends up in the blood. It is therefore normal for the blood metabolome or lipidome to be different between a breastfed child and a non-breastfed child. So at 3 months, the blood lipidome of children exclusively breastfed for 3 months is very different than receiving an infant formula (40), with differences to phosphatidylcholines, sphingomyelins, and triglycerides. This result is not necessarily linked to the difference in triglyceride composition between breast milk and infant formula but it may also be that the neonatal nutrition have had additional effects on lipid metabolism, which substantially modified the lipidome of the infant at 3 months.

The issue of breast milk in nutrition programming is really difficult to solve. In fact, the inter-individual variability of human milk, and the heterogeneity of breastfeeding times (dose effect) complicate the associations between a particular composition of breast milk and certain clinical parameters of the child who has

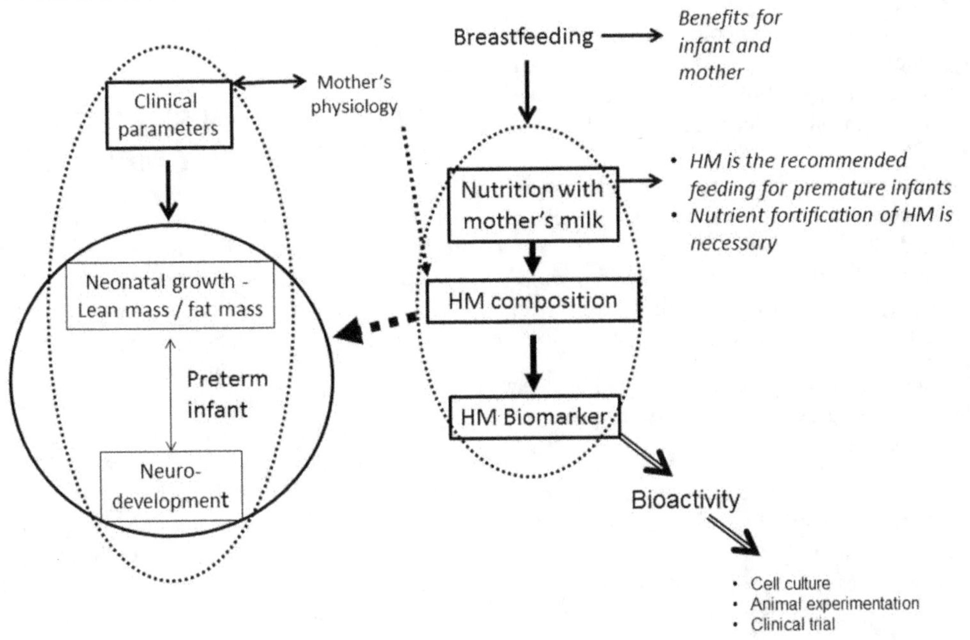

FIGURE 3 | Nutrition with human milk and preterm infant growth and neurodevelopment (HM, Human Milk).

received this milk. Among the retrospective studies that have addressed this issue, lipids and oligosaccharides in breast milk, as well as some micronutrients, have been the subject of recent publications.

Lipids in human milk are the second most important macronutrient in breast milk, and have been studied extensively since the 2000s (41–46). Human milk is rich in linoleic acid (LA) and α-linolenic acid (ALA) which are the precursors of long-chain polyunsaturated fatty acids (PUFAs) ω6 and ω3; these precursors are not synthesized *in vivo*, and breast milk is the only source of intake for the breastfed child. These PUFAs are essential for brain development, including DHA; breast milk is also rich in DHA and so it brings both DHA and its precursor ALA. As brain growth continues during the child's first weeks of life, especially for the premature infant, this intake of ALA and DHA is essential.

Associations have been sought between breast milk lipids and growth and development of the child. Several studies concern term infants (47, 48) but the development of preterm infants has also been studied. Mead acid (C20:3 n-9, an omega-9 fatty acid) in early breast milk is associated with general movement's score at 40 weeks of gestational age suggesting that increased concentration in mead acid influenced this score negatively (49). Similarly arachidonic acid was also negatively correlated with some behavioral assessment scores. These relatively simple associations reflect likely a more complex reality such as a shortage of fatty acids ω6 and ω3 or an imbalance between ω3 and ω6 fatty acids.

To better understand the role of different families of breast milk lipids, in a context of prematurity, we conducted a pilot study, on 2 groups of 11 mothers of infants born premature, and selected in the LACTACOL cohort (NCT01493063), on the basis of growth (rather good [difference between discharge and birthweight Z-score during neonatal hospitalization of −0.5] vs. rather poor [difference between discharge and birthweight Z-score during neonatal hospitalization of −1.5]) of their breastfed children. We found a strong relationship between the growth of these premature children during hospitalization and the presence of several lipid biomarkers in breast milk, identified by both targeted methods of fatty acid assays and non-targeted methods without *a priori* (lipidomic analysis). Based on the lipidomic profiles of breast milk, obtained after analysis by liquid chromatography coupled with mass spectrometry, and after using discriminating statistical tools, several lipid species have been selected for their ability to predict the weight growth of premature infants, during their first 4 weeks of life. The faster growth was associated with milk containing more medium chain saturated fatty acids and sphingomyelin, more phosphoethanolamine containing dihomo-ɣ-linolenic acid, and less oxylipines (50).

The oligosaccharides of human milk are present in high concentration (51–53) and have many functions:

- They have a "prebiotic" effect (54, 55) and can therefore be considered as non-digestible dietary components that beneficially affect the health of the host by selectively stimulating the colon, growth and/or activity of a species or a limited number of bacterial species (56). Several recent studies have shown a link between the presence of oligosaccharides and the microbiota of the newborn (22, 57–60).
- They participate in the inhibition of bacteria, viruses or even parasites (22, 61): by the similarity of their structure with the receptors present on the intestinal mucosa, they play a role of decoy, on which are fixed bacteria and

viruses. Many pathogens use lectins to attach to the glycans of the intestinal epithelium. Human oligosaccharides have structures close to those of cell surface glycans and pathogens bind with oligosaccharides instead of surface glycoproteins / glycolipids... but a human oligosaccharide cannot block all lectins alone!

- They would modulate certain immune reactions because certain human oligosaccharides interfere *in vitro* with cell-cell interactions mediated by selectins;
- They are rich in sialic acid found in brain glangliosides (62);
- They protect the premature newborn against necrotizing enterocolitis (NEC) (63, 64).

The oligosaccharides fraction of preterm breast milk is likely the most interesting one raising challenging scientific questions. This is due to several reasons:

- The increase in oligosaccharides diversity over time with 56 HMO present in mature milk at 40 weeks of post-menstrual age that were not present at birth (65) revealing a new aspect in immaturity of preterm human milk at the beginning of lactation with likely some consequences on infant's gut colonization;
- The presence of an α 1,2 linked fucosylated HMO, 2′ fucosyllactose (2′ FL) in human milk indicates that the mother is a secretor and 60 to 80% women are secretors. De Leoz et al. found an unexpectedly high number of apparent non-secretors among women delivering preterm and the lack of consistency in "milk secretor status" over time in a few women (65) with momentary strong decline in 2'FL concentration. However, these conclusions need to be confirmed by studies with larger sample size;
- The relationship between a secretor status and a protective effect against bacterial dysbiosis defined as a delayed maturation of infant microbiota and against NEC (66);
- The microbiome of children with large growth delays is not refractory to nutritional supplementation with oligosaccharides (67, 68). This opens interesting perspectives for the care of preterm infants.

Other milk compounds have also been tested for their ability to predict the clinical characteristics of the breastfed child but mainly for term infants [fructose (69), leptin (70), TNFα et IL6 (71)]. A very recent review completes all of these data (72). The difficulty of all these studies is that many of them are only proof of concept studies with small size samples that will need complementary trials.

In preterm infants the overall breast milk composition impacts the gut microbiota with a greater bacterial diversity and a more gradual acquisition of diversity in infants fed breast milk compared to infants fed infant formula (73). This could be explained by the presence in human milk of oligosaccharides, of a microbiome and of secretory IgA that protect infant against pathogenic bacteria. Since the developmental pattern of preterm infant microbiota is characterized by different phases (74), the association between macronutrient intake and growth appears very complex depending on the composition of the gut microbiota and differing between microbiota phases. This opens new opportunities to fortify human milk differently for each preterm infant in a precision medicine.

A BIOMARKER IN BREAST MILK DOES NOT NECESSARILY MEAN A BIOACTIVITY

All previous work demonstrates biomarkers of growth of the newborn in breast milk, and those we have described are essentially oligosaccharides or lipids. But a biomarker does not necessarily have a biological activity because it can only represent the product of a metabolism. To prove its bioactivity, it is necessary to use a cellular model (to test an activity in cell culture, including cell proliferation, differentiation, secretion of cytokines, or the expression of growth factors, etc.), animal experimentation or finally the clinical study (**Figure 3**): an infant formula is supplemented with the biomarker to test its bio-activity, for example its effect on the growth of the newborn. Many minor proteins, present in breast milk and absent in cow's milk, or present in high concentration compared to cow's milk, have been tested. This is the case of lactoferrin, which has antimicrobial activity (75), which acts on the absorption of iron (76) and is bifidogenic (77). Oral lactoferrin supplementation decreases late-onset sepsis, NEC, and "all-cause mortality" in preterm infants without adverse effects but authors conclude that the evidence is moderate- to low-quality (78).

Demmelmair et al. (14) recently identified these minor proteins that have been the subject of clinical studies:

- Lysozyme with a 1000 times higher concentration in human milk than in cow's milk;
- Osteopontin which is 10 times more concentrated in human milk than in cow's milk and which plays a role in the immunity of the child;
- Bile salt stimulated lipase, present in human milk, which would improve the digestibility of long-chain fatty acids. In a multi-center randomized trial, recombinant BSSL has been tested vs. placebo with a follow-up for 12 months; there was no improvement in weight growth in preterm infants except in the sub-group of Small for Gestational Age infants but with some imbalance in the adverse effects (79).
- α-lactalbumin, which improves the absorption of iron;
- Lactoferrin, about 20 times more concentrated in human milk compared to cow's milk, and whose functions have been mentioned above.

In addition to these minor proteins, a complex of proteins and lipids has been the subject of several clinical trials: these are Milk Fat Globule Membranes (MFGMs). The fat globules are surrounded by a triple membrane which is a complex construct. The outer membrane is hydrophilic and allows the dispersion of fat globules in milk which is an oil-water emulsion. These membranes contain cholesterol, glycerophospholipids, sphingolipids, and minor proteins (mucin 1, xanthine oxidoreductase, butyrophilin, lactadherin, adipophilin)(14). About 25–70% of these MFGMs are proteins. Infantile preparations enriched with MFGM or constituents of these MFGMs (phospholipids) have been tested in clinical trials with convincing results in terms of programming of immunity and cognitive functions.

These differences in composition between human and bovine milks highlight that human milk composition is very specific and certainly better adapted for preterm infants. Even if formula producers have improved their process to better mimic human milk, large discrepancies will continue to exist.

CONCLUSIONS

Breast milk is a "natural" and "sustainable" food, without any impact on the environment, with a strong symbolic value, since it represents the first "vector" of transmission of taste, rules governing the terms of the meal, and so of the food identity (80). It is a reference for the nutrition of the newborn, even if there is no ideal composition. It is best adapted to the nutrition of the newborn and breastfeeding is not recommended in a few rare diseases [in case of infection with HIV (AIDS virus), except in countries where access to infant formulas and especially to drinking water is difficult, and in case of galactosemia, a disease that does not allow the child to metabolize galactose]. The benefits of breastfeeding have been quantified economically and increased breastfeeding rates bring substantial savings for any health system (81).

Benefits of breastfeeding are recognized and although it must be admitted that breast milk is not always perfect, the benefit or risk balance is leaning on the benefits side, especially for preterm infants. The scientific consensus is that breast milk is the best food for preterm infants as soon as their digestive maturity allows them to digest proteins and lipids. In fact preterm mortality has decreased a lot during the past years because these infants are really better taken care in neonatology units. Better managing nutrition of these infants would likely improve their development. In order to improve milk fortification, we need to better know the complexity of nutritional composition and the relationship between this composition and infant physiology.

Although it contains macronutrients with a fairly stable concentration, breast milk has a very plastic micronutrient composition, which depends in particular on the physiology of the mother. The question of whether it has an adaptive composition, according to the needs of the child, remains to this day unanswered.

AUTHOR CONTRIBUTIONS

The author confirms being the sole contributor of this work and has approved it for publication.

ACKNOWLEDGMENTS

I thank Prof. Dominique Darmaun (Nantes University Hospital) for the fruitful discussions on this topic of breast milk in the situation of prematurity.

REFERENCES

1. Barker DJ, Hales CN, Fall CH, Osmond C, Phipps K, Clark PM. Type 2 (non-insulin-dependent) diabetes mellitus, hypertension and hyperlipidaemia (syndrome X): relation to reduced fetal growth. *Diabetologia* (1993) 36:62–7. doi: 10.1007/BF00399095
2. Godfrey KM, Barker DJ. Fetal nutrition and adult disease. *Am J Clin Nutr.* (2000) 71:1344S–52S. doi: 10.1093/ajcn/71.5.1344s
3. Victora CG, Bahl R, Barros AJ, Franca GV, Horton S, Krasevec J, et al. Breastfeeding in the 21st century: epidemiology, mechanisms, and lifelong effect. *Lancet* (2016) 387:475–90. doi: 10.1016/S0140-6736(15)01024-7
4. Jeeva SM, Bireshwar S, Ranadip C, Nita B, Sunita T, Jose M, et al. Optimal breastfeeding practices and infant and child mortality: a systematic review and meta-analysis. *Acta Paediatr.* (2015) 104:3–13. doi: 10.1111/apa.13147
5. Der G, Batty GD, Deary IJ. Effect of breast feeding on intelligence in children: prospective study, sibling pairs analysis, and meta-analysis. *BMJ* (2006) 333:945. doi: 10.1136/bmj.38978.699583.55
6. Rozé JC, Darmaun D, Boquien CY, Flamant C, Picaud JC, Savagner C, et al. The apparent breastfeeding paradox in very preterm infants: relationship between breast feeding, early weight gain and neurodevelopment based on results from two cohorts, EPIPAGE and LIFT. *BMJ Open* (2012) 2:e000834. doi: 10.1136/bmjopen-2012-000834
7. Bernard JY, De Agostini M, Forhan A, Alfaiate T, Bonet M, Champion V, et al. Breastfeeding duration and cognitive development at 2 and 3 years of age in the EDEN mother-child cohort. *J Pediatr.* (2013) 163:36–42.e31. doi: 10.1016/j.jpeds.2012.11.090
8. Vohr BR, Poindexter BB, Dusick AM, McKinley LT, Wright LL, Langer JC, et al. Beneficial effects of breast milk in the neonatal intensive care unit on the developmental outcome of extremely low birth weight infants at 18 months of age. *Pediatrics* (2006) 118:e115–23. doi: 10.1542/peds.2005-2382
9. Ehrenkranz RA, Dusick AM, Vohr BR, Wright LL, Wrage LA, Poole WK. Growth in the neonatal intensive care unit influences neurodevelopmental and growth outcomes of extremely low birth weight infants. *Pediatrics* (2006) 117:1253–61. doi: 10.1542/peds.2005-1368
10. Belfort MB, Anderson PJ, Nowak VA, Lee KJ, Molesworth C, Thompson DK, et al. Breast milk feeding, brain development, and neurocognitive outcomes: a 7-year longitudinal study in infants born at less than 30 weeks' gestation. *J Pediatr.* (2016) 177:133–9.e1. doi: 10.1016/j.jpeds.2016.06.045
11. Chowdhury R, Sinha B, Sankar MJ, Taneja S, Bhandari N, Rollins N, et al. Breastfeeding and maternal health outcomes: a systematic review and meta-analysis. *Acta Paediatr.* (2015) 104:96–113. doi: 10.1111/apa.13102
12. Gunderson EP, Lewis CE, Lin Y, Sorel M, Gross M, Sidney S, et al. Lactation duration and progression to diabetes in women across the childbearing years: the 30-year *CARDIA study. JAMA Int Med.* (2018) 178:328–37. doi: 10.1001/jamainternmed.2017.7978
13. Tackoen M. [Breast milk: its nutritional composition and functional properties]. *Rev Med Brux.* (2012) 33:309–17.
14. Demmelmair H, Prell C, Timby N, Lonnerdal B. Benefits of lactoferrin, osteopontin and milk fat globule membranes for infants. *Nutrients* (2017) 9:817. doi: 10.3390/nu9080817
15. Antignac JP, Main KM, Virtanen HE, Boquien CY, Marchand P, Venisseau A, et al. Country-specific chemical signatures of persistent organic pollutants (POPs) in breast milk of French, Danish and Finnish women. *Environ Pollut.* (2016) 218:728–38. doi: 10.1016/j.envpol.2016.07.069
16. Thomsen C, Stigum H, Froshaug M, Broadwell SL, Becher G, Eggesbo M. Determinants of brominated flame retardants in breast milk from a large scale Norwegian study. *Environ Int.* (2010) 36:68–74. doi: 10.1016/j.envint.2009.10.002
17. Weber JA, Baxter DH, Zhang S, Huang DY, Huang KH, Lee MJ, et al. The microRNA spectrum in 12 body fluids. *Clin Chem.* (2010) 56:1733–41. doi: 10.1373/clinchem.2010.147405
18. Alsaweed M, Hartmann PE, Geddes DT, Kakulas F. MicroRNAs in breastmilk and the lactating breast: potential immunoprotectors and developmental

regulators for the infant and the mother. *Int J Environ Res Public Health* (2015) 12:13981–4020. doi: 10.3390/ijerph121113981

19. Laubier J, Castille J, Le Guillou S, Le Provost F. No effect of an elevated miR-30b level in mouse milk on its level in pup tissues. *RNA Biol.* (2015) 12:26–9. doi: 10.1080/15476286.2015.1017212
20. Martin R, Jimenez E, Heilig H, Fernandez L, Marin ML, Zoetendal EG, et al. Isolation of bifidobacteria from breast milk and assessment of the bifidobacterial population by PCR-denaturing gradient gel electrophoresis and quantitative real-time PCR. *Appl Environ Microbiol.* (2009) 75:965–9. doi: 10.1128/AEM.02063-08
21. Hunt KM, Foster JA, Forney LJ, Schütte UME, Beck DL, Abdo Z. Characterization of the diversity and temporal stability of bacterial communities in human milk. *PLoS ONE* (2011) 6:e21313. doi: 10.1371/journal.pone.0021313
22. De Leoz ML, Kalanetra KM, Bokulich NA, Strum JS, Underwood MA, German JB, et al. Human milk glycomics and gut microbial genomics in infant feces show a correlation between human milk oligosaccharides and gut microbiota: a proof-of-concept study. *J Proteome Res.* (2015) 14:491–502. doi: 10.1021/pr500759e
23. Bauer J, Gerss J. Variability in human milk composition: benefit of individualized fortification in very-low-birth-weight infants. *Clin Nutr.* (2011) 30:215–20. doi: 10.1016/j.clnu.2010.08.003
24. Gidrewicz DA, Fenton TR. A systematic review and meta-analysis of the nutrient content of preterm and term breast milk. *BMC Pediatr.* (2014) 14:216. doi: 10.1186/1471-2431-14-216
25. Zhang Z, Adelman AS, Rai D, Boettcher J, Lonnerdal B. Amino acid profiles in term and preterm human milk through lactation: a systematic review. *Nutrients* (2013) 5:4800–21. doi: 10.3390/nu5124800
26. Mehta R, Petrova A. Biologically active breast milk proteins in association with very preterm delivery and stage of lactation. *J Perinatol.* (2011) 31:58–62. doi: 10.1038/jp.2010.68
27. Albenzio M, Santillo A, Stolfi I, Manzoni P, Iliceto A, Rinaldi M, et al. Lactoferrin levels in human milk after preterm and term delivery. *Am J Perinatol.* (2016) 33:1085–9. doi: 10.1055/s-0036-1586105
28. Koenig A, Albuquerque Diniz EM, Barbosa SFC, Vaz FAC. Immunologic factors in human milk: the effects of gestational age and pasteurization. *J Hum Lact.* (2005) 21:439–43. doi: 10.1177/0890334405280652
29. Garcia C, Duan RD, Brevaut-Malaty V, Gire C, Millet V, Simeoni U, et al. Bioactive compounds in human milk and intestinal health and maturity in preterm newborn: an overview. *Cell Mol Biol.* (2013) 59:108–31. doi: 10.1170/T952
30. Molinari CE, Casadio YS, Hartmann BT, Arthur PG, Hartmann PE. Longitudinal analysis of protein glycosylation and beta-casein phosphorylation in term and preterm human milk during the first 2 months of lactation. *Br J Nutr.* (2013) 110:105–15. doi: 10.1017/S0007114512004588
31. Kunz C, Meyer C, Collado MC, Geiger L, Garcia-Mantrana I, Bertua-Rios B, et al. Influence of gestational age, secretor, and lewis blood group status on the oligosaccharide content of human milk. *J Pediatr Gastroenterol Nutr.* (2017) 64:789–98. doi: 10.1097/MPG.0000000000001402
32. Bokor S, Koletzko B, Decsi T. Systematic review of fatty acid composition of human milk from mothers of preterm compared to full-term infants. *Ann Nutr Metabol.* (2007) 51:550–6. doi: 10.1159/000114209
33. Fily A, Pierrat V, Delporte V, Breart G, Truffert P. Factors associated with neurodevelopmental outcome at 2 years after very preterm birth: the population-based Nord-Pas-de-Calais EPIPAGE cohort. *Pediatrics* (2006) 117:357–66. doi: 10.1542/peds.2005-0236
34. Larroque B, Ancel PY, Marret S, Marchand L, Andre M, Arnaud C, et al. Neurodevelopmental disabilities and special care of 5-year-old children born before 33 weeks of gestation (the EPIPAGE study): a longitudinal cohort study. *Lancet* (2008) 371:813–20. doi: 10.1016/S0140-6736(08)60380-3
35. Larroque B, Ancel PY, Marchand-Martin L, Cambonie G, Fresson J, Pierrat V, et al. Special care and school difficulties in 8-year-old very preterm children: the Epipage cohort study. *PLoS ONE* (2011) 6:e21361. doi: 10.1371/journal.pone.0021361
36. Wood NS, Marlow N, Costeloe K, Gibson AT, Wilkinson AR. Neurologic and developmental disability after extremely preterm birth. EPICure Study Group. *N Engl J Med.* (2000) 343:378–84. doi: 10.1056/NEJM200008103430601
37. Hofman PL, Regan F, Jackson WE, Jefferies C, Knight DB, Robinson EM, et al. Premature birth and later insulin resistance. *N Engl J Med.* (2004) 351:2179–86. doi: 10.1056/NEJMoa042275
38. Stettler N, Zemel BS, Kumanyika S, Stallings VA. Infant weight gain and childhood overweight status in a multicenter, cohort study. *Pediatrics* (2002) 109:194–9. doi: 10.1542/peds.109.2.194
39. Agostoni C, Buonocore G, Carnielli VP, De Curtis M, Darmaun D, Decsi T, et al. Enteral nutrient supply for preterm infants: commentary from the European Society of Paediatric Gastroenterology, Hepatology and Nutrition Committee on Nutrition. *J Pediatr Gastroenterol Nutr.* (2010) 50:85–91. doi: 10.1097/MPG.0b013e3181adaee0
40. Prentice P, Koulman A, Matthews L, Acerini CL, Ong KK, Dunger DB. Lipidomic analyses, breast- and formula-feeding, and growth in infants. *J Pediatr.* (2015) 166:276–81.e6. doi: 10.1016/j.jpeds.2014.10.021
41. Innis SM. Polyunsaturated fatty acids in human milk: an essential role in infant development. *Adv Exp Med Biol.* (2004) 554:27–43. doi: 10.1007/978-1-4757-4242-8_5
42. Innis SM. Human milk: maternal dietary lipids and infant development. *Proc Nutr Soc.* (2007) 66:397–404. doi: 10.1017/S0029665107005666
43. Koletzko B, Lien E, Agostoni C, Bohles H, Campoy C, Cetin I, et al. The roles of long-chain polyunsaturated fatty acids in pregnancy, lactation and infancy: review of current knowledge and consensus recommendations. *J Perinat Med.* (2008) 36:5–14. doi: 10.1515/JPM.2008.001
44. Koletzko B, Agostoni C, Bergmann R, Ritzenthaler K, Shamir R. Physiological aspects of human milk lipids and implications for infant feeding: a workshop report. *Acta Paediatr.* (2011) 100:1405–15. doi: 10.1111/j.1651-2227.2011.02343.x
45. Innis SM. Impact of maternal diet on human milk composition and neurological development of infants. *Am J Clin Nutr.* (2014) 99:734S–41S. doi: 10.3945/ajcn.113.072595
46. Delplanque B, Gibson R, Koletzko B, Lapillonne A, Strandvik B. Lipid quality in infant nutrition: current knowledge and future opportunities. *J Pediatr Gastroenterol Nutr.* (2015) 61:8–17. doi: 10.1097/MPG.0000000000000818
47. Prentice P, Ong KK, Schoemaker MH, van Tol EA, Vervoort J, Hughes IA, et al. Breast milk nutrient content and infancy growth. *Acta Paediatr.* (2016) 105:641–7. doi: 10.1111/apa.13362
48. Bernard JY, Armand M, Peyre H, Garcia C, Forhan A, De Agostini M, et al. Breastfeeding, polyunsaturated fatty acid levels in colostrum and child intelligence quotient at age 5–6 years. *J Pediatr.* (2017) 183:43–50.e3. doi: 10.1016/j.jpeds.2016.12.039
49. Lundqvist-Persson C, Lau G, Nordin P, Strandvik B, Sabel KG. Early behaviour and development in breast-fed premature infants are influenced by omega-6 and omega-3 fatty acid status. *Early Hum Dev.* (2010) 86:407–12. doi: 10.1016/j.earlhumdev.2010.05.017
50. Alexandre-Gouabau MC, Moyon T, Cariou V, Antignac JP, Qannari EM, Croyal M, et al. Breast milk lipidome is associated with early growth trajectory in preterm infants. *Nutrients* (2018) 10:164. doi: 10.3390/nu10020164
51. Kunz C, Kuntz S, Rudloff S. Bioactivity of human milk oligosaccharides, In: Moreno FJ, Sanz MLE, editors. *Food Oligosaccharides: Production, Analysis and Bioactivity.* Chichester: Wiley-Blackwell (2014). P. 5–20. doi: 10.1002/9781118817360.ch1
52. Gabrielli O, Zampini L, Galeazzi T, Padella L, Santoro L, Peila C, et al. Preterm milk oligosaccharides during the first month of lactation. *Pediatrics* (2011) 128:e1520–31. doi: 10.1542/peds.2011-1206
53. Xu G, Davis JC, Goonatilleke E, Smilowitz JT, German JB, Lebrilla CB. Absolute quantitation of human milk oligosaccharides reveals phenotypic variations during lactation. *J Nutr.* (2017) 147:117–24. doi: 10.3945/jn.116.238279
54. Ward RE, Ninonuevo M, Mills DA, Lebrilla CB, German JB. *In vitro* fermentation of breast milk oligosaccharides by Bifidobacterium infantis and *Lactobacillus gasseri*. *Appl Environ Microbiol.* (2006) 72:4497–9. doi: 10.1128/AEM.02515-05
55. Ben XM, Li J, Feng ZT, Shi SY, Lu YD, Chen R, et al. Low level of galacto-oligosaccharide in infant formula stimulates growth of intestinal Bifidobacteria and Lactobacilli. *World J Gastroenterol.* (2008) 14:6564–8. doi: 10.3748/wjg.14.6564

56. Gibson GR, Roberfroid MB. Dietary modulation of the human colonic microbiota: introducing the concept of prebiotics. *J Nutr.* (1995) 125:1401–12. doi: 10.1093/jn/125.6.1401
57. Coppa GV, Gabrielli O, Zampini L, Galeazzi T, Ficcadenti A, Padella L, et al. Oligosaccharides in 4 different milk groups, Bifidobacteria, and Ruminococcus obeum. *J Pediatr Gastroenterol Nutr.* (2011) 53:80–7. doi: 10.1097/MPG.0b013e3182073103
58. Frese SA, Hutton AA, Contreras LN, Shaw CA, Palumbo MC, Casaburi G, et al. Persistence of supplemented *Bifidobacterium longum* subsp. *infantis* EVC001 in breastfed infants. *mSphere* (2017) 2:e00501-17. doi: 10.1128/mSphere.00501-17
59. Medina DA, Pinto F, Ovalle A, Thomson P, Garrido D. Prebiotics mediate microbial interactions in a consortium of the infant gut microbiome. *Int J Mol Sci.* (2017) 18:2095. doi: 10.3390/ijms18102095
60. Hoashi M, Meche L, Mahal LK, Bakacs E, Nardella D, Naftolin F, et al. Human milk bacterial and glycosylation patterns differ by delivery mode. *Reprod Sci.* (2016) 23:902–7. doi: 10.1177/1933719115623645
61. Bode L. Human milk oligosaccharides: every baby needs a sugar mama. *Glycobiology* (2012) 22:1147–62. doi: 10.1093/glycob/cws074
62. Wang B, McVeagh P, Petocz P, Brand-Miller J. Brain ganglioside and glycoprotein sialic acid in breastfed compared with formula-fed infants. *Am J Clin Nutr.* (2003) 78:1024–9. doi: 10.1093/ajcn/78.5.1024
63. Bode L. Recent advances on structure, metabolism, and function of human milk oligosaccharides. *J Nutr.* (2006) 136:2127–30. doi: 10.1093/jn/136.8.2127
64. Jantscher-Krenn E, Zherebtsov M, Nissan C, Goth K, Guner YS, Naidu N, et al. The human milk oligosaccharide disialyllacto-N-tetraose prevents necrotising enterocolitis in neonatal rats. *Gut* (2012) 61:1417–25. doi: 10.1136/gutjnl-2011-301404
65. De Leoz ML, Gaerlan SC, Strum JS, Dimapasoc LM, Mirmiran M, Tancredi DJ, et al. Lacto-N-tetraose, fucosylation, and secretor status are highly variable in human milk oligosaccharides from women delivering preterm. *J Proteome Res.* (2012) 11:4662–72. doi: 10.1021/pr3004979
66. Underwood MA, Gaerlan S, De Leoz MLA, Dimapasoc L, Kalanetra KM, Lemay DG, et al. Human milk oligosaccharides in premature infants: absorption, excretion, and influence on the intestinal microbiota. *Pediatr Res.* (2015) 78:670–7. doi: 10.1038/pr.2015.162
67. Charbonneau MR, O'Donnell D, Blanton LV, Totten SM, Davis JC, Barratt MJ, et al. Sialylated milk oligosaccharides promote microbiota-dependent growth in models of infant undernutrition. *Cell* (2016) 164:859–71. doi: 10.1016/j.cell.2016.01.024
68. Bashiardes S, Thaiss CA, Elinav E. It's in the milk: feeding the microbiome to promote infant growth. *Cell Metabol.* (2016) 23:393–4. doi: 10.1016/j.cmet.2016.02.015
69. Goran MI, Martin AA, Alderete TL, Fujiwara H, Fields DA. Fructose in breast milk is positively associated with infant body composition at 6 months of age. *Nutrients* (2017) 9:146. doi: 10.3390/nu9020146
70. Miralles O, Sanchez J, Palou A, Pico C. A physiological role of breast milk leptin in body weight control in developing infants. *Obesity* (2006) 14:1371–7. doi: 10.1038/oby.2006.155
71. Fields DA, Demerath EW. Relationship of insulin, glucose, leptin, IL-6 and TNF-alpha in human breast milk with infant growth and body composition. *Pediatr Obes.* (2012) 7:304–12. doi: 10.1111/j.2047-6310.2012.00059.x
72. Eriksen KG, Christensen SH, Lind MV, Michaelsen KF. Human milk composition and infant growth. *Curr Opin Clin Nutr Metab Care* (2018) 21:200–6. doi: 10.1097/MCO.0000000000000466
73. Gregory KE, Samuel BS, Houghteling P, Shan G, Ausubel FM, Sadreyev RI, et al. Influence of maternal breast milk ingestion on acquisition of the intestinal microbiome in preterm infants. *Microbiome* (2016) 4:68. doi: 10.1186/s40168-016-0214-x
74. Grier A, Qiu X, Bandyopadhyay S, Holden-Wiltse J, Kessler HA, Gill AL, et al. Impact of prematurity and nutrition on the developing gut microbiome and preterm infant growth. *Microbiome* (2017) 5:158. doi: 10.1186/s40168-017-0377-0
75. Arnold RR, Brewer M, Gauthier JJ. Bactericidal activity of human lactoferrin: sensitivity of a variety of microorganisms. *Infect Immun.* (1980) 28:893–8.
76. Fransson GB, Keen CL, Lonnerdal B. Supplementation of milk with iron bound to lactoferrin using weanling mice: L. Effects on hematology and tissue iron. *J Pediatr Gastroenterol Nutr.* (1983) 2:693–700. doi: 10.1097/00005176-198311000-00021
77. Liepke C, Adermann K, Raida M, Magert HJ, Forssmann WG, Zucht HD. Human milk provides peptides highly stimulating the growth of bifidobacteria. *Eur J Biochem.* (2002) 269:712–8. doi: 10.1046/j.0014-2956.2001.02712.x
78. Pammi M, Abrams SA. Oral lactoferrin for the prevention of sepsis and necrotizing enterocolitis in preterm infants. *Cochrane Database Syst Rev.* (2015):CD007137. doi: 10.1002/14651858.CD007137.pub5
79. Casper C, Hascoet JM, Ertl T, Gadzinowski JS, Carnielli V, Rigo J, et al. Recombinant bile salt-stimulated lipase in preterm infant feeding: a randomized phase 3 study. *PLoS ONE* (2016) 11:e0156071. doi: 10.1371/journal.pone.0156071
80. Debucquet G, Adt V. The naturalist discourse surrounding breastfeeding among french mothers. In: Cassidy T, El Tom A, editors. *Ethnographies of breastfeeding: Cultural contexts and confrontations*. London: Bloomsbury Publishing (2015).
81. Rollins NC, Bhandari N, Hajeebhoy N, Horton S, Lutter CK, Martines JC, et al. Why invest, and what it will take to improve breastfeeding practices? *Lancet* (2016) 387:491–504. doi: 10.1016/S0140-6736(15)01044-2

24

A New High Hydrostatic Pressure Process to Assure the Microbial Safety of Human Milk While Preserving the Biological Activity of its Main Components

Gérard Demazeau [1†], Adrien Plumecocq [1], Philippe Lehours [2], Patrice Martin [3], Leslie Couëdelo [4] and Claude Billeaud [5]*

[1] HPBioTECH, Gradignan, France, [2] Laboratoire de Bacteriologie, Centre Hospitalier Universitaire de Bordeaux, Bordeaux, France, [3] UMR1313 GABI, INRA, AgroParisTech, Université Paris-Saclay, Jouy-en-Josas, France, [4] Department Nutrition-Health & Lipid biochemistry of ITERG, Bordeaux, France, [5] Neonatology Nutrition, Lactarium Bordeaux-Marmande, CIC Pédiatrique 1401 Children's Hospital, Bordeaux, France

***Correspondence:**
Claude Billeaud
claude.billeaud@chu-bordeaux.fr

†Deceased

Background: The main process used to pasteurize human milk is the low-temperature, long-time Holder method. More recently, the high-temperature, short-time method has been investigated. Both processes lead to the appropriate inactivation of vegetative bacterial forms but are ineffective against bacterial spores.

Research Aims/Questions: We aimed to accomplish two main objectives: inactivation of all pathogens, including spores; and preservation of the activity of milk components.

Design/Methods: Recently, a novel high-hydrostatic pressure process has been developed by HPBioTECH. Using the same raw human milk samples, we compared the effects of this method with those of the Holder method on vegetative and spore forms of pathogens and on bioactive components (lipase activity, immunoproteins).

Results: Two main microbial strains were selected: *Staphylococcus aureus* (as a reference for vegetative forms) and *Bacillus cereus* (as a reference for spores). Use of the high-hydrostatic pressure process led to microbial decontamination of 6 log for both *S. aureus* and *B. cereus.* Additionally, the bioactivity of the main components of human milk was preserved, with activities of lipase, α-lactalbumin, casein, lysozyme, lactoferrin, and sIgA of ~80, 96–99, 98–100, 95–100, 93–97, and 63–64%, respectively.

Conclusions: Use of this novel high-hydrostatic pressure process to generate microbiologically safe human milk may provide important benefits for preterm infants, including improved assimilation of human milk (leading increased weight gain) and improved resistance to infections. Because 10% of all human milk collected is contaminated by *B. cereus*, use of this method will also prevent waste.

Keywords: human milk, HHP, pasteurization, human milk bank, spores, lipase, immune proteins, CMV

INTRODUCTION

Human milk is the appropriate standard nutrient for infant development (1) and is also given to preterm and very low birth weight infants (2, 3).

Two types of pathogens can contaminate such a medium: (i) endogenous pathogens from the mother and (ii) exogenous pathogens that mainly result from human milk collection by milk banks (4). Consequently, ensuring the safety and quality of donor human milk appears to be a crucial issue (5–8).

The main processes used for human milk pasteurization are based on thermal pathogen inactivation: (i) the low-temperature, long-time (LTLT) method (62.5°C; 30 min) (5, 6), which is also called the Holder method (traditionally developed in milk banks); and (ii) the high-temperature, short-time (HTST) method or flash heat pasteurization, which has been more recently investigated (9–13).

Regarding microbial safety, both processes (LTLT and HTST) lead to appropriate inactivation of the vegetative forms of pathogens; however, these methods are completely ineffective against bacterial spores from exogenous contamination. During the last few years, two other human milk treatments have been developed: UV (14–16) and ultrasound (17, 18).

In terms of preserving the activity of human milk after these pasteurization treatments, the LTLT process leads to many components (with nutritional enzymatic and immune properties) with reduced activity.

Over the last 25 years, high hydrostatic pressure (HHP) processes have been developed in food processing to mainly induce microbial safety (19–22), which also consequently increases shelf life. Because HHP processes apply weaker energy than thermal ones, their main advantage is the preservation of the intrinsic properties of the treated medium. More recently, HHP processes have been extended to biological applications (23–30).

The first industrial developments of HHP processes were established in Japan (1985–1990). In this first approach (called a "conventional approach"), HHP processes were defined by only three main parameters: pressure (**P**), temperature (**T**), and duration of treatment (**t**). When HHP processes are managed by only these three parameters, high pressure values (450–600 MPa) must be applied to ensure high microbial safety (31), which has a negative consequence of inducing the modification of biological components or organoleptic properties of the handled product (32). If high temperatures (80–120°C) are not used to induce detrimental modifications to biological activity, these HPP processes are ineffective at spore inactivation (33).

DEFINITION OF AN HHP PROCESS APPLIED TO HUMAN MILK

Different applications of this "conventional approach" to HHP treatment of human milk were tested with an emphasis on their ability to improve microbial safety. Viazis et al. (34) applied constant pressure (400 MPa) to human milk inoculated with different microorganisms [*Staphylococcus aureus* (ATCC 6538 and ATCC 25923), *Streptococcus agalactiae* (ATCC 12927), *Listeria monocytogenes* (ATCC 19115), and *Escherichia coli* (ATCC 25922)] to compare LTLT thermal pasteurization (Holder process) to high pressure treatment. The starting temperature was close to 21°C to reach a temperature of ~31°C due to adiabatic compression heating. Six- to eight-log reductions were observed in microbial populations during treatment. Unfortunately, this HHP treatment used a conventional approach and was ineffective against bacterial spores, particularly *Bacillus cereus* spores, which represent a microbial strain observed in the contamination of fresh milk, heat-treated milk and human milk (35, 36).

Research Aim

To establish an HHP process to inactivate both vegetative forms and bacterial spores contaminating human milk while preserving a substantial portion of the activity of milk components.

METHODS

Considering that high temperatures are rejected and that the pressure–temperature range required for spore inactivation would also lead to strong alterations of the biological activity of human milk components, an HHP process that could induce the germination of bacterial spores at lower pressure conditions (a moderate pressure value: $P \approx 350$ MPa) was needed to preserve the biological activity of human milk as required for infant feeding.

Recently, a new approach to HHP processes was established by Demazeau et al. (37), and this approach accounts for parameters that characterize pressure delivery. Specifically, the compression rate (**VA**) or decompression rate (**VD**), application mode (**MA**) (continuous or cyclic) and latency time ($\mathbf{t_l}$) between each cycle were defined.

Design

(i) To prove that this novel HHP was efficient for all pathogens with vegetative and spore forms, we performed a "challenge test." To validate this novel approach to HPP processes for the decontamination of human milk, we inoculated sterilized human milk at a level of 6 log with two main strains of microorganisms: *S. aureus* (ATCC 6538), which is a gram-positive vegetative bacterium resistant to pressure inactivation (38), and bacterial spores of *B. cereus* (ATCC 14579), a sporulated bacterial form that can induce severe intestinal infections (39).

After applying various optimization tests, we defined the HHP experimental conditions based on 6 parameters that can inactivate all vegetative forms and bacterial spores (such as *B. cereus* spores).

The set of optimized process parameters was as follows: Pressure = 350 MPa, temperature = 38°C, VA (application rate) = 1 MPa.s^{-1}, MA (application mode) with n_a (number of cycles) = 4 cycles and t_a (duration of each cycle) = 5 min, and t_l (latency time with normal pressure between each cycle) = 5 min.

(ii) To demonstrate the conservation of bioactive components of human milk, we compared raw human milk with pasteurized and HHP treatments of the same sample.

We measured the main biologic components of human milk, including lipase activity, lactoferrin, lysozyme, and IgA under either Holder pasteurization (62.5°C, 30 min) or novel high hydrostatic pressure.

Setting

The high-hydrostatic pressure machine is located at HPbioTech, which is situated 10 km from the Human Milk Bank (HMB) of Bordeaux-Marmande.

We used human milk after consent from the mother. Raw human milk is pasteurized and stored at −18°C at HMB; when transferred to HPbioTech, it is stored at −80°C until analysis.

Sample

The pasteurized human milk was used to set of optimized process parameters of HHP. Sterile human milk was inoculated with 5–6 log *S. aureus* or *B. cereus* and treated with the optimized set of HHP. This was termed the "Challenge test."

The raw human milk was treated with the optimized set of HHP to measure the biologic products of human milk, such as lipase activity and immune proteins lactoferrin, lysozyme, IgAs.

After HHP treatment, the challenge was employed to identify conditions that allow for destroying vegetative and spore forms of bacteria and preserving lipase activity and immune bioactive proteins.

Compared to Holder pasteurization, which destroyed 0 spores (see **Table 1**), the HHP sample size was determined to be 6 log of *B. cereus* spores and 6 log of *S. aureus*. The value obtained after Holder pasteurization showed no destruction of *B. cereus,* but no *B. cereus* was found after HHP treatment. Thus, very few samples are needed (see **Table 1**). We measured the reproducibility of destroying 6 log *B. cereus* in 3 repeated HHP treatments.

The Holder treatment destroyed all lipase activity (activity = 0), whereas between 70 and 100% of residual activity was found with the HHP treatment (see **Table 3**).

Data Analysis

We first verified the normality of the population and the homoscedasticity of variances. If verification was achieved, we used the Student *t* test to compare the two treatments (Holder vs. HHP); if not, we used the non-parametric test.

Two tailed $p < 0.05$ indicated significance.

Ethical Consideration

The milk used in this study was derived from the Human Milk Bank of Bordeaux-Marmande. Prior to donating milk, each mother signed a consent form indicating that any discarded milk could be used for research purposes. We therefore did not require approval for this study from the local Ethics Committee.

Moreover we can utilize human milk samples that cannot be used because the mother smokes or there are other contraindications to its donation.

TABLE 1 | Inactivation Efficiency (IE) of *B. cereus* (ATCC 14579) (as spores) and *Staphylococcus aureus* (ATCC 6538) after the new High Hydrostatic Pressure (HHP) treatment.

	N_i	N_{HHP}	IE
Microorganism (bacteria sporulated form)[a]			
B. cereus control D11	4.9	–	–
B. cereus HHP8 D11 n°1	4.9	0	4.9
B. cereus HHP8 D11 n°2	4.9	0	4.9
B. cereus HHP8 D11 n°3	4.9	0	4.9
Microorganism (vegetative form)[b]			
S. aureus control D11	5.7	–	–
S. aureus HHP8 D11 n°1	5.7	0	5.7
S. aureus HHP8 D11 n°2	5.7	0	5.7
S. aureus HHP8 D11 n°3	5.7	0	5.7

[a] *Inactivation Efficiency (IE) of B. cereus (ATCC 14579) (as spores) after the new HHP treatment. The inactivation efficiency of the HHP process for human milk inoculated with Staphylococcus aureus (ATCC 6538) and the evaluation of its reproducibility (n°1, n°2, n°3) are given on **Table 2**. N_i and N_{HHP} are respectively the initial (before the HHP treatment) and final (after the HHP treatment) microbial contamination. IE corresponds to the Inactivation Efficiency of the HHP treatment.*

[b] *Inactivation Efficiency (IE) of Staphylococcus aureus (ATCC 6538) after the new HHP treatment. The inoculation rate was limited to 5.7 log the initial contamination of human milk accepted for a decontamination treatment (as LTLT as the present time) by Staphylococcus aureus being limited to 4 log due to the release of toxins (40).*

MEASUREMENT

Protein and Lipid Analyses

Proteins

Caseins and the main soluble proteins were analyzed qualitatively and quantitatively using RP-HPLC coupled with Electro Spray Ionization-Mass Spectrometry (LC-MS); 50 samples of the same batch of raw HM (50), LTLTHM (50) and HPPHM (50) (INRA Jouy en Josas, Dr. P. Martin) were used (**Figure 1**).

Bioactive, antimicrobial and immune proteins: lactoferrin, lysozyme and IgA, showing more or less broad ranges of functions, were analyzed using Enzyme Linked ImmunoSorbent Assays (ELISAs) based on the sandwich technique; the antibody directed against the protein to analyze is pre-coated on the surface of microtiter wells. A biotinylated detection antibody is then added to the wells to bind to the captured protein. Streptavidin-conjugated horseradish peroxidase (SA-HRP) is then added to catalyze a colorimetric reaction with the chromogenic substrate 3,3′,5,5′-tetramethylbenzidine. The colorimetric reaction produces a blue product, which turns yellow when the reaction is terminated by addition of dilute sulfuric acid. The absorbance of the yellow product at 450 nm is proportional to the amount of protein present in the sample. The protein concentrations in the test samples can then be quantified by interpolating their absorbance from the standard curve generated in parallel with the samples (41).

Lipids

Lipase activity (Institut Biochimie Nutrition ITERG, Dr. C. Vaysse–Dr. L. Couedelo). The lipase activity compared to the substrate was monitored by quantitative release of fatty

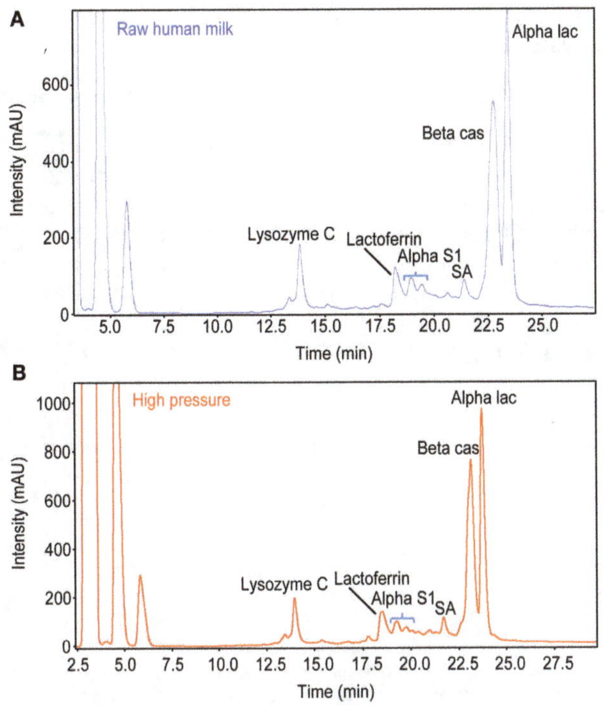

FIGURE 1 | Comparison of proteins profile between **(A)** Raw Human Milk and **(B)** HHP Human Milk. There is strictly the same proteins profile of Raw HM and HHP HM.

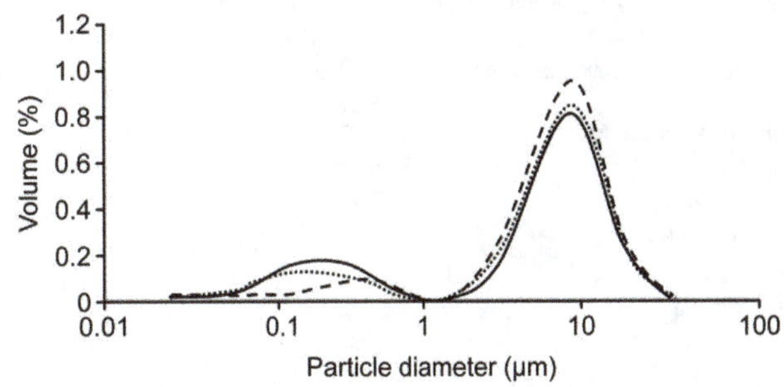

FIGURE 2 | Distribution of the volume size of milk fat globules (MFGs): raw (____) pasteurized (- - - -) or high pressure (.........). Evaluation of the size of MFGs showed that the population was bimodal he proportion of "small MFGs" was greater in raw milk and HHP-treated milk (d3.2 = 0.6 vs. 0.8 µm, respectively) compared to that in LTLT-pasteurized human milk (d3.2 = 3.1 µm). This result suggests that the size structure of raw breast milk is preserved by HHP treatment, whereas LTLT promotes coalescence and therefore increases the number of "large" MFGs.

acids and glycerol generated during the hydrolysis of TAG lipase. The hydrolysis reaction is automatically followed by pH measurements via neutralization of fatty acids liberated by the enzyme over time by a standard solution of sodium hydroxide (NaOH 25 mmol/L) at pH 8 ± 0.2.

The results are expressed as the in International Units as micromoles of fatty acids liberated per minute and per milliliter of breast milk.

We used the granulometry of lipid droplets of human milk: raw, pasteurized, and novel HHP of the same batch (**Figure 2**).

RESULTS

Microbial Spore and Vegetative Destruction

In these experimental conditions, total inactivation of the microbial contamination of human milk was possible in challenge tests with *S. aureus* and *B. cereus* spores.

The IE of the new HHP process for human milk inoculated with spores of *B. cereus* (ATCC 14579) and an evaluation of its reproducibility (n°1, n°2, and n°3) are provided in **Table 1**. N_i and N_{HHP} are, respectively, the initial (prior to HHP treatment) and final (after HHP treatment) microbial concentrations. IE is provided for HHP treatment

Tables 1, 2 provide the corresponding inactivation efficiency (IE) of each microorganism. The HHP experiment and microbial analysis were repeated 3 times (n°1, n°2, and n°3) for the same human milk samples, with parameters of New HHP-$P = 350$ MPa, $T = 38°C$, MA = 4 × 5 min, Tl = 5 min, VA = 1 MPa/s

The effect of HHP on 10 samples (1.5^E+06), whereby colonies of B. Cereus were all destroyed

i.e., 1.5E+06 Colonies Inactivation Efficiency (IE) = 6.18 Log

In addition, this HHP process was evaluated for the inactivation of cytomegalovirus (CMV). This virus was selected due to its risk of human milk contamination and risk of postnatal infection (40, 42–44).

Different attempts were made using a suspension of cytomegalovirus with an initial viral particle concentration of up to 7 log. After application of the HHP treatment, which was characterized by the optimized process parameters used for the inactivation study of either *S. aureus* or bacterial spores of *B. cereus*, total CMV inactivation was observed.

Activity Retention of the Main Constituents of Human Milk

As a first evaluation, three main types of human milk components were selected:

- A component with enzymatic properties (lipase),
- Components with antimicrobial properties (lysozyme and lactoferrin) or with immunological properties (IgA), and
- Components with nutritional properties.

Impact of the HHP Process on Lipase Activity

An evaluation of lipase activity was important to compare the biological effects of this HPP process with those of thermal LTLT treatment (induction of total inactivation). The experimental conditions of HHP treatment were the same as those used for microbial decontamination ($P = 350$ MPa, $T = 38°C$, VA = 1 MPa.s^{-1}, MA = 4 cycles of 5 min and $t_l \pm 5$ min).

Residual activities of the lipase enzyme in three samples (raw milk, LTLT-pasteurized milk and HHP-treated milk) and in three replicates (n°1, n°2, and n°3) for HHP treatment are provided in **Table 3**. Due to the variability of lipase activity in human milk,

TABLE 2 | The effect of High Hydrostatic Pressure (HHP) on 10 samples of (1.5 × 106) colonies of *Bacillus cereus*; HHP destroyed all the colonies, i.e., 1.5 × 106 colonies with Inactivation Efficiency (IE) = 6.18 Log.

Microorganism (spore form)	N (UFC/mL)	N (Log)	IE
HM B.cer control	1.5 × 106	6.18	–
HM B.cer 1 HP	0	0	6.18
HM B.cer 2 HP	0	0	6.18
HM B.cer 3 HP	0	0	6.18
HM B.cer 4 HP	0	0	6.18
HM B.cer 5 HP	0	0	6.18
HM B.cer 6 HP	0	0	6.18
HM B.cer 7 HP	0	0	6.18
HM B.cer 8 HP	0	0	6.18
HM B.cer 9 HP	0	0	6.18
HM B.cer 10 HP	0	0	6.18

***Tables 1, 2** provide the corresponding IE of each microorganism. The HHP experiment and microbial analysis were repeated 3 times (n°1, n°2, and n°3) for the same human milk samples, with parameters of New HHP-P = 350 MPa, T = 38°C, MA = 4 × 5 min, TI = 5 min, VA = 1 MPa/s.*

three different human milk samples (A, B, and C) were used. The lipase activity was completely destroyed (0% lipase activity) by LTLT, whereas lipase activity after the new HHP remained similar to its original value (Raw Human Milk) between 78.6 and 100% with a mean of 87.8% (Wilcoxon test $p = 0.25$) (**Table 3**).

The residual activity of the lipase enzyme after HHP processing of human milk was between 80 and 85% of the initial value of human milk treated at 38°C.

A comparison with the residual activity from the conventional HHP process [reproducing Viazis's et al. (34) HHP treatment] resulted in a residual lipase activity of close to 75%.

Impact of the HHP Process on the Activity of Different Components With Antibacterial or Immune Properties

The activity of biological components (lysozyme, lactoferrin, α-lactalbumin, and IgA) was also evaluated before and after HHP processing of human milk using the same set of experimental parameters (**Table 5; Figure 1**).

Considering the differences between our HHP process and those described in the literature for human milk, the following remarks can be made.

Impact of the HHP Process on Human Milk Components With Nutritional Properties Milk Fat Globule (MFG) Granulometry in Raw, LTLT-Pasteurized, and HHP-Treated Human Milk Using This Novel HHP Process

Evaluation of the size of MFGs showed that the population was bimodal with an approximately equivalent average diameter (d4.3) for all types of milk (raw milk: 5.5 μm; LTLT: 5.6 μm; and HHP: 5.4 μm). In addition, the proportion of "small MFGs" was greater in raw milk and HHP-treated milk (d3.2 = 0.6 vs. 0.8 μm, respectively) compared to that in LTLT-pasteurized human milk (d3.2 = 3.1 μm). This result suggests that the size structure of raw breast milk is preserved by HHP treatment, whereas LTLT promotes coalescence and therefore increases the

TABLE 3 | Lipase activity of raw human milk samples and milk samples after thermal "Low-Temperature, Long-Time" (LTLT) pasteurization and High Hydrostatic Pressure (HHP) processing.

Sample	Lipase activity	% Lipase activity
Raw milk A	0.57	100
Raw milk B	0.71	100
Raw milk C	0.70	100
LTLT-PASTEURIZED MILK		
Pasteurized A	0.00	0.00
Pasteurized B	0.00	0.00
Pasteurized C	0.00	0.00
HHP-TREATED MILK		
HHP A n°1	0.57	100
HHP A n°2	0.53	92.9
HHP A n°3	0.53	92.9
HHP B n°1	0.68	95.8
HHP B n°2	0.56	79
HHP B n°3	0.58	81.7
HHP C n°1	0.59	84.3
HHP C n°2	0.55	78.6
HHP C n°3	0.60	85.7

(A, B, and C correspond to 3 different human milk samples, and n°1, n°2, and n°3 correspond to HHP treatment reproducibility assays. Lipase activity of raw human milk samples and milk samples after thermal LTLT pasteurization and HHP processing (A, B, and C correspond to 3 different human milk samples, and n°1, n°2, and n°3 correspond to HHP treatment reproducibility assays) The lipase activity was completely destroyed (0% lipase activity) by LTLT, whereas lipase activity after the new HHP remained similar to its original value (Raw Human Milk) between 78.6 and 100% with a mean of 87.8% (Wilcoxon test p = 0.25).

number of "large" MFGs. In addition, the total fat content was similar regardless of the performed treatment (raw, LTLT and HHP: 34.0, 34.1, and 32.3 mg/mL milk, respectively) and of the fatty acid profile of the milk.

DISCUSSION

For the first time, this new HHP process for the microbial safety of human milk can irreversibly inactivate both the vegetative forms of microorganisms, such as gram-positive bacteria including *S. aureus*, and **bacterial spores**, such as those of the contaminant *B. cereus*, while preserving at least 80% of the biological activity of the main components. Previously reported works involving HHP treatments were based on so-called "conventional" approaches in which the applied pressure was not controlled (15). **Table 4** provides average values of the resulting microbial safety using three processes (LTLT, HTST and this new HHP) on human milk with *S. aureus* (gram-positive bacterium) and *B. cereus* (sporulated bacterium) as contamination references. Consequently, inactivation of bacterial spores, such as those of *B. cereus*, was not possible with a technique other than the new HHP.

The retention rates of the biological activity for different components with specific properties [BSSL lipase (with enzymatic properties), lysozyme and lactoferrin (characterized by antimicrobial properties), and IgA (with immunological properties)] are summarized in **Table 5**.

TABLE 4 | Average values of the resulting microbial safety using *Staphylococcus aureus* (Gram-Positive Bacterium) and *Bacillus cereus* (Sporulated Bacterium) as contamination references.

	Inactivation efficiency (IE)		
	LTLT[a]	HTST[b]	New HHP[c]
S. aureus	≈4	≈4	≈6
B. cereus spores	No effect	No effect	≈5

[a] *Higher contamination accepted for the Holder treatment (10^4 CFU /mL) due to toxin production by S. aureus.*
[b] *Giribaldi et al. (45).*
[c] *This paper.*

TABLE 5 | Average retention rates of biological activity for different components with specific properties after "Low-temperature, long-time" (LTLT), "High-temperature, short-time" (HTST) and the new "High Hydrostatic Pressure" (HHP) treatments were applied to human milk.

	Retention rates (% vs. the raw milk)		
	LTLT	HTST	New HHP
BSSL (lipase)	0–10 (45)	26 (45)	80–85 (this paper)
Lysozyme	52.3	48.8 (45)	> 95 (this paper)
Lactoferrin	≈ 20 (12)	30–40 (12)	93–97 (this paper)
IgA	46.3	78.9 (45)	64 (this paper)

Comparisons with the HTST process suggest that the retention rates of the biological activity of human milk components vary widely (particularly for BSSL) by author (9–13). In a recent paper by Giribaldi et al. (45), two aspects of the impact of the HTST process were evaluated: (i) microbial inactivation but not destruction of *B. cereus* and microbial spores and (ii) retention of the biological activity of human milk components using a specific HTST device for human milk pasteurization. Residual lysozyme activity was between 95% and 100% after application of our HHP process. Our value agrees with that reported by Viazis et al. (46) (96%) following HHP treatment of human milk at 400 MPa and 20°C. Viazis's et al. (34) HHP treatment resulted in a residual lipase activity of close to 75%.

Mayayo et al. (47) found that treatment at 300, 400, 500, and 600 MPa for 15 min and $T = 20°C$ using the "conventional approach" to HHP processes denatured 9, 23, 34, and 48% of lactoferrin, respectively. In our approach, the retention rate of lactoferrin was over 93% (denaturation was below 7%) despite using a temperature of 38°C to limit the germination of *B. cereus* spores.

The residual activity of IgA was comparable to that obtained by Delgado et al. (48) (47.5% at 300 MPa and 50°C). In an early paper, Viazis et al. (46) found that high-pressure processing of human milk using the "conventional approach" at 400 MPa for 30, 60, 90, and 120 min and at a treatment temperature close to 31°C resulted in 85.6, 87.1, 80.6, and 75.4% retention, respectively. Permanyer et al. (49) claimed that after a treatment at 400 MPa for 5 min at 12°C, 100% of IgA activity was maintained, whereas IgA retention was 87.9 and 69.3% at higher pressure conditions (500 and 600 MPa, respectively). Contador et al. (50) evaluated the retention activity of IgA after high-pressure treatment at different pressures (400 and 600 MPa) and different treatment durations (3 and 6 min) with an initial temperature of 10°C at 400 MPa for 6 min; the retention of IgA activity was close to 90%.

Comparisons of these research studies suggest that IgA activity mainly depends on both the pressure and temperature of high-pressure treatment.

The retention rates of the biological activity for different components with specific properties [BSSL lipase (with enzymatic properties), lysozyme and lactoferrin (characterized by antimicrobial properties), and IgA (with immunological properties)] are summarized in **Table 5**.

LIMITATIONS

The new HHP process requires 90 min to treat human milk vs. 60 min for the Holder method; however, the cost of the HHP device is more than is a conventional pasteurizer. However, the new HHP saves up to 10% of material contaminated by *B. cereus*. For example, the Bordeaux Human Milk Bank collects 11,000 liters of human milk per year; 10% of this amount (or 1,100 liters) is contaminated with *B. cereus* and therefore must be discarded (51). This represents 165000€ /year, lost with the conventional pasteurizer per year, which would not be rejected with the new HHP.

CONCLUSION

This new HHP process is promising for implementation in human milk banks based on a comparison of three processes for the microbial safety and retention of the biological activity of different milk components. This approach is the first process that can inactivate bacterial spores, such as those of *B. cereus*; this point is important due to the risks of bacterial spores to preterm or young infants (52).

AUTHOR CONTRIBUTIONS

GD and AP processed the human milk samples, and the results of bacteriological analyses were verified in double-blind experiments performed by PL of CHU. GD worked with AP to write the first version of the manuscript; unfortunately, GD is now deceased. PL performed a double-blind bacteriological study on the HHP samples from GD at the CHU. LC and PM performed the experiments, analyzed the data and wrote their part of manuscript and participated in revising the manuscript. Technis and results of Bacteriology was revised by PL and AP. The technics and results of Lipids by LC. The technics and results of proteins by PM. CB wrote the manuscript.

ACKNOWLEDGMENTS

The authors would like to acknowledge Dr. Delphine Lamireau and the technicians from the Bordeaux Human Milk Bank. We also thank LC, Carole Vaysse and Laurence Fonseca for performing the lipid assay and the technicians from ITERG, Bordeaux University, for performing lipid measurement. We thank PM, G. Miranda, Z. Krupova, and L. Bianchi for performing the protein assay UMR1313 GABI, INRA, AgroParisTech, Université Paris-Saclay, 78350 Jouy-en-Josas, France.

REFERENCES

1. Menon G, Williams TC. Human milk for preterm infants: why, what, when and how? *Arch Dis Child Fetal Neonatal Ed.* (2013) 98:F559–62. doi: 10.1136/archdischild-2012-303582
2. Chu CH. Breastfeeding: best for babies. *Pediatr Neonatol.* (2013) 54:351–2. doi: 10.1016/j.pedneo.2013.06.004
3. Tudehope DI. Human milk and the nutritional needs of preterm infants. *J Pediatr.* (2013) 162:S17–25. doi: 10.1016/j.jpeds.2012.11.049
4. Dewitte C, Courdent P, Charlet C, Dumoulin D, Courcol R, Pierrat V. [Contamination of human milk with aerobic flora: Evaluation of losses for a human milk bank]. *Arch Pediatr.* (2015) 22:461–7. doi: 10.1016/j.arcped.2015.02.011
5. ESPGHAN Committee on Nutrition, Arslanoglu S, Corpeleijn W, Moro G, Braegger C, Campoy C, et al. Donor human milk for preterm infants: current evidence and research directions. *J Pediatr Gastroenterol Nutr.* (2013) 57:535–42. doi: 10.1097/MPG.0b013e3182a3af0a
6. Corpeleijn WE, Vermeulen MJ, van Vliet I, Kruger C, van Goudoever JB. Human milk banking - facts and issues to resolve. *Nutrients* (2010) 2:762–9. doi: 10.3390/nu2070762
7. Peila C, Emmerik NE, Giribaldi M, Stahl B, Ruitenberg JE, van Elburg RM, et al. Human milk processing: a systematic review of innovative techniques to ensure the safety and quality of donor milk. *J Pediatr Gastroenterol Nutr.* (2017) 64:353–61. doi: 10.1097/MPG.0000000000001435
8. Picaud JC, Buffin R. Human milk - treatment and quality of banked human milk. *Clin Perinatol.* (2017) 44:95–119. doi: 10.1016/j.clp.2016.11.003
9. Baro C, Giribaldi M, Arslanoglu S, Giuffrida MG, Dellavalle G, Conti A, et al. Effect of two pasteurization methods on the protein content of human milk. *Front Biosci.* (2011) 3:818–29.
10. Dhar J, Fichtali J, Skura BJ, Nakai S, Davidson AGF. Pasteurization efficiency of a HTST system for human milk. *J Food Sci.* (1996) 61:569–73. doi: 10.1111/j.1365-2621.1996.tb13160.x
11. Goldblum RM, Dill CW, Albrecht TB, Alford ES, Garza C, Goldman AS. Rapid high-temperature treatment of human milk. *J Pediatr.* (1984) 104:380–5. doi: 10.1016/S0022-3476(84)81099-9
12. Klotz D, Joellenbeck M, Winkler K, Kunze M, Huzly D, Hentschel R. High-temperature short-time pasteurisation of human breastmilk is efficient in retaining protein and reducing the bacterial count. *Acta Paediatr.* (2017) 106:763–7. doi: 10.1111/apa.13768
13. Terpstra FG, Rechtman DJ, Lee ML, Hoeij KV, Berg H, Van Engelenberg FACV, et al. Antimicrobial and antiviral effect of high-temperature short-time (HTST) pasteurization applied to human milk. *Breastfeed Med.* (2007) 2:27–33. doi: 10.1089/bfm.2006.0015
14. Christen L, Lai CT, Hartmann B, Hartmann PE, Geddes DT. The effect of UV-C pasteurization on bacteriostatic properties and immunological proteins of donor human milk. *PLoS ONE* (2013) 8:e85867. doi: 10.1371/journal.pone.0085867
15. Gabriel AA, Marquez GGF. Inactivation behaviors of selected bacteria in ultraviolet-C-treated human breast milk. *Innov Food Sci Emerg Technol.* (2017) 41:216–23. doi: 10.1016/j.ifset.2017.03.010
16. Martysiak-Zurowska D, Puta M, Kotarska J, Cybula K, Malinowska-Panczyk E, Kołodziejska I. The effect of UV-C irradiation on lipids and selected biologically active compounds in human milk. *Int Dairy J.* (2017) 66:42–8. doi: 10.1016/j.idairyj.2016.10.009
17. Christen L, Lai CT, Hartmann PE. Ultrasonication and the quality of human milk: variation of power and time of exposure. *J Dairy Res.* (2012) 79:361–6. doi: 10.1017/S0022029912000246
18. Czank C, Simmer K, Hartmann PE. Simultaneous pasteurization and homogenization of human milk by combining heat and ultrasound: effect on milk quality. *J Dairy Res.* (2010) 77:183–9. doi: 10.1017/S0022029909990483
19. Huang H-W, Lung H-M, Yang BB, Wang C-Y. Responses of microorganisms to high hydrostatic pressure processing. *Food Control* (2014) 40:250–9. doi: 10.1016/j.foodcont.2013.12.007
20. Huang H-W, Wu S-J, Lu J-K, Shyu Y-T, Wang C-Y. Current status and future trends of high-pressure processing in food industry. *Food Control* (2017) 72:1–8. doi: 10.1016/j.foodcont.2016.07.019
21. Rastogi NK, Raghavarao KSMS, Balasubramaniam VM, Niranjan K, Knorr D. Opportunities and challenges in high pressure processing of foods. *Crit Rev Food Sci Nutr.* (2007) 47:69–112. doi: 10.1080/10408390600626420
22. Wang CY, Huang HW, Hsu CP, Yang BB. Recent advances in food processing using high hydrostatic pressure technology. *Crit Rev Food Sci Nutr.* (2016) 56:527–40. doi: 10.1080/10408398.2012.745479
23. Aertsen A, Meersman F, Hendrickx MEG, Vogel RF, Michiels CW. Biotechnology under high pressure: applications and implications. *Trends Biotechnol.* (2009) 27:434–41. doi: 10.1016/j.tibtech.2009.04.001
24. Demazeau G, Rivalain N. High hydrostatic pressure and biology: a brief history. *Appl Microbiol Biotechnol.* (2011) 89:1305–14. doi: 10.1007/s00253-010-3070-9
25. Demazeau G, Rivalain N. The development of high hydrostatic pressure processes as an alternative to other pathogen reduction methods. *J Appl Microbiol.* (2011) 110:1359–69. doi: 10.1111/j.1365-2672.2011.05000.x
26. Masson P, Tonello C, Balny C. High-pressure biotechnology in medicine and pharmaceutical science. *J Biomed Biotechnol.* (2001) 1:85–8. doi: 10.1155/S1110724301000158
27. Meyer-Pittroff R. High pressure applications in medecine. In: Winter R, editor. *Advances in High Pressure Bioscience and Biotechnology II.* New York,NY: Springer (2003). p. 295–305. doi: 10.1007/978-3-662-05613-4_53
28. Rigaldie Y, Demazeau G. [Contribution of high pressure to pharmaceutical and medical science]. *Ann Pharm Fr.* (2004) 62:116–27. doi: 10.1016/S0003-4509(04)94290-3
29. Rivalain N (2009). *Sur un Procédé Hautes Pressions de Sécurisation du Plasma Sanguin Humain.* Ph.D. thesis, University Bordeaux I, no. 3910.
30. Rivalain N, Roquain J, Demazeau G. Development of high hydrostatic pressure in biosciences: pressure effect on biological structures and potential applications in biotechnologies. *Biotechnol Adv.* (2010) 28:659–72. doi: 10.1016/j.biotechadv.2010.04.001
31. Huppertz T, Smiddy MA, Upadhyay VK, Kelly AL. High-pressure-induced changes in bovine milk: a review. *Int J Dairy Technol.* (2006) 59:58–66. doi: 10.1111/j.1471-0307.2006.00246.x
32. Lambert Y, Demazeau G, Largeteau A, Bouvier JM. Changes in aromatic volatile composition of strawberry after high pressure treatment. *Food Chem.* (1999) 67:7–16. doi: 10.1016/S0308-8146(99)00084-9
33. Sevenich R, Kleinstueck E, Crews C, Anderson W, Pye C, Riddellova K, et al. High-pressure thermal sterilization: food safety and food quality of baby food puree. *J Food Sci.* (2014) 79:M230–7. doi: 10.1111/1750-3841.12345
34. Viazis S, Farkas BE, Jaykus LA. Inactivation of bacterial pathogens in human milk by high-pressure processing. *J Food Prot.* (2008) 71:109–18. doi: 10.4315/0362-028X-71.1.109
35. Aires GSB, Walter EHM, Junqueira VCA, Roig SM, Faria JAF. *Bacillus cereus* in refrigerated milk submitted to different heat treatments. *J Food Prot.* (2009) 72:1301–5. doi: 10.4315/0362-028X-72.6.1301
36. Bartoszewicz M, Hansen BM, Swiecicka I. The members of the *Bacillus cereus* group are commonly present contaminants of fresh and heat-treated milk. *Food Microbiol.* (2008) 25:588–96. doi: 10.1016/j.fm.2008.02.001

37. Demazeau G, Rivalain N, Billeaud C. *Procédé de Traitement Sous Hautes Pressions d'un Milieu Pour L'inactivation des Spores Bactériennes*. Bordeaux: French Patent N° 12 60214. (p. 26/10/2012) (2012).
38. Patterson MF, Quinn M, Simpson R, Gilmour A. Sensitivity of vegetative pathogens to high hydrostatic pressure treatment in phosphate-buffered saline and foods. *J Food Prot*. (1995) 58:524–9. doi: 10.4315/0362-028X-58.5.524
39. Decousser JW, Ramarao N, Duport C, Dorval M, Bourgeois-Nicolaos N, Guinebretière MH, et al. *Bacillus cereus* and severe intestinal infections in preterm neonates: putative role of pooled breast milk. *Am J Infect Control* (2013) 41:918–21. doi: 10.1016/j.ajic.2013.01.043
40. Kim JH, Chung E-J, Park HK, Moon SJ, Choi S-M, Oh SH. Postnatal cytomegalovirus infection in an extremely premature infant transmitted via breast milk: a case report. Korean *J Pediatr*. (2009) 52:1053–8. doi: 10.3345/kjp.2009.52.9.1053
41. Miranda G, Krupova Z, Bianchi L, Martin P. A novel LC-MS protein profiling method to characterize and quantify individual milk proteins and multiple isoforms. In: *10th Annual Symposium of the International Milk Genomics Consortium*. Davis, CA: University of California, Davis Conference Center, (2013).
42. Kurath S, Halwachs-Baumann G, Müller W, Resch B. Transmission of cytomegalovirus via breast milk to the prematurely born infant: a systematic review. *Clin Microbiol Infect*. (2010) 16:1172–8. doi: 10.1111/j.1469-0691.2010.03140.x
43. Lawrence RM. Cytomegalovirus in human breast milk: risk to the premature infant. *Breastfeed Med*. (2006) 1:99–107. doi: 10.1089/bfm.2006.1.99
44. Numazaki K. Human cytomegalovirus infection of breast milk. *FEMS Immunol Med Microbiol*. (1997) 18:91–8. doi: 10.1111/j.1574-695X.1997.tb01032.x
45. Giribaldi M, Coscia A, Peila C, Antoniazzi S, Lamberti C, Ortoffi M, et al. Pasteurization of human milk by a benchtop high-temperature short-time device. *Innov Food Sci Emerg Technol*. (2016) 36:228–33. doi: 10.1016/j.ifset.2016.07.004
46. Viazis S, Farkas BE, Allen JC. Effects of high-pressure processing on immunoglobulin A and lysozyme activity in human milk. *J Hum Lact*. (2007) 23:253–61. doi: 10.1177/0890334407303945
47. Mayayo C, Montserrat M, Ramos SJ, Martínez-Lorenzo MJ, Calvo M, Sánchez L, et al. Kinetic parameters for high-pressure-induced denaturation of lactoferrin in human milk. *Int Dairy J*. (2014) 39:246–52. doi: 10.1016/j.idairyj.2014.07.001
48. Delgado FJ, Contador R, Álvarez-Barrientos A, Cava R, Delgado-Adámez J, Ramírez R. Effect of high pressure thermal processing on some essential nutrients and immunological components present in breast milk. *Innov Food Sci Emerg Technol*. (2013) 19:50–6. doi: 10.1016/j.ifset.2013.05.006
49. Permanyer M, Castellote C, Ramírez-Santana C, Audí C, Pérez-Cano FJ, Castell M, et al. Maintenance of breast milk immunoglobulin A after high-pressure processing. *J Dairy Sci*. (2010) 93:877–83. doi: 10.3168/jds.2009-2643
50. Contador R, Delgado-Adámez J, Delgado FJ, Cava R, Ramírez R. Effect of thermal pasteurisation or high pressure processing on immunoglobulin and leukocyte contents of human milk. *Int Dairy J*. (2013) 32:1–5. doi: 10.1016/j.idairyj.2013.03.006
51. Rigourd V, Barnier J, Ferroni A, Nicloux M, Hachem T, Magny J, et al. Recent actuality about *Bacillus cereus* and human milk bank: a new sensitive method for microbiological analysis of pasteurized milk. *Eur J Clin Microbiol Infect Dis*. (2018) 37:1297–303. doi: 10.1007/s10096-018-3249-z
52. Sousa SG, Delgadillo I, Saraiva JA. Human milk composition and preservation: evaluation of high-pressure processing as a nonthermal pasteurization technology. *Crit Rev Food Sci Nutr*. (2016) 56:1043–60. doi: 10.1080/10408398.2012.753402

25

Donor Human Milk: Effects of Storage and Heat Treatment on Oxidative Stress Markers

Enrico Bertino [1], Chiara Peila [1,2], Francesco Cresi [1], Elena Maggiora [1], Stefano Sottemano [1], Diego Gazzolo [3], Sertac Arslanoglu [4] and Alessandra Coscia [1]*

[1] Neonatology Unit, Department of Public Health and Pediatrics, Università degli Studi di Torino, Turin, Italy, [2] Department of Maternal, Fetal and Neonatal Health, Azienda Ospedaliera Nazionale SS. Antonio e Biagio e Cesare Arrigo, Alessandria, Italy, [3] Neonatal Intensive Care Unit, Università degli Studi G. d'Annunzio Chieti e Pescara, Chieti, Italy, [4] Department of Pediatrics, Division of Neonatology, Istanbul Medeniyet University Goztepe Education and Research Hospital, Istanbul, Turkey

***Correspondence:**
Chiara Peila
peila.chiara@gmail.com

Mother's own milk is the first choice for the feeding and nutrition of preterm and term newborns. When mother's own milk is unavailable or in short supply donor human milk (DM) could represent a solution. Heat treatment and cold storage are common practices in Human Milk Banks (HMBs). Currently, Holder pasteurization process is the recommended heat treatment in all international guidelines. This method is thought to lead to a good compromise between the microbiological safety and nutritional/biological quality of DM. Moreover, storage of refrigerated milk is a common practice in HMBs and in NICUs. Depending on the length and on the type of storage, human milk may lose some important nutritional and functional properties. The available data on oxidative stress markers confirm that pasteurization and refrigeration affected this important elements to variable degrees, even though it is rather difficult to quantify the level of deterioration. Nonetheless, clinical practice demonstrates that many beneficial properties of human milk are preserved, even after cold storage and heat treatment. Future studies should be focused on the evaluation of new pasteurization techniques, in order to achieve a better compromise between biological quality and safety of DM.

Keywords: donor human milk, human milk, human milk bank, oxidative stress, heat treatment, refrigeration, pasteurization

INTRODUCTION

Human milk (HM) is the gold standard for feeding and nutrition for preterm and term newborns. Mother's own milk is the first choice for improving short and long-term outcomes for all neonates (1–3). HM benefits are mediated by different components, including specific and immunomodulatory molecules and species-specific factors. Breastmilk could be considered as a dynamic system and species-specific nourishment for newborns (4). Human Donor Milk (DM) can replace breastmilk when unavailable or lacking, although safe procedures for milk storage and conservation are required (5, 6). Currently, several reviews that show the advantages of donor milk, the World Health Organization and the American Academy of Pediatrics suggest the use of DM as a substitute of mother milk (1, 3).

Heat treatment on milk delivered to Human Milk Banks (HMBs) is critical for milk safety: pasteurization, indeed, inactivates bacterial and viral agents (5). Pasteurization is a process consisting of three main phases: rapid heating, stationary temperature phase and rapid cooling. Currently, the Holder Pasteurization (HoP) method, providing a temperature of 62,5°C for 30 min, is fundamental for HMBs constitution and its use is suggested by international guidelines (5, 6) as HoP represents the best compromise between nutritional and biological characteristics and microbiological safety (7–11).

Cold storage of HM is a routine not only in HMB but also at home and in the hospitals, especially in Neonatal Intensive Care Units. According to the length and on the typology of storage, HM may lose some significant nutritional and functional characteristics. The maximum refrigeration time for human milk ranges between 24 h and 8 days, according to the current advices on safe HM storage (12–14). Such variability replicates the heterogeneity of the scientific sources, which is ascribable to differences in the study design and in methodological approach (5, 14, 15). Recently, Slutzah et al. concluded that HM may be stored for 96 h at 4°C without affecting the overall milk integrity, as determined by bacterial growth, white cell count, pH, osmolality, and concentration of selected biological factors (sIgA, lactoferrin, total fat, and total proteins) (16, 17).

On the other hand, detailed data on the effects of storage, in terms of oxidative stress markers, on mother's milk are still lacking. Thus, the present paper is aimed at reviewing published evidences, and at comparing results on the effects of HoP and the refrigerated storage on the oxidative stress markers of human milk.

SEARCH METHODOLOGY

The literature review was performed by electronic searches of MEDLINE, EMBASE, CINHAL, and the Cochrane Library. The electronic search used the following keywords and MeSH terms: donor milk, banked milk, milk bank, milk banking, (human milk OR donor milk) AND Holder pasteurization AND oxidative stress, (human milk OR donor milk) AND pasteurization AND oxidative stress, (human milk OR donor milk) AND storage AND oxidative stress, (human milk OR donor milk) AND heat treatment AND oxidative stress, (human milk OR donor milk) AND cold treatment AND oxidative stress, (human milk OR donor milk) AND refrigeration AND oxidative stress(donor milk OR Holder pasteurization) AND oxidative stress, (donor milk OR cold storage) AND oxidative stress, (donor milk OR cold storage) AND oxidative stress.

The research was performed in December 2017 and no limits concerning publication date were set.

Considering differences between the research protocols published to date, we focused our review on studies with an experimental design that:

- define exactly the pasteurization method (62.5–63°C for 30 min)
- define exactly the refrigeration method (4°C for maximum 96 h)
- compare the same samples of HM before and after the heat or the cold treatments.

HEAT TREATMENT

The effects of HoP on oxidative stress markers are evaluated only in three studies.

Oxidative status was assessed, on raw and pasteurized breastmilk, by the evaluation of oxidants molecules and the activity of oxidants scavengers. Silvestre et al. showed that HoP does not significantly influence the levels of malondialdehyde while glutathione peroxidase activity, glutathione concentrations and total antioxidant capacity result seriously compromised. This result shows a reduction on oxidative scavenging systems of HM (18). Other authors (19) did not find changes in hexanal and malondialdehyde concentration and in the total antioxidant capacity (measured by means of oxygen radical absorbance capacity essay) thus meaning no lipid oxidation neither contraction of antioxidant systems.

Moreover, Peila et al. analyzed the effects of HoP on an emergent oxidative stress marker of the HM: the hemeoxygenase-1 (HO-1) (20). HO-1 is a stress-inducible rate-limiting enzyme and it is involved in different cytoprotective effects, due to its multiple catalytic by-products. HO-1 is active in HM and shows no significant reduction in its activity after HoP process, even after being corrected for milk maturation degree and gestational age (20). The protective effect of HO-1, similarly to other milk antioxidant scavenger systems, could be found in its antioxidant activity which induces the conversion of free heme into three final products: (i) biliverdin, which is metabolized in bilirubin that shows antioxidant activity), (ii) carbon monoxide, a neurotransmitter and vasodilator with antiapoptotic and anti-inflammatory activities, and (iii) iron (Fe^{2+}) which is bound by specific proteins (20–24). Furthermore, HO-1 could have an immunoregulatory role in addition to its enzymatic activity, related to its capacity to bind specific receptors and to modulate the immune response (20). Indeed, extracellular stress proteins, including Heat Shock Proteins (HSP), rise as fundamental mediators of signaling and transport (25, 26). Behavioral stress influences the release of this proteins by the cell as well as the exposition to immunological "danger signals" (24). HSP released into extracellular fluid can bind receptors exposed by adjacent cells and begin the signal transduction cascades, likewise, the transport of molecules like antigenic peptides and chaperokines with immunomodulatory effect (20, 27). In particular, Li Volti et al. through a molecular modeling approach, found an important immunoregulatory receptor that could be the natural ligands of HO-1(20, 28). Nevertheless, the integration of experimental data with informatics data shows HO-1 role in the modulation of immune system (28).

Considering the various functions of HO-1 in the body, data reported in literature showing underlying a reduction in NEC incidence in preterm fed with DM compared to those fed with formula (7–11) and, the unclear pathophysiology of NEC (immature gastrointestinal epithelium, impaired immunological defenses, enteral feeding, and bacterial colonization), it is possible to argue that human milk HO-1 may play a role in the development and regulation of the immune system of the gastrointestinal tract (20).

Over the past decades the food industry and, in particular, the dairy industry tested innovative alternatives to standard pasteurization in an effort to maximize the preservation of food taste and nutritional features. Alternative processing techniques that are currently being tested to investigate their effect on HM include high-temperature–short-time pasteurization (HTST), high pressure processing (HPP), ultraviolet (UV) irradiation and (thermo-) ultrasonic processing (29).

HTST is a thermal pasteurization method that is well established in the dairy industry ("fresh" bovine milk is usually pasteurized by means of HTST). The method involves a thin layered milk flow being heated rapidly to 72°C and being kept at this temperature for a few seconds (usually 15 s), and then immediately cooled down. This method preserves most of the sensory features and nutritional values of the milk, and ensures a lower degradation of proteins and vitamins (29). Silvestre et al. (18) investigated oxidative stress markers (reduced glutathione, glutathione peroxidase activity, malondialdehyde, and total antioxidant capacity), and showed that the pasteurization of HM implies a decrease in its antioxidant properties, especially in the glutathione balance, but HTST caused a smaller loss in antioxidant potential than HoP.

COLD STORAGE

The effects of refrigerated storage at 4°C on oxidative stress markers are evaluated only in four studies.

Concerning the insurgence of lipid peroxidation and the creation of oxidation molecules, contrasting data have been reported in literature (30–32). Some studies reveal that cold storage of HM may reduce its antioxidants capacity (32) and increase malondialdehyde concentration (30). On the other hand, the study of Giribaldi et al. showed that the refrigerated storage at 4°C for 96 h did not affect the oxidative status of HM, evaluating the total antioxidant capacity, conjugated dienes, thiobarbituric acid reactive species and malondialdehyde concentration (14, 17). Their results did not indicate any evidence of lipid peroxidation, same Michalski et al reported (17, 31). The oxidative status of the HM during cold storage is particularly relevant for preterm newborns whose disorders are mainly due to disequilibrium between antioxidant capacity and oxidative stress, having a reduced antioxidant capacity and being often exposed to oxidant stress (32, 33). Moreover, the recent study of Peila et al. evaluated the effects of prolonged refrigerated storage on an important marker in HM: Adrenomedullin (AM) (34). AM is a C-amidated peptide, implicated in response to hypoxia and inflammation, which are linked also with neovascularization. Recent studies indicate that AM is synthesized also in the mammary gland and secreted in breast milk (35–37). AM levels in preterm milk (milk produced to mother who have delivered preterm, Gestational Age <37 weeks) are significant higher compared to term milk (milk produced to mother who have delivered at term, Gestational Age >37 weeks). This protein is not thermostable at 4°C: AM is significant reduced (56%) at 24 h and is nearly undetectable at 96 h (34). AM is a regulatory peptide and its expression was demonstrated in several tissues and biologic fluids such as plasma, cerebro-spinal fluid, sweat, amniotic fluid and urine (38–40). AM has been involved in the modulation of several physiological functions including cardiovascular tone, central brain activity (41–44), bronchodilation, renal function, hormone secretion, cell growth-differentiation, and immune response(45–52). Moreover, AM has been tested for its connection to ischemia-reperfusion injury whilst in healthy infants has been proved to contribute in the cascade of events sustaining fetal/neonatal cardiovascular adaptation (43–47). AM has been also taken into consideration for the analysis of beneficial/side-effects of *in-utero* vasodilation therapeutic strategies in pregnancies complicated by fetal chronic hypoxia (43–47). Concerning this, relation with AM and the occurrence of adverse neurological outcome has been reported in infants with congenital heart disease (47). Considering these important functions, it is possible to hypothesize that the existence of the active peptide AM in HM, and its variability in concentrations throughout different milk maturation degrees, gestational pathologies and gestational age at delivery, could have some direct impact in infants development due to the various physiological activities that have been related to it. In the gastrointestinal tract, immunoreactive AM has been found in human stomach, duodenum, jejunum, ileum and colon (47, 53, 54), and specific binding sites have been also found in rat stomach (54). This arrangement supposes a role for AM in the regulation of secretory-motor functions in the gastrointestinal tract, as well as in its development during the embryogenesis and the period immediately following birth. Since the developing intestine in the neonate is believed considered to be one of the main target organs for the growth factors present in human milk, Pio et al. proved that milk has a growth-promoting function on human small intestinal epithelial cell line (Int-407) (35, 36). These authors hypothesize that since MoAb-G6 partially blocks the milk-induced growth, AM may be one of the growth factors present in milk (35, 36). AM has also been characterized as an agent with antimicrobial activity against gastrointestinal microorganisms (36, 51, 52). This activity could be relevant for the protection of the neonate against gastroenteritis produced by intestinal pathogens. Eventually, since some peptides are absorbed from the neonatal gastrointestinal tract and appear intact in plasma (36, 55), AM could also exercise an activity in the modulation of tissue growth as well as in the regulation of the immune system (36, 55).

CONCLUSION

Multiple studies have been conducted to evaluate the effects of pasteurization and cold storage on breast milk and the results indicate that these treatments affect the concentration and activity of the constituents of HM to varying degrees. However, many studies show the persistence of the benefits of donated milk compared to artificial milk in the nutrition of preterm infants. With regard to the effects on oxidative stress markers, the data are currently lacking and contrasting. Many questions remain to be answered in particular, future studies will have to be conducted to clarify the aspects not yet investigated on the markers of oxidative stress and on biological properties in relation to the

HoP and cold treatments of breast milk. Future investigations must be aimed at improving the biological quality and safety of DM and should be: (i) designed to investigate the pre-analytical stability of these components according to storage procedures; (ii) intended to evaluate innovative test technologies, such as metabolomics; (iii) focused on new pasteurization techniques (high-temperature short-term pasteurization, thermoultrasonic treatment, high-pressure processing, and Ohmic heat treatment); (iv) aimed to evaluate analytical techniques able to assess the protein changes due to thermic treatments, as well as their interaction with sugars and lipids; (v) evaluated the effects of HoP on other biomarkers involved in growth and developing of newborns.

Moreover further studies will aimed at elucidating the protein stability during industrial processes for the preparation of artificial milk such as pasteurization and spray-drying, which have already been shown to affect milk composition and properties.

AUTHOR CONTRIBUTIONS

EB, CP, and AC contributed conception and design of the review. CP wrote the first draft of the manuscript. CP, EM and SS wrote sections of the manuscript. All authors contributed to manuscript revision, read, and approved the submitted version.

REFERENCES

1. American Academy of Paediatrics. Breastfeeding and use of human milk. *Pediatrics* (2012) 129:e827. doi: 10.1542/peds.2011-3552
2. Hamosh M. Protective function of proteins and lipids in human milk. *Biol Neonate* (1998) 74:163–76.
3. Horta BL, Victora CG, World Health Organization. *Long-Term Effects of Breastfeeding: A Systematic Review*. Geneva: WHO Library (2013).
4. Newman J. How breast milk protects newborns. *Sci Am.* (1995) 273:76–9.
5. Italian Association of Human Milk Banks, Arslanoglu S, Bertino E, Tonetto P, De Nisi G, Ambruzzi AM, et al. Guidelines for the establishment and operation of a donor human milk bank. *J Matern Fetal Neonatal Med.* (2010) 23:1–20. doi: 10.3109/14767058.2010.512414
6. Human Milk Banking Association of North America In: Tully MR, editors. *Guidelines for the Establishment and Operation of a Donor Human Milk Bank.* 9th ed. Raleigh, NC: Human Milk Banking Association of North America (2000). Available online at: www.hmbana.org (Accessed May 14, 2018).
7. Boyd CA, Quigley MA, Brocklehurst P. Donor breast milk versus infant formula for preterm infants: systematic review and meta-analysis. *Arch Dis Child Fetal Neonatal Ed.* (2007) 92:F169–7. doi: 10.1136/adc.2005.089490
8. McGuire W, Anthony MY. Donor human milk versus formula for preventing necrotising enterocolitis in preterm infants: systematic review. *Arch Dis Child Fetal Neonatal Ed.* (2003) 88:F11–4. doi: 10.1136/fn.88.1.F11
9. Quigley MA, Henderson G, Anthony MY, Mc Guire W. Formula milk versus donor breast milk for feeding preterm or low birth weight infants. *Cochrane Database Syst Rev.* (2007) 4:CD002971. doi: 10.1002/14651858.CD002971
10. Rønnestad A, Abrahamsen TG, Medbø S, Reigstad H, Lossius K, Kaaresen PI, et al. Late onset septicemia in a Norwegian national cohort of extremely premature infants receiving very early full human milk feeding. *Pediatrics* (2005) 115:269–76. doi: 10.1542/peds.2004-1833
11. Schanler RJ, Lau C, Hurst NM, Simth EO. Randomized trial of donor human milk versus preterm formula as substitutes for mothers' own milk in the feeding of extremely premature infants. *Pediatrics* (2005) 116:400–6. doi: 10.1542/peds.2004-1974
12. La Leche League International web site. *Storage Guidelines* (2012). Available online at: https://www.llli.org/breastfeeding-info/storingmilk/
13. Academy of Breastfeeding Medicine. ABM Clinical Protocol #8: human milk storage. Information for home use for full-term infants. *Breastfeed Med.* (2010) 5:127–30. doi: 10.1089/bfm.2017.29047.aje
14. Bertino E, Marzia G, Baro C, Giancotti V, Pazzi M, Peila C, et al. Effect of prolonged refrigeration on the lipid profile, lipase activity, and oxidative status of human milk. *J Pediatr Gastroenterol Nutr.* (2013) 56:390–6. doi: 10.1097/MPG.0b013e31827af155
15. Davanzo R, Travan L, Demarini S. Storage of human milk: accepting certain uncertainties. *J Hum Lactat.* (2010) 26:233–4. doi: 10.1177/0890334410374601
16. Slutzah M, Codipilly CN, Potak D, Clark RM, Schanler RJ. Refrigerator storage of expressed human milk in the neonatal intensive care unit. *J Pediatr.* (2010) 156:26–8. doi: 10.1016/j.jpeds.2009.07.023
17. Giribaldi M, Ortoffi MF, Giuffrida MG, Gastaldi D, Peila C, Coscia A, et al. Effect of prolonged refrigeration on the protein and microbial profile of human milk. *Int Dairy J.* (2013) 31:121–6. doi: 10.1016/j.idairyj.2013.01.006
18. Silvestre D, Miranda M, Muriach M, Almansa I, Jareno E, Romero FJ. Antioxidant capacity of human milk: effect of the thermal conditions for the pasteurization. *Acta Paediatr.* (2008) 97:1070–4. doi: 10.1111/j.1651-2227.2008.00870.x
19. Elisia I, Kitts DD. Quantification of hexanal as an index of lipid oxidation in human milk and association with antioxidant components. *J Clin Biochem Nutr.* (2011) 49:147–52. doi: 10.3164/jcbn.10-142
20. Peila C, Coscia A, Bertino E, Li Volti G, Barbagallo I, Visser GHA, et al. Heme oxygenase-1 in donor human milk. *Curr Pediatr Res.* (2016) 20:304–8. Available online at: www.currentpediatrics.com
21. Stocker, R., Yamamoto, Y., McDonagh, A.F., Glazer, A.N., Ames, B.N. (1987) Bilirubin is an antioxidant of possible physiological importance. *Science* 235(4792):1043–6.
22. Ryter SW, Alam J, Choi AM. Heme oxygenase-1/carbon monoxide: from basic science to therapeutic applications. *Physiol Rev.* (2006) 86:583–650. doi: 10.1152/physrev.00011.2005
23. Ghosh S, Mukherjee A, Sadler PJ, Verma S. Periodic iron nanomineralization in human serum transferrin fibrils. *Angew Chem Int Ed.* (2008) 47:2217–21. doi: 10.1002/anie.200705723
24. Maines MD. The heme oxygenase system: a regulator of second messenger gases. *Annu Rev Pharmacol Toxicol.* (1997) 37:517–54.
25. Calderwood SK, Mambula SS, Gray PJ Jr, Theriault JR. Extracellular heat shock proteins in cell signaling. *FEBS Lett.* (2007) 581:3689–94. doi: 10.1016/j.febslet.2007.04.044
26. Macario AJ, Conway DM. Molecular chaperones: multiple functions, pathologies, and potential applications. *Front Biosci.* (2007) 12:2588–600. doi: 10.2741/2257
27. Calderwood SK, Theriault J, Gray PJ, Gong J. Cell surface receptors for molecular chaperones. *Methods* (2007) 43:199–206. doi: 10.1016/j.ymeth.2007.06.008
28. Li Volti G, Galvano F, Frigiola Guccione S, Di Giacomo C, Forte S, et al. Potential immunoregulatory role of hemeoxygenase-1 in human milk: a combined biochemical and molecular modeling approach. *J Nutr Biochem.* (2010) 21:865–71. doi: 10.1016/j.jnutbio.2009.06.011
29. Peila, C., Emmerik. N.E., Giribaldi, M., Stahl, B., Ruitenberg, J.E., van Elburg, R.M., et al. (2017) Human milk processing: a systematic review of innovative techniques to ensure the safety and quality of donor milk. *J Pediatr Gastroenterol Nutr.* 6:353–61. doi: 10.1097/MPG.0000000000001435
30. Miranda, M., Muriach, M., Almansa, I., Jareño, E., Bosch-Morell, F., Romero, F.J., et al.,(2004) Oxidative status of human milk and its variations during cold storage. *Biofactors* 20:129–37. doi: 10.1002/biof.5520200302
31. Michalski MC, Calzada C, Makino A, Michaud S, Guichardant M. Oxidation products of polyunsaturated fatty acids in infant formulas compared to human milk—a preliminary study. *Mol Nutr Food Res.* (2008) 52:1478–85. doi: 10.1002/mnfr.200700451

32. Hanna N, Ahmed K, Anwar M, Petrova A, Hiatt M, Hegyi T. Effect of storage on breast milk antioxidant activity. *Arch Dis Child Fetal Neonatal Ed.* (2004) 89:F518–20. doi: 10.1136/adc.2004.049247
33. Thibeault DW. The precarious antioxidant defenses of the preterm infant. *Am J Perinatol.* (2000) 17:167–81. doi: 10.1055/s-2000-9422
34. Peila C, Coscia A, Bertino E, Li Volti G, Galvano F, Barbagallo I, et al. Human Milk adrenomedullin is unstable during cold storage at 4°C. *Breastfeed Med.* (2017) 12:561–5. doi: 10.1089/bfm.2017.0072
35. Pio R, Martínez A, Elsasser TH, Cuttitta F. Presence of immunoreactive adrenomedullin in human and bovine milk. *Peptides* (2000) 21:1859–63. doi: 10.1016/S0196-9781(00)00341-7
36. Cekmen MB, Balat A, Balat O, Aksoy F, Yurekli M, Erbagci AB, et al. Decreased adrenomedullin and total nitrite levels in breast milk of preeclamptic women. *Clin Biochem.* (2004) 37:146–8. doi: 10.1016/j.clinbiochem.2003.10.010
37. Ohta N, Tsukahara H, Ohshima Y, Nishii M, Ogawa Y, Sekine K, et al. Nitric oxide metabolites and adrenomedullin in human breast milk. *Early Hum Dev.* (2004) 78:61–5. doi: 10.1016/j.earlhumdev.2004.04.002
38. Montuenga LM, Marti'nez A, Miller MJ, Garayoa M, Elsasser T, Cuttitta F. Expression of adrenomedullin and PAMP in normal adult and developing mammals. In: Marti'nez A, Cuttitta F, editors. *Adrenomedullin.* Washington, DC: IOS Press (1998) p. 49–68.
39. Sato K, Hirata Y, Imai T, Iwashina M, Marumo F. Characterization of immunoreactive adrenomedullin in human plasma and urine. *Life Sci.* (1995) 57:189–94.
40. Takahashi K, Sone M, Satoh F, Murakami O, Totsune K, Tanji H, et al. Presence of adrenomedullin-like immunoreactivity in the human cerebrospinal fluid. *Peptides* (1997) 18:459–61.
41. Eto T, Kitamura K, Kato J. Biological and clinical roles of adrenomedullin in circulation control and cardiovascular diseases. *Clin Exp Pharmacol Physiol.* (1999) 26:371–80.
42. Allen M, Smith PM, Ferguson AV. Adrenomedullin microinjection into the area postrema increases blood pressure. *Am J Physiol.* (1997) 272:R1698–703.
43. Gazzolo D, Abella R, Frigiola A, Giamberti A, Tina G, Nigro F, et al. Neuromarkers and unconventional biological fluids. *J Matern Fetal Neonatal Med.* (2010) 23:66–9. doi: 10.3109/14767058.2010.507960
44. Florio P, Abella R, Marinoni E, Di Iorio R, Li Volti G, Galvano F,et al. Biochemical markers of perinatal brain damage. *Front Biosci.* (2010) 2:47–72. doi: 10.2741/s45
45. Gazzolo D, Abella R, Marinoni E, Di Iorio R, Li Volti G, Galvano F, et al. New markers of neonatal neurology. *J Matern Fetal Neonatal Med.* (2009) 22:57–61. doi: 10.1080/14767050903181468
46. Kanazawa H, Kurihara N, Hirata K, Kudoh S, Kawaguchi T, Takeda T. et al. Adrenomedullin, a newly discovered hypotensive peptide, is a potent bronchodilator. *Biochem Biophys Res Commun.* (1994) 205:251–4.
47. Serpero LD, Bellissima V, Colivicchi M, Sabatini M, Frigiola A, Ricotti A, et al. Next generation biomarkers for brain injury. *J Matern Fetal Neonatal Med.* (2013) 26:44–9. doi: 10.3109/14767058.2013.829688
48. Jougasaki M, Wei CM, Aarhus LL, Heublein DM, Sandberg SM, Burnett JCJr. Renal localization and actions of adrenomedullin: a natriuretic peptide. *Am J Physiol.* (1995) 268:657–63.
49. Wong HK, Tang F, Cheung TT, Cheung B. Adrenomedullin and diabetes. *World J Diabetes* (2014) 5:364–71. doi: 10.4239/wjd.v5.i3.364
50. Allaker RP, Kapas S. Adrenomedullin and mucosal defence: interaction between host and microorganism. *Regul Pept.* (2003) 112:147–52. doi: 10.1016/S0167-0115(03)00033-8
51. Walsh T, Marti'nez A, Peter J. Antimicrobial activity of adrenomedullin and its gene related peptides. *Clin Infect Dis.* (1996) 23:877–9.
52. Allaker RP, Zihni C, Kapas S. An investigation into the antimicrobial effects of adrenomedullin on members of the skin, oral, respiratory tract and gut microflora. *FEMS Immunol Med Microbiol.* (1999) 23:289–93.
53. Kitani M, Sakata J, Asada Y, Kitamura K, Eto T. Distribution and expression of adrenomedullin in human gastrointestinal tissue. *Ann Clin Biochem.* (1999) 35:643–8. doi: 10.1177/000456329803500508
54. Owji AA, Smith DM, Coppock HA, Morgan DG, Bhogal R, Ghatei MA. et al. An abundant and specific binding sitefor the novel vasodilator adrenomedullin in the rat. *Endocrinology* (1995) 136:2127–34.
55. Thornburg W, Matrisian L, Magun B, Koldovsky O. Gastrointestinal absorption of epidermal growth factor in suckling rats. Am J Physiol. (1984) 246:80–5.

26

Individualized Target Fortification of Breast Milk: Optimizing Macronutrient Content using Different Fortifiers and Approaches

Stephanie Fusch[1,2]*, Gerhard Fusch*[3]*, Efrah I. Yousuf*[3]*, Markus Rochow*[4]*, Hon Yiu So*[5]*, Christoph Fusch*[3,6] *and Niels Rochow*[3,6,7*]

[1] *Department of Pediatrics, University Medicine Greifswald, Greifswald, Germany,* [2] *Department of Pediatrics, Kantonsspital Aarau AG, Aarau, Switzerland,* [3] *Department of Pediatrics, McMaster University, Hamilton, ON, Canada,* [4] *Carl-Thiem-Hospital, Cottbus, Germany,* [5] *Department of Mathematics and Statistics, Oakland University, Rochester, MI, United States,* [6] *Department of Pediatrics, General Hospital, Paracelsus Medical University, Nuremberg, Germany,* [7] *Department of Pediatrics, Rostock University Medical Center, Rostock, Germany*

Correspondence:
Niels Rochow
rochow@npmmcmaster.ca

Background: Native breast milk composition displays significant inter- and intra-individual variation which persists after standard fortification with fixed doses and challenges target fortification. This study aims to analyze the macronutrient composition of different commercially available fortifiers and the effect of different fortification strategies on nutritional intake of preterm infants.

Methods: In 103 preterm infants, native breast milk samples were collected from 24-h feeding batches (n = 3,338) and fat, protein and carbohydrate contents were analyzed. Nutrient content was compared for breast milk that had undergone either (i) standard fortification, (ii) targeted fortification, (iii) selective batching according to breast milk composition, or (iv) partial lyophilization. For (i) eight commercially available standard fortifiers were tested. Targeted fortification (ii) involved the addition of single component modulars of either protein, fat or carbohydrates to standard fortified breast milk. Using a mathematical growth model, the combined effect of protein, fat and carbohydrate intake on growth was assessed. The best composition of standard fortifiers as the initial step for target fortification was explored assuming three clinical scenarios for milk analysis.

Results: Macronutrient content was highly variable between native breast milk samples, and this variation was still present after standard fortification, however at elevated macronutrient levels. Standard fortification, breast milk batching, as well as partial lyophilization of human milk resulted in deficient and imbalanced enteral intakes in a significant proportion of infants. Target fortification reduced this variation in a, respectively, higher percentage of samples. The effect size was dependent on the number of measurements per week. The optimum composition of standard fortifiers was dependent on the clinical scenario (measurement frequency) for target fortification.

Conclusions: To provide precise and accurate intakes of macronutrients, breast milk should be target fortified. Standard fortified breast milk can result in excess above recommended intakes of some macronutrients which limits the efficiency of target fortification. Standard fortifiers with improved composition are needed for target fortification.

Keywords: human milk, milk analysis, standard fortification, fat, carbohydrates, protein, preterm infants, growth

INTRODUCTION

Between 43 and 97% of preterm infants experience postnatal growth restriction (1, 2). Adequate nutrition of preterm infants is known to improve neurodevelopmental outcomes in later life and to reduce the risk of chronic cardiovascular and metabolic diseases in adulthood (3–8). For term infants, breast milk is considered as the optimal source of nutrition. It provides macronutrients such as proteins, fat, carbohydrates (carbs), as well as micronutrients that include vitamins and minerals. Breast milk is also known to have positive immunomodulatory and psychological effects and reduces the risk of developing many diseases like respiratory tract infections and allergic diseases (9, 10). Preterm infants fed breast milk during hospitalization in neonatal intensive care units (NICUs) have a lower risk of developing infections and necrotizing enterocolitis (4, 11–18). However, for preterm infants to reach intrauterine growth rates (19), in general higher amounts of nutrients are needed, which cannot be obtained solely from native breast milk [**Figure 1**] (1).

Fortification of native breast milk is routinely used to meet clinical recommendations of enteral nutrient intake (20). Various types of fortification methods are used to increase the macronutrient content of breast milk. Standard fortification assumes an average composition of breast milk and aims to improve nutrient intake by adding a fixed dose of fortifier to native breast milk (**Figure 1**). However, because native breast milk shows significant inter- and intraindividual variation of nutrient contents, this fortification strategy is frequently leading to an unbalanced intake (21–23). This will result in suboptimal growth, but in clinical routine it usually will take a few days to recognize and adjust intake—valuable time that is lost for appropriate growth. Adjustable fortification is an alternative approach originally reported to adjust protein intake based on blood urea nitrogen levels. However, the adjustment of deficient nutrients is delayed because it reacts on dynamics of metabolic response to an inappropriate supply (24, 25). Conversely, target fortification aims to provide infants with fortified breast milk that adheres to current clinical recommendations for macronutrient intake. Based on actual measurements of macronutrient contents in native breast milk, one-component modulars of either protein, fat or carbs are added to standard fortified breast milk to reach targeted macronutrient levels (**Figure 1**). While this process is the most accurate and allows infants to be fed the prescribed dose of macronutrients, it is also the most time-consuming method (26–28).

In the current paper, we examine differences in macronutrient contents of native breast milk samples and the impact of standard and targeted fortification on this variation when using different standard fortifiers and analysis schedules. Further, in this study we aimed (1) to identify the best composition of a standard fortifier for three clinical scenarios for target fortification; (2) to analyze the effect of fortification on infant's growth based on established growth models; and (3) to study pre-fortification approaches to optimize the macronutrient content by batching and lyophilization.

MATERIALS AND METHODS

Study Design and Study Population

This modeling study is a secondary analysis of a dataset obtained during a randomized controlled clinical trial (RCT) which was conducted between November 2012 and July 2016 at the Division of Neonatology (Level-III NICU) at McMaster Children's Hospital (Hamilton, Ontario, Canada) (28). The purpose of this RCT was to study the effect of target fortification of breast milk on growth, metabolism and neurodevelopmental outcomes using three single macronutrient modular products and compare it to standard fortification. The study was approved by Research Ethics Board of McMaster University (#12-109). All parents gave informed written consent prior to inclusion into the study. The flowchart of performed experiments is outlined in **Figure 2**.

Sample Collection and Breast Milk

Samples were collected from pooled batches ($n = 3{,}338$) of 24-h feedings before breast milk was fortified. Batches were usually prepared from frozen milk of the own mother (MOM) and—depending on the level of available MOM—supplemented with pasteurized frozen human donor milk. Data from 103 preterm infants born at a mean gestational age of 27.0 ± 1.5 weeks (birth weight 980 ± 240 g, head circumference 25.1 ± 2.7 cm, and length 34.7 ± 3.3 cm) were available. Fortification (and subsequent collection of breast milk samples) began at day of life 21 ± 6 and continued over an average period of 33 days ± 10 days. Each study participant provided samples covering at least 14 consecutive days. The native breast milk samples were stored at −20°C until milk analysis.

Breast milk samples were analyzed using validated methods. Samples were thawed and homogenized using a sonicator for 15 s (VCX 130; Chemical Instruments AB, Sollentuna, Sweden). Content of true protein and fat was determined by a validated near-infrared milk analyzer (SpectraStar; Unity Scientific, Brookfield, Connecticut) (29, 30). Lactose was measured using an established reference method (UPLC-MS/MS) in order to avoid crossover from non-digestible carbohydrates, i.e., human oligosaccharides (31).

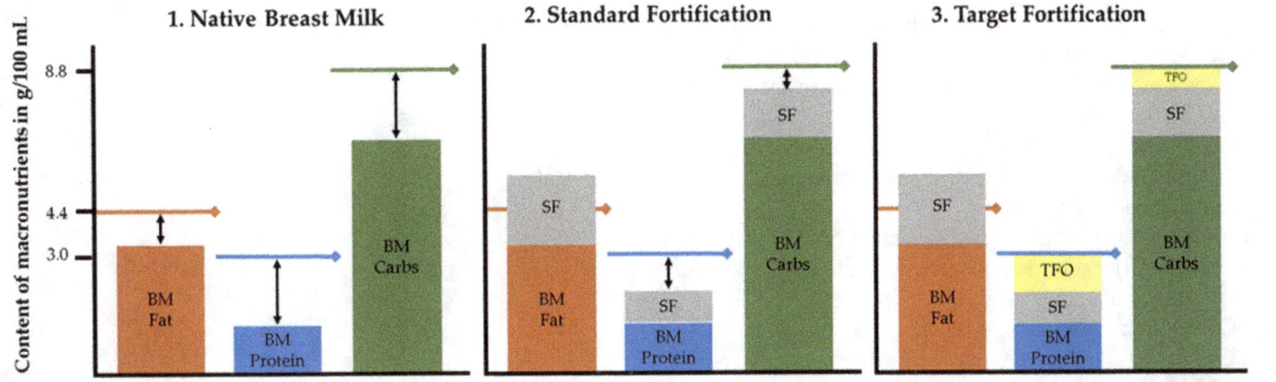

FIGURE 1 | Macronutrient content in native breast milk, standard fortified and target fortified breast milk. Lines represent recommended macronutrient contents of 4.4 g fat, 8.8 g carbs, and 3.0 g protein per 100 mL to reach ESPGHAN recommended intakes assuming an average fluid intake of 150 mL/kg/d leading to a total daily intake of 6.6, 13.2, and 4.5 g/kg/d for fat, carbs, and protein, respectively. BM, native breast milk; Carbs, carbohydrates; SF, standard fortification; TFO, target fortification. Under certain conditions single nutrient levels can exceed ESPGHAN recommendations already after standard fortification.

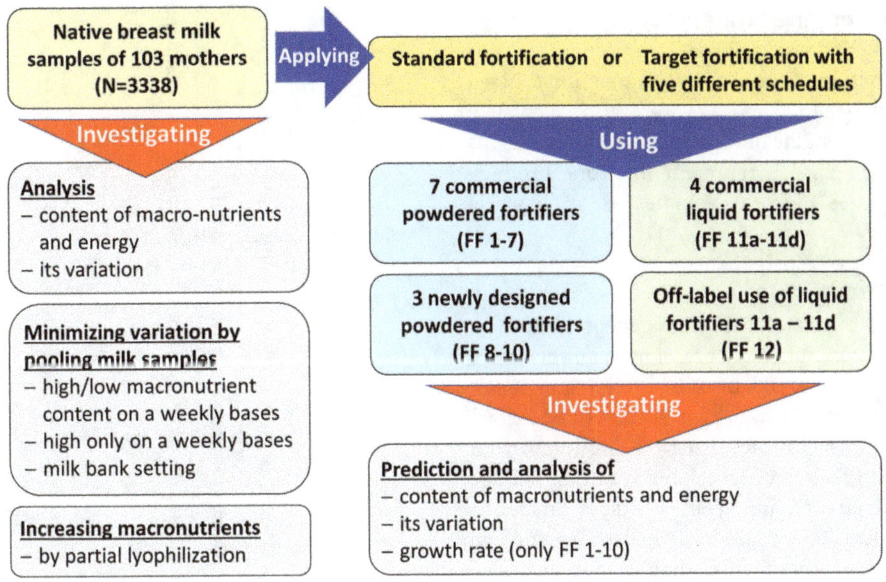

FIGURE 2 | Workflow of experiments (FF, fortifier).

Descriptive Analysis of Breast Milk Content and Macronutrient Targets After Fortification

Levels of fat, protein, carbohydrate, and lactose [g/100 mL] were measured in all native breast milk samples. The energy content (kcal/100 mL) was calculated using energy equivalents which assume that protein and carbs yield 4 kcal/g and that fat yields 9 kcal/g of energy, respectively (Atwater factor) (32). Additionally, the protein-to-energy ratio (P:E ratio, [g protein/100 kcal]) (33) and the ratio of total carbohydrate energy vs. non-protein energy was calculated (carbs/NPE, %) (34) for native breast milk as well as for all fortified variations.

Target macronutrient intake for preterm infants <1,000 g of birth weight were defined according to the guidelines of the European Society for Pediatric Gastroenterology Hepatology and Nutrition (ESPGHAN): 4.5 g/kg/d protein, 6.6 g/kg/d fat, and 13.2 g/kg/d carbs (20). With an assumed daily fluid intake of 150 mL/kg/d, nutrient contents of enteral feeds then translate to 3 g of protein, 4.4 g of fat, 8.8 g of carbohydrates per 100 mL of feeds. Achieving the recommended amounts of macronutrients would result in 87 kcal/100 mL, a protein -to-energy (P:E) ratio of 3.5 g/100 kcal and carbohydrate-to-NPE ratio of 47%.

Standard Fortifier

In this study, seven commercially available multicomponent powdered standard fortifiers (fortifiers 1–7) with different compositions were used. Each of them provides 1.0–1.5 g of extra protein per 100 ml thereby comprising comparable energy intakes. Based on their non-protein composition, they can be divided into three groups: (i) low-fat/high-carbohydrate, (ii) medium-fat/medium-carbohydrate, and (iii) high-fat/low-carbohydrate content (**Table 1**). For each 24 h-feeding, final macronutrient levels, energy content and corresponding ratios were calculated for all fortifiers.

In a second step, the optimum macronutrient composition for standard fortification was identified based on three different scenarios for milk analysis as described below (fortifiers 8–10). Composition was optimized for each macronutrient to minimize the deviation between fortified breast milk content and ESPGHAN recommended intake by minimizing the residual sum of squares. In a next step, the performance of fortifiers was evaluated for the three different measurement scenarios. Fortifier 8 represents a fortifier that was optimized for standard fortification only, i.e., no measurement of macronutrients in native breast milk. Fortifiers 9 and 10 were optimized for target fortification using either one breast milk analysis per week (occurring on Monday) or three breast milk analyses per week (occurring on Monday, Wednesday, Friday), respectively.

Further, the macronutrient intake for human milk based liquid fortifiers (fortifiers 11a-d and 12) were also calculated. Fortifiers 11a to 11d represent the different preparation strengths (20–50 mL). Fortifiers 11 and 12 represent the same product, however, fortifier 12 uses different volumes as an off-label clinical approach.

Target Fortification

Target fortification was calculated using three steps (**Figure 1**). First, macronutrient contents of native breast milk samples were analyzed (methods see paragraph Sample Collection and Breast Milk). In a second step, a standard fortifier (as described below) was added to native 24-h breast milk batches. Third, based on the measurement of the macronutrient content of breast milk, single component modulars containing either protein, fat and/or carbohydrates were added to standard fortified breast milk to achieve the recommended enteral macronutrient intake. The amount of required modulars was calculated by subtracting the standard fortified breast milk content for fat, protein, and carbs from the ESPGHAN recommended targets (20, 26). Further details and a model calculation have been previously described (28). In cases where the amount of a macronutrient already exceeded the recommendations after standard fortification, this macronutrient was not further fortified; the others were adjusted through the addition of modular products.

Schedules for Target Fortification

For the target fortification approach, we tested five different schedules for milk analysis and simulated the resulting macronutrient concentrations using fortifiers 1–12 (**Table 2**).

Target Fortification With Liquid Fortifier

Macronutrient intakes achieved by using commercially available human milk based liquid fortifiers were also investigated. Different from powdered fortifiers, all liquid fortifiers inherently

TABLE 1 | Macronutrients added at recommended doses of fortifiers to obtain 100 mL of ready-to-feed breast milk, *g per portion, $^{\$}$kcal per portion (carbs, carbohydrates; LF, liquid fortifier).

Fortifier group	Standard multicomponent powdered fortifie							Optimized standard fortifier			Liquid fortifier based on human milk			
	Low-fat/high-carbs		Medium-fat/medium-carbs			High-fat/low-carbs								
Fortifier #	**1**	**2**	**3**	**4**	**5**	**6**	**7**	**8**	**9**	**10**	**11a**	**11b**	**11c**	**11d**
Ratio of LF: breast milk	–	–	–	–	–	–	–	–	–	–	20:80	30:70	40:60	50:50
Fat (g/100 mL)	0	0.02	0.72	0.36	0.7	0.7	1	0.77	0	0	1.8*	2.7*	3.6*	4.5*
Protein (g/100 mL)	1.1	1	1.4	1	1.3	1.5	1.1	1.85	1.54	1.26	1.2*	1.8*	2.4*	3*
Carbohydrates (g/100 mL)	2.7	3.3	1.3	1.8	1.5	0.01	0.4	2.13	0.99	0.45	1.8*	2.8*	3.6*	4.6*
Energy (kcal/100 mL)	15	18	17	14	17	13	14	23	10	7	28$^{\$}$	42$^{\$}$	56$^{\$}$	71$^{\$}$

TABLE 2 | Different schedules of target fortification analysis and recipe adjustment (BM—pooled native breast milk batch for 24 h feeding).

Approach		Monday BM batch	Tuesday BM batch	Wednesday BM batch	Thursday BM batch	Friday BM batch	Saturday BM batch	Sunday BM batch
1/week	Analysis	X						
	Recipe	Mo	Mo	Mo	Mo	Mo	Mo	Mo
2/week	Analysis	X			X			
	Recipe	Mo	Mo	Mo	Th	Th	Th	Th
3/week	Analysis	X		X		X		
	Recipe	Mo	Mo	We	We	Fr	Fr	Fr
5/week	Analysis	X	X	X	X	X		
	Recipe	Mo	Tu	We	Th	Fr	Fr	Fr
7/week	Analysis	X	X	X	X	X	X	X
	Recipe	Mo	Tu	We	Th	Fr	Sa	Su

"X" indicates the day of milk analysis. Same colors indicate the same recipe for target fortification.

will replace a specific volume of native breast milk. For example, for a final feeding volume of 100 mL, 20 mL of fortifier product will be added to 80 mL breast milk. To achieve higher strengths of fortification the ratio of fortifier-to-breast milk needs to be increased (from 20:80 to 30:70, 40:60, or 50:50 v/v e.g.). In this study, four different fortifier strengths were studied consisting of the following composition per 100 ml of ready-to-feed-batches: 20 mL (fortifier 11a), 30 mL (fortifier 11b), 40 mL (fortifier 11c), and 50 mL (fortifier 11d). All four different liquid fortifier products contain identical macronutrient concentrations (g/mL). The 10 mL- increase in the volume ratio of fortifier to breast milk leads to an incremental increase in protein by ~0.6 g, fat by ~0.9 g, and carbohydrates by ~1.0 g per 10 mL of fortifier.

The following approaches were applied and referred to as fortifier 11 in the analyses: (1) Standard fortification with liquid fortifier: an average protein content of 1.2 g/100 mL in native breast milk was assumed. Fortifier 11b (30:70 v/v ratio) which increases the protein content by 1.8 g/100 mL was chosen as reference fortifier because it represents the fortifier which is most frequently used in clinical routine. (2) For target fortification: Breast milk analysis was performed and the extra protein content needed to reach 3 g/100 mL was calculated. Based on the analysis, the fortifier (11a to 11d) was chosen that was most appropriate to reach the protein target range of 2.8–3.4 g/100 mL. In the final step, fat and carbohydrate content—if below target—were adjusted by adding single component modular products to meet ESPGHAN recommended intake (20).

Off-Label Use of Liquid Fortifier for Target Fortification

Switching between the four different strengths of the HM based liquid fortifiers (11a, 11b, 11c, and 11d) will lead to stepwise increase of protein and macronutrients intake. To allow a more continuous increase fortifiers were dosed in an off-label approach to achieve ESPGHAN recommendations. This approach is categorized as fortifier 12.

For this off-label approach, target fortification was performed by measuring breast milk macronutrient content and native breast milk batches were adjusted to final target protein concentration of 3 g/100 mL. For native breast milk with a protein content of ≥1.8 g/100 mL, liquid fortifier 11a was used as a 20: 80 ratio (i.e., ratio of fortifier: native BM). For native breast milk with a protein content of ≥1.2 to 1.8, the liquid fortifier was 11a was used as the base component and fortifier 11b was added to reach a protein content of 3 g/100 mL. In this case, the ratio between the volume of fortifier 11a and 11b was 2:3 or, as expressed in volume referred to a ready to feed volume of 100 mL, 20 ml of fortifier 11a would be replaced by 15 ml of fortifier 11b, consequently, the volume of native milk needs to be reduced by this amount. For native breast milk with a protein content of ≥0.6 to <1.2 g/100 mL, fortifier 11b constituted the base fortifier and fortifier 11c was added in a ratio of 3:4. For native breast milk with a protein content of ≥0 to <0.6 g/100 mL, fortifier 11c formed the base component and fortifier 11d was added in a ratio of 4:5 (**Figure 3**).

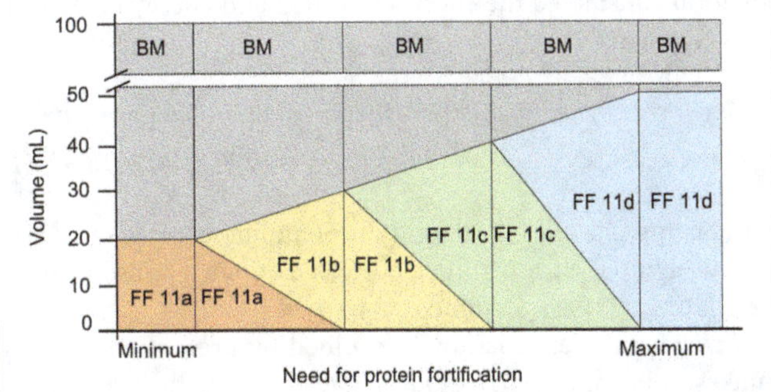

FIGURE 3 | Off-label approach for target fortification with liquid fortifier based on the need of protein fortification in native breast milk (BM, breast milk; FF, fortifier).

After target fortification of protein, the final step of adjusting fat to 4.4 g/100 mL and carbs to 8.8 g/100 mL was performed using modular products.

Identification of Feeds With Insufficient Macronutrient Intake

Because of the natural intra- and interindividual variation of breast milk macronutrient composition standard fortification (i.e., without milk analysis) will always result in over- or under-fortification of a significant number of breast milk samples. To investigate the magnitude of this inherent weakness feeds with inappropriate macronutrient composition shall be identified applying principles of nutritional physiology. Levels of all three macronutrients and energy as well as ratios of protein-to-energy as well as carbohydrate energy-to-non-protein energy were incorporated into an established prediction equation for growth velocity (33–35). Feeds resulting in growth deviating for more than 1 g/kg/d from expected target weight gain velocity would be considered as inappropriate (33–35). To calculate the daily growth of the study infants depending on the nutritional intake routine feeding volumes of 150 mL/kg/d were assumed and the weight gain velocity was calculated per body weight (g/kg body weight per day).

Two nutritional physiological approaches were considered. The base equation was derived from Kashyap et al. (35). This equation considered the effects of protein and energy on growth rates (Equation 1).

$$\textit{weight gain velocity} = 0.095 \cdot \textit{energy intake} + 3.6 \cdot \textit{protein intake} - 0.00468 \cdot BW + 1.699 \quad (1)$$

with energy intake as [kcal/kg/d], protein intake as [g/kg/d] and birth weight (BW) as (g). For our calculations a constant birth weight of 1,000 g was assumed.

Growth rates are mainly determined by protein and energy intakes, but nutritional studies have shown that variations of the carbohydrate-to-non-protein energy ratio significantly modulate growth rates (33, 34). This impact is quantified by using a metabolic factor given in Equation (2). The equation was obtained from regression analysis performed on previously published growth data of preterm infants fed with same amount of protein and calories, however with different carbohydrate to non-protein energy ratios (33, 34). Combining both equations into one leads to Equation (3) combining the impact of all three macronutrients on weight gain

$$\textit{Metabolic factor} = 0.7757 + \left(0.47 \cdot \frac{\textit{Carbs energy}}{\textit{NPE energy}}\right) \quad (2)$$

$$\textit{Target weight gain velocity} = \left(0.095 \cdot \textit{Energy intake} + 3.6 \cdot \textit{Protein intake} - 0.00468 \cdot BW + 1.699\right) \cdot \left(0.7757 + \left(0.47 \cdot \frac{\textit{Carbs energy}}{\textit{NPE energy}}\right)\right) \quad (3)$$

Target weight gain velocity was defined using (Equation 3) thereby assuming ESPGHAN recommended intakes for an infant with a body weight of 1,000 g (4.5 g/150 mL protein, 6.6 g/150 mL fat, and 13.2 g/150 mL carbohydrate), the target weight gain velocity was defined. Macronutrient composition of single feeds was considered as "inadequate" if the estimated weight gain velocity was >1 g/kg/d above or below the target weight.

Human milk based liquid fortifiers were not included in this analysis due to insufficient reference data. Additionally, the fat phase from human milk might have different physiological effects when compared with fat in formula (36).

Optimization of Macronutrient Content in Native Breast Milk to Reduce the Variation

Simulation of Selection and Combination of Specific Native Breast Milk Samples

To investigate whether the natural variation of breast milk can be reduced, pairs of breast milk samples from the same mother with matching macronutrient content shall be pooled. Length of pooling intervals was set to alternating between $n = 6$ and $n = 8$ days (~1 week) to allow paired matching. The interval length was chosen assuming a minimum number of frozen milk samples during the major part of a NICU stay available to prepare feedings. Within each group BM samples were sorted by one macronutrient (either fat, protein, carbs) or by energy content in ascending order. Assuming identical volumes (e.g., 100 mL), as a next step two or three samples were pooled using two different approaches:

(i) *Averaging macronutrient by combining breast milk samples with high and low macronutrient content:* According to the selected macronutrient, pairs of samples (the highest and the lowest value, the second highest and second lowest, proceeding continuously) were pooled. Pooled samples were split into two of equal volume.

(ii) *Combining breast milk samples with the highest macronutrient content:* The three samples containing the highest amounts of the selected macronutrient were mixed and divided into equal samples containing a volume of 100 mL each. The remaining three or five batches were not included into further analysis (see discussion).

The content and variation of fat, protein, carbohydrates, and energy were calculated for each of the resulting batches.

Random Milk Pooling to Reduce the Variation of Macronutrients

This simulation addresses the question whether random pooling of native breast milk samples will be able to reduce the variability of macronutrients and, if so, which would be the most efficient set size. For this purpose, a defined number of native breast milk batches were randomly drawn from the original data set of 3,338 batches, were pooled and the resulting content of protein, fat, and carbohydrates was calculated. For any given set size, this step of random allocation was repeated 1,000 times and mean and SD were calculated to serve as an estimate of the most likely distribution of nutrient contents after pooling. Set size started at $n = 1$ and was increased up to $n = 996$ with increments of $n = 5$. Cut-off criterium for efficiency was the minimum set size needed to reduce protein content below 10% variability.

Optimizing Macronutrient Content by Lyophilization (Freeze-Drying)

This simulation uses partial lyophilization to up-concentrate the breast milk content. Separate analyses were done for protein, fat, and carbohydrates as the leading macronutrient to determine

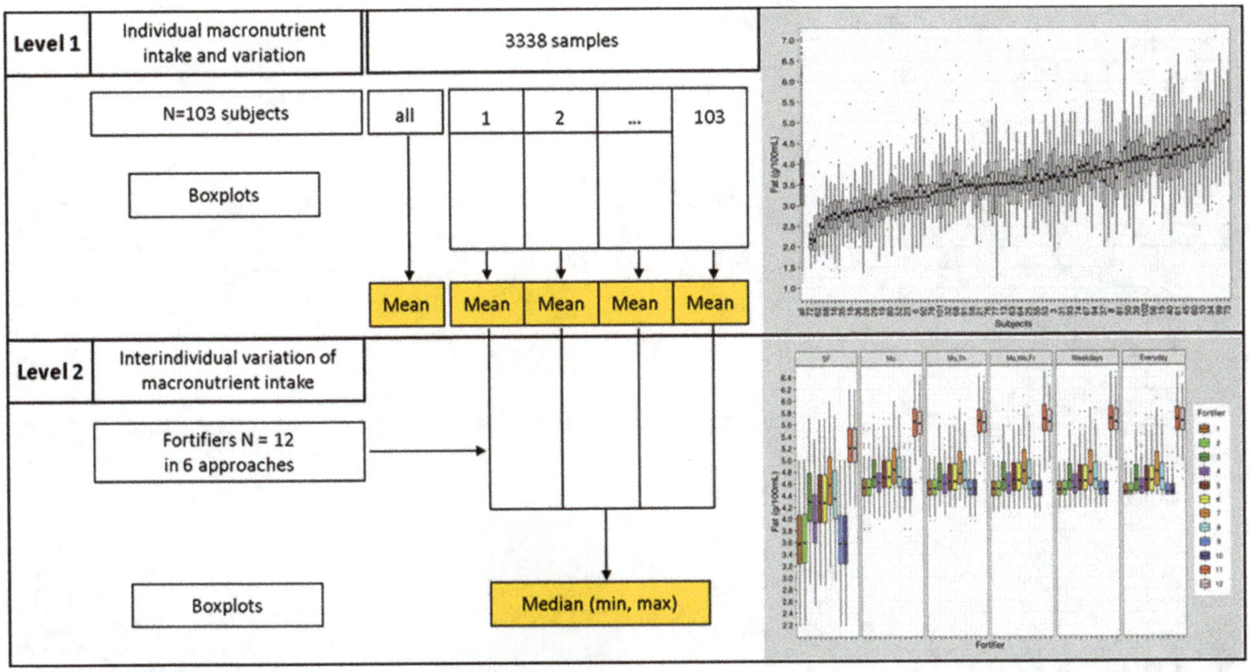

FIGURE 4 | Statistical analyses process; Level 1 analysis—presentation of individual data, Level 2 analysis—inter-individual comparison.

the amount of water to be removed to meet ESPGHAN recommendations at a h feeding volume of 150 mL/kg/d (20). Up-concentrated compositions of the other two macronutrients were calculated using the "new" hydration factor.

Statistics

Descriptive statistics for the macronutrient content of native breast milk and the different approaches to target fortification were calculated using R version 3.5.3 (2019-03-11, R Development Core Team 2019).

Level 1 analysis analyzed individual data. For each subject ($n = 103$), mean, standard deviation, median, interquartile range, quantile distance $Q_{0.1}$-$Q_{0.9}$, and boxplots were calculated (**Figure 4**).

Level 2 analysis employed an interindividual analysis. Results from "Level 1 analysis" were used to assess interindividual differences (**Figure 4**). Level 2 analysis compared and evaluated means and quantile distances from each subject ($n = 103$) of the "Level 1 analysis." Boxplots and descriptive statistics were generated.

RESULTS

Native Breast Milk Analysis and Description

Overall, the fat, protein, and lactose content of native breast milk showed high inter- and intra-individual variation and a high range of macronutrient content or composition (**Table 3**).

At the intra-individual level, native breast milk samples from the same mother were also found to vary in macronutrient composition (**Figure 5**). Boxplots depicting infant macronutrient content were sorted in ascending order of the subject's median fat, protein, and lactose content. The order of subject IDs was found to be different between the three macronutrients (**Figure 5**). This suggests that fat, protein and lactose content were not correlated with one another. For instance, mothers who had breast milk with high levels of fat did not necessarily have high protein or lactose content in their milk.

In addition to the variation in median macronutrients, the range of macronutrient content was also highly variable between individuals. Independent of the median macronutrient concentration, breast milk samples with low median protein content could have large interquartile ranges, while breast milk samples with high median

TABLE 3 | Macronutrient content of $n = 3{,}338$ native breast milk samples from $n = 103$ subjects.

	Mean ± *SD*	Range
Fat (g/100 mL)	3.6 ± 0.9	1.5–7
Protein (g/100 mL)	1.1 ± 0.3	0.3–2.5
Lactose (g/100 mL)	6.7 ± 0.8	4.0–9.0
Energy (kcal/100 mL)	64 ± 9	40–95
Protein:Energy (g/100 kcal)	1.8 ± 0.4	0.8–3.3
Carbs/NPE (%)	46 ± 7	25–70

Carbs, carbohydrate; NPE, non-protein energy; Carbs/NPE, carbohydrate energy/carbohydrate energy + fat energy.

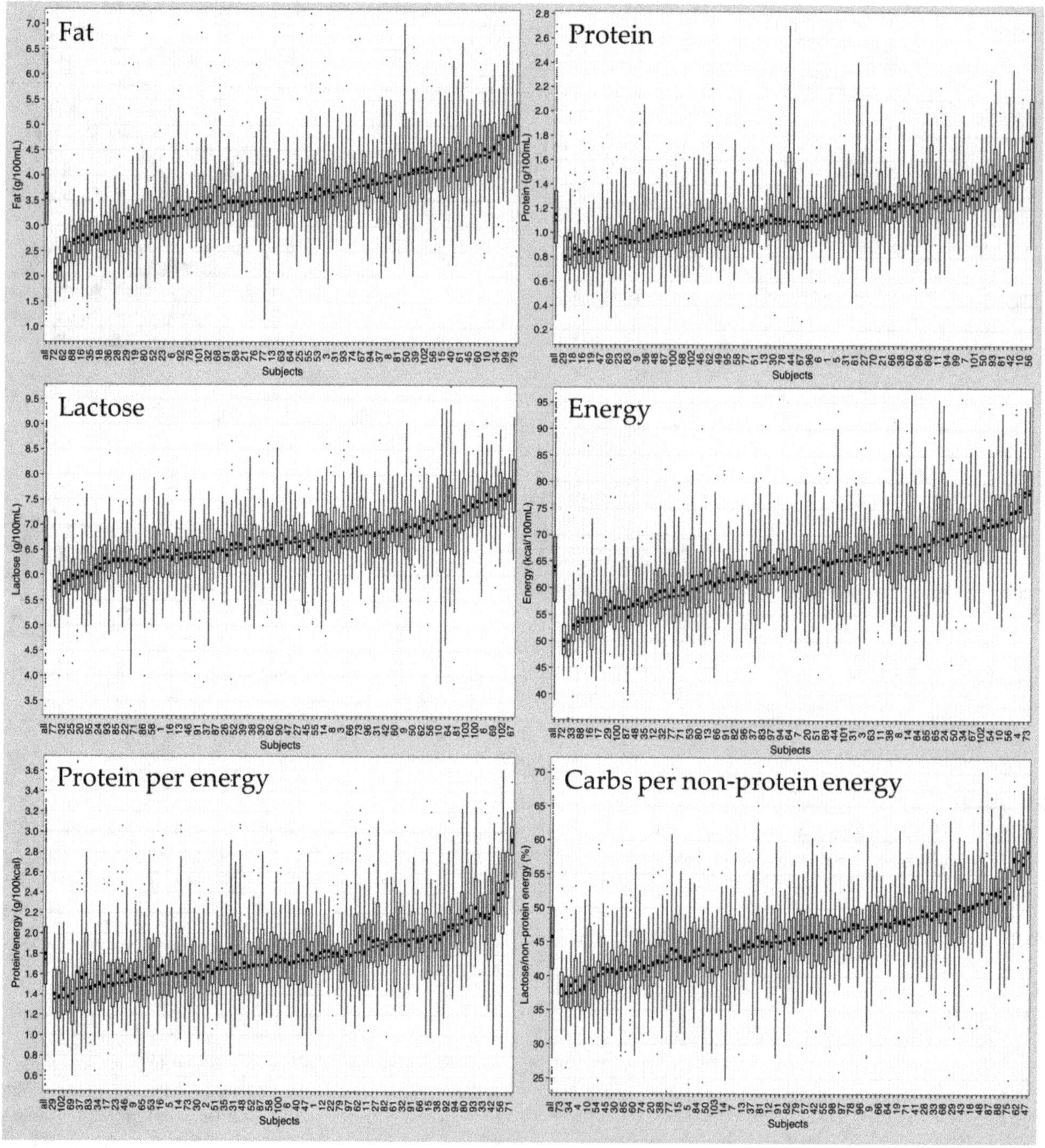

FIGURE 5 | Composition of native breast milk presented in ascending order of median nutrient content per subject. Boxplots display median values of all subjects (left boxplot) and of individual subjects (103 boxplots). Circles represent mean values, dots represent outliers.

protein content could show small interquartile ranges or vice versa.

Moreover, the high variation was also observed in calculated parameters like "Protein to Energy Ratio" and "Carbohydrate Energy per Non-Protein Energy" (**Supplementary Tables 1, 2**).

Commercially Available Multicomponent Standard Fortifier (Fortifier 1–7 and 11)

Standard fortified breast milk. Overall, all commercially available standard fortifiers did not meet recommended nutrient intakes for preterm infants (**Figure 6**). In most cases, the protein content

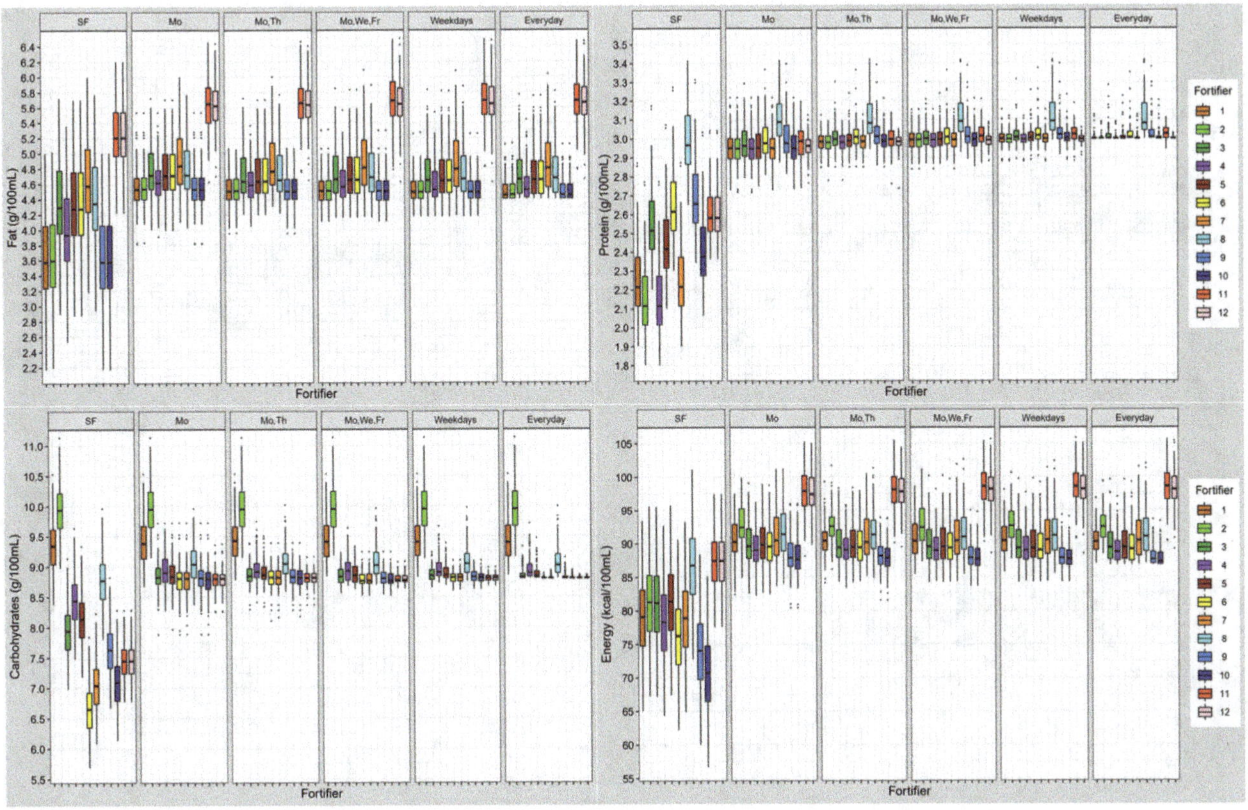

FIGURE 6 | Macronutrient (fat, protein, carbohydrates) and energy content of fortified breast milk with 12 fortifiers using different schedules for milk analysis. Boxplots display the distribution of the mean intake of $n = 103$ subjects. Dots represent outliers (SF, standard fortification; Mo, Monday; We, Wednesday; Th, Thursday; Fr, Friday; SF, fortifier 11 and 12 are identical due to following standard fortification protocol).

was below the target (median of 2.1–2.6 g/100 mL instead of 3.0 g/100 mL). For fat and carbohydrate levels results were dependent from the type of fortifier used. For low-fat/high-carbohydrates fortifiers (fortifiers #1 and #2) breast milk batches ended up with median fat levels below 3.6 g/100 mL, and with median carbohydrate levels from 9.3 to 9.9 g/100 mL thus exceeding ESPGHAN recommendations. For medium-fat/medium-carbohydrate fortifiers (fortifiers #3, #4, and #5), median fat and carbohydrate contents were in the range of the recommended intake, however, a significant number of batches still had insufficient carbohydrate content In the high-fat/low-carbohydrates group (fortifiers #6 and #7), median fat content exceeded recommendations (4.3–4.6 g/100 mL), while median carbohydrate content ranged between 6.7 and 7.1 g/100 mL. i.e., below the recommendations (**Figure 7**). Median energy intake as well as protein to energy ratio (P:E ratio) were also below the targets. The percentage of carbohydrate energy per non-protein energy (Carbs/NPE) was lowest in the high-fat/low-carbs group (fortifiers #6 and #7) (**Table 4**). Further details are presented in the **Supplementary Figures 1, 3.**

When using the liquid fortifier (#11b), the median fat content exceeded the recommended intake by ~0.8 g/100 mL (**Figure 6**) while median protein (2.6 g/100 mL) and carbohydrate (7.5 g/100 mL) content were close to ESPGHAN recommendations. However, the median energy content (88 kcal/100 mL) was higher compared to standard powder fortified breast milk (76–81 kcal/100 mL).

Overall, breast milk standard fortified with fortifier 11 still showed a high individual variation of macronutrients. The individual variation (Quantile range $Q_{0.1}$-$Q_{0.9}$) was 0.6 g/100 mL for protein, 1.5 g/100 mL for fat, 1.3 g/100 mL for carbohydrates, and 15 kcal/100 mL for energy. Due to the volume displacement, the use of liquid fortifier (#11b) decreased the variation of macronutrients (protein: 0.4; fat: 1.1; carbohydrates: 0.9 g/100 mL; and energy: 11 kcal/100 mL) when compared to powdered fortifiers (**Figure 7**).

Optimized Standard Fortifier (Fortifiers #8, #9, and #10)

Using the macronutrient data obtained from all 3,338 breast milk samples, the optimum composition of a standard fortifier for three given measurement schedules (none vs. once vs. three times per week) was calculated (fortifier 8–10). For all three measurement schedules final macronutrient content of breast milk batches fortified with the corresponding optimized fortifier were then computed (**Table 1**). Macronutrient composition was found to be different for each of the three optimized fortifiers. Fortifier 8 (standard fortification, no measurements) had the

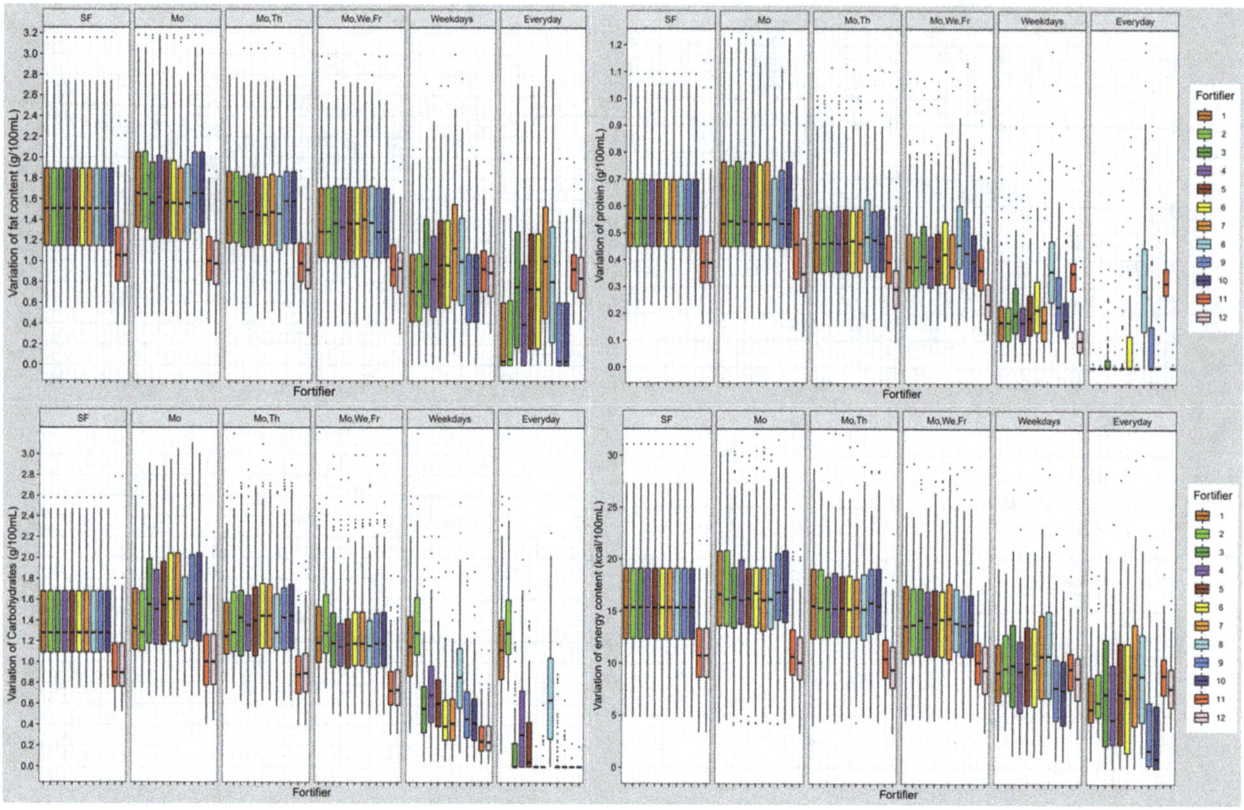

FIGURE 7 | Variation of macronutrient (fat, protein, carbohydrates) and energy content in fortified breast milk using 12 fortifiers with different schedules for milk analysis. Boxplots show the distribution of quantile distances ($Q_{0.1}$-$Q_{0.9}$) of n = 103 subjects (SF, standard fortification; Mo, Monday; We, Wednesday; Th, Thursday; Fr, Friday).

TABLE 4 | Energy ratio of standard fortified breast milk (median) compared to ESPGHAN recommendation achieved with *150 mL/kg/d milk intake, carbs, carbohydrate; P:E ratio, protein to energy ratio; Carbs/NPE, carbohydrate energy per non-protein energy.

	ESPGHAN targets	Standard fortifier by non-protein composition		
		Low-fat/high-carbs	Medium-fat/medium-carbs	High-fat/low-carbs
Energy (kcal)*	130	119–122	117–122	114–119
P:E ratio (g/100 kcal)	3.5	2.6–2.8	2.7–3.2	2.8–3.5
Carbs/NPE (%)	47	54–55	45–49	41

highest macronutrient and energy content (fat 0.8 g, protein 1.9 g, carbs 2.1 g, energy 23 kcal) and on average provided ESPGHAN recommended intakes. However, intra- and interindividual variation of standard fortified breast milk remained unchanged compared to that of native breast milk. As a result, many breast milk batches had macronutrient compositions that were above or below recommendations or had unbalanced ratios, i.e., P:E or carbohydrate-to-non-protein-energy.

Fortifiers 9 and 10 shall serve as base fortifiers for target fortification with either one measurement per week or 3 measurements per week, respectively. Macronutrient levels decreased with increasing measurement frequency. Interestingly, they did not require the addition of fat. Since fat content was highly variable and exceeded recommendations in a significant number of breast milk batches routinely adding more fat seems to be quite unreasonable. As a consequence of this approach, administering any extra fat by single macronutrient modular is not required in ~40% of the feeds. Compared to fortifier 9, fortifier 10 added lower amounts of protein (1.3 vs. 1.5 g) and carbohydrates (0.5 vs. 1.0 g).

Target Fortified Breast Milk

Overall, target fortification was able to achieve ESPGHAN recommended intakes. Target fortification based on just one breast milk analysis per week provided a median macronutrient intake that met recommended levels. However, some residual day-to-day variation remained. A clinically significant reduction

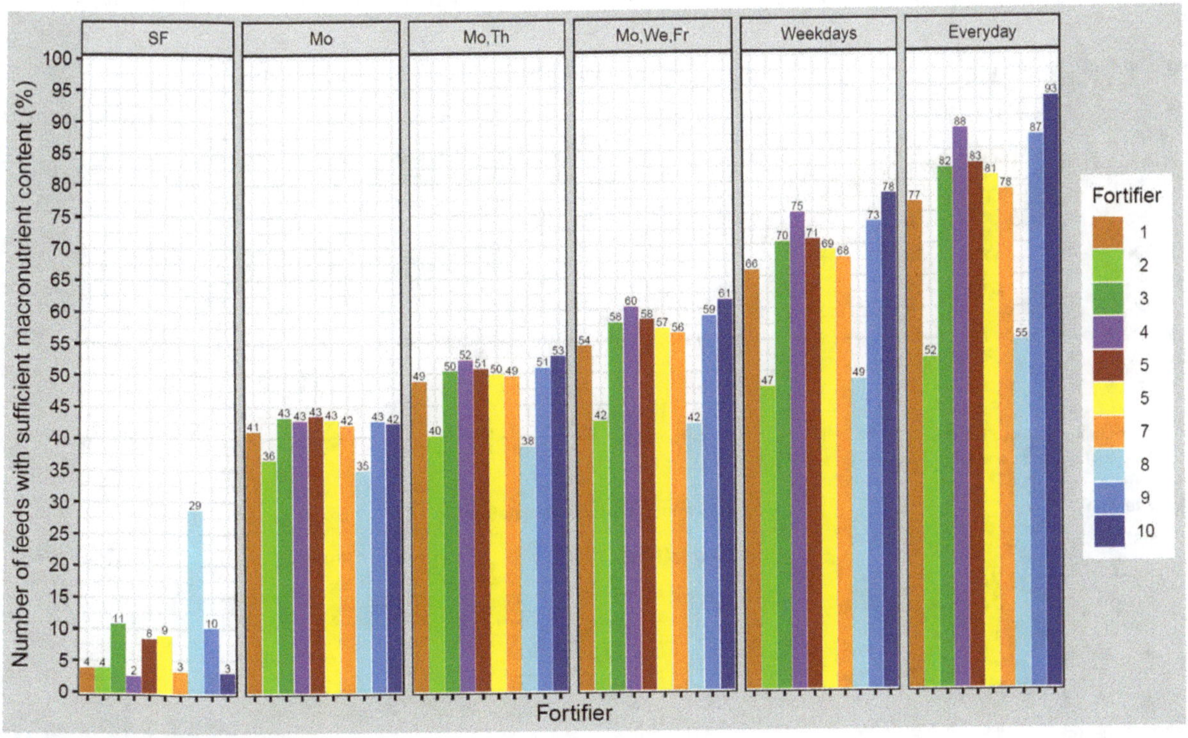

FIGURE 8 | Percentage of feeds with appropriate macronutrient content to achieve growth rates in a range of ±1.0 g/kg/d from estimated target weight gain velocities. Ten different fortifiers in six different scenarios/schedules to measure breast milk macronutrient content were studied (SF, standard fortification; Mo, Monday; We, Wednesday; Th, Thursday; Fr, Friday). The number of fortifiers refers to **Table 1**.

in macronutrient variation was found when target fortification was based on three or more measurements per week (**Figure 7**).

Target fortification using low-fat/high-carbohydrate standard fortifiers (fortifiers #1 and #2) led to some milk samples exceeding the recommended carbohydrate content without extra modular macronutrients being added, while the use of high-fat/low-carbs fortifiers (fortifiers #6 and #7) resulted in fat levels that exceeded recommendations. In these samples target fortification was not able to reduce the macronutrient variation as well as to achieve recommended intakes. The fortifier optimized for three measurements (fortifiers #10) came the closest to ESPGHAN recommended intakes for three or more measurements. The highest precision and accuracy of nutrient intake was reached with daily measurements.

The use of the liquid fortifier (#11) led to median fat (5.6 g/100 mL) and energy (97 kcal/100 mL) levels that were above the recommended intake. The use of liquid fortifier also reduced the variability of macronutrient content due to volume displacement [see also last paragraph of chapter Commercially Available Multicomponent Standard Fortifier (Fortifier 1–7 and 11)] One measurement per week for target fortification achieved a lower variation when compared with powdered fortifiers.

Detailed data about energy intake, protein per energy ratio as well as carbohydrate energy per non-protein energy are presented in **Supplementary Figures 2–4**.

Assessment of Achieved Macronutrient Intake at Standardized Tolerance Range

In a next step, we were aiming to evaluate the quality of nutrient supply provided by the different fortification regimes. For this purpose, rather than assess the quality of each single nutrient intake separately, we focused on the effect of the composite intake on growth. Growth is a function of the intake of all three macronutrients therefore we applied an established growth model to estimate ELBW infant growth rates assuming a fixed intake of 150 mL/kg/d for all fortification approaches (20, 33–35). Growth rates achieved by ESPGHAN recommended intakes were considered to be the reference data.

Applying standard fortification, most samples led to growth rates below the defined tolerance range of ±1 g/kg/d. The optimized standard fortifier, i.e., no breast milk analysis (fortifier 8) lead to adequate growth in about 30% of the feeds. Using target fortification, a higher number of fortified batches met the tolerance range as the number of measurements per week increased. About 40% were inside the growth range when applying one measurement per week. The percentage of appropriately fortified samples increased in increments of ~10% along with the number of measurements per week. The highest accuracy hit the optimized fortifier with one (fortifier 9) or three (fortifier 10) measurements per week of 87–93% (**Figure 8**).

TABLE 5 | Reduction of variation of fat in native breast milk samples of $n = 103$ subjects, when matching native breast milk batches containing the highest and the lowest macronutrient content, the second highest and the second lowest values, proceeding continuously were combined.

Matching criterium	Variation of macronutrient content in batched native breast milk			
	Fat (g/100 mL)	Protein (g/100 mL)	Lactose (g/100 mL)	Energy (kcal/100 mL)
None	1.5 (0.5, 3.4)	0.6 (0.2, 1.6)	1.3 (0.7, 4.0)	15 (5, 31)
Fat	0.7 (0.5, 1.0)	0.4 (0.3, 0.6)	1.0 (0.8, 1.2)	7.8 (6.2, 10.2)
Protein	1.0 (0.8, 1.4)	0.3 (0.2, 0.5)	0.9 (0.8, 1.2)	10.7 (8.8, 13.9)
Lactose	1.1 (0.8, 1.4)	0.4 (0.3, 0.6)	0.6 (0.5, 0.8)	10.8 (8.2, 14.3)
Energy	0.8 (0.6, 1.0)	0.4 (0.3, 0.6)	0.9 (0.8, 1.2)	7.4 (5.2, 9.9)

Data show median and interquartiles of ranges $Q_{0.1}$-$Q_{0.9}$ (quantile) (level 2 analysis). Colors highlight the effect of matching on the selected macronutrient compared with native breast milk, yellow - fat, red - protein, green - lactose, blue - energy.

TABLE 6 | Increase of the macronutrient content in native breast milk samples of $n = 103$ subjects, breast milk samples were selected in groups of 6 or 8 consecutive samples and ordered by either energy, fat, protein, and lactose content.

Matching criterium	Macronutrient content in native breast milk batches			
	Fat (g/100 mL)	Protein (g/100 mL)	Lactose (g/100 mL)	Energy (g/100 mL)
None	3.5 (3.0, 4.1)	1.1 (0.9, 1.3)	6.7 (6.2, 7.2)	63 (57, 70)
Fat	4.1 (3.6, 4.6)	1.2 (1.1, 1.3)	6.6 (6.3, 7.0)	69 (64, 73)
Protein	3.7 (3.3, 4.2)	1.3 (1.1, 1.4)	6.6 (6.3, 6.9)	65 (62, 71)
Lactose	3.6 (3.1, 4.1)	1.1 (1.0, 1.3)	7.0 (6.7, 7.4)	65 (60, 70)
Energy	4.0 (3.6, 4.6)	1.2 (1.1, 1.3)	6.8 (6.4, 7.1)	69 (64, 73)

Samples containing the three highest values were combined. Values present median and interquartiles (Q_{25}, Q_{75}) of mean macronutrient of native breast milk (Level 2 analysis). Colors highlight the effect of matching on the selected macronutrient compared with native breast milk, yellow - fat, red - protein, green - lactose, blue - energy.

Optimization of Macronutrient Content in Native Breast Milk to Reduce the Variation

Selection and Combination of Specific Native Breast Milk Samples

Combining samples with opposite extremes [see Methods section Simulation of Selection and Combination of Specific Native Breast Milk Samples (i)] based on one macronutrient (fat, protein, or lactose) or on energy resulted in a decrease in variation of more than 50% for the selected macronutrient, while the other macronutrients showed a smaller decrease in variation. When samples were combined according to energy content, the variation for fat, protein and carbohydrates decreased by 47, 33, and 31%, respectively (**Table 5**).

For the second approach, i.e., pooling breast milk samples with the highest content of either protein or carbohydrates or fat [see Methods section Simulation of Selection and Combination of Specific Native Breast Milk Samples (ii)] increased the selected macronutrient content by 9–15%. However, when ordered by energy or fat, the average macronutrient intake improved for the other macronutrients by 9–13% (**Table 6**). This approach showed only a minimal reduction in macronutrient variation (data not shown).

Simulation of a Milk Bank Setting by Pooling Native Breast Milk

Pooling of at least 150 random breast milk samples is needed to reduce the variation of macronutrients to below ±10% (~0.3 g). **Figure 9** shows the effects on the variation of fat. Similar effects were observed for protein, carbohydrates, and energy (**Supplementary Figure 5**).

Optimizing Macronutrient Content by Partial Lyophilization (Freeze-Drying)

Various factors for partial lyophilization were tested by up-concentrating native breast milk samples to achieve recommended ESPGHAN intakes for macronutrients and energy (**Table 7**). No lyophilization factor (i.e., hydration factor) could be identified which would achieve recommended levels for all macronutrients in individual batches by using native breast milk. When protein is adjusted to the target level, fat and carbohydrate intakes will be by far too high (energy content of 262 kcal/100 mL). When carbohydrate levels are adjusted to target levels, fat intake will be too high whereas protein intakes would be too low.

DISCUSSION

This study confirms the presence of considerable intra- and inter-individual variation of native breast milk composition with no relationship between macronutrients. This challenges the ability of fortification strategies to achieve recommended intakes. While standard fortification with fixed doses increases the macronutrient content of native breast milk, it does not reduce its variation and the associated risk of unbalanced intakes. Only target fortification, based on at least two breast milk analyses per week in combination with an optimized standard

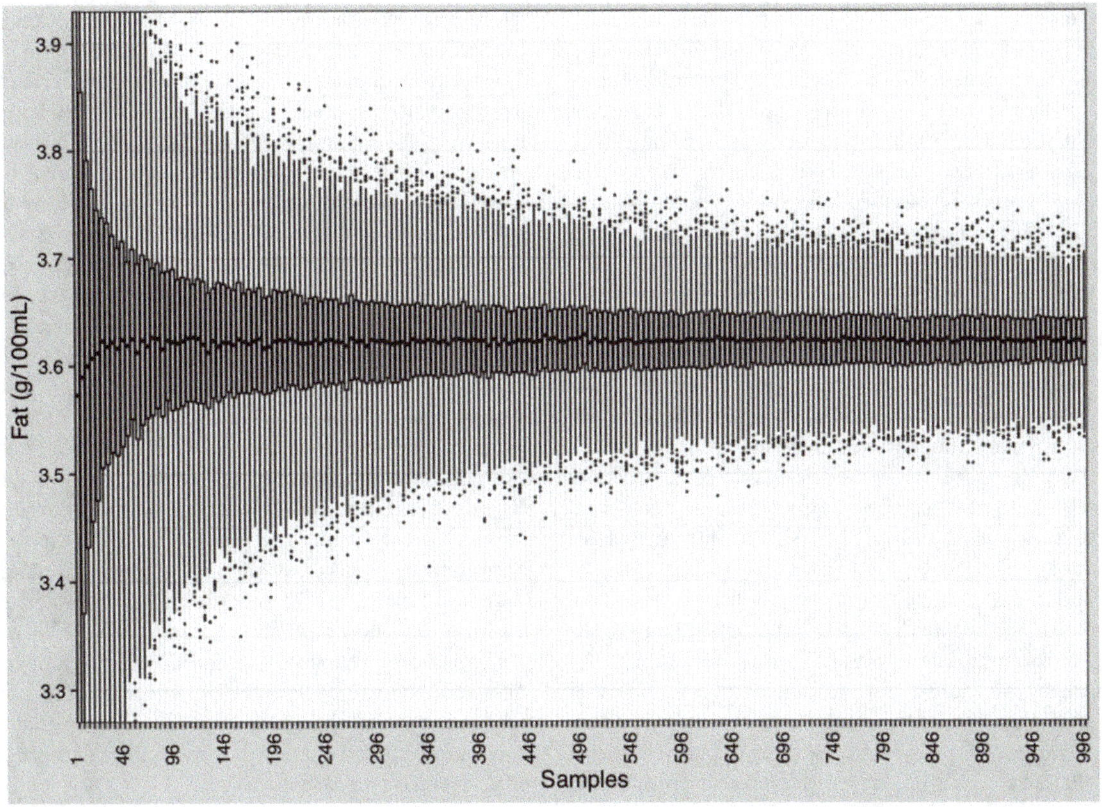

FIGURE 9 | Reduction of the variation of macronutrients and energy in native breast milk. Randomly selection and batching of breast milk samples by stepwise increase from 1 to 996 samples in increments of 5. Each step was repeated 1,000 times and mean and standard deviation were calculated.

TABLE 7 | Macronutrient levels in native breast milk (BM) in 150 mL fluid intake.

	Lyophilization factor	Final macronutrient level			
		Fat (g)**	**Protein (g)****	**Carbs (g)****	**Energy (kcal)****
Native breast milk/ESPGHAN	1.0	5.4	1.7	10.1	96
Target macronutrient per kg/d					
Fat [6.6 g*]	1.2	6.6	2.0	12.3	117
Protein [4.5 g*]	2.7	14.7	4.5	27.4	262
Carbs [13.2 g*]	1.3	7.1	2.2	13.2	126
Energy 135 [kcal*]	1.4	7.6	2.3	14.1	135

Recommended nutritional intake based on ESPGHAN guidelines reached applying freeze-drying by required lyophilization factor. BM, breast milk; carbs, carbohydrates. A green cell indicates the parameter used for adjustment.

**Target intake per kg per day.*

***Amount per 150 mL breast milk.*

Blue—values below ESPGHAN targets for macronutrient content, red—values above targets, and green—within targets.

fortifier (fortifiers #9, #10), was able to provide macronutrient intakes that adhered to the recommendations of nutritional committees (20).

Evaluation of milk analysis of 3,338 samples and eight commercially available fortifier shows that standard fortified breast milk meets nutritional requirements as suggested by ESPGHAN in <12% of all feeds. Based on our data, we suggest a "new" optimized standard fortifier in order to meet these recommendations [see chapter Optimized Standard Fortifier (fortifiers #8, #9, and #10)]. The composition of this fortifier differs from current commercially available fortifiers. The optimized fortifier increases the number of appropriately fortified batches; however, 70% of feeds will still have a more or less unbalanced composition of fat, protein, or carbohydrates. In conclusion, standard fortification is not suited to reduce the significant macronutrient variation of breast milk for all preterm infants, and instead transfers the degree of imbalance to higher macronutrient levels (27, 30, 37). It is of interest to note that liquid fortifiers, as opposed to powdered fortifiers, will reduce macronutrient variation: replacement of up to 50% of the volume of breast milk using a fortifier with defined composition will reduce the natural variability to the same degree.

Target fortification reduces the high macronutrient variation of standard fortified breast milk and improves deficient macronutrient content depending on the frequency of native breast milk measurements per week: one measurement per week will allow fortified breast milk to reach the average recommended macronutrient intake, although some intra-individual variation remained. Two or more measurements per week decrease the variation significantly. The best performance was achieved by daily measurements, however, with significantly increased clinical workload. This finding is comparable to our recently published randomized controlled trial, which also suggested to perform two or more weekly breast milk measurements to meet recommended macronutrient intakes and reduce variation (27).

The efficiency of target fortification depends on the composition of the standard product used as base fortifier (**Figure 1**). Target fortification reduces macronutrient deficiencies in breast milk by adding modular macronutrient products to standard fortified breast milk based on breast milk analysis. However, target fortification cannot reduce a macronutrient that exceeds target levels already after standard fortification as observed for lactose and fat (see **Figure 6**; lactose: fortifier #1 and #2; fat: fortifier #6, #7, and #8). This has important implications for the nutrient profile of standard fortifiers used in clinical scenarios with target fortification. All commercially available standard fortifiers add between 1 and 1.5 g protein to 100 mL of human milk which rarely leads to protein levels above target leaving room for fine-tuning by adding extra protein. However, their impact on fat, carbohydrate, and eventually energy levels is less consistent because their non-protein composition is quite heterogeneous. Basically, commercially available standard fortifiers can be classified into (i) low-fat/high-carbohydrate, (ii) medium-fat/medium-carbs, or (iii) high-fat/low-carbohydrate containing products. Hence, each group of fortifiers presents a different likelihood for inadequate or excessive intake of macronutrients. Fortifiers with medium-fat/medium-carbs composition provide the most balanced results. In many samples, high-fat/low-carbs fortifiers achieved fat levels above the recommended intake and low carbs levels, whereas low-fat/high-carbs fortifiers provided carbs levels above the recommendations and low-fat intakes (**Figure 6**).

In this present study, we propose an optimized composition for base fortifiers to reach recommended intakes with feeding volumes of 150 mL/kg/d of milk for most of the batches. The macronutrient composition of these optimized base fortifiers was different if developed for standard (no analysis) or for target (one to three analyses per week) fortification. Neither base fortifier for target fortification should contain fat. Additionally, the composition of the base fortifier for target fortification was determined by the frequency of breast milk analyses. With three measurements per week, the optimized base fortifier had a lower macronutrient content than the fortifier based on one measurement per week. In an individualized approach with more frequent measurements such lower macronutrient levels are needed to prevent overfortification of native breast milk. Conversely, deficient samples will be corrected by individually adding modular single macronutrient products. In an ideal scenario, milk analysis and adjustment by target fortification would occur daily. Hence, the development of a general base fortifier for target fortification would be oriented to adequately fortify samples with higher macronutrient levels (as this is already the case for protein) and thus contain rather low amounts of non-protein components. Besides that base fortifiers would also focus on the important role to provide preterm infants with micronutrients, electrolytes, vitamins, phosphate, and trace elements. The required fine-tuning with macronutrients (fat, protein, carbs), could then individually be made by single macronutrient modulars only according to the breast milk analysis. Consequently, a modern fortification concept for use in clinical routine would aim to standardize intake on the basis of a biologically valuable base liquid with random composition effect by applying real-time component analysis followed by base fortification with (full) micro- and (partial) macronutrients using an optimized base fortifier plus fine-tuning with three modular for protein, fat and carbohydrates.

Our study demonstrated that the commercial liquid fortifier based on human milk provides higher amounts of fat than powdered standard fortifiers. Most of the samples fortified with the liquid fortifier had a higher fat content than recommended by ESPGHAN. However, from a nutritional point of view, the quality of fat from human milk sources cannot directly be compared to fat from non-human milk. The fat fraction of human milk has a particular composition and is constituted by specific fat globules. These fat globules contain glycerophospholipids, sphingolipids, cholesterol, and proteins (36, 38), which may serve as building blocks for cell membranes and cellular structures and also act as bioactive properties supporting the maturation of the gut and the immune system (36). Further, clinical studies have shown that preterm infants fed a human milk diet, containing human milk fat globules, demonstrate body composition, and neurodevelopmental outcomes comparable to term infants (39). While there seem to be benefits of an exclusive human milk diet for preterm infants, there are no studies that have compared the effects of fat derived from human milk to fat from non-human milk on growth and development of preterm infants.

In the present study we were able to show that selective batching of corresponding breast milk batches and/or up-concentrating by partial freeze drying are not appropriate to reduce the variation in the composition of breast milk and to meet the needs of preterm infants. Two main factors limit the effectiveness of these approaches. First, there is only a weak correlation between fat, protein, and carbs (30). Therefore, when breast milk is optimized for one macronutrient, the other two macronutrients may not necessarily reach recommended targets. Secondly, the ratio between macronutrients in native breast milk is different compared to the ratio resulting from adhering to recommendations for preterm infants. In native breast milk, the ratio for protein to fat is 1:3.2 and the ratio for protein to carbohydrates is 1:6.1, while nutritional guidelines suggest a ratio for protein to fat of 1:1.5 and for protein to carbohydrates of 1:2.9. Such differences cannot be overcome by simply up-concentrating batches.

These findings have implications for breast milk preparation. Our data show that on a large scale, like in a milk bank setting, batching of a high number of milk samples (>150) has a high likelihood of creating large volume batches with a similar composition and less macronutrient variation. However, even considering that our sample set might provide a higher variability due to early milk vs. mature milk that a milk bank would have in stock, batch sizes would exceed reasonable numbers. However, on an individual level, mixing, and batching of a small number of breast milk batches only from one mother is unlikely to make a difference of clinical significance. To attain an exclusively human milk diet from mother's own milk by freeze-drying is also infeasible: we were able to demonstrate that the lyophilized human milk concentrates generated in this study fail to provide recommended intakes. The degree of up-concentrating native breast milk to optimize protein intake would lead to a significant over-fortification (more than double) of fat and carbohydrates. Further, freeze-drying could negatively affect infant's intake of vitamins and micronutrients (40) and increase the concentration of environmental pollutants (41, 42).

This study suggests that individualized target fortification of breast milk is able to provide an adequate intake of nutrients at recommended intakes with reduced macronutrient variability. In contrast, current practice of standard fortification provides an uncertain, probably sometimes even unsafe intake of imprecisely defined amounts of macronutrients, unlike the administration of parenteral nutrition or medications which requires accurate dosage and where such practice of random composition would be considered as unacceptable. Unbalanced or excessively high or low intakes of macronutrients may only be recognized by growth failure or metabolic disturbances and hence there inherently is a delay in detection. However, an optimal macronutrient composition is needed to achieve desired body composition outcomes. Recent studies have demonstrated that optimized nutrition leads to higher percentages of fat free mass, which is associated with faster neuronal processing, larger brain size and improved motor development (43–46). Unbalanced macronutrient intake, or under- and over-fortification would result in suboptimal utilization of nutrients and increased risk for adverse long-term health and neurodevelopmental outcomes (33, 47–50).

Strengths of this study include the high number of breast milk batches and mothers ($n = 3{,}338$ of $n = 103$ subjects), the daily sample collection for a minimum period of 15 days during the NICU stay, and the use of validated methods to precisely measure macronutrient content of breast milk (28–31). Unlike other studies which often present total carbohydrates only (sum of lactose and oligosaccharides), we precisely measured lactose in breast milk using UPLC-MS-MS, allowing us to calculate energy intake without confounding by oligosaccharides. Further, we followed good clinical and laboratory practices guidelines (GCPL) for milk collection, storage, and analysis (28, 51). However, our study also had limitations. Based on the recommendations for macronutrient intake for ELBW infants (birth weight <1,000 g), we studied the achieved nutrient levels using different fortification approaches. However, VLBW infants (i.e., birth weight <1,500 g), intrauterine growth restriction or bronchopulmonary dysplasia may have different nutritional needs, but would be similarly affected by the natural variation of breast milk. Clinical studies are required to explore the effects of fortification approaches on growth for different groups of preterm infants. Another limitation of this study is that we collected milk samples from milk batches which were prepared for 24-h feedings as opposed to collecting samples from individual pumping sessions, which may show greater variation in macronutrient content. Our study did not include data about the quality of macronutrients (human milk protein vs. cow's milk protein), fat (human milk fat globules vs. oil from different sources), and carbs (lactose or glucose polymers). Approaches to reduce the macronutrient variation or improve macronutrient content were performed by theoretical calculation and did not consider the effects of sample preparation and workload. Further, we focused on macronutrients and did not consider micronutrients, vitamins, electrolytes, or trace elements.

CONCLUSIONS

The macronutrient composition of native breast milk varies widely and frequently does not meet the nutritional needs of preterm infants. Batching of native breast milk by using selective strategies as well as concentrating the macronutrients by removing water with freeze-drying is not able to provide the recommended macronutrient intake to all preterm infants. Most commercial standard fortifiers do not achieve ESPGHAN recommended intakes. An optimized fortifier for standard fortification could only reach recommended intake in 30% of feeds. Target fortification reduces the inter- and intraindividual macronutrient variation and can achieve recommended ESPGHAN intake for individual infants. However, the composition of the base fortifier needs to be adjusted for best practice target fortification and is different from a fortifier originally developed for standard fortification. More frequent breast milk measurements and recipe refinement for fortifiers (and modular) to be used in target fortification would improve the macronutrient intake and thus growth.

AUTHOR CONTRIBUTIONS

CF and NR: conceptualization, methodology. HS, MR, and NR: formal analysis. GF and SF: milk analysis. GF, NR, and SF: data curation. EY, NR, and SF: writing—original draft preparation. CF, MR, NR, and SF: visualization. NR: supervision. CF: project administration. All authors writing—review and editing. All authors have read and agreed to the published version of the manuscript.

ACKNOWLEDGMENTS

This paper is dedicated to Dr. Adrien Charles Moessinger (1944–2021), Professor Emeritus (CHUV, Lausanne, Switzerland), Former Director of the Neonatal Intensive Care Units at CHUV (Lausanne) and at Inselspital (Berne) with great respect for his outstanding life work on lung development, introducing nasal CPAP into clinical routine in Central Europe and for planting seeds in young doctors how important nutrition is for positive long-term neurodevelopmental outcome. We would like to thank Tanja Pfitzenmaier for editorial support.

REFERENCES

1. Cooke RJ, Ainsworth SB, Fenton AC. Postnatal growth retardation: a universal problem in preterm infants. *Arch Child Fetal Neonatal Ed.* (2004) 89:F428–30. doi: 10.1136/adc.2001.004044
2. Su BH. Optimizing nutrition in preterm infants. *Pediatr Neonatol.* (2014) 55:5–13. doi: 10.1016/j.pedneo.2013.07.003
3. Barker DJP. The fetal and infant origins of adult disease. *BMJ.* (1990) 301:1111.
4. Lucas A, Morley R, Cole TJ, Gore SM, Lucas PJ, Crowle P, et al. Early diet in preterm babies and developmental status at 18 months. *Lancet.* (1990) 335:1477–81.
5. Leon DA, Lithell HO, Vagero D, Koupilova I, Mohsen R, Berglund L, et al. Reduced fetal growth rate and increased risk of death from ischaemic heart disease: cohort study of 15 000 Swedish men and women born 1915-29. *BMJ.* (1998) 317:241–5.
6. Lucas A, Morley R, Cole TJ. Randomised trial of early diet in preterm babies and later intelligence quotient. *BMJ.* (1998) 317:1481–7.
7. Eriksson JG, Forsen T, Tuomilehto J, Osmond C, Barker DJ. Early growth and coronary heart disease in later life: longitudinal study. *BMJ.* (2001) 322:949–53. doi: 10.1136/bmj.322.7292.949
8. Ehrenkranz RA, Dusick AM, Vohr BR, Wright LL, Wrage LA, Poole WK. Growth in the neonatal intensive care unit influences neurodevelopmental and growth outcomes of extremely low birth weight infants. *Pediatrics.* (2006) 117:1253–61. doi: 10.1542/peds.2005-1368
9. Greer FR, Sicherer SH, Burks AW, Committee on Nutrition and Section on Allergy and Immunology. The effects of early nutritional interventions on the development of atopic disease in infants and children: the role of maternal dietary restriction, breastfeeding, hydrolyzed formulas, and timing of introduction of allergenic complementary foods. *Pediatrics.* (2019) 143:e20190281. doi: 10.1542/peds.2019-0281
10. Section on Breastfeeding. Breastfeeding and the use of human milk. *Pediatrics.* (2012) 129:e827–41. doi: 10.1542/peds.2011-3552
11. Lucas A, Cole TJ. Breast milk and neonatal necrotising enterocolitis. *Lancet.* (1990) 336:1519–23.
12. Lonnerdal B. Nutritional and physiologic significance of human milk proteins. *Am J Clin Nutr.* (2003) 77:1537–43s. doi: 10.1093/ajcn/77.6.1537S
13. Ip S, Chung M, Raman G, Chew P, Magula N, DeVine D, et al. Breastfeeding and maternal and infant health outcomes in developed countries. *Evid Rep Technol Assess Full Rep.* (2007) 1–186.
14. Gartner LM, Morton J, Lawrence RA, Naylor AJ, O'Hare D, Schanler RJ, et al. Breastfeeding and the use of human milk. *Pediatrics.* (2005) 115:496–506. doi: 10.1542/peds.2004-2491
15. O'Connor DL, Gibbins S, Kiss A, Bando N, Brennan-Donnan J, Ng E, et al. Effect of supplemental donor human milk compared with preterm formula on neurodevelopment of very low-birth-weight infants at 18 months: a randomized clinical trial. *JAMA.* (2016) 316:1897–905. doi: 10.1001/jama.2016.16144
16. Quigley M, Embleton ND, McGuire W. Formula versus donor breast milk for feeding preterm or low birth weight infants. *Cochrane Database Syst Rev.* (2018) 6:CD002971. doi: 10.1002/14651858.CD002971.pub4
17. Chetta KE, Schulz EV, Wagner CL. Outcomes improved with human milk intake in preterm and full-term infants. *Semin Perinatol.* (2021) 45:151384. doi: 10.1016/j.semperi.2020.151384
18. Miller J, Tonkin E, Damarell RA, McPhee AJ, Suganuma M, Suganuma H, et al. A systematic review and meta-analysis of human milk feeding and morbidity in very low birth weight infants. *Nutrients.* (2018) 10:E707. doi: 10.3390/nu10060707
19. Arslanoglu S, Moro GE, Ziegler EE. Preterm infants fed fortified human milk receive less protein than they need. *J Perinatol.* (2009) 29:489–92. doi: 10.1038/jp.2009.50
20. Agostoni C, Buonocore G, Carnielli VP, De Curtis M, Darmaun D, Decsi T, et al. Enteral nutrient supply for preterm infants: commentary from the European society of paediatric gastroenterology, hepatology and nutrition committee on nutrition. *J Pediatr Gastroenterol Nutr.* (2010) 50:85–91. doi: 10.1097/MPG.0b013e3181adaee0
21. Weber A, Loui A, Jochum F, Buhrer C, Obladen M. Breast milk from mothers of very low birthweight infants: variability in fat and protein content. *Acta Paediatr.* (2001) 90:772–5. doi: 10.1111/j.1651-2227.2001.tb02803.x
22. Sauer CW, Boutin MA, Kim JH. Wide variability in caloric density of expressed human milk can lead to major underestimation or overestimation of nutrient content. *J Hum Lact.* (2017) 33:341–50. doi: 10.1177/0890334416672200
23. Fusch G, Mitra S, Rochow N, Fusch C. Target fortification of breast milk: levels of fat, protein or lactose are not related. *Acta Paediatr.* (2015) 104:38–42. doi: 10.1111/apa.12804
24. Arslanoglu S, Moro GE, Ziegler EE. Adjustable fortification of human milk fed to preterm infants: does it make a difference? *J Perinatol.* (2006) 26:614–21. doi: 10.1038/sj.jp.7211571
25. Rochow N, Landau-Crangle E, Fusch C. Challenges in breast milk fortification for preterm infants. *Curr Opin Clin Nutr Metab Care.* (2015) 18:276–84. doi: 10.1097/mco.0000000000000167
26. Rochow N, Fusch G, Choi A, Chessell L, Elliott L, McDonald K, et al. Target fortification of breast milk with fat, protein, and carbohydrates for preterm infants. *J Pediatr.* (2013) 163:1001–7. doi: 10.1016/j.jpeds.2013.04.052
27. Rochow N, Fusch G, Zapanta B, Ali A, Barui S, Fusch C. Target fortification of breast milk: how often should milk analysis be done? *Nutrients.* (2015) 7:2297–310. doi: 10.3390/nu7042297
28. Rochow N, Fusch G, Ali A, Bhatia A, So HY, Iskander R, et al. Individualized target fortification of breast milk with protein, carbohydrates, and fat for preterm infants: a double-blind randomized controlled trial. *Clin Nutr Edinb Scotl.* (2021) 40:54–63. doi: 10.1016/j.clnu.2020.04.031
29. Choi A, Fusch G, Rochow N, Sheikh N, Fusch C. Establishment of micromethods for macronutrient contents analysis in breast milk. *Matern Child Nutr.* (2015) 11:761–72. doi: 10.1111/mcn.12053
30. Fusch G, Rochow N, Choi A, Fusch S, Poeschl S, Ubah AO, et al. Rapid measurement of macronutrients in breast milk: how reliable are infrared milk analyzers? *Clin Nutr.* (2015) 34:465–76. doi: 10.1016/j.clnu.2014.05.005
31. Fusch G, Choi A, Rochow N, Fusch C. Quantification of lactose content in human and cow's milk using UPLC-tandem mass spectrometry. *J Chromatogr B Anal Technol Biomed Life Sci.* (2011) 879:3759–62. doi: 10.1016/j.jchromb.2011.09.053
32. Carpenter KJ. A short history of nutritional science: part 2 (1885-1912). *J Nutr.* (2003) 133:975–84. doi: 10.1093/jn/133.4.975
33. Kashyap S, Ohira-Kist K, Abildskov K, Towers HM, Sahni R, Ramakrishnan R, et al. Effects of quality of energy intake on growth and metabolic response of enterally fed low-birth-weight infants. *Pediatr Res.* (2001) 50:390–7. doi: 10.1203/00006450-200109000-00015
34. Kashyap S, Towers HM, Sahni R, Ohira-Kist K, Abildskov K, Schulze KF. Effects of quality of energy on substrate oxidation in enterally fed, low-birth-weight infants. *Am J Clin Nutr.* (2001) 74:374–80. doi: 10.1093/ajcn/74.3.374
35. Kashyap S, Schulze KF, Ramakrishnan R, Dell RB, Heird WC. Evaluation of a mathematical model for predicting the relationship between protein and energy intakes of low-birth-weight infants and the rate and composition of weight gain. *Pediatr Res.* (1994) 35:704–12. doi: 10.1203/00006450-199406000-00017
36. Lee H, Padhi E, Hasegawa Y, Larke J, Parenti M, Wang A, et al. Compositional dynamics of the milk fat globule and its role in infant development. *Front Pediatr.* (2018) 6:313. doi: 10.3389/fped.2018.00313

37. Gidrewicz DA, Fenton TR. A systematic review and meta-analysis of the nutrient content of preterm and term breast milk. *BMC Pediatr.* (2014) 14:216. doi: 10.1186/1471-2431-14-216
38. Michalski MC, Briard V, Michel F, Tasson F, Poulain P. Size distribution of fat globules in human colostrum, breast milk, and infant formula. *J Dairy Sci.* (2005) 88:1927–40. doi: 10.3168/jds.S0022-0302(05)72868-X
39. Bergner EM, Shypailo R, Visuthranukul C, Hagan J, O'Donnell AR, Hawthorne KM, et al. Growth, body composition, and neurodevelopmental outcomes at 2 years among preterm infants fed an exclusive human milk diet in the neonatal intensive care unit: a pilot study. *Breastfeed Med.* (2020) 15:304–11. doi: 10.1089/bfm.2019.0210
40. Gross SJ, David RJ, Bauman L, Tomarelli RM. Nutritional composition of milk produced by mothers delivering preterm. *J Pediatr.* (1980) 96:641–4. doi: 10.1016/S0022-3476(80)80729-3
41. Hesse V. Insektizide und Polychlorierte Biphenyle (PCBs) in der Muttermilch, Kuhmilch und Milchprodukten in Deutschand-Ost und -West vor und nach der Wiedervereinigung - ein Vergleich mit der aktuellen Situation. *Acta Acad Sci.* (2019) 17:29–56.
42. Pajewska-Szmyt M, Sinkiewicz-Darol E, Gadzała-Kopciuch R. The impact of environmental pollution on the quality of mother's milk. *Environ Sci Pollut Res.* (2019) 26:7405–27. doi: 10.1007/s11356-019-04141-1
43. Pfister KM, Gray HL, Miller NC, Demerath EW, Georgieff MK, Ramel SE. Exploratory study of the relationship of fat-free mass to speed of brain processing in preterm infants. *Pediatr Res.* (2013) 74:576–83. doi: 10.1038/pr.2013.138
44. Bell KA, Matthews LG, Cherkerzian S, Palmer C, Drouin K, Pepin HL, et al. Associations of growth and body composition with brain size in preterm infants. *J Pediatr.* (2019) 214:20–26.e2. doi: 10.1016/j.jpeds.2019.06.062
45. Ramel SE, Gray HL, Christiansen E, Boys C, Georgieff MK, Demerath EW. Greater early gains in fat-free mass, but not fat mass, are associated with improved neurodevelopment at 1 year corrected age for prematurity in very low birth weight preterm infants. *J Pediatr.* (2016) 173:108–15. doi: 10.1016/j.jpeds.2016.03.003
46. Pfister KM, Zhang L, Miller NC, Ingolfsland EC, Demerath EW, Ramel SE. Early body composition changes are associated with neurodevelopmental and metabolic outcomes at 4 years of age in very preterm infants. *Pediatr Res.* (2018) 84:713–8. doi: 10.1038/s41390-018-0158-x
47. Singhal A, Cole TJ, Fewtrell M, Kennedy K, Stephenson T, Elias-Jones A, et al. Promotion of faster weight gain in infants born small for gestational age: is there an adverse effect on later blood pressure? *Circulation.* (2007) 115:213–20. doi: 10.1161/CIRCULATIONAHA.106.617811
48. Min JW, Kong KA, Park BH, Hong JH, Park EA, Cho SJ, et al. Effect of postnatal catch-up growth on blood pressure in children at 3 years of age. *J Hum Hypertens.* (2007) 21:868–74. doi: 10.1038/sj.jhh.1002215
49. Ong KK, Kennedy K, Castañeda-Gutiérrez E, Forsyth S, Godfrey KM, Koletzko B, et al. Postnatal growth in preterm infants and later health outcomes: a systematic review. *Acta Paediatr.* (2015) 104:974–86. doi: 10.1111/apa.13128
50. Kashyap S, Forsyth M, Zucker C, Ramakrishnan R, Dell RB, Heird WC. Effects of varying protein and energy intakes on growth and metabolic response in low birth weight infants. *J Pediatr.* (1986) 108:955–63.
51. Kwan C, Fusch G, Rochow N, Fusch C, Kwan C, Fusch G, et al. Milk analysis using milk analyzers in a standardized setting (MAMAS) study: a multicentre quality initiative. *Clin Nutr.* (2020) 39:2121–8. doi: 10.1016/j.clnu.2019.08.028

27

Tailoring Human Milk Oligosaccharides to Prevent Necrotising Enterocolitis among Preterm Infants

Safiyyah Abbas[1], *Amy K. Keir*[1,2,3,4], *Maria Makrides*[2,4], *Laura D. Klein*[5], *Luke E. Grzeskowiak*[2,6], *Andrew J. McPhee*[2] *and Alice R. Rumbold*[2,3,4*]

[1] Women's and Children's Health Network, Adelaide, SA, Australia, [2] SAHMRI Women and Kids, South Australian Health and Medical Research Institute, Adelaide, SA, Australia, [3] Adelaide Medical School, The University of Adelaide, Adelaide, SA, Australia, [4] Robinson Research Institute, The University of Adelaide, Adelaide, SA, Australia, [5] Business Growth and Innovation, Australian Red Cross Lifeblood, Sydney, NSW, Australia, [6] College of Medicine and Public Health, Flinders University, Adelaide, SA, Australia

Correspondence:
Alice R. Rumbold
alice.rumbold@sahmri.com

Necrotising enterocolitis (NEC) is a devastating disease affecting preterm infants, with little improvement in mortality rates and treatment strategies in the last 30 years. Human milk oligosaccharides (HMOs) are emerging as a potential preventive therapy, with multiple protective functions postulated. Our aim is to summarise the evidence concerning the role of HMOs in NEC development and emerging strategies to tailor the delivery of HMOs to preterm infants. Most research efforts to date have focused on supplementing preterm infants with simple oligosaccharides, which are structurally different to HMOs and derived mainly from plants. Clinical trials demonstrate limited benefits for NEC prevention arising from the use of these supplements. Alternative strategies under investigation include optimising HMOs for infants receiving donor human milk, concentrating oligosaccharides from donor human milk and from animal milks, as well as more sophisticated synthetic oligosaccharide production strategies. Critically, high quality evidence to support implementation of any of these approaches in the neonatal unit is lacking. Whether it is a specific HMO alone or a combination of HMOs that exert protective effects remains to be elucidated. Further challenges include how best to manufacture and administer oligosaccharides whilst retaining bioactivity and safety, including evaluation of the long-term effects of altering the balance of HMOs and gut microbiota in preterm infants. While several human clinical trials are underway, further research is needed to understand whether a tailored approach to oligosaccharide supplementation is beneficial for preterm infants.

Keywords: preterm (birth), neonatal nutrition, oligosaccharides, breast milk, very low birth weight infants, necrotising enterocolitis

INTRODUCTION

Human milk oligosaccharides (HMOs) are complex carbohydrates that comprise the third most abundant solid component of human milk (1–5). Synthesised in the mammary gland, the basic HMO structure consists of a single glucose molecule at the reducing end attached to galactose, forming a lactose core (2, 6). Variation results from additional N-acetylglucosamine and galactose residues, and fucose or sialic acid at the non-reducing end (7–9). Over 200 structurally unique HMOs have been identified (2, 5, 10) and range in size from 3 to 32 sugars (6).

The three major classes of HMOs are fucosylated neutral HMOs, non-fucosylated neutral HMOs and sialylated acidic HMOs (11). Breast milk contains 80% neutral HMOs (12). Of these, 2′-fucosyllactose (2′-FL) (fucosylated) and Lacto-N-neotetraose (LNnT) (non-fucosylated) are the most abundant structures (13).

The amount and diversity of HMOs vary significantly based on the mother's stage of lactation, an infant's gestation at birth, and maternal genetic factors (1). HMOs are maximally concentrated in colostrum compared with mature milk (2, 14, 15). The ratio of fucosylated α1-2-linked HMOs to non-fucosylated HMOs changes from 5:1 to 1:1 over the first year of lactation (2). Variation in HMO composition is postulated to have crucial functional implications (9).

Milk from mothers delivering preterm contains a significantly greater concentration of HMOs than more mature milk, but there is great variation in concentration between mothers (6, 8, 14) and the HMO content is also less diverse (16). For example, compared with milk from mothers delivering at term, lacto-N-tetraose is generally more abundant (9), fucosylation is not as well-regulated (7, 9), and sialic acid content in the initial month postpartum is greater (7). However, these findings are not consistent across all studies of preterm and term milk (17).

Maternal "secretor" status and Lewis blood group are strong genetic determinants of HMO production, particularly concerning fucosylated HMOs, imparting four patterns of HMO fucosylation (1, 2, 5, 6, 18). Over 70% of women are "secretors," meaning they express the α1-2fucosyltranferase *FUT2* gene, and produce α1-2fucosylated HMOs, such as 2'-fucosyllactose (2'FL) or lacto-N-fucopentaose 1 (LNFP1). "Non secretor" women, who have homozygous mutations in *FUT2* and comprise 20% of Caucasian populations, do not produce these HMOs (2, 5, 13, 14, 19).

Lewis positive blood group women express α1-3/4-fucosyltransferase FUT3, producing α1-4-fucosylated HMOs such as LNFP2 (14). Combining Lewis blood group and secretor status has important implications. For example, Lewis blood group (a+b–) "non-secretor" milk contains 35–45% less total HMO amount than Lewis (a–b+) "secretor" milk (17).

ROLE AND FUNCTIONS OF HMOS

Due to the unique design of HMOs, their role in infant health and development has been under intense investigation during the past decade (8). HMOs are non-digestible sugars that are nutritionally beneficial not for the infant but for the bacteria residing in their gut (10, 20). A small proportion of HMOs are absorbed into the systemic circulation (5) and excreted through the urinary tract (10). The majority of HMOs that reach the gut are either passed in the stool or fermented in the intestine to short-chain fatty acids (SCFA) and lactic acids, creating an acidic environment unfavourable for many pathogenic microbes (2, 12, 18). HMOs selectively enhance the growth of beneficial bacteria, resulting in a healthy gut microbiome (21). Of the various gut microbiota species, only bifidobacteria and bacteroides can digest HMOs (21). Certain *Bifidobacterium* and *Bacteroides* species have been shown to efficiently utilise HMOs due to genes encoding specific enzymes involved with cleavage and transport of HMOs, in marked contrast other bacterial species (22, 23). *In-vitro* studies indicate LNnT, LNT, LNFP and 2'FL are preferentially digested by *Bifidobacterium longum* subsp. *infantis (B. infantis)*, and, to a lesser extent, *Bifidobacterium bifidum*. In contrast, pathogenic bacterial species show variation in HMO consumption. *Bacteroides fragilis* and *vulgatus* consume HMOs, but *Lactobacillus acidophilus, Clostridium perfringens, E. coli, Eubacterium rectale, Streptococcus thermophiles, E. faecalis,* and *Veillonella parvula* show limited or no utilisation of HMOs (8). Thus, the presence of HMOs, particularly fucosylated and sialylated HMOs, is thought to reduce the nutrients available for pathogenic bacteria, thus reducing their growth (19, 24, 25). "Secretor" milk may promote bifidobacteria species and protect against infant diarrhoea (13).

In addition to shaping the intestinal microbiota, evidence suggests additional antimicrobial and immunomodulatory roles of HMOs.

First, HMOs act as decoy receptors, competitively binding to pathogens by mimicking structurally homologous intestinal epithelial receptors, thus preventing pathogen attachment and invasion of the intestinal epithelium (2, 6, 8, 10). Sialylated HMOs, such as 3'SL, inhibit the binding of enteropathogenic *E. coli* (EPEC) (2, 18) in intestinal epithelial cells and uropathogenic *E. coli* (UPEC) in bladder epithelial cells (24). α1-2-fucosylated HMOs, such as 2'FL or LNFP1, inhibit the attachment of *C. jejuni* to the intestinal epithelium (14).

Second, HMOs may directly modulate immune cell responses to pathogens (14) and act as signalling molecules (24). For example, 2'FL directly inhibits lipopolysaccharide-mediated inflammation during *E. coli* invasion of intestinal epithelial cells (24). Other possible roles include leukocyte-endothelial cell and platelet-neutrophil interactions (2, 10), effects at the level of gut-associated lymphoid tissue (2), and interaction with selectins, integrins, and toll-like receptors (2, 26).

Third, HMOs affect intestinal epithelial cells, such as triggering intracellular processes such as differentiation and apoptosis, and reducing intestinal permeability in preterm infants during the first month of life (2, 14). In addition, HMOs may have other extraintestinal, indirect innate immune system effects, protecting against late-onset sepsis and urinary tract infections (6). Various other possible roles for HMOs have been postulated, including anti-allergic effects (2), and a role in growth and metabolism in the liver, muscle, and brain (2, 7, 10, 14, 19).

Research is needed to clarify the specific roles of HMOs and elucidate whether effects are due to one specific HMO, or a combination of HMOs interacting together (5). While speculative, it is highly likely that the beneficial effects of HMOs are dependent on several factors including total HMO amount, structural characteristics of individual HMOs, and abundance of specific HMOs (14).

HMOs are significantly more concentrated and structurally complex than milk oligosaccharides of any other species, including cow, sheep, goat, and non-human primates (2, 5, 6, 27). HMOs show greater complexity and diversity than non-human primate oligosaccharides, which are in turn more diverse than non-primates (28). Dairy animal milks contain more sialylated oligosaccharides, whereas fucosylated oligosaccharides predominate in human milk (4, 6, 10).

IMPORTANCE OF HMOS FOR PRETERM INFANT HEALTH AND DEVELOPMENT

Prematurity is associated with a higher risk of mortality and significant morbidities in infancy. HMOs may have a critical role in promoting a healthy gut microbiome and preventing bowel diseases such as necrotising enterocolitis (NEC).

NEC is a potentially life-threatening disease that affects 2–10% of very low birth weight (VLBW, i.e., <1,500 g) infants (7, 8). Characterised by intestinal inflammation, NEC can lead to bowel necrosis and perforation requiring surgery, with chronic complications including short gut syndrome, malabsorption, and neurodevelopmental delay (8, 29). Little has changed in NEC mortality rates—which can be as high as 25% in severe cases (8)—and treatment strategies over the last three decades (30).

The main risk factors for NEC are prematurity, pathogenic bacterial colonisation, and formula feeding (30). The premature gut is immature in several ways, with gut epithelium predisposed to mounting an exaggerated inflammatory response to pathogenic bacteria, resulting in the mucosal damage and impaired mesenteric perfusion implicated in the pathogenesis of NEC (8, 30). Increased toll-like receptor 4 (TLR4) signalling plays a role in this exaggerated inflammatory response (30–32). A bloom of pathogenic organisms, such as *γ-Proteobacteria,* is seen just before NEC onset (24, 25).

The most successful preventive strategies for NEC include feeds containing maternal milk and/or donor human milk, and probiotics (20). Preterm infants receiving their mother's milk are at six to ten times reduced risk of developing NEC than their formula-fed counterparts (3, 7). Suggested mechanisms behind the protective effect of breast milk against NEC include inhibition of TLR4 signalling (30), reduction of intestinal permeability (33), and promotion of a healthy gut microbiome through HMOs' selective enhancement of healthy bacteria (6, 10, 21).

The composition of the infant gut microbiome is strongly implicated in the development of NEC. Development of the gut microbiome occurs mainly due to breastfeeding (2). Various factors contribute to gut dysbiosis, including mode of delivery, antibiotic use, acid suppression, degree of prematurity, intestinal immaturity, lack of fresh breast milk, delayed introduction of enteral feeds, maternal gut microbiome composition, post-birth environment, and prolonged hospital stay with greater exposure to opportunistic infections (4, 5, 20, 25, 34).

The gut microbiota profile shows wide variability from the day after birth. Breastfed infants mainly show significant individual variation, and gut microbiota composition increases in amount and diversity with age (4). Compared with term infants, the preterm gut microbiota has low bacterial diversity, more potentially pathogenic gut flora strains, lower levels of *Bifidobacterium* and *Bacteroides*, immature digestive processes, and an immature mucosal barrier vulnerable to bacterial invasion and toxin damage (5, 8, 19, 34). All of these factors have been implicated in the development of NEC and sepsis (19, 24).

Animal studies suggest that disialyllacto-N-tetraose (DSLNT) (14) and 2'-fucosyllactose (2'FL) may be protective against NEC (35). Human observational studies support this with Autran et al. (3) and Van Niekerk et al. (1) finding breast milk low in DSLNT concentration was associated with an increased risk of NEC in the recipient preterm infants. Masi et al. (36) similarly found that DSLNT was significantly lower in maternal milk received by infants with NEC than age-matched controls. Infants who received milk with low DSLNT had lower relative abundance of *Bifidobacterium* spp. Further, Wejryd et al. reported lower HMO diversity and Lacto-N-difucohexaose I (which is only produced by secretor and Lewis positive mothers) levels in mothers of NEC cases, compared with non-NEC infants (37). There is evidence that preterm infants of "non-secretor" mothers show higher levels of *Proteobacteria*, which includes pathogens associated with NEC and sepsis (24). However, Demmert et al. demonstrated no differences in late onset sepsis or NEC in VLBW infants based on *FUT2* genotype (38).

This emerging evidence linking the HMO profile of maternal breast milk with risk of NEC has led to intense interest in understanding ways to improve the delivery of HMOs to vulnerable infants as a preventive strategy against NEC. Altering the profile of HMOs in maternal breast milk is difficult to achieve, as it is primarily determined by genetic factors and gestation at birth. Nevertheless, there are several possibilities regarding the use of donor human milk.

OPTIMISING HMOS FOR INFANTS RECEIVING DONOR HUMAN MILK

Donor milk is the preferred source of nutrition when sufficient maternal milk is not available (39, 40). While donor milk is associated with better health outcomes for preterm infants than infant formula, outcomes for donor milk-fed infants are not equivalent to those receiving maternal breast milk (41). This may be due to losses in milk nutrients or bioactives during storage and processing, or a mismatch in milk composition due to differences between donor and maternal lactation stage and/or maturity of the mammary gland (42). However, HMOs are one of few human milk components whose content and composition is unaltered by Holder pasteurisation (43).

Donor milk is typically prioritised for very preterm infants and used in the first weeks of life, when recipients would usually receive maternal colostrum or transitional milk. Yet donor milk is often mature milk from mothers who have given birth at term (29). The proportion of preterm donations to milk banks can vary considerably. For example, 65% of donors to an Indian milk bank had preterm births (44), compared with 10% of Taiwanese donors (45). This has important implications for preterm infants receiving donor milk, containing fewer HMOs than typical of breast milk from mothers who give birth preterm (14).

Donor and recipient matching may improve the nutrition and bioactives that infants receive. In a small observational study, Sánchez Luna et al. (46) observed a decrease in NEC rates in very preterm infants and late onset sepsis after implementing a personalised nutrition program that matches donor milk to recipient infants by gestational age and stage of lactation. While promising, donor milk matching programs require availability of milk from preterm donors, which may require targeted recruitment to increase the proportion of preterm donors, and staff resources to support labelling and matching. Increasing preterm donors could also increase similarities between donors' and recipient mothers' HMO profiles. However, this cannot be assumed given the variability in HMO content from mothers who deliver preterm (6, 8, 14). Additional studies are needed to compare nutrition and bioactives from gestational and lactation stage-matched donor milk to standard donor milk and to robustly evaluate the health benefits of such programs.

Matching donor milk to maternal secretor status may be a potential strategy to personalise donor milk, and provide infants of non-secretor mothers with milk from a secretor donor. An ongoing clinical trial is evaluating the impact of this on the gut microbiome among very preterm infants (47). Alternatively, increasing the diversity of HMOs in donor milk may be beneficial, for example, to include fucosylated HMOs (19, 25) and HMOs found in secretor milk (48). Pooling milk from multiple donors is already recommended to reduce variation in the macronutrient content of donor milk (49). More data about the composition and concentrations of key HMOs for preventing complications such as NEC or improving growth will be required to inform optimal milk pooling practises.

DEVELOPING CONCENTRATED HMO SUPPLEMENTS FROM DONOR MILK

The development of human milk-derived supplements for preterm infants has been an area of intensive research and commercial interest, resulting in the use of at least one commercially available human-milk derived fortifier in neonatal units in the US (50, 51), used predominantly to increase protein intake. While there has been limited independent evaluation of the HMO content of this product, its product description states that the HMO content is similar to fresh milk (52). Meta-analysis of the evidence from the two published trials evaluating this product indicates the risk of NEC is reduced when this product is used compared with a bovine milk-based fortifier product. However, the overall quality of evidence was rated as low (53).

To date, there has been one published randomised trial of a supplement designed explicitly to produce a concentrated HMO product from donated human milk. The trial by Underwood et al. (20) examined two strategies. The first involved comparing infants fed formula supplemented with increasing doses of either a synthetic oligosaccharide product or an experimental donor human milk product containing concentrated HMOs. The second involved comparing infants fed maternal milk fortified with a commercially available human milk fortifier or a bovine milk fortifier. None of the interventions resulted in significant increases in faecal bifidobacteria, and there was a trend towards increased γ-Proteobacteria in the two experimental groups. The study was limited by the small sample population ($n = 27$ in total) precluding examination of clinical outcomes, and the high use of antibiotics in one of the human milk groups. Thus, the evidence for supplements that pool human milk oligosaccharides remains limited and in need of further investigation. Ongoing studies of new human milk-derived products are underway (54, 55).

OLIGOSACCHARIDE SUPPLEMENTS DERIVED FROM DAIRY SPECIES

Concentrating non-human sources of oligosaccharides have been proposed as an alternative supplementation strategy for preterm infants, but species specificity and lower concentrations of oligosaccharides in dairy animal milks pose challenges for development (2, 5, 6). For example, humans only produce one sialic acid residue, N-acetyl neuraminic acid (Neu5Ac), whereas other species produce other sialic acids (10). Studies focused on developing bovine milk oligosaccharides (BMO) reveal low concentrations of sialic acid overall, which is thought to be important to neurodevelopment and immunity (2), as well as lower HMO complexity (18). Further, most HMOs are fucosylated, which is not observed in BMOs (6).

Nevertheless, in animal models, BMOs are well-tolerated. They have been associated with increased stool frequency, softer stools, and greater bifidobacteria numbers, but may have limited benefits for gastrointestinal infections, respiratory infections, allergic responses, and growth (56). Goat milk oligosaccharides are another option, with greater concentrations of oligosaccharides than bovine milk (2). At present, there are no published trials involving animal-derived oligosaccharides given to human preterm infants, and there is limited evidence from trials examining the effects of BMOs given to healthy term infants (57).

SYNTHETIC OLIGOSACCHARIDE PRODUCTS

Years of commercial interest have resulted in commercially available oligosaccharides produced from plants or lactose, many of which are now added to infant formula for term and preterm infants. Long-chain fructo-oligosaccharides (lcFOS) contain fructose and are derived from inulin. Neutral short-chain galacto-oligosaccharides (scGOS) include galactose polymers from different fungi, yeast, and bacteria. Commercially available preparations often include a mixture of 90% scGOS and 10% lcFOS, which is proposed to mimic the prebiotic effect of neutral HMOs (12). Another type is pectin-derived acidic oligosaccharides (pAOS) (2, 20, 34). Reported side effects are attributed mainly to scFOS and are mild, such as flatulence (12), but overall these synthetic oligosaccharides appear to be well-tolerated (58).

The most recent systematic review of human clinical trials of synthetic oligosaccharides supplements (largely scGOS and lcFOS) in preterm infants was published in 2019 by Chi et al.

(34). Meta-analyses revealed supplementation was associated with significant decreases in the incidence of sepsis, mortality, length of hospital stay, and time to full enteral feeding; but no significant difference in the risk of NEC or feeding intolerance.

Trials of synthetic oligosaccharides may show a lack of effect on NEC because lcFOS and scGOS are structurally much simpler than HMOs, and lack the diversity and unique effects of HMOs, such as bacterial specificity (2, 20, 59). Further, the current body of evidence is limited by major variation in the way these oligosaccharides are delivered to preterm infants. For example, trials have been undertaken comparing the addition of supplements among exclusively formula fed infants, whereas others have been restricted to exclusively breastfed infants or infants fed a mixture of breast milk and formula. Thus, it has not been possible to reliably tease out the effects of the supplement *per se*, from the effects of increased breast milk intake or complete removal of formula from the diet. In addition, most studies have been small and may therefore lack statistical power to show important effects with regard to NEC. Ongoing studies evaluating oligosaccharide products in preterm infants are underway and may help to shed light on these issues (60).

Results of animal studies have generally been mixed. In neonatal rat studies, the HMO disialyllacto-N-tetraose (DSLNT) (61) and enzymatically sialylated GOS or 2'FL (62) demonstrated protection against NEC. Further, 2'-FL and/or 6'-SL reduced NEC in mice and piglet models, and inhibited TLR4 signalling in human intestinal cells *in vitro* (31). Preterm pigs showed no benefit from oligosaccharides in terms of clinical outcome, systemic immunity, or gut function, flora or health (56, 63), which may suggest that HMO effects are seen only when the gut attains a certain degree of development (29). In a mouse model, pooled HMOs decreased EPEC attachment to and invasion of epithelial cells, but scGOS did not (8).

Other data suggest that some synthetic oligosaccharides can successfully act as decoy receptors. *In vitro* studies show that synthetic 2'FL and 3FL decrease adhesion of *C. jejuni*, *Pseudomonas*, *EPEC*, and *Salmonella enterica* serovar Fyris to Caco-2-cells (8). Additionally, scGOS can mimic the protective effect HMOs have on intestinal epithelial cells against *Entamoeba histolytica* cytotoxicity (8).

More recently, there have been advances in producing synthetic oligosaccharide structures that are identical in structure to those in human milk. To date, less than ten of the many hundreds of HMOs have been able to be replicated using chemical processes and microbial production (64). While this represents an exciting advancement in the field, trials proving safety and efficacy in preterm infants have not yet been undertaken.

DISCUSSION

Foremost, strategies to support mothers of preterm infants to breastfeed must be paramount given the clear evidence of benefit of maternal breast milk for NEC prevention and infant growth and development. Beyond this, other methods to optimise intake of HMOs lack evidence of efficacy for NEC prevention and safety. Nevertheless, HMOs have plausible roles in protection against NEC and sepsis in preterm infants that warrant further investigation (**Figure 1**). For infants that lack access to maternal

HMOs

- Third most abundant solid component of human milk
- Species-specific, therefore unique to humans
- Structure and amount influenced by gestational and maternal factors
- 3 major classes: fucosylated neutral, non-fucosylated neutral, sialylated acidic
- Maternal genetic factors influence production ("secretor" status, Lewis blood group)

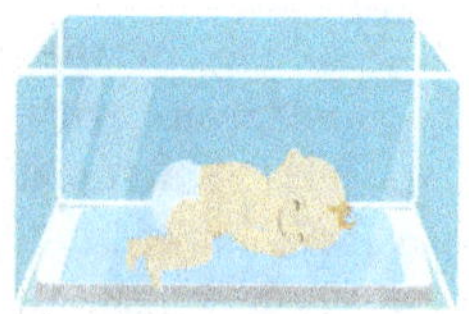

Putative roles of HMOs in ↓ NEC

- ↑ growth of beneficial bacteria
- ↑ differentiation and apoptosis of intestinal epithelial cells
- ↓ nutrients available for growth of pathogenic bacteria (e.g. Proteobacteria)
- ↓ pathogen binding
- ↓ intestinal permeability
- ↓ inflammation (including through ↓TLR4 signalling)

Potential interventions

- Donor milk matching based on maternal status
- Multiple donor pooling (↑ diversity of HMOs)
- HMO concentrates derived from human milk (↑ concentration of HMOs, match diversity of HMOs found in maternal milk)
- Concentrate oligosaccharides from dairy animal species – replicate some benefits of HMOs
- Synthetic HMOs – mimic protective effects and structures of some HMOs

FIGURE 1 | Potential HMO mechanisms and interventions to prevent NEC in preterm infants.

milk, altering the profile of donor milk, either via matching donor and recipients based on gestation or secretor status or by pooling donor milk, could increase HMO intake, but to date, all of these strategies lack rigorous evaluation.

Supplementation with synthetic oligosaccharides, predominantly scGOS and lcFOS, suggests benefits for some neonatal morbidities but trials have failed to demonstrate conclusive evidence that the risk of NEC is reduced. The relatively simple structure of scGOS and lcFOS suggest that they may be unlikely to mimic the complex functions of HMOs. The production of synthetic oligosaccharides identical in structure to HMOs also appears promising but all are yet to be tested in trials with preterm infants. Also lacking are studies of optimal dosing.

A critical limitation of research efforts to date is the focus on a limited number of oligosaccharide structures (7), thus negating the potential benefits of the wide variety of HMOs structures in existence. HMOs are produced as complex mixtures with possible synergistic mechanisms of action against NEC and infection (65). There is also a risk that supplementing feeds with just one or two of the many HMOs may cause an unwanted effect on the balance of the gut microbiome population and/or the immune system, with potential long-term implications.

Isolating HMOs from human milk would capture the diversity and complexity of HMOs and may be possible with the growth in human milk banking worldwide but presents other challenges. Products derived from donated breast milk are often processed to reduce risk for medically fragile infants. While low-temperature pasteurisation does not impact the amount or structure of HMOs, high-temperature sterilisation reduces HMOs (9, 66, 67). Heat treatment may also reduce the amount and activity of other milk components (e.g., B and T cells, soluble CD14, growth factors, vitamins, SIgA, lysozyme, Lactoferrin) (8, 9, 29) and it remains essential to ascertain whether the loss of the original human milk composition also results in functional changes to early microbial-HMO interactions (68).

Further, high quality research is needed that focuses on elucidating the mechanisms underlying the specific and synergistic effects of HMOs to inform the development of therapeutic applications. Any future HMO therapies require rigorous testing in trials that are of sufficient size to detect differences in NEC and other important clinical outcomes, to ensure there is robust evidence of efficacy and safety.

AUTHOR CONTRIBUTIONS

AR and SA conceptualised the paper and wrote the first draft, with input from AK and LK. All authors contributed to reviewing drafts and refining the paper and agree to be accountable for the content of the work.

REFERENCES

1. Niekerk EV, Autran CA, Nel DG, Kirsten GF, Blaauw R, Bode L. Human milk oligosaccharides differ between HIV-infected and HIV-uninfected mothers and are related to necrotizing enterocolitis incidence in their preterm very-low-birth-weight infants. *J Nutr.* (2014) 144:1227–33. doi: 10.3945/jn.113.187799
2. Chichlowski M, German B, Lebrilla CB, Mills DA. The influence of milk oligosaccharides on microbiota of infants: opportunities for formulas. *Annu Rev Food Sci Technol.* (2011) 2:331–51. doi: 10.1146/annurev-food-022510-133743
3. Autran CA, Kellman BP, Kim JH, Asztalos E, Blood AB, Spence ECH, et al. Human milk oligosaccharide composition predicts risk of necrotising enterocolitis in preterm infants. *Gut.* (2018) 67:1064–70. doi: 10.1136/gutjnl-2016-312819
4. Chong CYL, Bloomfield FH, O'Sullivan JM. Factors affecting gastrointestinal microbiome development in neonates. *Nutrients.* (2018) 10:274. doi: 10.3390/nu10030274
5. Moukarzel S, Bode L. Human milk oligosaccharides and the preterm infant: a journey in sickness and in health. *Clin Perinatol.* (2017) 44:193–207. doi: 10.1016/j.clp.2016.11.014
6. Perrone S, Longini M, Zollino I, Bazzini F, Tassini M, Vivi A, et al. Breast milk: to each his own. From metabolomic study, evidence of personalized nutrition in preterm infants. *Nutrition.* (2019) 62:161–8. doi: 10.1016/j.nut.2018.12.015
7. Austin S, Castro CAD, Sprenger N, Binia A, Affolter M, Garcia-Rodenas CL, et al. Human milk oligosaccharides in the milk of mothers delivering term versus preterm infants. *Nutrients.* (2019) 11:1282. doi: 10.3390/nu11061282
8. Pacheco AR, Barile D, Underwood MA, Mills DA. The impact of the milk glycobiome on the neonate gut microbiota. *Annu Rev Anim Biosci.* (2015) 3:419–445. doi: 10.1146/annurev-animal-022114-111112
9. Leoz MLAD, Gaerlan SC, Strum JS, Dimapasoc LM, Mirmiran M, Tancredi DJ, et al. Lacto-N-tetraose, fucosylation, and secretor status are highly variable in human milk oligosaccharides from women delivering preterm. *J Proteome Res.* (2012) 11:4662–72. doi: 10.1021/pr3004979
10. Smilowitz JT, Lebrilla CB, Mills DA, German JB, Freeman SL. Breast milk oligosaccharides: structure-function relationships in the neonate. *Annu Rev Nutr.* (2014) 34:143–69. doi: 10.1146/annurev-nutr-071813-105721
11. Ray C, Kerketta JA, Rao S, Patel S, Dutt S, Arora K, et al. Human milk oligosaccharides: the journey ahead. *Int J Pediatr.* (2019) 2019:2390240. doi: 10.1155/2019/2390240
12. Fanaro S, Boehm G, Garssen J, Knol J, Mosca F, Stahl B, et al. Galacto-oligosaccharides and long-chain fructo-oligosaccharides as prebiotics in infant formulas: a review. *Acta Paediatr Suppl.* (2005) 94:22–6. doi: 10.1111/j.1651-2227.2005.tb02150.x
13. Vandenplas Y, Berger B, Carnielli VP, Ksiazyk J, Lagström H, Luna MS, et al. Human milk oligosaccharides: 2'-fucosyllactose (2'-FL) and lacto-N-neotetraose (LNnT) in infant formula. *Nutrients.* (2018) 10:1161. doi: 10.3390/nu10091161
14. Marx C, Bridge R, Wolf AK, Rich W, Kim JH, Bode L. Human milk oligosaccharide composition differs between donor milk and mother's own milk in the NICU. *J Hum Lact.* (2014) 30:54–61. doi: 10.1177/0890334413513923
15. Sundekilde UK, Downey E, O'Mahony JA, O'Shea C-A, Ryan CA, Kelly AL, et al. The effect of gestational and lactational age on the human milk metabolome. *Nutrients.* (2016) 8:304. doi: 10.3390/nu8050304
16. Lewis ED, Richard C, Larsen BM, Field CJ. The importance of human milk for immunity in preterm infants. *Clin Perinatol.* (2017) 44:23–47. doi: 10.1016/j.clp.2016.11.008
17. Kunz C, Meyer C, Collado MC, Geiger L, García-Mantrana I, Bertua-Ríos B, et al. Influence of gestational age, secretor, and lewis blood group status on the oligosaccharide content of human milk. *J Pediatr Gastroenterol Nutr.* (2017) 64:789–798. doi: 10.1097/MPG.0000000000001402
18. Kunz C, Rudloff S. Biological functions of oligosaccharides in human milk. *Acta Paediatr.* (1993) 82:903–12. doi: 10.1111/j.1651-2227.1993.tb12597.x
19. Underwood MA, Davis JCC, Kalanetra KM, Gehlot S, Patole S, Tancredi DJ, et al. Digestion of human milk oligosaccharides by bifidobacterium breve in the premature infant. *J Pediatr Gastroenterol Nutr.* (2017) 65:449–55. doi: 10.1097/MPG.0000000000001590
20. Underwood MA, Kalanetra KM, Bokulich NA, Mirmiran M, Barile D, Tancredi DJ, et al. Prebiotic oligosaccharides in premature infants. *J Pediatr Gastroenterol Nutr.* (2014) 48:352–60. doi: 10.1097/MPG.0000000000000211
21. Underwood MA. Impact of probiotics on necrotizing enterocolitis. *Semin Perinatol.* (2017) 41:41–51. doi: 10.1053/j.semperi.2016.09.017

22. Marcobal A, Barboza M, Froehlich JW, Block DE, German JB, Lebrilla CB, et al. Consumption of human milk oligosaccharides by gut-related microbes. *J Agric Food Chem.* (2010) 58:5334–40. doi: 10.1021/jf9044205
23. Marcobal A, Sonneburg JL. Human milk oligosaccharide consumption by intestinal microbiota. *Clin Microbiol Infect.* (2012) 18 (Suppl. 4):12–5. doi: 10.1111/j.1469-0691.2012.03863.x
24. Underwood MA, Gaerlan S, Leoz MLAD, Dimapasoc L, Kalanetra KM, Lemay DG, et al. Human milk oligosaccharides in premature infants: absorption, excretion, and influence on the intestinal microbiota. *Pediatr Res.* (2015) 78:670–7. doi: 10.1038/pr.2015.162
25. Underwood MA, Kalanetra KM, Bokulich NA, Lewis ZT, Mirmiran M, Tancredi DJ, et al. A comparison of two probiotic strains of bifidobacteria in premature infants. *J Pediatr.* (2013) 163:1585–91.e1589. doi: 10.1016/j.jpeds.2013.07.017
26. Modi N, Uthaya S, Fell J, Kulinskaya E. A randomized, double-blind, controlled trial of the effect of prebiotic oligosaccharides on enteral tolerance in preterm infants (ISRCTN77444690). *Pediatr Res.* (2010) 68:440–5. doi: 10.1203/PDR.0b013e3181f1cd59
27. Jacobi SK, Odle J. Nutritional factors influencing intestinal health of the neonate. *Adv Nutr.* (2012) 3:687–96. doi: 10.3945/an.112.002683
28. Tao N, Wu S, Kim J, An HJ, Hinde K, Power ML, et al. Evolutionary glycomics: characterization of milk oligosaccharides in primates. *J Proteome Res.* (2011) 2011:4. doi: 10.1021/pr1009367
29. Bering SB. Human milk oligosaccharides to prevent gut dysfunction and necrotizing enterocolitis in preterm neonates. *Nutrients.* (2018) 10:1461. doi: 10.3390/nu10101461
30. Niño DF, Sodhi CP, Hackam DJ. Necrotizing enterocolitis: new insights into pathogenesis and mechanisms. *Nat Rev Gastroenterol Hepatol.* (2016) 13:590–600. doi: 10.1038/nrgastro.2016.119
31. Sodhi CP, Wipf P, Yamaguchi Y, Fulton WB, Kovler M, Niño DF, et al. The human milk oligosaccharides 2'-fucosyllactose and 6'-sialyllactose protect against the development of necrotizing enterocolitis by inhibiting toll-like receptor 4 signaling. *Pediatr Res.* (2021) 89:91–101. doi: 10.1038/s41390-020-0852-3
32. Hackam DJ, Sodhi CP. Toll-like receptor-mediated intestinal inflammatory imbalance in the pathogenesis of necrotizing enterocolitis. *Cell Mol Gastroenterol Hepatol.* (2018) 6:229–38.e221. doi: 10.1016/j.jcmgh.2018.04.001
33. Taylor SN, Basile LA, Ebeling M, Wagner CL. Intestinal permeability in preterm infants by feeding type: mother's milk versus formula. *Breastfeed Med.* (2009) 4:11–5. doi: 10.1089/bfm.2008.0114
34. Chi C, Buys N, Li C, Sun J, Yin C. Effects of prebiotics on sepsis, necrotizing enterocolitis, mortality, feeding intolerance, time to full enteral feeding, length of hospital stay, and stool frequency in preterm infants: a meta-analysis. *Eur J Clin Nutr.* (2019) 73:657–70. doi: 10.1038/s41430-018-0377-6
35. Good M, Sodhi CP, Yamaguchi Y, Jia H, Lu P, Fulton WB, et al. The human milk oligosaccharide 2′-fucosyllactose attenuates the severity of experimental necrotising enterocolitis by enhancing mesenteric perfusion in the neonatal intestine. *Br J Nutr.* (2016) 116:1175–87. doi: 10.1017/S0007114516002944
36. Masi AC, Embleton ND, Lamb CA, Young G, Granger CL, Najera J, et al. Human milk oligosaccharide DSLNT and gut microbiome in preterm infants predicts necrotising enterocolitis. *Gut.* (2020). doi: 10.1136/gutjnl-2020-322771. [Epub ahead of print].
37. Wejryd E, Martí M, Marchini G, Werme A, Jonsson B, Landberg E, et al. Low diversity of human milk oligosaccharides is associated with necrotising enterocolitis in extremely low birth weight infants. *Nutrients.* (2018) 10:1556. doi: 10.3390/nu10101556
38. Demmert M, Schaper A, Pagel J, Gebauer C, Emeis M, Heitmann F, et al. FUT 2 polymorphism and outcome in very-low-birth-weight infants. *Pediatr Res.* (2015) 77:586–90. doi: 10.1038/pr.2015.1
39. American Academy of Pediatrics. *Breastfeeding and the Use of Human Milk.* Available online at: https://pediatrics.aappublications.org/content/pediatrics/129/3/e827.full.pdf. Published 2012 (accessed 30 June, 2021).
40. Australian Breastfeeding Association. *Position Statement on Donor Milk.* (2014). Available online at: https://www.breastfeeding.asn.au/system/files/content/POL-StatementonDonorMilk-V3-201803.pdf (accessed 30 June, 2021).
41. Ford SL, Lohmann P, Preidis GA, Gordon PS, O'Donnell A, Hagan J, et al. Improved feeding tolerance and growth are linked to increased gut microbial community diversity in very-low-birth-weight infants fed mother's own milk compared with donor breast milk. *Am J Clin Nutr.* (2019) 109:1088–97. doi: 10.1093/ajcn/nqz006
42. Meier P, Patel A, Esquerra-Zwiers A. Donor human milk update: evidence, mechanisms, and priorities for research and practice. *J Pediatr.* (2017) 180:15–21. doi: 10.1016/j.jpeds.2016.09.027
43. Bakar SYBA, Salim M, Clulow AJ, Nicholas KR, Boyd BJ. Human milk composition and the effects of pasteurisation on the activity of its components. *Trends Food Sci Technol.* (2021) 111:166–74. doi: 10.1016/j.tifs.2021.02.055
44. Nangia S, Ramaswamy VV, Bhasin M. The profile of donors to a human milk bank in a developing nation. *Breastfeed Med.* (2020) 15:135–9. doi: 10.1089/bfm.2019.0212
45. Chang FY, Cheng SW, Wu TZ, Fang LJ. Characteristics of the first human milk bank in Taiwan. *Pediatr Neonatol.* (2013) 54:28–33. doi: 10.1016/j.pedneo.2012.11.004
46. Sánchez Luna M, Martin SC, Gómez-de-Orgaz CS. Human milk bank and personalized nutrition in the NICU: a narrative review. *Eur J Pediatr.* (2021) 180:1327–33. doi: 10.1007/s00431-020-03887-y
47. Azad M. *Matching Donor Human Milk On Maternal Secretor Status (MMOMSS) Study (MMOMSS).* (2021). Available online at: https://clinicaltrials.gov/ct2/show/NCT04130165?term=human$+$milk$+$oligosaccharide&draw=5 (accessed 30 June, 2021).
48. Morrow AL, Ruiz-Palacios GM, Altaye M, Jiang X, Guerrero ML, Meinzen-Derr JK, et al. Human milk oligosaccharides are associated with protection against diarrhea in breast-fed infants. *J Pediatr.* (2004) 145:297–303. doi: 10.1016/j.jpeds.2004.04.054
49. Friend LL, Perrin MT. Fat and protein variability in donor human milk and associations with milk banking processes. *Breastfeed Med.* (2020) 15:370–6. doi: 10.1089/bfm.2020.0046
50. Sullivan S, Schanler RJ, Kim JH, Patel AL, Trawöger R, Kiechl-Kohlendorfer U, et al. An exclusively human milk-based diet is associated with a lower rate of necrotizing enterocolitis than a diet of human milk and bovine milk-based products. *J Pediatr.* (2010) 154:562–7. doi: 10.1016/j.jpeds.2009.10.040
51. Assad M, Elliot MJ, Abraham JH. Decreased cost and improved feeding tolerance in VLBW infants fed an exclusive human milk diet. *J Perinatol.* (2016) 36:216–20. doi: 10.1038/jp.2015.168
52. Prolacta Bioscience. *Humavant Human Milk Fortifier (Human, Pasteurized).* (2013–2021). Available online at: http://prolacta.asia/products/human-milk-fortifier. Published 2013-2021 (accessed 30 June, 2021).
53. Grace E, Hilditch C, Gomersall J, Collins CT, Rumbold A, Keir A. Safety and efficacy of human milk-based fortifier in enterally fed preterm and/or low birthweight infants: a systematic review and meta-analysis. *Arch Dis Child Fetal Neonatal Ed.* (2021) 106:137–42. doi: 10.1136/archdischild-2020-319406
54. Abrahamsson T. *Human Milk Fortification in Extremely Preterm Infants (N-forte).* (2021). Available online at: https://clinicaltrials.gov/ct2/show/NCT03797157?term=human+milk+oligosaccharide&draw=5 (accessed 30 June, 2021).
55. Shama S, Unger S, Pouliot Y, Doyen A, Suwal S, Pencharz P, et al. A human milk-based protein concentrate developed for preterm infants retains bioactive proteins and supports growth of weanling rats. *J Nutr.* (2021) 151:840–7. doi: 10.1093/jn/nxaa383
56. Obelitz-Ryom K, Rendboe AK, Nguyen DN, Rudloff S, Brandt AB, Nielsen DS, et al. Bovine milk oligosaccharides with sialyllactose for preterm piglets. *Nutrients.* (2018) 10:1489. doi: 10.3390/nu10101489
57. Meli F, Puccio G, Cajozzo C, Ricottone GL, Pecquet S, Sprenger N, et al. Growth and safety evaluation of infant formulae containing oligosaccharides derived from bovine milk: a randomized, double-blind, noninferiority trial. *BMC Pediatr.* (2014) 14:306. doi: 10.1186/s12887-014-0306-3
58. Srinivasjois R, Rao S, Patole S. Prebiotic supplementation in preterm neonates: updated systematic review and meta-analysis of randomised controlled trials. *Clin Nutr.* (2013) 32:958–65. doi: 10.1016/j.clnu.2013.05.009
59. Jost T, Lacroix C, Braegger C, Chassard C. Impact of human milk bacteria and oligosaccharides on neonatal gut microbiota establishment and gut health. *Nutr Rev.* (2015) 73:426–37. doi: 10.1093/nutrit/nuu016
60. Nestle. *Use of a Liquid Supplement Containing 2 Human Milk Oligosaccharides (HMOs) in Preterm Infants.* (2021). Available online at: https://clinicaltrials.gov/ct2/show/NCT03607942?cond=human+milk+oligosaccharides&draw=2 (accessed 30 June, 2021).
61. Jantscher-Krenn E, Zherebtsov M, Nissan C, Goth K, Guner YS, Naidu N, et al. The human milk oligosaccharide disialyllacto-N-tetraose prevents necrotising enterocolitis in neonatal rats. *Gut.* (2012) 61:1417–25. doi: 10.1136/gutjnl-2011-301404

62. Autran CA, Schoterman MHC, Jantscher-Krenn E, Kamerling JP, Bode L. Sialylated galacto-oligosaccharides and 2′-fucosyllactose reduce necrotising enterocolitis in neonatal rats. *Br J Nutr.* (2016) 116:294–9. doi: 10.1017/S0007114516002038
63. Rasmussen SO, Martin L, Østergaard MV, Rudloff S, Roggenbuck M, Nguyen DN, et al. Human milk oligosaccharide effects on intestinal function and inflammation after preterm birth in pigs. *J Nutr Biochem.* (2017) 40:141–54. doi: 10.1016/j.jnutbio.2016.10.011
64. Ravindran S. *Producing Human Milk Sugars for Use in Formula. SPLASH! Milk Science Update: October 2015.* (2015) Available online at: https://milkgenomics.org/article/producing-human-milk-sugars-for-use-in-formula/ (accessed 30 June, 2021).
65. Bührer C, Fischer HS, Wellmann S. Nutritional interventions to reduce rates of infection, necrotizing enterocolitis and mortality in very preterm infants. *Pediatr Res.* (2019) 87:371–7. doi: 10.1038/s41390-019-0630-2
66. Meredith-Dennis L, Xu G, Goonatilleke E, Lebrilla CB, Underwood MA, Smilowitz JT. Composition and variation of macronutrients, immune proteins, and human milk oligosaccharides in human milk from nonprofit and commercial milk banks. *J Hum Lact.* (2018) 34:120–9. doi: 10.1177/0890334417710635
67. Bertino E, Coppa GV, Giuliani F, Coscia A, Gabrielli O, Sabatino G, et al. Effects of holder pasteurization on human milk oligosaccharides. *Int J Immunopathol Pharmacol.* (2008) 21:381–5. doi: 10.1177/039463200802100216
68. Neu J. Preterm infant nutrition, gut bacteria, and necrotizing enterocolitis. *Curr Opin Clin Nutr Metab Care.* (2015) 18:285–8. doi: 10.1097/MCO.0000000000000169

28

Successful Full Lactation Achieved by Mothers of Preterm Infants using Exclusive Pumping

Xifang Ru[†], Xiaofang Huang[†] and Qi Feng[*]

Department of Pediatrics, Peking University First Hospital, Beijing, China

***Correspondence:**
Qi Feng
fengqizf@126.com

[†] These authors have contributed equally to this work*

Background: Some mothers of preterm infants suffer from difficulties in initiating and maintaining adequate milk production. This study was designed to investigate the milk production in mothers of preterm infants using hospital-grade breast pumps and to study the nutrient content of their milk.

Methods: This was an observational prospective study. Mothers of preterm infants with gestational age < 32 weeks or birth weight < 1,500 g who were admitted to our hospital from August 2016 to December 2017 were recruited. A pumping diary and a questionnaire were completed by mothers ($n = 30$). Milk samples from before, during, and after each pumping session on days 7 and 14 postpartum were analyzed.

Results: The median time to onset of lactogenesis II was 75.4 h. Mean milk output increased gradually, meeting key thresholds of 350 g/d on day 6, 500 g/d on day 8, and close to 750 g/d on day 14. Then, all mean milk outputs were over 750 g/d. The mean milk output exceeded the mean feeding volume on days 7, 14, 21, 28, 35, and 42. Mothers using hospital-grade breast pumps had more cumulative milk production compared with mothers using hand expression. The milk yield on days 7 and 14 were positively correlated to that on days 21, 28, 35, and 42. Milk outputs on days 7, 14, and 42 of mothers with a pumping frequency of ≥ 6 times/d were greater than mothers with a pumping frequency of < 6 times/d. Threshold values for milk output on day 7 (cut-off, 406.8 g/d; sensitivity, 68.2%; specificity, 100%) and day 14 (cut-off, 518.0 g/d; sensitivity, 81.8%; specificity, 100%) were identified as predicting a milk output of more than 750 g/d on day 42. Fat and energy levels were higher in hind-milk than fore- or mixed-milk on days 7 and 14. Those who pumped ≥ 6 times/d had higher levels of fat, carbohydrate, and energy in their milk on day 7.

Conclusion: Most preterm infants' mothers using a hospital-grade pump with a pumping frequency of ≥ 6 times/d can reach full lactation successfully. Nutrient analysis of the human milk should be performed.

Keywords: human milk production, breastfeeding, breast pump, lactation, prematurity, nutrition

INTRODUCTION

Human milk, especially mother's own milk, is highly recommended for preterm infants due to the beneficial effects it has on their development and health (1). Feeding with mother's own milk is now considered to be the best practice for preterm infants to reduce the risk of necrotizing enterocolitis and is believed to have a dose-dependent effect on neurodevelopmental improvement (2).

Unlike term infants, most preterm infants are unable to feed directly at the breast due to immaturity, illness, maternal-infant separation, etc. Under such circumstances, mothers are breast pump-dependent and often suffer from difficulties in initiating and maintaining adequate milk production. However, many mothers feel that the provision of milk is the only positive contribution they can make to the growth of their babies in this critical period, and failing to do so increases maternal anxiety (3). Therefore, establishing lactation (in the absence of direct breastfeeding) and developing an adequate expressing regime (method and schedule) are essential for the well-being of both mother and infant.

For mothers of preterm infants globally, insufficient milk volume remains a concern (4). Studies have demonstrated that the first 2 weeks after birth are a critical period for the initiation and development of lactation, during which mammary epithelial cells appear to undergo programming processes that regulate long-term milk synthesis (5, 6).

There is strong evidence that, for pump-dependent mothers, using a hospital-grade electric breast pump results in greater milk output than other expression methods (6–8). Many different recommendations are available in the literature regarding the use of a breast pump and the development of expression schedules (frequency) for the expressing mother. Current recommendations suggest that breast pumping should be performed with the same frequency as breastfeeding of a full term infant, i.e., every 3 h, night break of no more than 5 h, milk expression at least five times each day, and cumulative time at the breast pump of more than 100 min per day (9, 10).

However, these are generalized recommendations with no regard to the individual differences between mothers. In order to make individualized recommendations and to maximize milk output, it is necessary to identify the major determinants of milk production and to understand how these vary between individual mothers. Although it is challenging to establish milk supply in mothers of very-low-birth-weight (VLBW) infants early in the postpartum period, its importance should be emphasized.

The primary aim of this study was to investigate the initiation of lactation and the milk production with the help of hospital-grade breast pumps in mothers who were separated from their preterm infants in our neonatal intensive care unit (NICU). The secondary aim was to study the effect of breast pumping frequency on the volume and nutrient content of expressed milk.

MATERIALS AND METHODS

Study Setting

Mothers who planned on breastfeeding and their preterm infants who were admitted to our NICU from August 2016 to December 2017 were involved in our study.

This was an observational prospective study carried out in the NICU of our hospital. The hospital was a Baby-Friendly Hospital, lactation services, such as breastfeeding knowledge and skills education, were available from obstetricians, obstetric nurses, and NICU team during hospitalization and the postpartum period. In our hospital, mothers were unable to stay with their preterm babies in the NICU, and no donor milk bank was available. The only way for mothers to breastfeed their preterm infants was to provide their own expressed milk. The obstetric nurses instructed each mother on the technique for milk expression through educational video, verbal instruction, and hands-on support for first milk expression. All participating mothers received standardized instructions on breast pumping by NICU doctors specializing in breast milk consultation several hours after delivery. Key recommendations, including starting pumping as soon as possible after delivery (target was within 6 h after delivery) and pumping every 2–3 h with no more than a 5-h break during the night, were communicated to the mothers. All mothers were seen daily by doctors and nurses during hospitalization to review milk expression techniques and to answer questions. Our breastfeeding hotline was open day and night to answer breastfeeding related inquiries.

A hospital-grade electric breast pump (Symphony, Medela AG, Switzerland) was provided to each mother immediately after enrollment. The pump was provided free of charge for the first 42 days postpartum, and all related disposable devices and milk containers were provided, whether in the hospital or at home. Mothers had the option to rent the pump if it was still needed after the 42-day period. Detailed information on breastfeeding was distributed and instructions on pump usage were given by the researchers. Before the onset of lactogenesis II (OOL-II), the initiation program (initiation breast pump suction patterns, I-BPSP) was selected for each pumping session. Once the OOL-II occurred as determined by the mother expressing a volume of 20 mL for three consecutive pumping sessions, the pumping program was switched to the maintenance program (standard breast pump suction patterns, S-BPSP). Mothers continued pumping for an additional 2 min after the last droplets of milk were noted to ensure that breasts were sufficiently drained. Mothers were encouraged to express their breast milk using the maximum comfortable vacuum as determined according to the mothers' own preferences. The maximum comfortable vacuum was determined by slowly increasing the vacuum until it felt slightly uncomfortable (not painful) and then decreasing it slightly. The selected pressure was then maintained over the course of the study.

Inclusion and Exclusion Criteria

The inclusion criteria for enrollment included: (a) infants' gestational age (GA) < 32 weeks or birth weight < 1,500 g; (b) infants admitted to the NICU within the first 12 h of birth; (c) mothers over 18 years old; (d) mothers willing to breastfeed; (e) mothers joining our study within 24 h postpartum. The exclusion criteria were: (a) preterm infants who were very critical with unstable vital signs; (b) preterm infants or their mothers who had breastfeeding contraindications; (c) hospitalization for < 2 weeks or discharged against medical advice.

Measurements

Daily milk output was defined as the cumulative milk volume from both left and right breasts from midnight to midnight. Milk output was measured by an electronic digital scale to the nearest 0.1 g. The time to the OOL-II was defined as the time point whenever milk output ≥ 20 g for three consecutive pumping sessions.

A dedicated human milk pumping diary recording pumping frequency and duration and milk output for each pumping session was completed for this study over the first 14 days, and on the 21st, 28th, 35th, and 42nd days postpartum. All mothers completed a questionnaire 5–7 days after enrollment.

Three characteristics of the OOL-II were measured: time to establish OOL-II; number of pumping sessions from birth to the OOL-II; and cumulative duration of pumping until the OOL-II.

Milk samples were collected from the mothers who were enrolled from September 2017 to December 2017. Milk (~1 mL) was taken from each breast before (fore), during (mixed), and after (hind) each pumping session on days 7 and 14 postpartum. Milk samples were collected in plastic tubes (with scale lines), stored at −18°C, and transferred to the hospital as soon as possible. Consultations on milk pumping and sampling were provided by the researchers around the clock. Phone call reminders for sample collections were made on days 6 and 13, 1 day before each milk sampling.

A human milk analyzer (HMA, Miris®, Sweden) was used for macronutrient analysis, as per the manufacturer's instructions. Briefly, the frozen milk samples were thawed at 40°C, stirred, and homogenized with ~2 mL (mixture of 1 mL from each breast) of milk used per analysis.

TABLE 1 | The characteristics of the study population, pumping performance and OOL-II related information.

Characteristics	n	Mean ± SD, M (P_{25}, P_{75}) or n (%)
Mothers' age (years)	30	32.9 ± 4.5
Cesarean delivery	30	19 (63.3)
After IVF-ET	30	7 (23.3)
Multipara	30	9 (30.0)
Gestational ages (weeks)	30	29.7 ± 1.8
Birth weight (g)	37	1235.7 ± 260.8
Multiple birth	30	7 (23.3)
Pre-pregnancy BMI (kg/m^2)	30	24.1 ± 4.5
Weight gain during pregnancy (kg)	30	8.0 ± 4.2
Drinking alcohol or smoking during pregnancy or lactation	30	0 (0.0)
Maternal risk factor for preterm birth	30	28 (93.3)
Premature rupture of membranes	30	5 (16.7)
Pre-eclampsia/eclampsia	30	3 (10.0)
Maternal diabetes	30	1 (3.3)
Infection	30	3 (10.0)
Placenta previa, vaginal bleeding	30	1 (3.3)
Placental abruption	30	1 (3.3)
≥ 2 maternal risk factors	30	14 (46.7)
Breast inflamation or surgery	30	0 (0.0)
Gestational ages ≤ 30 weeks	37	22 (59.5)
Birth weight < 1,500 g	37	28 (75.8)
First pumping postpartum (h)	30	7.6 (4.6, 10.3)
Time to establish OOL-II		
After birth (h)	30	75.4 (60.7, 83.9)
After 1st pumping (h)	30	65.8 (56.6, 76.5)
Number of pumping sessions from birth to the OOL-II (times)	30	16.0 (13.8, 21.0)
Cumulative duration of pumping until the OOL-II (h)	30	4.0 (3.4, 5.3)
Breast pumping frequency (times/d, within 42 d after delivery)	30	6.7 ± 0.7

IVF-ET, in vitro fertilization and embryo transfer; BMI, body mass index; OOL-II, onset of lactogenesis II.

Data Collection

Data were collected and collated by designated well-trained researchers. The dedicated human milk pumping diaries were requested. Milk nutritional data were recorded in the data system in a timely manner. Data were kept secure under the rigorous management of our hospital. Original data collected from the diaries were archived for quality control in a well-protected data system. The data were not permitted to be utilized for commercial purposes.

Data Analysis

Data analysis was performed using Statistical Package for the Social Sciences (SPSS) software for Windows version 20.0 (SPSS Inc, Chicago, IL, USA). Data with normal distribution were expressed as mean ± standard deviation (SD). Comparison of the various continuous parameters was performed using univariate analysis of variance and t-test. Non-normal data were expressed as M (P_{25}, P_{75}) and compared with non-parametric test. Correlation analysis was performed using Pearson correlation. Receiver operating characteristic (ROC) curves were drawn using SPSS to explore the predictive value of milk output of more than 750 g or 1,000 g on day 42. A P-value of < 0.05 was considered to be statistically significant.

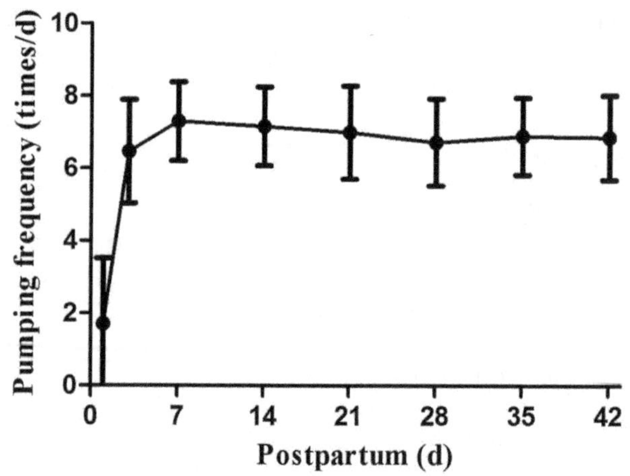

FIGURE 1 | Pumping frequency during study period.

RESULTS

Characteristics of the Study Population and Pumping Sessions

Initially, 33 mothers of preterm infants who met the inclusion criteria were included. However, three were later excluded from our study, as one found it difficult to keep up with the pumping and two did not keep records as we requested. The characteristics of the study population were shown in **Table 1**. The mean age of the mothers was 32.9 ± 4.5 years, 19 underwent cesarean sections, 9 were multiparous, and 7 had multiple births. The mean GA was 29.7 ± 1.8 weeks, and the mean birth weight was 1235.7 ± 260.8 g. The GA of 22 (59.5%) infants was <= 30 weeks, and 28 (75.8%) infants were VLBW infants (< 1,500 g). None of the mothers smoked or drank during pregnancy or lactation, and 14 mothers had ≥ 2 maternal risk factors for preterm birth.

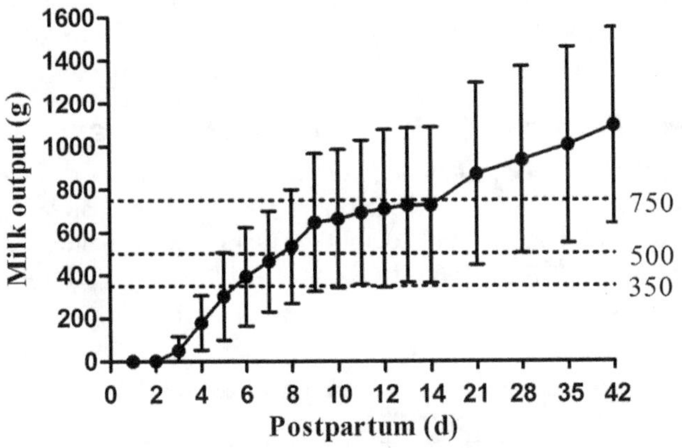

FIGURE 2 | Daily maternal milk output in 1st 42 days postpartum.

TABLE 2 | Daily maternal milk output ≥ 350 g/d, 500 g/d and 750 g/d (*n*, %).

Milk output	D7	D14	D21	D28	D35	D42
≥ 350 g/d	17 (56.7)	28 (93.3)	28 (93.3)	28 (93.3)	28 (93.3)	28 (93.3)
≥ 500 g/d	13 (43.3)	19 (63.3)	24 (80.0)	26 (86.7)	28 (93.3)	28 (93.3)
≥ 750 g/d	5 (16.7)	11 (36.7)	16 (53.3)	19 (63.3)	20 (66.7)	22 (73.3)

Onset of Lactogenesis II

The median time from delivery to starting pumping was 7.6 h. The median time from delivery to OOL-II was 75.4 (60.7, 83.9) h (**Table 1**). Of these, 40% (12/30) of mothers reached the OOL-II within the recommended 72 h, with a mean time of 57.5 h (ranging from 44.6 to 72.0 h), while a delayed onset of lactogenesis II (DOL-II) occurred in 60% (18/30) of the participants. Moreover, two mothers failed to reach the OOL-II throughout the 42-day study period.

Pumping Frequency

The mean frequency of pumping sessions within 42 days after delivery was 6.7 times/d. In the first 7 days postpartum, maternal pumping frequency gradually increased; after day 7, pumping frequency remained relatively stable at ~6–8 times/d (**Figure 1**).

Daily Human Milk Output

Daily Milk output of preterm infants' mothers increased steadily from the OOL-II establishment until 6 weeks postpartum, with a particularly rapid increase from day 7 to day 28 (**Figure 2**). Large variations in milk output were found among the mothers throughout the study, and the disparity became more apparent as time went by, e.g., 107.3 g/d vs. 1,850.0 g/d on day 42. Mean milk output increased as the study progressed, meeting key thresholds of 350g/d on day 6, 500 g/d on day 8, and close to 750 g/d on day 14. Then, all mean milk outputs were over 750 g/d. The percentage of daily milk output ≥ 350 g/d, ≥ 500 g/d, and ≥ 750 g/d are shown in **Table 2**. On day 42, only 2 mothers (6.7%) did not reach 350 g/d or 500 g/d, and 8 mothers (26.7%) did not reach 750 g/d.

The mean milk output of mothers of single birth on day 1 was less than the mean feeding volume of their babies ($P < 0.001$, **Figure 3**). The mean milk output gradually increased and

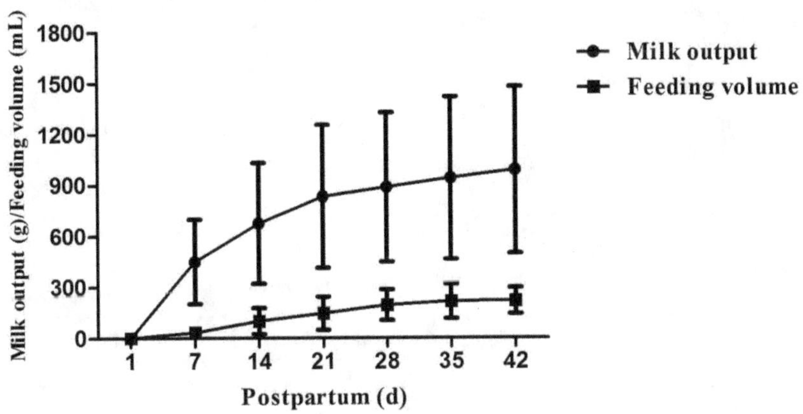

FIGURE 3 | Milk output and feeding volume on days 7, 14, 21, 28, 35 and 42 (all $P < 0.001$).

exceeded the mean feeding volume on days 7, 14, 21, 28, 35, and 42 ($P < 0.001$, **Figure 3**). The percentages of milk output in mothers of single birth exceeding feeding volume of their infants were 43.5% on day 1, 100% on days 7, 14, and 21, 95.6% on days 28 and 35, and 91.3% on day 42, respectively.

The milk output of mothers using hospital-grade breast pumps in this study were compared with that of mothers of VLBW infants with early exclusive hand expression in the literature (8). Except for the first 2 days after birth, mothers using hospital-grade breast pumps in this study had significantly ($P < 0.05$, **Table 3**) more cumulative daily milk production throughout the first 14 days postpartum compared with mothers using exclusive hand expression in the literature.

Correlations Between Milk Output on Days 7 and 14 With That on Other Days

Pearson correlation analysis was used to analyze the correlations of milk output on days 7 and 14 with that on other days (**Table 4**). Milk yield on day 7 was positively correlated to those on days 14, 21, 28, 35, and 42. Milk yield on day 14 also had positive correlations with those on days 21, 28, 35, and 42. As the study progressed, the correlation gradually weakened (day 7 with day 14, $r = 0.886$; day 7 with day 42, $r = 0.756$; day 14 with day 21, $r = 0.951$; day 14 with day 42, $r = 0.843$; all $P < 0.001$).

Factors Affecting Milk Output

Mothers were assigned to one of two groups based on their mean pumping frequency. On days 7, 14, and 42, the mean milk output of mothers with a pumping frequency of ≥ 6 times/d was greater than that of mothers with a pumping frequency of < 6 times/d. On postpartum day 42, this difference was statistically significant ($t = -2.828$, $P = 0.009$, **Table 5**). On days 7, 14, and 42, mothers who started pumping within 6 h after delivery ($n = 12$) had the same milk output as those who started pumping after 6 h or more ($n = 18$). The time from delivery to the OOL-II was also associated with milk output. Mothers who reached the OOL-II within 72 h had significantly higher milk output on postpartum days 7, 14, and 42 ($P < 0.001$, **Table 5**).

The mean milk output of mothers who had multiple births was not significantly different from that of mothers who had single births ($P > 0.05$). On postpartum days 7, 14, and 42, the mean milk output of mothers with GA ≥ 30 weeks vs. < 30 weeks were not significantly different ($P > 0.05$).

Predictors of Milk Output > 750 g/d and > 1,000 g/d on Day 42

As shown in **Figure 4**, ROC curves were used to analyze the predictive value of milk output on days 7 and 14 for milk output > 750 g/d (**Figure 4A**) and > 1,000 g/d (**Figure 4B**)

TABLE 3 | Comparison of mothers with hospital-grade breast pump in this study vs. mothers with hand expression in the literature.

	This study (hospital-grade breast pump, g, *n* = 30)	The literature (hand expression, mL, *n* = 12)	*Z*	*P*-value
Cumulative milk output after				
D1	0.0 (0.0, 0.0)	0.1 (0.0, 2.6)	0	<0.001
D2	0.0 (0.0, 0.6)	0.25 (0, 11)	201.0	0.493
D3	28.8 (3.0, 82.9)	15 (0.3, 41)	355.0	0.012
D4	173.3 (94.6, 360.5)	119 (6, 167)	371.0	0.004
D5	428.8 (269.7, 828.5)	216 (28, 267)	416.0	<0.001
D6	820.0 (482.3, 1308.8)	359 (59, 594)	440.0	<0.001
D7	1139.3 (827.1, 1289.3)	456 (104, 866)	456.0	<0.001
D14	5802.6 (3630.5, 8406.7)	2,387 (1,196, 3,952)	453.0	<0.001
Cumulative milk output between				
D8-14	4560.8 (2866.4, 6646.7)	1,789 (957, 3,320)	453.0	<0.001

TABLE 5 | Milk output with different pumping frequency, first pumping time or OOL-II time.

	n	Milk output (g/d)		
		D7	D14	D42
Pumping frequency				
< 6 times/d	4	299.5 ± 213.1	447.5 ± 361.3	557.5 ± 308.2
≥ 6 times/d	26	490.1 ± 231.0	768.5 ± 348.2	1178.7 ± 419.4
t-test		−1.549	−1.71	−2.828
P-value		0.133	0.098	0.009
First pumping time (h)				
≤ 6 h	12	480.3 ± 239.2	794.1 ± 420.9	1096.9 ± 551.4
> 6 h	18	454.2 ± 237.9	680.0 ± 319.6	1095.2 ± 396.8
t-test		0.294	0.843	0.010
P-value		0.771	0.406	0.992
Time to reach OOL-II				
≤ 72 h	12	654.6 ± 183.0	1028.5 ± 252.1	1436.9 ± 278.4
> 72 h	18	344.0 ± 183.7	523.8 ± 270.8	868.6 ± 409.0
t-test		4.412	5.137	4.197
P-value		< 0.001	< 0.001	< 0.001

TABLE 4 | Correlations between milk output on days 7 and 14 and other days.

	D14		D21		D28		D35		D42	
	r	*P*-value	*r*	*P*-value	*r*	*P*-value	*r*	*P*-value	*r*	*P*-value
D7	0.886	< 0.001	0.847	< 0.001	0.813	< 0.001	0.841	< 0.001	0.756	< 0.001
D14	1		0.951	< 0.001	0.925	< 0.001	0.877	< 0.001	0.843	< 0.001

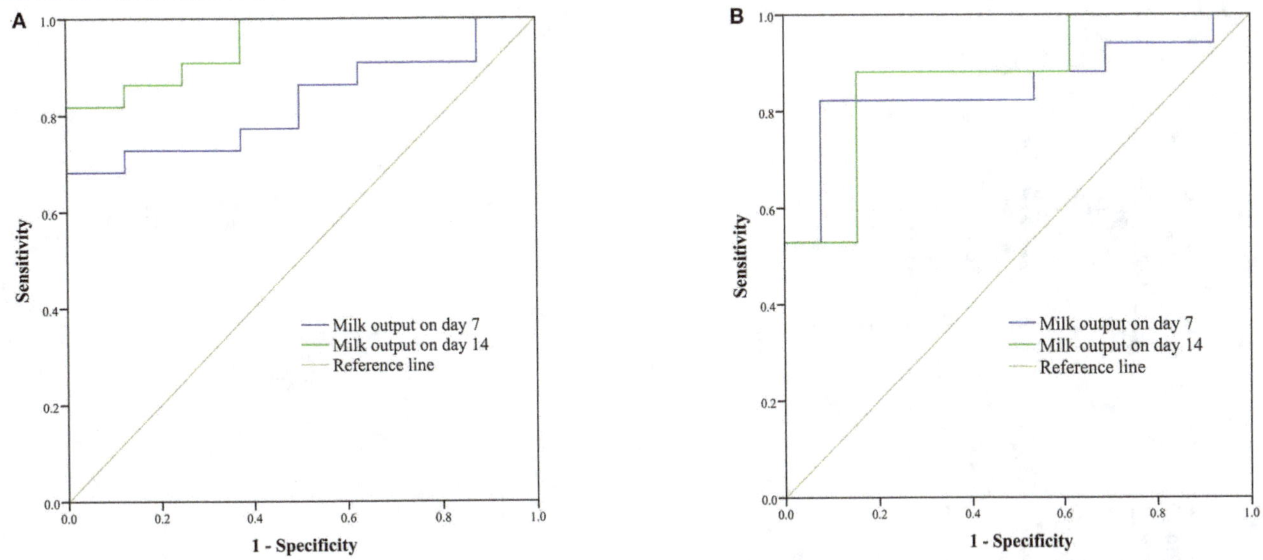

FIGURE 4 | Receiver operating characteristic (ROC) curves of milk output on days 7 and 14 for prediction of milk output > 750 g/d **(A)** and > 1,000 g/d **(B)** on day 42. **(A)** For the cut-off values of 406.8 g/d on day 7 [the area under the curve (AUC) was 0.824; 95% *CI* was 0.678–0.970; $P = 0.008$; sensitivity was 68.2%; specificity was 100%] and 518.0 g/d on day 14 (AUC was 0.949; 95% *CI* was 0.875–1.000; $P < 0.001$; sensitivity was 81.8%; specificity was 100%) were selected to predict the milk output being more than 750 g/d on day 42. **(B)** For the cut-off values of 406.8 g/d on day 7 (AUC was 0.851; 95% *CI* was 0.705–0.996; $P = 0.001$; sensitivity was 82.4%; specificity was 94.3%) and 600.9 g/d on day 14 (AUC was 0.873; 95% *CI* was 0.745–1.000; $P = 0.001$; sensitivity was 88.2%; specificity was 84.6%) were selected to predict the milk output being more than 1,000 g/d on day 42.

TABLE 6 | Nutrients in human milk on days 7 and 14.

		Fat (g/100 mL)	Protein (g/100 mL)	Carbohydrate (g/100 mL)	Energy (Kcal/100 mL)
D7	*n*	56	56	56	56
	Fore-milk	3.31 ± 0.80	1.94 ± 0.19	7.33 ± 0.43	68.43± 7.77
	Mixed-milk	3.62 ± 0.73	1.96 ± 0.21	7.43 ± 0.32	71.77 ± 7.16
	Hind-milk	4.14 ± 1.24	1.94 ± 0.25	7.35 ± 0.43	76.34 ± 11.57
	F	10.945	0.115	1.067	10.798
	P-value	< 0.001	0.892	0.346	< 0.001
D14	*n*	47	47	47	47
	Fore-milk	3.6 ± 1.1	1.73 ± 0.16	7.64 ± 0.31	71.47 ± 10.84
	Mixed-milk	4.6 ± 0.9	1.69 ± 0.16	7.61 ± 0.18	80.68 ± 8.78
	Hind-milk	5.2 ± 1.1	1.67 ± 0.18	7.51 ± 0.27	86.49 ± 10.42
	F	28.693	1.667	3.391	26.689
	P-value	< 0.001	0.193	0.036	< 0.001

on day 42. Cut-off values of milk output on day 7 (406.8 g/d) and day 14 (518.0 g/d) were identified as predicting milk output of more than 750 g/d on day 42. Cut-off values for milk output on day 7 (406.8 g/d) and day 14 (600.9 g/d) were identified as predicting milk output of more than 1,000 g/d on day 42.

Milk Composition

A total of 309 samples from 8 participants were analyzed with the Miris HMA. Of these, 168 samples were colostrum, with 56 sets of fore-, mixed-, and hind-milk samples, and 141 samples were transitional milk, with 47 sets of fore-, mixed-, and hind-milk samples.

Fat and energy levels were higher in hind-milk than fore- or mixed-milk on days 7 and 14 ($P < 0.001$, **Table 6**). Fat and energy levels varied greatly over 24 h on day 7, but protein and carbohydrate levels remained relatively stable (**Figure 5**). Variation in nutrients on day 14 showed the same trends.

Those who pumped 6 times/d or more had higher fat, carbohydrate, and energy levels in their milk on day 7 (**Figure 6**: A, fat; B, protein; C, carbohydrate; D, energy). However, these differences were no longer present on day 14.

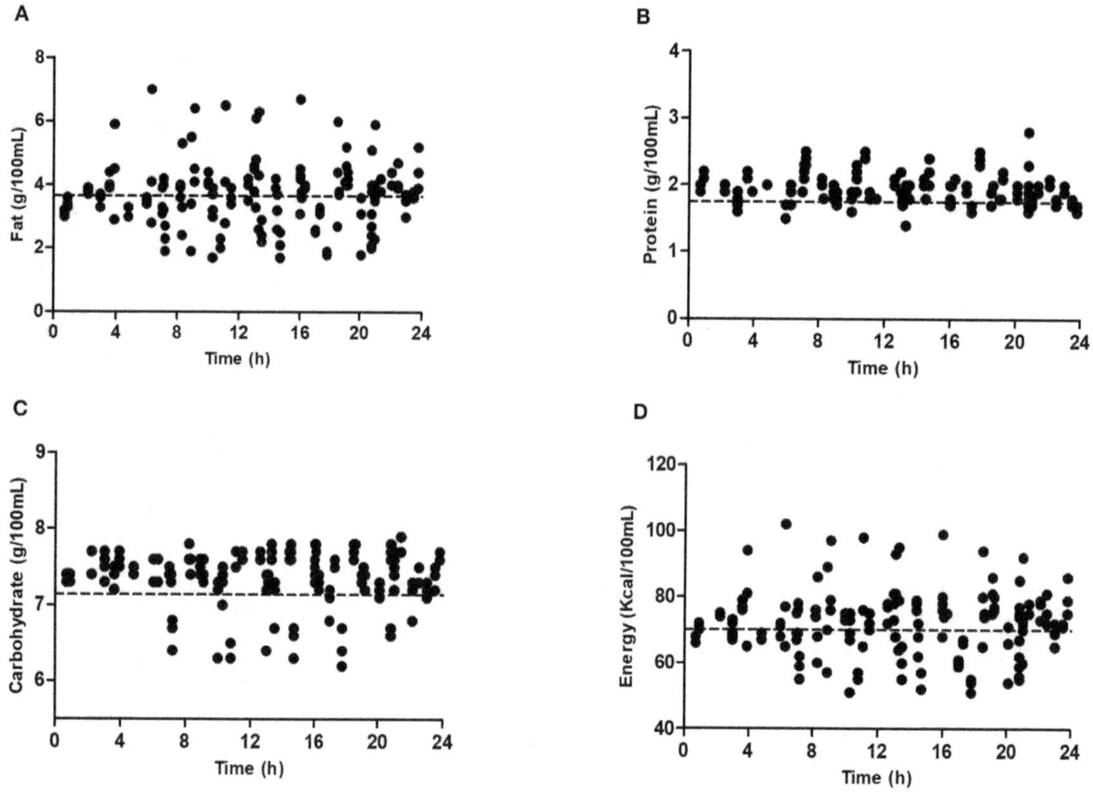

FIGURE 5 | Nutrients in milk sample on day 7. **(A)** Fat; **(B)** protein; **(C)** carbohydrate; **(D)** energy.

DISCUSSION

This research was conducted to investigate the breast pumping practices, milk production, milk nutrient content in mothers separated from their preterm infants using hospital-grade breast pumps. These data will be used to establish a baseline for the initiation and maintenance of lactation in mothers of preterm infants, and adds to the limited published literature on the concentration of macronutrients in the milk of mothers of VLBW infants.

In this study, the mean pumping frequency of preterm infants' mothers was 6.7 times per day, with 40% (12/30) of mothers starting pumping within 6 h postpartum, and 83.3% (25/30) of mothers starting pumping within 12 h. The median time from delivery to starting pumping was 7.6 h. Reasons for a delay in pumping (more than 6 h) may include pumps not being available prior to entering the study, insufficient support from family and staff, time-consuming transfers of infants to our hospital, and insufficient preparation for breast feeding sick infants.

The OOL-II typically occurs within 48–72 h after birth. Some researchers defined DOL-II as lactation onset occurring after 72 h postpartum (11, 12). DOL-II was a common issue occurring in mothers of preterm infants (4, 13). The definition of OOL-II in this study is a pragmatic approach similar to that reported by Meier et al. (14). The incidence of DOL-II (60%) in our study was higher than that reported in other Chinese literature (36%) (15), however, the GA and birthweight in our study were lower than that in the Chinese literature. In addition, the mean time to reach the OOL-II in this study (75.4 h) was shorter than that reported in mothers of VLBW infants (97.15 h) (16).

Linked to eventual milk output and duration of lactation, the successful completion of the transition from initiation to maintenance is a critical process (17). Preterm expressing mothers often suffer from inadequate milk supply (4). The minimum milk volume needed by preterm infants were 350 mL/d, 500 mL/d, and 750 mL/d when they are in the NICU, discharged from the NICU, and several months post-birth, respectively (18). These data showed that 56.7% and 43.3% of participants with hospital-grade breast pump produced milk output $\geq$ 350 g/d and 500 g/d on day 7. This rose to 63.3% on day 14 and 93.3% on day 42, similar to the percentage reported by Post et al. (19) in 2016 (91% in $<$ 34 w group using I-BPSP). With the help of hospital-grade breast pump, mothers had more cumulative daily milk production than using exclusive hand expression in the literature (8). In addition, on days 7, 14, 21, 28, 35, and 42 postpartum, the mean milk output was all greater than the feeding volume of their babies. Furthermore, milk output on day 21 (870.7 $\pm$ 423.5 g/d) was greater than that reported by Parker et al. (20) in 2012 for VLBW infants' mothers with early initiation (within 1 h) or late initiation (1–6 h) pump (613.0 mL and 267.2 mL, respectively). In our study, highly positive correlations were found among the week-to-week milk

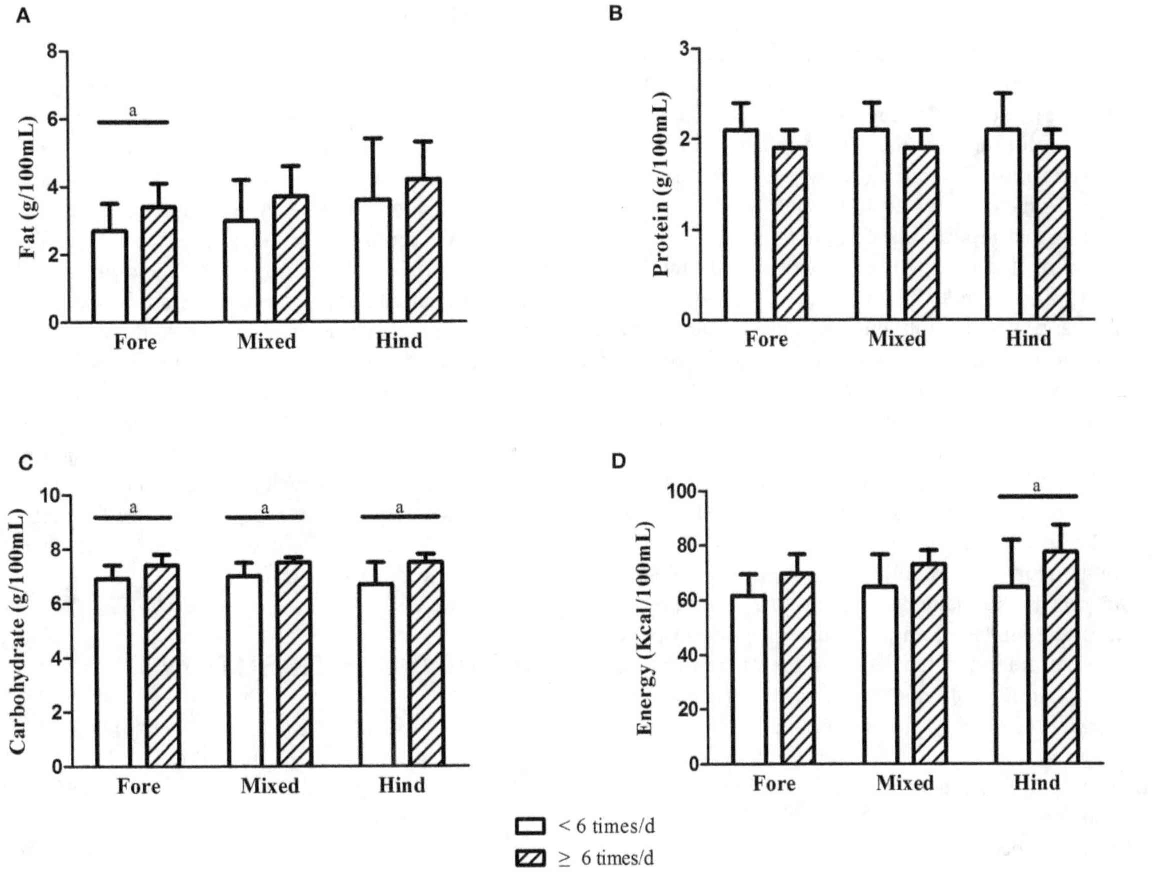

FIGURE 6 | Comparison of nutrients of breastmilk with different pumping frequency on day 7. **(A)** Fat; **(B)** protein; **(C)** carbohydrate; **(D)** energy (a, $P < 0.05$).

output, similar to previous studies (4, 21). Moreover, milk output on day 7 (area under the curve (AUC) = 0.824; $P = 0.008$) and day 14 (AUC = 0.949; $P < 0.001$) both predicted milk output (> 750 g/d) on day 42 with a high level of significance. These data suggest that milk output ≥ 406.8 g/d on day 7 and ≥ 518.0 g/d on day 14 is the most significant value for predicting milk adequacy on day 42.

Associations have been established by many previous studies between pumping initiation, pumping frequency, and milk output (20, 22). In this study, pumping frequency and milk output on day 42 were positively correlated. Compared with those who pumped <6 times/d, mothers who pumped ≥ 6 times/d produced significantly more milk on day 42 ($P = 0.009$). This suggests that pumping at least 6 times/d can help improve milk output on day 42, which is consistent with the results of previous research (9). The current study did not find significant associations between early initiation of milk expression and milk output, differing from previous studies (8, 20). Possible explanations are that the early-initiation mothers in our study may not have initiated pumping early enough to make a difference, e.g., < 1 h postpartum (20) or that the number of participants in this study was too small. The difference in milk output between the multiple birth group and the non-multiple birth group was not significant. Compared with mothers of infants with GA of < 30 w, the GA ≥ 30 w group did not show significant differences in milk output throughout the postpartum period.

The HMA (Miris) was considered to be a convenient and precise instrument for analysis of the macronutrient levels in breast milk (22). Menjo et al. (23) used an HMA to test fat and protein levels of diluted human milk. They proved four-time dilution to be acceptable. However, others have shown that dilution might affect the performance of the device (24, 25). In our study, we used undiluted breast milk for measurement. We analyzed milk samples collected over 24 h, including fore-, mixed- and hind- milk. This approach helped us more clearly distinguish the differences among milk samples within a single pumping session. Our milk sample collection method was in line with that in the existing literature (26) but differed from that of Valentine et al. (27). In agreement with other research (22), large variations in the fat and energy content of milk were found in this study both within and between mothers of preterm infants on days 7 and 14. Nevertheless, protein and carbohydrate content remained relatively stable. On day 7, a mean milk fat concentration of 3.31 g/100 mL was observed in fore-milk, 3.62 g/100 mL in mixed-milk and 4.14 g/100 mL in hind-milk. On day 14, fat concentration increased to 3.60 g/100 mL in fore-milk, 4.60 g/100 mL in mixed-milk and 5.20 g/100 mL in hind-milk. These results confirm earlier findings that, as lactation progressed and the breast emptied, the fat content of human milk increased (26, 28), and that fat concentrations were consistently higher in hind-milk than in fore-milk samples from the same pumping session (29). However, the degree of increase in fat concentration from fore-milk to hind-milk on day 7 was not as significant as that reported by Saarela et al. (28) in mothers of term infants or that reported by Bishara et al. in mothers of VLBW infants of <28 weeks' gestation (1.7-fold) (30). The same phenomenon appeared in milk energy concentration patterns. For protein and carbohydrate concentrations, only very slight changes were detected among fore-, mixed-, and hind-milk. Milk protein concentration decreased as time went by. The mean protein concentrations on day 7 for fore-milk and hind-milk were both 1.94 g/100 mL, higher than the values reported by Saarela et al. (28) for protein in full-term fore-milk (1.68 g/100 mL) and hind-milk (1.64 g/100 mL) (28).

According to previous studies (26, 31, 32), the degree of breast emptying is the major factor explaining variance in fat concentrations of milk within women. For pump-dependent mothers of preterm infants, the degree of breast emptying could be decided by pumping frequency/interval and emptying the breasts to highly consistent degrees in each pumping session. In this study, we found that those who pumped 6 or more times/d had significantly higher fat, carbohydrate, and energy levels in their fore-milk on day 7.

This was a prospective observational cohort study to assess the initiation of lactation, milk production and milk nutrient content with the help of hospital-grade breast pumps in mothers who were separated from their preterm infants. With the help of a hospital-grade pump, most preterm infants' mothers can start lactation and reach full lactation successfully. The recommended pumping frequency is at least 6 times/d. There is great variation in the nutrient levels of milk from mothers of preterm infants, so nutrient analysis of breast milk is needed. These results are critical for mothers of preterm infants and every NICU workers. Based on our research, we can provide professional lactation support for mothers of preterm infants. Further research involving mothers of VLBW infants is needed to determine early intervention measures that may improve milk output of mothers at risk of lactation failure.

This study had some limitations. The number of participants was small due to the heavy participation requirements of this study. We did not document the specific nutritional habits of the mothers, which might somehow affect milk contents, especially fat content. However, the study was carried out in a tertiary university teaching hospital, all mothers received regular prenatal examinations and detailed nutritional guidance during pregnancy and after delivery. The mother's nutritional status was relatively balanced. In addition, this was an observational cohort, meaning that it was the first step in a longer program of research, a multi-center research will be carried out in the future. As our study was carried out in a tertiary university teaching hospital, it is possible that the conclusions drawn from it may only be applicable to other similar hospitals.

AUTHOR CONTRIBUTIONS

XR, XH, and QF designed the study and analyzed the data. XR and XH acquired the data, organized the database, and drafted the manuscript. QF read and revised the manuscript. All authors contributed to all study data, write and approved the final version of the manuscript.

ACKNOWLEDGMENTS

We would like to express our gratitude to all the mothers who spared time to take part in this research and provided milk samples to make the analyses possible. Additional thanks go to Dr. Mitoulas L. R. for the guidance of the study.

REFERENCES

1. Lechner BE, Vohr BR. Neurodevelopmental outcomes of preterm infants fed human milk: a systematic review. *Clin Perinatol.* (2017) 44:69–83. doi: 10.1016/j.clp.2016.11.004
2. Vohr BR, Poindexter BB, Dusick AM, McKinley LT, Higgins RD, Langer JC, et al. Persistent beneficial effects of breast milk ingested in the neonatal intensive care unit on outcomes of extremely low birth weight infants at 30 months of age. *Pediatrics.* (2007) 120:e953–9. doi: 10.1542/peds.2006-3227
3. Park J, Thoyre S, Estrem H, Pados BF, Knafl GJ, Brandon D. Mothers' psychological distress and feeding of their preterm infants. *MCN Am J Matern Child Nurs.* (2016) 41:221–9. doi: 10.1097/NMC.0000000000000248
4. Hill PD, Aldag JC, Chatterton RT, Zinaman M. Comparison of milk output between mothers of preterm and term infants: the first 6 weeks after birth. *J Hum Lact.* (2005) 21:22–30. doi: 10.1177/0890334404272407
5. Neville MC. Anatomy and physiology of lactation. *Pediatr Clin North Am.* (2001) 48:13–34. doi: 10.1016/S0031-3955(05)70283-2
6. Meier PP, Patel AL, Hoban R, Engstrom JL. Which breast pump for which mother: an evidence-based approach to individualizing breast pump technology. *J Perinatol.* (2016) 36:493–9. doi: 10.1038/jp.2016.14
7. Parker LA, Krueger C, Sullivan S, Kelechi T, Mueller M. Effect of breast milk on hospital costs and length of stay among very low-birth-weight infants in the NICU. *Adv Neonatal Care.* (2012) 12:254–9. doi: 10.1097/ANC.0b013e318260921a
8. Lussier MM, Brownell EA, Proulx TA, Bielecki DM, Marinelli KA, Bellini SL, et al. Daily breastmilk volume in mothers of very low birth weight neonates: a repeated-measures randomized trial of hand expression versus electric breast pump expression. *Breastfeed Med.* (2015) 10:312–7. doi: 10.1089/bfm.2015.0014
9. Furman L, Minich N, Hack M. Correlates of lactation in mothers of very low birth weight infants. *Pediatrics.* (2002) 109:e57. doi: 10.1542/peds.109.4.e57
10. Hill PD, Aldag JC, Chatterton RT. Initiation and frequency of pumping and milk production in mothers of non-nursing preterm infants. *J Hum Lact.* (2001) 17:9–13. doi: 10.1177/089033440101700103
11. Preusting I, Brumley J, Odibo L, Spatz DL, Louis JM. Obesity as a predictor of delayed lactogenesis II. *J Hum Lact.* (2017) 33:684–91. doi: 10.1177/0890334417727716
12. Rocha BO, Machado MP, Bastos LL, Barbosa Silva L, Santos AP, Santos LC, et al. Risk factors for delayed onset of lactogenesis II among primiparous mothers from a brazilian baby-friendly hospital. *J Hum Lact.* (2019) 36:146–56. doi: 10.1177/0890334419835174
13. Alves E, Magano R, Amorim M, Nogueira C, Silva S. Factors influencing parent reports of facilitators and barriers to human milk supply in neonatal intensive care units. *J Hum Lact.* (2016) 32:695–703. doi: 10.1177/0890334416664071
14. Meier PP, Engstrom JL, Janes JE, Jegier BJ, Loera F. Breast pump suction patterns that mimic the human infant during breastfeeding: greater milk

output in less time spent pumping for breast pump-dependent mothers with premature infants. *J Perinatol.* (2012) 32:103–10. doi: 10.1038/jp.2011.64

15. Yu X, Li J, Lin X, Luan D. Association between delayed Lactogenesis II and early milk volume among mothers of preterm infants. *Asian Nurs Res (Korean Soc Nurs Sci).* (2019) 13:93–8. doi: 10.1016/j.anr.2019.02.001
16. Parker LA, Sullivan S, Krueger C, Mueller M. Association of timing of initiation of breastmilk expression on milk volume and timing of lactogenesis stage II among mothers of very low-birth-weight infants. *Breastfeed Med.* (2015)10:84–91. doi: 10.1089/bfm.2014.0089
17. Neville MC, Morton J, Umemura S. Lactogenesis. The transition from pregnancy to lactation. *Pediatr Clin North Am.* (2001) 48:35–52. doi: 10.1016/S0031-3955(05)70284-4
18. Meier PP, Brown LP, Hurst NM. Breastfeeding the preterm infant. In: Riordan J, Auerbach KG, editors. *Breastfeeding and Human Lactation.* Boston, MA: Jones and Bartlett (1999). p. 449–81.
19. Post ED, Stam G, Tromp E. Milk production after preterm, late preterm and term delivery; effects of different breast pump suction patterns. *J Perinatol.* (2016) 36:47–51. doi: 10.1038/jp.2015.152
20. Parker LA, Sullivan S, Krueger C, Kelechi T, Mueller M. Effect of early breast milk expression on milk volume and timing of lactogenesis stage II among mothers of very low birth weight infants: a pilot study. *J Perinatol.* (2012) 32:205–9. doi: 10.1038/jp.2011.78
21. Hill, PD, Aldag, JC, Chatterton, RT. Effects of pumping style on milk production in mothers of non-nursing preterm infants. *J Hum Lact.* (1999) 15:209–16. doi: 10.1177/089033449901500310
22. Maastrup R, Hansen BM, Kronborg H, Bojesen SN, Hallum K, Frandsen A, et al. Factors associated with exclusive breastfeeding of preterm infants. Results from a prospective national cohort study. *PLoS ONE.* (2014) 9:e89077. doi: 10.1371/journal.pone.0089077
23. Menjo A, Mizuno K, Murase M, Nishida Y, Taki M, Itabashi K, et al. Bedside analysis of human milk for adjustable nutrition strategy. *Acta Paediatr.* (2009) 98:380–4. doi: 10.1111/j.1651-2227.2008.01042.x
24. Murase M, Miyazawa T, Taki M, Hibino S, Sasaki H, Watanabe T, et al. ACCURACY OF HUMAN MILK ANALYSER. *Arch Dis Child.* (2008) 93(Suppl. 2):30.
25. Casadio YS, Williams TM, Lai CT, Olsson SE, Hepworth AR, Hartmann PE. Evaluation of a mid-infrared analyzer for the determination of the macronutrient composition of human milk. *J Hum Lact.* (2010) 26:376–83. doi: 10.1177/0890334410376948
26. Daly SE, Di Rosso A, Owens RA, Hartmann PE. Degree of breast emptying explains changes in the fat content, but not fatty acid composition, of human milk. *Exp Physiol.* (1993) 78:741–55. doi: 10.1113/expphysiol.1993.sp003722
27. Valentine CJ, Hurst NM, Schanler RJ. Hindmilk improves weight gain in low-birth-weight infants fed human milk. *J Pediatr Gastroenterol Nutr.* (1994) 18:474–7. doi: 10.1097/00005176-199405000-00013
28. Saarela T, Kokkonen J, Koivisto M. Macronutrient and energy contents of human milk fractions during the first six months of lactation. *Acta Paediatr.* (2005). 94:1176–81. doi: 10.1111/j.1651-2227.2005.tb02070.x
29. Charpak N, Ruiz JG, KMC Team. Breast milk composition in a cohort of preterm infants' mothers followed in an ambulatory programme in Colombia. *Acta Paediatr.* (2007) 96:1755–9. doi: 10.1111/j.1651-2227.2007.00521.x
30. Bishara R, Dunn MS, Merko SE, Darling P. Nutrient composition of hindmilk produced by mothers of very low birth weight infants born at less than 28 weeks' gestation. *J Hum Lact.* (2008) 24:159–67. doi: 10.1177/0890334408316085
31. Jackson DA, Imong SM, Silprasert A, Ruckphaopunt S, Woolridge MW, Baum JD et al. Circadian variation in fat concentration of breast-milk in a rural northern Thai population. *Br J Nutr.* (1988) 59:349–63. doi: 10.1079/BJN19880044
32. Miller EM. What is significant about a single nursing session? An exploratory study. *Am J Hum Biol.* (2017) 29:e23004. doi: 10.1002/ajhb.23004

29

Human Milk-Based or Bovine Milk-Based Fortifiers Differentially Impact the Development of the Gut Microbiota of Preterm Infants

Miriam Aguilar-Lopez[1], *Christine Wetzel*[2], *Alissa MacDonald*[2], *Thao T. B. Ho*[3] *and Sharon M. Donovan*[1*]

[1] Division of Nutritional Sciences, University of Illinois Urbana-Champaign, Urbana, IL, United States, [2] Carle Hospital, Urbana, IL, United States, [3] Department of Pediatrics, Morsani College of Medicine, University of South Florida, Tampa, FL, United States

***Correspondence:**
Sharon M. Donovan
sdonovan@illinois.edu

Background: Preterm infants are exposed to different dietary inputs during their hospitalization in the neonatal intensive care unit (NICU). These include human milk (HM), with a human milk-based (HMF) or a bovine milk-based (BMF) fortifier, or formula. Milk consumption and the type of fortification will cause changes in the gut microbiota structure of preterm infants. This study aimed to characterize the gut microbiota of PT infant according to the type of feeding and the type of HM fortification and its possible association with infant's growth.

Methods: Ninety-seven infants born ≤33 wks of gestation or <1,500 g were followed during the hospitalization period in the NICU after birth until discharge. Clinical and dietary information was collected, including mode of delivery, pregnancy complications, mechanical ventilation, use of antibiotics, weight, and type and amount of milk consumed. To characterize the gut microbiota composition, weekly stool samples were collected from study participants. The V3–V4 region of the 16S rRNA bacterial gene was Sequenced using Illumina MiSeq technology.

Results: After birth, black maternal race, corrected gestational age (GA) and exposure to pregnancy complications, had a significant effect on gut microbial diversity and the abundance of *Enterococcus*, *Veillonella*, *Bifidobacterium*, *Enterobacter*, and *Bacteroides*. Over the course of hospitalization, corrected GA and exposure to chorioamnionitis remained to have an effect on gut microbial composition. Two different enterotypes were found in the gut microbiota of preterm infants. One enriched in *Escherichia-Shigella*, and another enriched in uncharacterized *Enterobacteriaceae*, *Klebsiella* and *Clostridium sensu stricto 1*. Overall, HM and fortification with HMF were the most common feeding strategies. When consuming BMF, PT infants had higher growth rates than those consuming HMF. Milk and type of fortification were significantly associated with the abundance of *Clostridium sensu stricto 1*, *Bifidobacterium* and *Lactobacillus*.

Conclusions: This observational study shows the significant association between milk consumption and the exposure to HMF or BMF fortification in the fecal microbiota composition of preterm infants. Additionally, these results show the effect of other perinatal factors in the establishment and development of PT infant's gut microbiota.

Keywords: gut microbiota, milk fortifiers, preterm infant, growth, enterotype

INTRODUCTION

The development of the gut microbiota during the neonatal period plays a key role in the characteristics of this ecosystem later in life and affects growth, immune and cognitive development, and risk of infection (1). Microbial colonization of preterm (PT) infants born at $\leq$37 wks gestational age (GA) is affected by a complex interaction of clinical and iatrogenic factors, including exposure to prolonged rupture of membranes [rupture of membranes >18 h (PROM)], Cesarean-section (C-section) delivery, antibiotic exposure, and hospitalization (2). In addition, genetics influences microbiome composition, as demonstrated by greater similarity among PT multiplets than singletons (3).

In both term and PT infants, diet is one of the major drivers of the gut microbiota composition and function. Consumption of human milk (HM) vs. infant formula results in significant differences in the infant gut microbiota composition (4). Mother's own milk (MOM) is the preferred source of nutrition for PT infants. When MOM is unavailable, donor human milk (DHM) is recommended, followed by specialized formula for PT infants (5). Neither unfortified MOM or unfortified DHM are nutritionally sufficient to meet the nutritional needs of the PT infant (6) so they need fortification to achieve an adequate macronutrient and micronutrient content (7).

Previous studies have documented differences in the fecal microbiota of PT fed MOM or DHM vs. infant formula (2). Less evidence exists related to the potential differences in the microbiota of PT infants fed HM supplemented with a human milk-based fortifier (HMF) compared to a bovine milk-based fortifier (BMF). A prior study with a small sample size (<10 infants) did not identify significant differences between the gut microbiota of PT infants consuming HM with HMF or BMF (8). Furthermore, infants can transition from one type of feeding to another, thus, being exposed to HM, infant formula, and different types of fortifiers over the course of their hospitalization in the NICU. Thus, the goal of this study was to analyze the potential effect of different types of feeding (HM or PT formula) and type of fortifiers on the gut microbiota composition of PT infants, while considering other perinatal factors, the exposure to antibiotics and the effect of postnatal age. This study also sought to evaluate the impact of milk fortifiers on the growth velocity of hospitalized PT infants and associations with characteristics of the PT infant gut microbiota. We hypothesized that gut microbial characteristics of PT infants fed primarily HM and a HMF would significantly differ from those fed HM supplemented with a BMF or PT formula.

Abbreviations: BMF, bovine milk-based fortifier; GA, gestational age; HM, human milk; HMF, human milk-based fortifier; HMOs, human milk oligosaccharides; LEFSE, linear discriminant analysis effect size; MaASLin2, microbiome multivariate association linear models; NICU, neonatal intensive care unit; OTU, operational taxonomic unit; PROM, premature rupture of membranes; PT, preterm.

MATERIALS AND METHODS

Study Participants

This cohort study was conducted between 2016 and 2018 at Carle Hospital in Urbana, IL. The study protocol was approved by the Institutional Review Board Committee of this same hospital (9, 10). Preterm infants were enrolled at birth and followed until discharge from the NICU. Participants were included if they were born <33 wks of gestation or <1,500 g at birth, and that were <72 h-old on admission to Carle Hospital. Infants were excluded if they had any major or lethal congenital anomalies or abdominal wall or intestinal defects. Informed consent was obtained from each infant's parent(s) or care provider(s) before study enrollment. Diagnoses of pregnancy complications, including clinical chorioamnionitis (bacterial infection of the membranes of the placenta and amniotic fluid) and PROM, were obtained from the mother's clinical chart. Additionally, maternal race, mode of delivery, GA, exposure to antibiotics, birth complications, head circumference, and weight (weekly) were retrieved from the medical records of each infant. Weight and head circumference Z-scores were calculated at birth and at discharge using the Fenton growth charts (11). Nursing staff from the NICU collected dietary information, including total daily feeding volume, volume of MOM, DHM, or PT formula, use of HMF (Prolact+H^{2}MF® [Prolacta Bioscience, Industry, CA]) and use of BMF (Similac® human milk fortifier-hydrolyzed protein concentrated liquid [Abbott Nutrition, Columbus, OH]). The fortification protocol at Carle Hospital consists of exclusively HM (raw MOM or pasteurized DHM) supplemented with a fortifier according to a standardized fortification regimen. Human milk is fortified with HMF in infants born <28 GA, and after 32 wks corrected GA, BMF can be introduced. In infants born between 28 and 34 wks GA, HM is supplemented with BMF. After 34 wks corrected GA, infants can to PT formula if HM is not available. The weekly proportion of each specific type of milk was calculated and based on intake, infants were assigned as exclusively fed MOM, exclusively fed DHM, exclusively fed PT formula, or mixed fed. In the latter case, it was calculated what type of milk (MOM, DHM, or infant formula) they were predominantly fed. A freshly voided stool was collected from the infant's diaper by the nursing staff on a weekly or bi-weekly basis. After collection, samples were placed into coolers with dry ice, picked-up by research staff and stored at −80°C until further processing.

DNA Extraction

Stool samples collected during the first days after birth are characterized by low bacterial DNA concentration (12). For this reason, bacterial DNA was extracted using two different commercial kits to optimize DNA yield. The Power Fecal DNA Isolation Kit (QIAGEN, Valencia, CA) was used for the first stool sample collected according to the manufacturer's instructions, with some modifications, including using a different bead beating tube, the mechanical lysis method, and the incubation temperature. Briefly, a total of 250 μg of stool (wet weight) were placed into a 2 mL Lysing Matrix E tube (MP Biomedicals. Santa Ana, CA). The stool sample and 600 μL of the C1 solution were then heated at 70°C for 10 min. Tubes were then shaken using the FastPrep-24 (MP Biomedicals. Santa Ana, CA) at 6.5 m/s for 45. The remaining steps were performed according to manufacturer's instructions. Bacterial DNA from the subsequent stool samples collected was extracted using the QIAamp Fast DNA Stool Mini Kit (QIAGEN, Valencia, CA), as previously described (3).

Sequencing and Bioinformatics Analysis

The V3–V4 region of the 16S rRNA gene was amplified with the forward F357 (5′-CCTACGGGNGGCWGCAG-3′) and reverse R805 (5′- GACTACHVGGGTATCTAATCC-3′) primers. DNA was amplified through PCR reactions using the AccuPrime Taq DNA Polymerase System (Life Technologies, Carlsbad, CA) in a DNA Engine (Bio-Rad, Hercules, CA). Amplicons were mixed in equimolar concentration and submitted for sequencing at the Roy J. Carver Biotechnology Center at the University of Illinois Urbana-Champaign. Sequencing was performed using the Illumina MiSeq platform using v3 paired-reads (2 × 250 bp) (San Diego, CA). Sequencing files were processed using QIIME2 (13) version 2018.6. Samples were demultiplexed using the demux emp-paired plugin. Data was denoised by identifying and removing chimeras using the Divisive amplicon De-noising Algorithm 2 pipeline (14). Reads were trimmed at 17 and 21 bp in the forward and reverse reads, respectively. A phylogenetic tree of the samples was constructed using the QIIME2 recommended plugins. Operational Taxonomic Units (OTUs) were characterized to single nucleotide variants, and a representative sequence was used to taxonomically characterize the sequence using a Naïve Bayes classifier trained in the V3–V4 region against the Silva 132 database (15). Alpha diversity metrics (Observed OTUs and Shannon), and beta diversity metrics were calculated at an even sampling depth of 23,098 reads. Alpha diversity describes the species diversity withing a sample, while beta diversity measures the dissimilarity between communities (16).

Statistical Analysis

Analyses were performed using RStudio V.1.3.1093. Taxonomic abundances (relative abundance) were transformed using the arcsine square root method. Linear mixed-effect models were used to estimate the effect of perinatal, anthropometric, and dietary factors on alpha diversity estimates. These variables were used to estimate their association with the taxonomic composition using Microbiome Multivariable Association Linear Models (MaASLin2) (9) with the Benjamin-Hochberg false discovery rate (FDR) correction. Perinatal, anthropometric, and dietary factors were included as fixed effects in the model, and each infant was included as random effects. Differences in beta diversity were calculated based on the Unweighted and Weighted UniFrac distances using permutational multivariable analysis of variance (Adonis) with 999 permutations using the vegan package (17).

Taxonomic composition at genus level was used to determine if any gut enterotypes existed in the PT infant gut across time. Analysis was performed as described by Arumugam et al. (18). First, sample clustering was done using the Jensen-Shannon divergence index and the Partitioning Around Medoids (PAM) syntax. Ideal number of clusters was determined using the Calinski-Harabasz index, this number was validated using the Silhouette Validation Technique. Following this, each stool sample was assigned to a specific enterotype. To evaluate the differential taxonomic abundance of each enterotype, Linear Discriminant Analysis (LDA) Effect Size (LefSe) (19) was conducted using the web-based Galaxy platform (http://huttenhower.sph.harvard.edu/galaxy).

Growth curves were calculated based on weight gain velocity (g/d) and corrected GA (GA at birth + postnatal age) using non-linear mixed-effects models from the nlme package (20).

TABLE 1 | Characteristics of study participants.

Characteristic	Birth $n = 97$	End of follow-up $n = 97$
Maternal race, *n* (%)		
Black	26 (26.8)	–
White	71 (73.2)	–
Chorioamnionitis, *n* (%)	18 (18.6)	–
PROM, *n* (%)	15 (15.5)	–
Infant sex, *n* (%)		
Female	61 (62.9)	–
Male	36 (37.1)	–
Mode of delivery, *n* (%)		
Vaginal	21 (21.6)	–
C-section	76 (78.3)	–
Gestational age, weeks	29 (4)	–
Prematurity category*, *n* (%)		
Extremely PT	26 (26.8)	–
Very PT	56 (55.7)	–
Moderate to Late PT	17 (17.5)	–
Postnatal age, weeks	–	6 (4)
Corrected GA, weeks	–	35 (2)
Weight, g	1,242 (636)	2,327 (799)
Weight *Z*-score	0.2 (1.26)	−0.49 (1.16)
Weight *Z*-score, percentile	58 (46)	31 (37)
Head circumference, cm	33 (2.5)	33 (2.5)
HC *Z*-score	0.07 (1.55)	−0.51 (1.24)
HC *Z*-score, percentile	57.8 (46)	31 (42)
Mechanical ventilation, *n* (%)	25 (25.8)	0
Use of antibiotics, *n* (%)	22 (22.7)	4 (4.12)

Data presented as n (%) for categorical data or median (IQR) for numerical data.
**Extremely PT: <28 wks GA; Very PT: 28–32 wks GA; Moderate to Late PT: 32–37 wks GA. GA, gestational age; HC, head circumference; PROM, premature rupture of membranes; PT, preterm infant.*

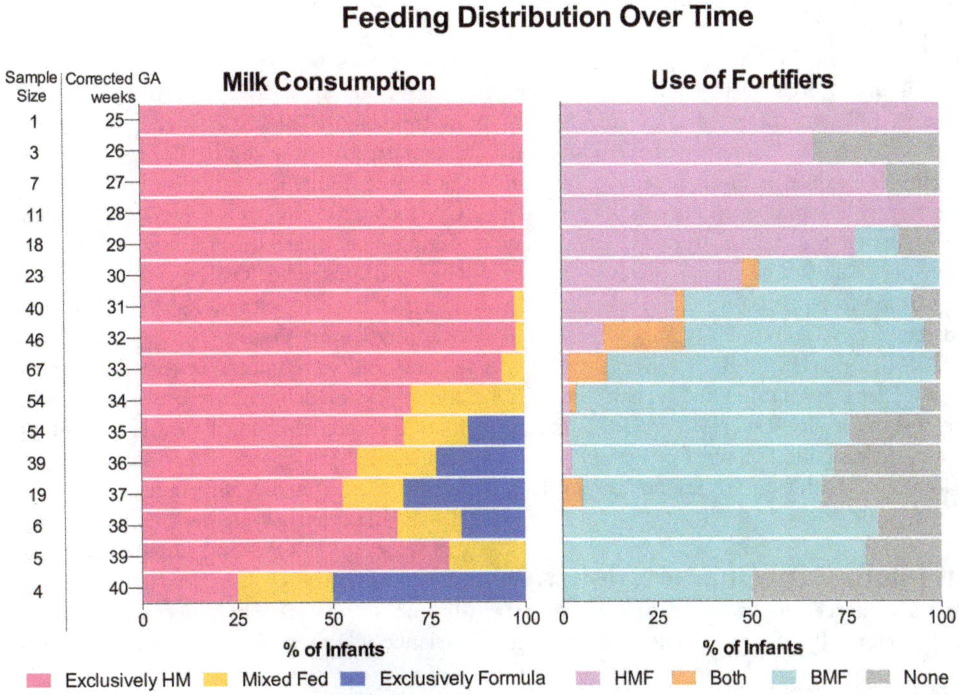

FIGURE 1 | Feeding distribution of preterm infants during hospitalization period at the neonatal intensive care unit. Consumption of milk and use of fortifiers over time. Human milk and the use of a BMF was the most common regimen. HM, Human milk; HMF, human milk-based fortifier; BMF, bovine milk-based fortifier.

The intercept and slope were set as fixed effects, variance of the intercept and the slope as random effects, and the grouping parameter was each infant. Spearman correlation was used to assess the association between weight gain velocity and bacterial abundance.

RESULTS

A total of 102 PT infants were enrolled in the study. However, five infants died during the study and were excluded from the analysis; thus, the final analysis was done with a sample size of 97 PT infants. **Table 1** shows the demographic characteristics of the included participants. According to the medical records, 18.6 and 15.5% of the infants were exposed to chorioamnionitis and PROM, respectively. A total of 62.9% were female, most infants were born *via* C-section (78.3%), and maternal race was predominantly white (73.2%). On average, infants were born at 28.9 ± 2.45 wks of gestation, weighed 1,273 ± 427 g, and had a head circumference of 26.3 ± 3.08 cm. A total of five infants (5.2%) had a birthweight *Z*-score below the 10th percentile, 12 infants (12.3%) fell below the 10th percentile for the head circumference *Z*-score. In the immediate postpartum period, 22.7% of participants were administered antibiotics, and 25.8% required mechanical ventilation. On average, the hospitalization period was 6.54 ± 3.10 wks (range: 1–16 wks). Infants were discharged at 35 ± 1.91 wks corrected GA, with a weight of 2,270 ± 556 g. At discharge, 17 (17.5%) and 24 (24.7%) infants fell below the 10th percentile for weight and head circumference, respectively. On average, 5 samples were collected per infant (range: 1–16).

TABLE 2 | Feeding categories.

Category	Milk	Fortifier
Human milk - none	Exclusively human milk or Mixed fed with >50% HM	None
Human milk + HMF	Exclusively human milk or Mixed fed with >50% HM	HMF
Human milk + BMF	Exclusively human milk or Mixed fed with >50% HM	BMF
Human milk + both	Exclusively human milk or Mixed fed with >50% HM	HMF + BMF
Formula + BMF	Exclusively formula or Mixed fed with >50% formula	BMF
Formula	Exclusively formula or Mixed fed with >50% formula	None

HMF, human milk-based fortifier; BMF, bovine milk-based fortifier.

Feeding Characteristics

To evaluate the effect of the dietary exposures on the gut microbiota composition, feeding categories were created based on the type of milk consumed and the type of HM fortifier used. Donor human milk was provided when MOM was insufficient or not available. Only 17.5% infants ($n = 17$) were fed DHM at some point during their NICU stay (**Supplementary Table 1**). For this reason, DHM and MOM were combined into one group described as HM for all the analysis presented in this study. As shown in **Figure 1**, exclusively HM was consumed by the most PT infants (25 wks corrected GA) until 30 wks corrected GA. At this point, PT formula was introduced in combination with HM (mixed fed). Over time, the number of infants that were mixed fed, or fed exclusively PT formula increased. However, most of the infants were fed exclusively HM. The use of fortifiers followed a similar pattern. Human milk-based fortifier was fed from birth until a BMF fortification started at 30 wks corrected GA. Overall, PT infants, were fed the combination of both of fortifiers (HMF+BMF during most of the hospitalization period). Using the amount and type of feed (HM or formula) and the type of fortification (HMF or BMF), feeding categories were created to examine the effect of dietary factors on the gut microbiota composition of PT infants as shown in **Table 2**.

Early-Life Gut Microbiota Characteristics

Only 29 infants had a collected stool sample during the first week postpartum. Therefore, the first available stool sample was used to characterize the "early-life" gut microbiota of all study participants, which on average, was collected at 2.16 ± 1.13 wks postnatal age (31.1 ± 2.25 wks corrected GA). Analyses of alpha diversity revealed that PT infants from black mothers had significantly higher number observed OTUs than infants from white mothers (23.3 ± 10.3 vs. 17.5 ± 11). This difference remained significant after adjusting for corrected GA and exposure to antibiotics (**Supplementary Figure 1A**). Additionally, there was a linear relationship between corrected GA and observed OTUs ($p = 0.02$), when analysis was adjusted for infant's weight and exposure to antibiotics (**Supplementary Figure 1B**). No statistically significant associations were found between the number of observed OTUs and mode of delivery, exposure to chorioamnionitis, PROM, infant's sex, or mechanical ventilation (**Supplementary Table 2**). Similarly, there was no effect of any of these perinatal factors on the Shannon diversity index. Beta diversity, measured by Unweighted and Weighted UniFrac distances showed that exposure to PROM and infant's sex, each explained 2.3% of the variance of the Unweighted and Weighted UniFrac distances ($p < 0.05$). Maternal race explained 2.1% of the variance of the Weighted UniFrac distances ($p = 0.021$)

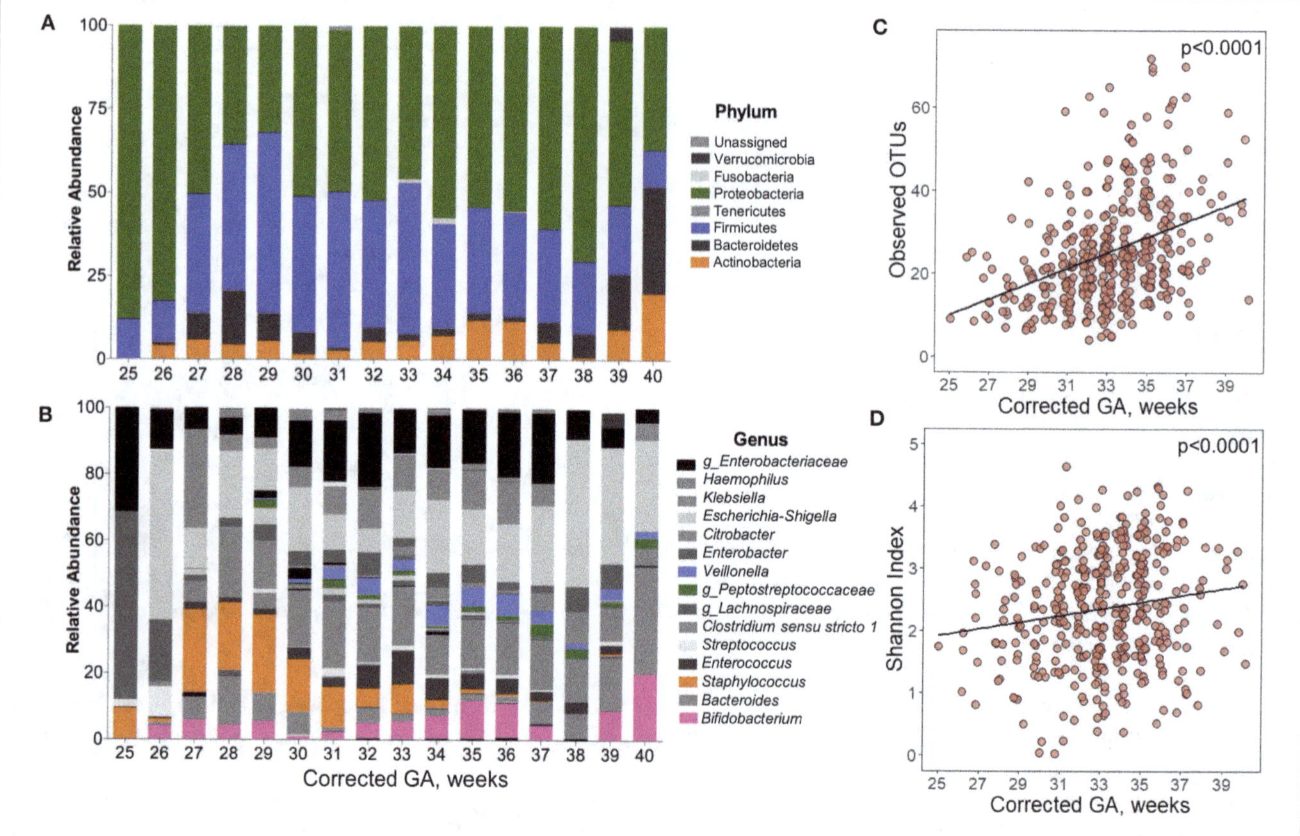

FIGURE 2 | Postpartum development of the gut microbiota composition of preterm infants. Over time, there were significant changes in the composition of the gut microbiota of preterm infants. Taxonomical composition at **(A)** phylum and **(B)** genus level. Highlighted in color are the bacteria that significantly changed over time ($q < 0.05$). Differences calculated using Microbiome Multivariable Association Linear Models (MaASLin2) with infants as a random effect term. **(C)** Observed OTUs and **(D)** Shannon diversity Index significantly increased over time. Differences calculated using linear mixed-effect model with infants as a random effect term. Adjusted for antibiotic use. Corrected GA: gestational age at birth + postnatal age. GA, gestational age.

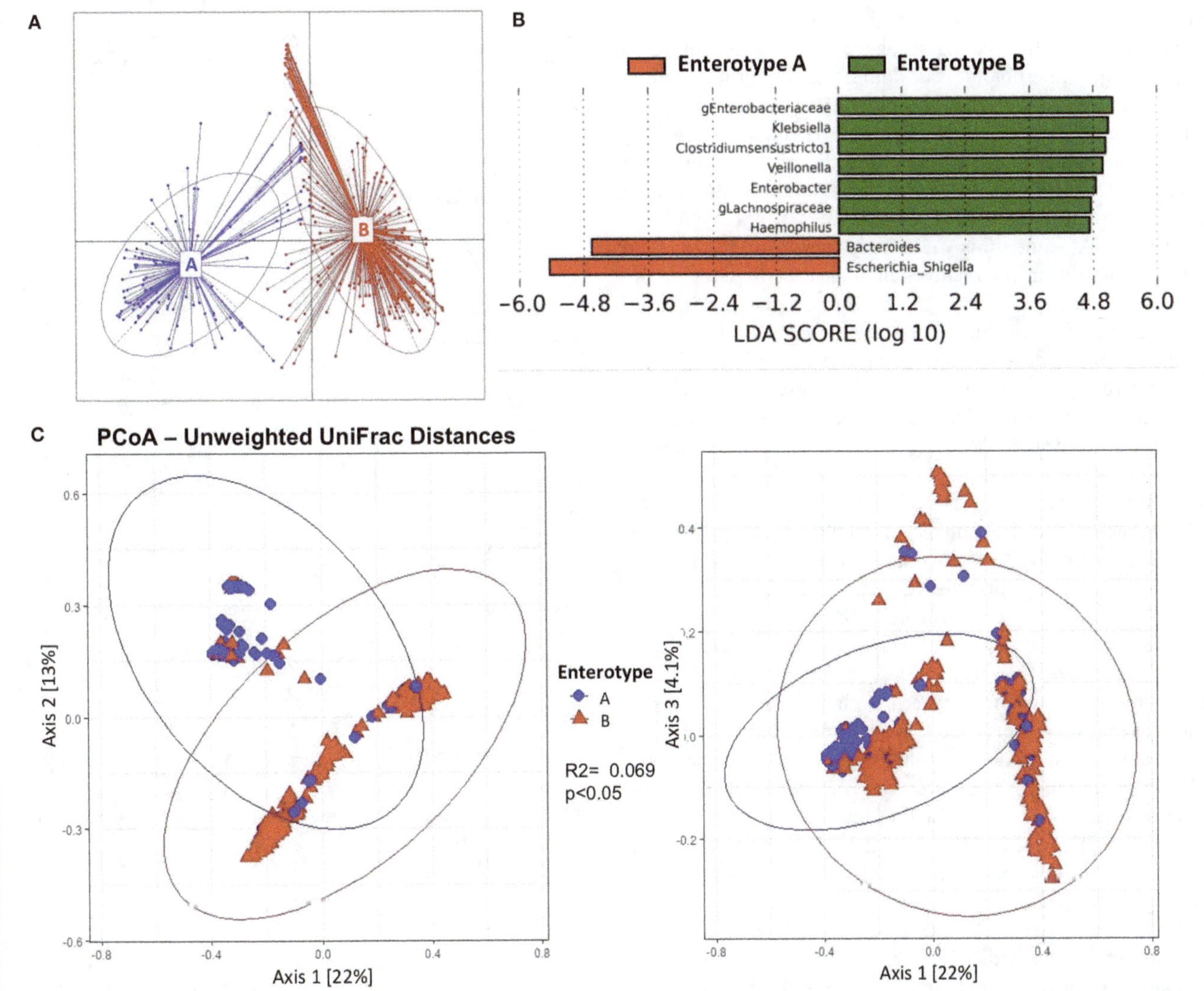

FIGURE 3 | Beta diversity and enterotypes characteristics of gut microbiota from preterm infants. Beta diversity was significantly associated to two different enterotypes. **(A)** Two different enterotypes (Enterotype A and Enterotype B) were characterized. The majority of the samples belonged to Enterotype B. **(B)** Discriminative genera determined by linear discriminant analysis (LDA) showed bacteria that *Bacteroides* and *Escherichia-Shigella* were enriched in Enterotype A; whereas uncharacterized *Enterobacteriaceae*, *Klebsiella*, *Clostridium sensu stricto 1*, *Veillonella*, *Enterobacter*, uncharacterized *Lachnospiraceae* and *Haemopohilus* were enriched in Enterotype B. **(C)** Principal coordinate representation of Unweighted UniFrac Distances (Axis 1 vs. Axis 2, and Axis 1 vs. Axis 3) of the two enterotypes. Enterotypes explained 6.9% of the variance of the Unweighted UniFrac Distances.

(**Supplementary Table 3**). There were no other associations between beta diversity metrics and delivery mode, exposure to chorioamnionitis, use of mechanical ventilator and exposure to antibiotics.

Taxonomical analysis revealed significant differences in the early-life microbiota based on perinatal characteristics. There was a positive association between corrected GA and the abundance of *Enterococcus* and *Veillonella* ($p = 0.0003$, $q = 0.01$; $p = 0.001$, $q = 0.018$, respectively); analysis was performed adjusting for exposure to antibiotics (**Supplementary Figure 2**). Infants that were vaginally delivered had higher abundance of *Bacteroides* (8.76%) than infants born *via* C-section (1.63%); $p = 0.05$, $q = 0.08$. Infants that were exposed to chorioamnionitis during pregnancy had higher relative abundances of *Bifidobacterium* and *Enterobacter* (7.19 and 8.04%) compared to those that were not exposed (6.05 and 3.02%). PROM was significantly associated with higher abundances of *Bacteroides* (8.79 vs. 1.0%; $p = 0.0001$, $q = 0.03$). There were no statistically significant differences between infant's sex, maternal race, use of mechanical ventilation, infant's weight, and exposure to antibiotics with the early-life gut microbial composition.

Changes in Gut Microbiota During the NICU Admission

Over the course of their hospitalization, changes in gut microbial alpha diversity, beta diversity and taxonomic composition were observed. Significant changes in the abundance of the phyla Proteobacteria, Firmicutes, and Actinobacteria were found (**Figure 2A**). At the youngest ages (25–26 wks corrected GA), the gut microbiota was dominated by Proteobacteria with a mean relative abundance <85% ± 10.2 of total reads. After 27 wks corrected GA, the relative abundance of Proteobacteria started to decrease, and the relative abundance of Firmicutes increased. At corrected GA<27 wks, the relative abundance of Firmicutes was 12% ± 10.6 (25–26 wks corrected GA), and this increased over the NICU stay. Across time, the mean relative abundance of bacteria of the phylum Actinobacteria was 7% ± 13.2. At the genus level, statistically significant differences were found over time in the abundance of *Bifidobacterium*, *Staphylococcus*, uncharacterized *Peptostreptococcaceae*, and *Veillonella* (**Figure 2B**). In infants with <32 wks corrected GA, the average relative abundance of *Bifidobacterium* was 3.5% ± 6.7, which increased over time to 8.82% ± 12. The abundance of *Staphylococcus* had a significant decrease with greater corrected GA. From 25 to 30 wks corrected GA, the mean relative abundance of *Staphylococcus* was 16% ± 22, which was followed by a dramatic decrease in its abundance to 3% ± 1.27 by 34 wks corrected GA. The genera uncharacterized *Peptostreptococcaceae* and *Veillonella* reached a mean relative abundance >1% up to 29 and 31 wks corrected GA, respectively.

Time also had a significant effect on alpha diversity. There was a linear relationship between both Observed OTUs and Shannon Index with corrected GA, even after accounting for the use of antibiotics. On average, there was a 7.97 increment per week in the number of Observed OTUs (**Figure 2C**). Similarly, Shannon Index increased 0.095 units per week corrected GA (**Figure 2D**). During the hospitalization, multiple factors influenced beta diversity. Around 50% of the variation of the Unweighted and Weighted UniFrac distances was explained by each infant. Chronological variables (GA, postnatal age, and corrected GA) had a significant effect on beta diversity (**Supplementary Table 4**). Delivery mode explained 0.07 and 1.3% of the Unweighted and Weighted UniFrac distances, respectively. Exposure to chorioamnionitis had a significant effect on both Unweighted and Weighted UniFrac distances. Lastly, exposure to PROM, use of mechanical ventilation, and exposure to antibiotics had a significant effect only in Unweighted UniFrac distances.

When beta diversity was explored to assess the changes over time, the samples clustered into two distinct groups. For this reason, enterotype analysis was performed and two different enterotypes were found (Enterotype A and Enterotype B) (**Figure 3A**). Overall, 175 samples (32.8%) belonged to Enterotype A, whereas 358 samples (67.2%) were assigned to Enterotype B. To further understand the characteristics of the two clusters, LefSe analysis was performed. Enterotype A had enriched abundance of bacteria from the genus *Bacteroides* and *Escherichia-Shigella*. While bacteria from the genus uncharacterized *Enterobacteriaceae*, *Klebsiella*, *Clostridium sensu stricto 1*, *Veillonella*, *Enterobacter*, *g_Lachnospiraceae*, and *Haemophilus* were enriched in Enterotype B (**Figure 3B**). The most striking difference between the enterotypes was the relative abundance of *Escherichia-Shigella*; which was 45.4% in samples belonging to Enterotype A compared to 1.47% in samples belonging to Enterotype B (**Supplementary Figure 3**). Other genera that showed significant differences between the enterotypes were *Clostridium sensu stricto 1* (26.7% difference) and *g_Enterobacteriaceae* (25.9% difference). Furthermore, alpha diversity indices revealed that Enterotype B was more diverse than Enterotype A (**Supplementary Figure 4**). Samples from Enterotype B had 26.5 ± 13.1 Observed OTUs, and a Shannon diversity Index of 2.61 ± 0.78 compared to 23.2 ± 12.9 Observed OTUs and 1.9 ± 0.95 Shannon Index in samples belonging to Enterotype A which was statistically significant. The enterotype clustering explained 6.9% of the variance from the Unweighted UniFrac distances ($p < 0.05$) (**Figure 3C**), and 2.5% of the Weighted UniFrac distances; however, the latter was not statistically significant. Furthermore, when clinical characteristics were compared between the enterotypes, more samples from infants exposed to chorioamnionitis belonged to Enterotype B (25.7 vs. 17.1%). In Enterotype A, there was a significantly higher percentage of samples from infants consuming BMF (72 vs. 62%) (**Table 3**).

From the total sample size ($n = 97$), 42 infants (43.3%) changed from one enterotype to another over the course of

TABLE 3 | Characteristics of stool samples belonging to each enterotype.

Variable	Enterotype A $n = 175$ samples	Enterotype B $n = 358$ samples	p*
Maternal race, *n* (%)			
Black	32 (12.3)	81 (22.6)	0.26
White	143 (81.7)	277 (77.4)	
Chorioamnionitis, *n* (%)	30 (17.1)	92 (25.7)	0.028
PROM, *n* (%)	45 (25.7)	75 (20.9)	0.22
Infant sex, *n* (%)			
Female	114 (65.1)	229 (63.9)	0.84
Male	61 (34.8)	129 (36.0)	
Mode of delivery, *n* (%)			
Vaginal	46 (26.3)	87 (24.3)	0.67
C-section	129 (73.7)	271 (75.7)	
Corrected GA, weeks	33 (4)	33 (3)	0.90
Weight, g	1,758 (1,044)	1,744 (786)	0.94
Use of antibiotics, *n* (%)	16 (9.14)	27 (7.54)	0.51
Milk consumed, *n* (%)			
Human milk	164 (93.7)	322 (89.9)	0.19
Formula	11 (6.28)	36 (10.0)	
Fortifier consumed, *n* (%)			
None	16 (9.14)	49 (13.7)	0.15
HMF	24 (13.7)	68 (18.9)	0.14
BMF	126 (72.0)	222 (62.0)	0.025
Both	9 (5.14)	19 (5.31)	0.9
Change enterotype, *n* (%)	116 (66.3)	138 (38.5)	<0.001

Data presented as n (%) for categorical data or median (IQR) for numerical data.
PROM, premature rupture of membranes; GA, gestational age; HMF, human milk-based fortifier; BMF, bovine milk-based fortifier.
**Differences based on Fisher's exact test for categorical variables or Kruskal-Wallis test for numerical variables.*

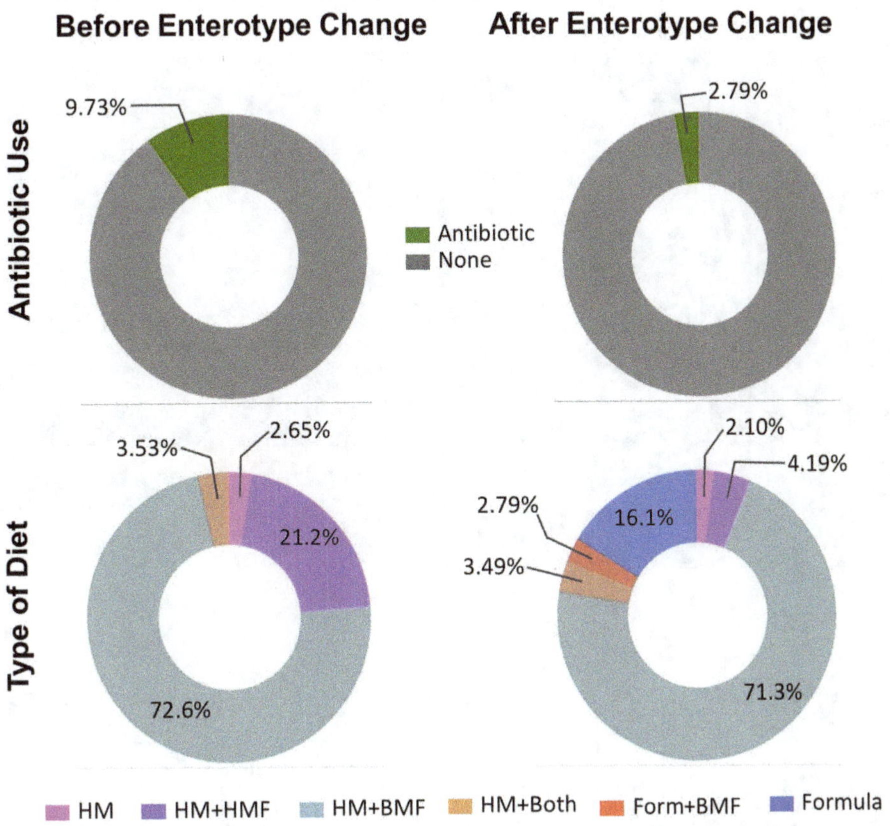

FIGURE 4 | Characteristics before and after change in enterotype. Percentage of antibiotic use and diet category of infants prior moving from on enterotype to another. Before the change of the enterotype, there was a greater use of antibiotics, and HM in combination with fortifiers was the main diet category. Stool samples after they changed to another enterotype were associated with less antibiotic use, and with the introduction to formula feeding. HM, human milk; HMF, human milk-based fortifier; BMF, bovine milk-based fortifier; Form, formula.

hospitalization. From the total number of samples belonging to Enterotype A, 116 samples (66.3%) moved to Enterotype B, compared to 138 samples (38.5%) that belonged to Enterotype B and moved to Enterotype A. Out of 97 studied infants, stool samples from 14 infants (14.4%) were associated exclusively to Enterotype A, samples from 41 infants (42.3%) exclusively to Enterotype B, and 42 infants (43.3%) had stool samples (254 stool samples) that changed from one enterotype to another. There were no statistically significant differences in the perinatal characteristics among infants exclusively belonging to one enterotype or infants that changed enterotypes (**Supplementary Table 4**). To further explore the possible variables associated to the change from one enterotype to another, chronological variables, use of antibiotics, and type of diet were assessed before and after samples changed to another enterotype. The mean corrected GA and body weight were significantly higher after enterotype change (31.7 wks corrected GA vs. 34.7 wks corrected GA and 1,578 g vs. 2,091 g, respectively; $p < 0.05$) (**Supplementary Table 5**). As shown in **Figure 4**, there was a higher percentage of antibiotics use prior to changing from one enterotype to another (9.73 vs. 2.79%, $p = 0.037$). There were significant associations in the dietary regimen and the change from one enterotype to another. Prior to the change to another enterotype, only HM with or without fortifiers was consumed. There was a higher percentage of HM+BMF use (72.6%), followed by HM+HMF (21.2%) and by the combination of both (HM+Both fortifiers: 3.53%) (**Figure 4**), there was no consumption of PT formula during this period. After changing to another enterotype, the use of infant formula increased to 16.1%. and HM+BMF remained as the most common feeding strategy.

Another goal of this study was to evaluate the associations between perinatal factors, use of antibiotics, growth, and dietary exposures with the taxonomic composition over the course of the NICU stay. Multivariate analyses revealed that exposure to chorioamnionitis was associated with higher relative abundance of *Enterobacter* (7.07%) over time compared to infants never exposed to chorioamnionitis (3.86%). Other associations were found between perinatal factors and taxonomic composition, including a higher abundance of *Negativicoccus* in male PT infants, higher abundance of uncharacterized *Peptostreptococcaceae* with the use of mechanical ventilation, lower abundance of *Anaerococcus* when exposed to chorioamnionitis, and lower abundance of *Veillonella* when infants needed mechanical ventilation. During the hospitalization period, the only bacterium that seem to be

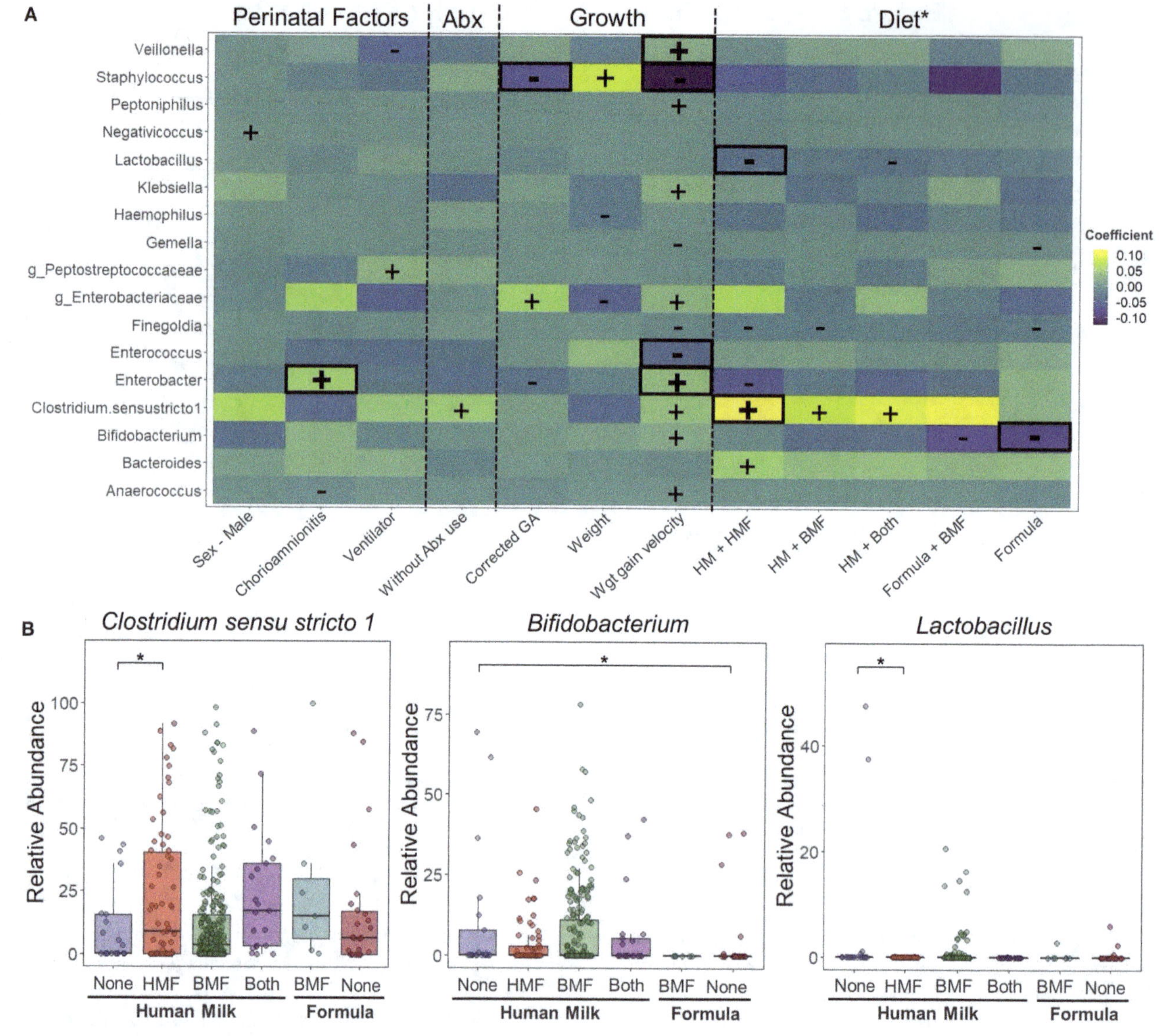

FIGURE 5 | Changes in taxonomic composition during hospitalization period at the neonatal intensive care unit. Taxonomical changes associated to different perinatal factors. **(A)** Heatmap of associations between bacterial genera and perinatal factors, use of antibiotics, growth and diet. Positive (+) and negative (–) signs denote significant associations ($p < 0.05$). Highlighted in red are the associations that remained significant after false discovery rate adjustment ($q < 0.05$). Differences calculated using Microbiome Multivariable Association Linear Models (MaASLin2). Model included infant sex, exposure to chorioamnionitis, use of mechanical ventilation, exposure to antibiotics, corrected GA, body weight, weight gain velocity, and type of milk and fortifier consumed. Infant was included as a random effect term. **(B)** Bacteria significantly affected by dietary factors. *HM without fortification as control group. Corrected GA: gestational age at birth + postnatal age. Abx, antibiotic; PROM, premature rupture of membranes; GA, gestational age; HM, human milk; HMF, human milk-based fortifier; BMF, bovine milk-based fortifier; Wgt, Weight.

affected by the use of antibiotics was *Clostridium sensu stricto 1*. However, these associations were no longer significant after FDR adjustment ($p < 0.05$ and $q > 0.05$) (**Figure 5A**). Growth variables [corrected GA, weight, and weight gain velocity (g/d)] were also analyzed in the multivariate analysis. Corrected GA and weight gain velocity were negatively associated with the abundance of *Staphylococcus* ($q < 0.01$). Another bacterium that was negatively associated with weight gain velocity was *Enterococcus* ($q < 0.01$). In contrast, there was a positive association between weight gain velocity and the abundance of *Veillonella* and *Enterobacter* ($q < 0.01$).

Dietary exposures were included in the multivariate analysis to evaluate their association with the taxonomic characteristics of study participants (**Figure 5A**). When different combinations of milk and milk fortifiers (HM-None, HM+HMF, HM+BMF, HM+Both, Formula+BMF, and Formula) were explored, 10 different associations with a $p < 0.05$ and $q > 0.05$ were found. Compared to HM consumption without any milk

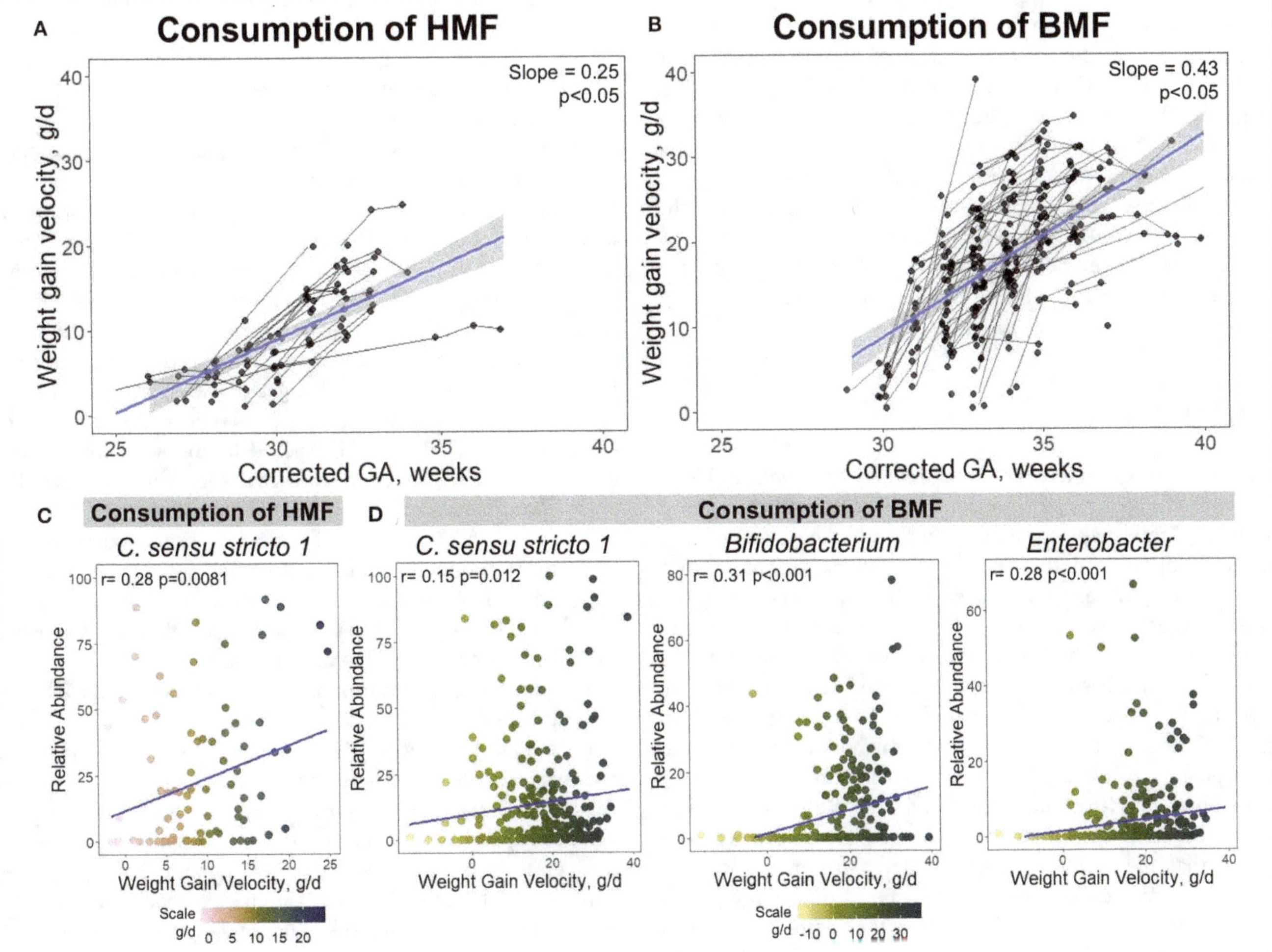

FIGURE 6 | Associations between growth velocity, use of fortifiers and taxonomic composition. The use of HMF and BMF are associated with the infant's growth and their taxonomic composition. **(A)** Growth curves of PT infants when consuming HMF, or **(B)** BMF. Spearman correlations showing positive associations between *Clostridium sensu stricto 1*, *Bifidobacterium*, and *Enterobacter* with weight gain velocity when infants were exposed to **(C)** HMF or **(D)** BMF. Corrected GA: gestational age at birth + postnatal age. GA, gestational age; HMF, human milk-based fortifier; BMF, bovine milk-based fortifier.

fortifier (HM-None), infants consuming HM+HMF had higher abundances of *Bacteroides*, and lower abundances of *Finegoldia* and *Enterobacter*. Infants consuming HM+BMF had higher abundance of *Clostridium sensu stricto 1*, and lower abundance of *Finegoldia*. When infants were exposed to HM with the combination of both fortifiers (HM+Both) they showed higher abundances of *Clostridium sensu stricto 1*, and lower abundances of *Lactobacillus* when comparing to HM-None. The consumption of PT formula alone or with BMF decreased the abundance of *Gemella*, *Finegoldia*, and *Bifidobacterium*. Overall, only three associations remained significant ($p < 0.05$ and $q < 0.05$) (**Figure 5B**). Compared to infants consuming HM-None, infants consuming HM with a HMF had higher abundances of *Clostridium sensu stricto 1* (HM-None: 10.8%; HM-HMF: 22.2%) and lower abundance of *Lactobacillus* (HM-None: 4.13%; HM-HMF <0.1%). Compared to consuming HM-None, infants consuming formula had significantly lower levels of *Bifidobacterium* (HM-None: 9.82%; Formula: 4.28%).

Effect of Milk Fortifiers on Growth Rates

A goal of HM fortification is to increase the macro and micronutrient content to ensure appropriate growth in PT infants. The HMF was used in PT infants <29 wks corrected GA. BMF was initiated around 29 weeks corrected GA and was the most commonly used fortification strategy in this study. Both fortifiers had a significant effect on the growth rate, measured by weight gain velocity (g/d). The overall growth rate in the study participants was 15 ± 9.76 g/d. This rate had a 0.39 increment per week, which was lower (0.25 g/d) when infants consumed a HMF (**Figure 6A**), and it was higher (0.43 g/d) when BMF was used (**Figure 6B**).

Next, associations between dietary intake, growth and microbial taxa were investigated. As previously mentioned, bacteria that were significantly associated with growth and/or dietary factors were *Clostridium sensu stricto 1*, *Bifidobacterium*, and *Enterobacter* (**Figure 5A**). Correlation analysis was performed between these bacteria abundances and weight gain velocity when infants were consuming either a HMF or BMF. There was a significant association between the abundance of *Clostridium sensu stricto 1* and weight gain velocity when fortification with a HMF was used (rho = 0.28, p = 0.0081) (**Figure 6C**). During the fortification with BMF, positive correlations were found between weight gain velocity and the abundance of *Clostridium sensu stricto 1* (rho = 0.15, p = 0.012), *Bifidobacterium* (rho = 0.31, $p < 0.001$), and *Enterobacter* (rho = 0.28, $p < 0.001$) (**Figure 6D**). There were no significant correlations between *Bifidobacterium* or *Enterobacter* abundance and weight gain velocity during fortification with HMF.

DISCUSSION

Differences in gut microbial structure associated with different perinatal and dietary characteristics were identified in this study. In the first collected stool sample after birth, the gut microbiota of infants of black mothers had a more diverse gut microbiota, which was significantly associated with beta diversity metrics. This could be due to characteristics of the maternal vaginal and cervical microbiota during pregnancy. The vertical transmission of microbes has been previously described (21). Mitchell et al. reported that seeding of maternal microbiota to the newborn's gut can be attributed to mother's rectal microbiota and not from the vaginal microbiota (22). However, PT infants are more likely to be born *via* C-section, a trend ($q > 0.05$) also observed in this study. While it remains controversial, some studies have shown that the womb is not a sterile environment, and the exposure to maternal microbes might initiate during pregnancy (23). Previous studies have shown that the vaginal microbiota of African American and Hispanic mothers had significantly higher alpha diversity compared to Asian and Caucasian mothers (24). Non-Hispanic black pregnant women have a more diverse cervical microbiota than pregnant white women (25). This effect of maternal race on infant gut microbial composition should be further explored.

Pregnancy complications were significantly associated with the gut microbiota of PT infants. Exposure to PROM significantly increased the abundance of *Bacteroides,* which could be associated with the maternal vaginal microbiota. There is a higher risk of PROM in pregnant women with bacterial vaginosis (26), which is characterized by lower *Lactobacillus* abundance and a bloom of other bacteria, including *Bacteroides* (27, 28). In the present study, PT infants exposed to chorioamnionitis had higher abundances of *Bifidobacterium* and *Enterobacter,* and the association between chorioamnionitis and *Enterobacter* abundance remained significant over the duration of the study. *Enterobacter* is a Gram-negative bacterium, which is a common early colonizer of the PT gut (29). Chorioamnionitis is an infection of the placenta membranes and the amniotic fluid. Evidence has suggested that there is an association between chorioamnionitis and the presence of *Enterobacteriaceae* (30), particularly of *Enterobacter* species (31) in placental tissues. In comparison to PROM, chorioamnionitis had a longer effect on the gut microbiota of PT infants, since it continued to have an association throughout the duration of hospitalization in the NICU.

After delivery, PT infants face a number of medical conditions secondary to prematurity, such as respiratory distress syndrome due to surfactant deficiency in the lungs. The most common treatment for this condition is mechanical ventilation. Bacteria of the genus *Veillonella* tended to be lower in infants exposed to respiratory support. *Veillonella*, an anaerobic bacterium, is a common colonizer of the newborn gut (10). This bacterium utilizes lactate from carbohydrate fermentation (10) and is able to produce propionate (32), which could be beneficial for the host. Another common medical treatment in PT infants is the use of antibiotics immediately after birth and during the hospitalization. Thus, we investigated the effect of antibiotics on the PT gut. Although it failed to remain significant after FDR correction, infants not exposed to antibiotics had higher abundances of *Clostridium sensu stricto 1*, which suggests the effect of antibiotics on PT gut microbiome. Members from the cluster of *Clostridium sensu stricto 1* have been associated with prematurity and increased incidence of necrotizing enterocolitis (33). Although the associations mentioned above failed to remain significant, it is important to point out these differences so further studies can be conducted looking at these factors.

Chronological and anthropometric variables such as corrected GA and body weight, are also associated with PT gut colonization. Herein, a positive association was observed between diversity metrics, taxonomic composition and corrected GA. Relative abundance of *Staphylococcus*, a facultative anaerobe, significantly decreased over the course of hospitalization, which is a common feature reported in PT infants (34–36). Higher abundance of *Staphylococcus* has been associated with C-section delivery (37), breastfeeding, and HM feeding (38, 39), suggesting that the source can be the mother's skin and/or the milk microbiota. The decrease in the relative abundance of *Staphylococcus* coincided with an increase abundance of other common colonizers of the newborn gut, including *Veillonella* and *Bifidobacterium*. In PT infants, there is a delayed colonization with *Bifidobacterium* (40, 41), but this increases over time (35, 42–44). The concurrent increase of *Veillonella* and *Bifidobacterium* could be attributed to their mutualistic relationship. As mentioned above, *Veillonella* metabolizes lactate for propionate production. *Bifidobacterium* is a strict anaerobe capable of digesting complex carbohydrates, such as human milk oligosaccharides (HMOs) and producing acetate, formate (45) and lactate (46), which then is utilized by *Veillonella*.

Enterotype analysis revealed that stool samples from PT infants clustered into two distinct groups (Enterotype A and Enterotype B). Enterotype A was characterized by a lower diversity, and enrichment of *Bacteroides* and *Escherichia-Shigella*. In contrast, stool samples in Enterotype B had greater diversity and higher abundances of members from the phyla Proteobacteria (*Enterobacteriaceae/Enterobacter*, *Haemophilus*, and *Klebsiella*) and Firmicutes (*Clostridium sensu stricto 1*, *g_Lachnospiraceae*, and *Veillonella*). Enterotypes were first characterized by Arumugam and coworkers in 2011, by describing three fecal enterotypes in adult populations: *Bacteroides*-enriched, *Prevotella*-enriched, and

Ruminococcus-enriched, which were strongly associated to the dietary habits (18). In pediatric populations, authors have described the existence of enterotypes. Zhong et al. analyzed the gut microbiota of school-age children and found three enterotypes: *Bacteroides*-dominated, *Prevotella*-dominated, and *Bifidobacterium*-dominated (47). A recent study reported that the gut microbiome of infants aged 0–6 months was characterized by three enterotypes: *Bifidobacteriaceae*-dominated, *Enterobacteriaceae*-dominated, and *Bacteroidaceae*-dominated (48). The enterotype enriched in *Bifidobacteriaceae* was characterized by an increased capacity of HMO utilization (48). In a similar analysis, Tauchi et al. (41) analyzed stool samples of PT and full-term infants using Weighted UniFrac distances to characterize the gut microbiota composition. These authors found three different clusters: *Bifidobacteriaceae*-dominated, *Enterobacteriaceae*-dominated and Gram-positive bacilli cocci (*Staphylococcaceae*, *Streptococcaceae*, or *Enterococcaceae*)-dominated. However, they reported that no cluster that was significantly associated exclusively to PT infants (41). Compared to adults, the gut microbiota of newborns is highly variable, changes drastically during the first weeks after birth, and could be affected by the environment the infant is developing (49). This could explain the variability and the lack of consistency in studies analyzing enterotypes in a pediatric population.

In this study, around 40% of the stool samples transitioned from one enterotype to another. The main factors associated with this transition were corrected GA, body weight, use of antibiotics and dietary characteristics. About 70% of the samples transitioned from Enterotype A (*Bacteroides* and *Escherichia-Shigella*-dominated) to Enterotype B (Proteobacteria and Firmicutes-dominated). Prior to the change from one enterotype to another, infants were receiving more antibiotics, and consuming primarily HM plus fortification (HMF and/or BMF), and there was no exposure to PT formula. After the transition to another enterotype, there was less exposure to antibiotics and the consumption of PT formula increased. The use of antibiotics in PT infants has been associated with higher abundances of *Bacteroides* (50) and *Escherichia-Shigella* (51). Additionally, Ma et al. reported that in full-term infants, *Bacteroides* abundance was significantly higher in breast-fed compared to formula-fed infants (52). Bacteria enriched in Enterotype B (*Enterobacteriaceae*, *Klebsiella*, *Clostridium sensu stricto 1*, *Veillonella*, *Enterobacter*, uncharacterized *Lachnospiraceae*, and *Haemophilus*) have been previously associated to the gut microbiota of PT infants. Evidence has shown that *Enterobacteriaceae*/*Enterobacter* increase with postnatal age in PT infants (41, 44, 53–55). Moreover, two different studies have suggested that the gut microbiota composition of PT infants, transitions over time from a *Staphylococcus* dominated (56) or Gram-positive bacilli cocci dominated (41), to an *Enterobacteriaceae*/*Enterobacter* dominated. Abundances of *Klebsiella* (55), *Clostridium* (57) and *Veillonella* (34, 57) have been found to increase with postnatal age in the gut of PT infants. Changes from one enterotype to another might not be attributed to a specific factor (e.g., greater use of infant formula). Instead, it might be the combination of multiple characteristics (clinical and dietary) contributing to the modification of the gut microbiota. The effect of the feeding type (human milk, infant formula, and type of fortifiers) and their association with the gut microbiota of PT infants is understudied. Furthermore, studies using clustering techniques such as enterotypes to assess the gut microbiota in a PT population are scarce. Hence, there is insufficient evidence on the clinical relevance of PT infants belonging or transitioning from one enterotype to another. Therefore, more research is needed to fully understand the implications of the gut microbiota clustering and feeding types in PT infants.

This study also explored the associations between taxonomic composition and dietary distribution over the course of hospitalization in the NICU. When perinatal and chronological indicators, as well as antibiotic exposure were considered, three different bacteria were significantly associated with the type of milk and/or fortifier consumed: *Clostridium sensu stricto 1*, *Bifidobacterium*, and *Lactobacillus*. Compared to HM alone, the consumption of HM with a HMF was associated with higher abundances of *Clostridium sensu stricto 1* and lower abundances of *Lactobacillus*, and consumption of infant formula was associated with lower abundances of *Bifidobacterium*. Evidence about the effect of milk fortifiers on the gut microbiota composition is scarce. Underwood and co-workers conducted a longitudinal study evaluating the effect of a HMF or BMF added to HM in the PT gut microbial composition. Over time, the abundance of the genus *Lactobacillus* decreased with the use of HMF (8). Additionally, prior studies have suggested that HM consumption (MOM or DHM) is associated with higher abundances of *Clostridium* in PT infants (58, 59). However, these studies consisted of only one time point analysis (59), or had small sample sizes (8, 58). In PT infants, the effect of HM consumption on *Lactobacillus* needs further exploration. Studies have reported both increased (59) and decreased (60) abundance of this microbe with the consumption of HM compared to specialized PT infant formula. *Lactobacillus* is a common colonizer of the gut microbiota capable of metabolizing carbohydrates to produce lactic acid (61). Supplementation of members of *Lactobacillus* to PT infants is associated with a reduction in the abundance of *Clostridium histolyticum* (62), and with an increase in beneficial bacteria such as *Bifidobacterium* (63) compared to those infants not receiving probiotic supplementation. The observed difference in fecal *Bifidobacterium* abundance between infants fed HM vs. PT formula in this study is consistent with the published literature in preterm (44, 59) and full-term infants (64).

Lastly, this study aimed to identify possible associations between the use of milk fortifiers and grow indicators. Weight gain velocity, commonly expressed as g/d, is used to estimate growth and development of PT infants. In the present study, over the course of hospitalization there was a linear growth trajectory. However, when infants were consuming a BMF, weight gain velocity was significantly faster compared to when infants were consuming HMF (5). The use of milk fortifiers (HMF or BMF) are recommended in PT infants fed HM due to the insufficient macro- (particularly protein) and micronutrient (particularly calcium and phosphate) content of HM compared to the PT infant's growth requirements (7). The amount of fortification with either of these two fortifiers depends on the infant's requirements, and similar protein concentration can be achieved either of both fortifiers (65). Thus, differences in growth trajectories might be associated to the types of protein in HM and bovine milk. Zhang and collaborators demonstrated that there are around 33 proteins associated with the milk fat globule membrane, and 16 whey proteins, that are significantly different between HM and bovine milk (66). On the other hand, PT birth is often associated with restricted growth (67). After birth, around 90% of infants with restricted growth exhibit a catch-up growth trajectory, during which, weight gain increases to the expected growth curve (68). However, a meta-analysis conducted by Martin and collaborators analyzing the health impacts of catch-up growth trajectory in low-birth weight infants suggested that while rapid growth might have beneficial outcomes in the short-term, there might be adverse long-term outcomes associated with catch-up growth (69). This suggests that future studies should assess the weight gain velocities of low-birth-weight infants, particularly when fed HMF or BMF. Evidence of the association between growth trajectories and the gut microbial composition in infants is limited. A recent study revealed that gut microbial diversity and taxonomic characteristics are associated with the growth trajectories from 1 to 5 years of age (70). Prospective studies assessing the relationships between diet, growth and gut microbiota could serve to develop biomarkers to predict the possible infant's growth characteristics.

This study longitudinally analyzed the development of the gut microbiota of PT infants and compared different feeding types and milk fortifiers, however, there are some potential limitations worth mentioning. First, a pregnancy complication included in this study and significantly associated with the gut microbiota composition was chorioamnionitis. However, this affection was clinically diagnosed and not confirmed by culture or histologic tests. Another limitation in this study is that the only information available from the infant's mother was race. Additional data related to maternal health status could help find possible links between the infant's gut microbiota and maternal characteristics. Next, multiple stool samples were collected during the time infants were hospitalized in the NICU; however, the time point and the time interval when the stool samples were collected was not consistent across participants. In the same manner, another limitation is that the gut microbiota characteristics after birth were evaluated based on the first stool sample available, which was about 2 weeks after birth. Moreover, given the nature of the study, the results presented here might be biased toward associations mostly related to infants very-low birth weight infants (smaller GA and lower birth weight) which are more likely to be exposed to different milk fortifiers (HMF and BMF) to have longer hospitalization periods and a larger number of stool samples collected. Another limitation is the sample size. Albeit having a sample size of 97 PT infants with multiple sample collection, gut microbiome studies analyzing a large number of variables related to diversity and taxonomic composition could be underpowered. This could explain why some associations failed to remain significant after FDR correction. Lastly, we didn't account for the effects of the environment surrounding infants hospitalized in the NICU that could affect their gut microbiome (2). These factors include transition from incubators to open cribs and skin-to-skin care. Therefore, future longitudinal studies should aim to characterize the gut microbiota of PT infants based on their feeding type with larger sample sizes and considering the effect of other environmental aspects.

CONCLUSION

This study found that PT infants from Black or Hispanic mothers have a distinct gut microbiota soon after birth, but these differences do not persist over time. Pregnancy complications, particularly chorioamnionitis, can have a long-term effect on the fecal taxonomic composition. The use of HM with a HMF, and infant formula consumption significantly modified the abundances of *Clostridium sensu stricto 1* and *Bifidobacterium*. The use of HMF or BMF contributes to weight gain velocity, the latter associated with a more rapid weight gain. Also, these fortifiers were positively correlated with the abundance of *Clostridium sensu stricto 1*, *Bifidobacterium* and *Enterobacter*. Lastly, two different enterotypes associated with PT infants were characterized. The difference between these enterotypes was mainly in diversity metrics, and enrichment of *Bacteroides*, *Escherichia-Shigella*' uncharacterized *Enterobacteriaceae*, *Klebsiella*, *Clostridium sensu stricto 1*, *Veillonella*, *Enterobacter*, uncharacterized *Lachnospiraceae* and *Haemophilus*. A significant proportion of infants changed from one enterotype to another, which was associated with corrected GA, body weight, administration of antibiotics and consumption of different HM or infant formula and different types of fortifiers. More studies are needed to further explore the effect of not only HM or formula but also HMF vs. BMF on the gut microbiota composition of PT infant.

AUTHOR CONTRIBUTIONS

TH, CW, and SD conceived the study. TH and SD designed the study. TH, CW, and AM collected samples analyzed in the study. CW and AM collected the clinical data for this study. MA-L analyzed the fecal microbiome and conducted bioinformatic and statistical analyses. MA-L, TH, CW, and SD wrote the manuscript. All authors approved the final manuscript prior publication.

ACKNOWLEDGMENTS

Authors thank all the nurses and staff from the NICU at Carle Hospital for their help and support in sample collection.

REFERENCES

1. Robertson RC, Manges AR, Finlay BB, Prendergast AJ. The human microbiome and child growth – first 1000 days and beyond. *Trends Microbiol.* (2019) 27:131–47. doi: 10.1016/j.tim.2018.09.008
2. Aguilar-Lopez M, Dinsmoor AM, Ho TTB, Donovan SM. A systematic review of the factors influencing microbial colonization of the preterm infant gut. *Gut Microbes.* (2021) 13:1–33. doi: 10.1080/19490976.2021.1884514
3. Lim SJ, Aguilar-Lopez M, Wetzel C, Dutra SVO, Bray V, Groer MW, et al. The effects of genetic relatedness on the preterm infant gut microbiota. *Microorganisms.* (2021) 9:278. doi: 10.3390/microorganisms9020278
4. Ho NT, Li F, Lee-Sarwar KA, Tun HM, Brown BP, Pannaraj PS, et al. Meta-analysis of effects of exclusive breastfeeding on infant gut microbiota across populations. *Nat Commun.* (2018) 9:4169. doi: 10.1038/s41467-018-06473-x
5. Quigley M, Embleton ND, McGuire W. Formula versus donor breast milk for feeding preterm or low birth weight infants. *Cochrane Database Syst Rev.* (2019) 7:CD002971. doi: 10.1002/14651858.CD002971.pub5
6. Hay WW, Thureen P. Protein for preterm infants: how much is needed? How much is enough? How much is too much? *Pediatr Neonatol.* (2010) 51:198–207. doi: 10.1016/S1875-9572(10)60039-3
7. Arslanoglu S, Boquien CY, King C, Lamireau D, Tonetto P, Barnett D, et al. Fortification of human milk for preterm infants: update and recommendations of the European Milk Bank Association (EMBA) working group on human milk fortification. *Front Pediatr.* (2019) 7:76. doi: 10.3389/fped.2019.00076
8. Underwood MA, Kalanetra KM, Bokulich NA, Mirmiran M, Barile D, Tancredi DJ, et al. Prebiotic oligosaccharides in premature infants. *J Pediatr Gastroenterol Nutr.* (2014) 58:352–60. doi: 10.1097/MPG.0000000000000211
9. Mallick H, Rahnavard A, McIver LJ, Ma S, Zhang Y, Nguyen LH, et al. Multivariable association discovery in population-scale meta-omics studies. *bioRxiv [Preprint].* (2021). doi: 10.1101/2021.01.20.427420
10. Milani C, Duranti S, Bottacini F, Casey E, Turroni F, Mahony J, et al. The first microbial colonizers of the human gut: composition, activities, and health implications of the infant gut microbiota. *Microbiol Mol Biol Rev.* (2017) 81:e00036-17. doi: 10.1128/MMBR.00036-17
11. Fenton TR. A new growth chart for preterm babies: Babson and Benda's chart updated with recent data and a new format. *BMC Pediatr.* (2003) 3:13. doi: 10.1186/1471-2431-3-13
12. Kalyuzhanaya MG, Waite DW, Roose-Amsaleg CL, Payne MS, Stinson LF, Keelan JA. Comparison of meconium DNA extraction methods for use in microbiome studies. *Front Microbiol.* (2018) 9:270. doi: 10.3389/fmicb.2018.00270
13. Bolyen E, Rideout JR, Dillon MR, Bokulich NA, Abnet CC, Al-Ghalith GA, et al. Reproducible, interactive, scalable and extensible microbiome data science using QIIME 2. *Nat Biotechnol.* (2019) 37:852–7. doi: 10.1038/s41587-019-0209-9
14. Allali I, Arnold JW, Roach J, Cadenas MB, Butz N, Hassan HM, et al. A comparison of sequencing platforms and bioinformatics pipelines for compositional analysis of the gut microbiome. *BMC Microbiol.* (2017) 17:194. doi: 10.1186/s12866-017-1101-8
15. Quast C, Pruesse E, Yilmaz P, Gerken J, Schweer T, Yarza P, et al. The SILVA ribosomal RNA gene database project: improved data processing and web-based tools. *Nucleic Acids Res.* (2013) 41:D590–6. doi: 10.1093/nar/gks1219
16. Jurasinski G, Retzer V, Beierkuhnlein C. Inventory, differentiation, and proportional diversity: a consistent terminology for quantifying species diversity. *Oecologia.* (2009) 159:15–26. doi: 10.1007/s00442-008-1190-z
17. Jari Oksanen F, Blanchet G, Friendly M, Kindt R, Legendre P, McGlinn D, et al. *vegan: Community Ecology Package.* (2020). Available online at: https://cran.r-project.org/package=vegan
18. Arumugam M, Raes J, Pelletier E, Le Paslier D, Yamada T, Mende DR, et al. Enterotypes of the human gut microbiome. *Nature.* (2011) 473:174–80. doi: 10.1038/nature09944
19. Segata N, Izard J, Waldron L, Gevers D, Miropolsky L, Garrett WS, et al. Metagenomic biomarker discovery and explanation. *Genome Biol.* (2011) 12:R60. doi: 10.1186/gb-2011-12-6-r60
20. Pinheiro J, Bates D, DebRoy S, Sarkar D, RCT. *nlme: Linear and Nonlinear Mixed Effects Modelse.* (2021). Available online at: https://cran.r-project.org/package=nlme
21. Asnicar F, Manara S, Zolfo M, Truong DT, Scholz M, Armanini F, et al. Studying vertical microbiome transmission from mothers to infants by strain-level metagenomic profiling. *MSYSTEMS.* (2017) 2:e00164.16. doi: 10.1128/mSystems.00164-16
22. Mitchell CM, Mazzoni C, Hogstrom L, Bryant A, Bergerat A, Cher A, et al. Delivery mode affects stability of early infant gut microbiota. *Cell Rep Med.* (2020) 1:100156. doi: 10.1016/j.xcrm.2020.100156
23. Walker RW, Clemente JC, Peter I, Loos RJF. The prenatal gut microbiome: are we colonized with bacteria in utero? *Pediatr Obes.* (2017) 12:3–17. doi: 10.1111/ijpo.12217
24. Hyman RW, Fukushima M, Jiang H, Fung E, Rand L, Johnson B, et al. Diversity of the vaginal microbiome correlates with preterm birth. *Reprod Sci.* (2014) 21:32–40. doi: 10.1177/1933719113488838
25. Wheeler S, Pryor K, Antczak B, Truong T, Murtha A, Seed P. The relationship of cervical microbiota diversity with race and disparities in preterm birth. *J Neonatal Perinatal Med.* (2018) 11:305–10. doi: 10.3233/NPM-17111
26. McGregor JA, French JI, Seo K. Premature rupture of membranes and bacterial vaginosis. *Am J Obstet Gynecol.* (1993) 169:463–6. doi: 10.1016/0002-9378(93)90342-G
27. Witkin SS. The vaginal microbiome, vaginal anti-microbial defence mechanisms and the clinical challenge of reducing infection-related preterm birth. *BJOG.* (2015) 122:213–8. doi: 10.1111/1471-0528.13115
28. Onderdonk AB, Delaney ML, Fichorova RN. The human microbiome during bacterial vaginosis. *Clin Microbiol Rev.* (2016) 29:223 LP–38. doi: 10.1128/CMR.00075-15
29. Groer MW, Luciano AA, Dishaw LJ, Ashmeade TL, Miller E, Gilbert JA. Development of the preterm infant gut microbiome: a research priority. *Microbiome.* (2014) 2:38. doi: 10.1186/2049-2618-2-38
30. Doyle RM, Harris K, Kamiza S, Harjunmaa U, Ashorn U, Nkhoma M, et al. Bacterial communities found in placental tissues are associated with severe chorioamnionitis and adverse birth outcomes. *PLoS ONE.* (2017) 12:e0180167. doi: 10.1371/journal.pone.0180167
31. Prince AL, Ma J, Kannan PS, Alvarez M, Gisslen T, Harris RA, et al. The placental membrane microbiome is altered among subjects with spontaneous preterm birth with and without chorioamnionitis. *Am J Obstet Gynecol.* (2016) 214:627.e1–16. doi: 10.1016/j.ajog.2016.01.193
32. Scheiman J, Luber JM, Chavkin TA, MacDonald T, Tung A, Pham LD, et al. Meta-omics analysis of elite athletes identifies a performance-enhancing microbe that functions via lactate metabolism. *Nat Med.* (2019) 25:1104–9. doi: 10.1038/s41591-019-0485-4
33. Schönherr-Hellec S, Klein GL, Delannoy J, Ferraris L, Rozé JC, Butel MJ, et al. Clostridial strain-specific characteristics associated with necrotizing enterocolitis. *Appl Environ Microbiol.* (2018) 84:e02428-17 doi: 10.1128/AEM.02428-17
34. Chernikova DA, Koestler DC, Hoen AG, Housman ML, Hibberd PL, Moore JH, et al. Fetal exposures and perinatal influences on the stool microbiota of premature infants. *J Matern Neonatal Med.* (2016) 29:99–105. doi: 10.3109/14767058.2014.987748
35. Sim K, Shaw AG, Randell P, Cox MJ, McClure ZE, Li MS, et al. Dysbiosis anticipating necrotizing enterocolitis in very premature infants. *Clin Infect Dis.* (2015) 60:389–97. doi: 10.1093/cid/ciu822
36. Costello EK, Carlisle EM, Bik EM, Morowitz MJ, Relman DA. Microbiome assembly across multiple body sites in low-birthweight infants. *mBio.* (2013) 4:e00782-13 doi: 10.1128/mBio.00782-13
37. Reyman M, van Houten MA, van Baarle D, Bosch AATM, Man WH, Chu MLJN, et al. Impact of delivery mode-associated gut microbiota dynamics on health in the first year of life. *Nat Commun.* (2019) 10:4997. doi: 10.1038/s41467-019-13373-1
38. Soeorg H, Metsvaht T, Eelmäe I, Merila M, Treumuth S, Huik K, et al. The role of breast milk in the colonization of neonatal gut and skin with coagulase-negative staphylococci. *Pediatr Res.* (2017) 82:759–67. doi: 10.1038/pr.2017.150
39. Murphy K, Curley D, O'Callaghan TF, O'Shea CA, Dempsey EM, O'Toole PW, et al. The composition of human milk and infant faecal microbiota over the first three months of life: a pilot study. *Sci Rep.* (2017) 7:40597. doi: 10.1038/srep40597
40. Forsgren M, Isolauri E, Salminen S, Rautava S. Late preterm birth has direct and indirect effects on infant gut microbiota development during the first six months of life. *Acta Paediatr.* (2017) 106:1103–9. doi: 10.1111/apa.13837

41. Tauchi H, Yahagi K, Yamauchi T, Hara T, Yamaoka R, Tsukuda N, et al. Gut microbiota development of preterm infants hospitalised in intensive care units. *Benef Microbes.* (2019) 10:641–51. doi: 10.3920/BM2019.0003
42. Korpela K, Blakstad EW, Moltu SJ, Strømmen K, Nakstad B, Rønnestad AE, et al. Intestinal microbiota development and gestational age in preterm neonates. *Sci Rep.* (2018) 8:2453. doi: 10.1038/s41598-018-20827-x
43. Arboleya S, Sánchez B, Milani C, Duranti S, Solís G, Fernández N, et al. Intestinal microbiota development in preterm neonates and effect of perinatal antibiotics. *J Pediatr.* (2015) 166:538–44. doi: 10.1016/j.jpeds.2014.09.041
44. Biagi E, Aceti A, Quercia S, Beghetti I, Rampelli S, Turroni S, et al. Microbial community dynamics in mother's milk and Infant's mouth and gut in moderately preterm infants. *Front Microbiol.* (2018) 9:2512. doi: 10.3389/fmicb.2018.02512
45. Lawson MAE, O'neill IJ, Kujawska M, Gowrinadh Javvadi S, Wijeyesekera A, Flegg Z, et al. Breast milk-derived human milk oligosaccharides promote Bifidobacterium interactions within a single ecosystem. *ISME J.* (2020) 14:635–48. doi: 10.1038/s41396-019-0553-2
46. Devika NT, Raman K. Deciphering the metabolic capabilities of Bifidobacteria using genome-scale metabolic models. *Sci Rep.* (2019) 9:18222. doi: 10.1038/s41598-019-54696-9
47. Zhong H, Penders J, Shi Z, Ren H, Cai K, Fang C, et al. Impact of early events and lifestyle on the gut microbiota and metabolic phenotypes in young school-age children. *Microbiome.* (2019) 7:2. doi: 10.1186/s40168-018-0608-z
48. Casaburi G, Duar RM, Brown H, Mitchell RD, Kazi S, Chew S, et al. Metagenomic insights of the infant microbiome community structure and function across multiple sites in the United States. *Sci Rep.* (2021) 11:1472. doi: 10.1038/s41598-020-80583-9
49. Xiao L, Wang J, Zheng J, Li X, Zhao F. Deterministic transition of enterotypes shapes the infant gut microbiome at an early age. *Genome Biol.* (2021) 22:243. doi: 10.1186/s13059-021-02463-3
50. Zhu D, Xiao S, Yu J, Ai Q, He Y, Cheng C, et al. Effects of one-week empirical antibiotic therapy on the early development of gut microbiota and metabolites in preterm infants. *Sci Rep.* (2017) 7:8025. doi: 10.1038/s41598-017-08530-9
51. Zou ZH, Liu D, Li HD, Zhu DP, He Y, Hou T, et al. Prenatal and postnatal antibiotic exposure influences the gut microbiota of preterm infants in neonatal intensive care units. *Ann Clin Microbiol Antimicrob.* (2018) 17:9. doi: 10.1186/s12941-018-0264-y
52. Ma J, Li Z, Zhang W, Zhang C, Zhang Y, Mei H, et al. Comparison of gut microbiota in exclusively breast-fed and formula-fed babies: a study of 91 term infants. *Sci Rep.* (2020) 10:15792. doi: 10.1038/s41598-020-72635-x
53. Zwittink RD, van Zoeren-Grobben D, Martin R, van Lingen RA, Groot Jebbink LJ, Boeren S, et al. Metaproteomics reveals functional differences in intestinal microbiota development of preterm infants. *Mol Cell Proteomics.* (2017) 16:1610–20. doi: 10.1074/mcp.RA117.000102
54. Younge NE, Newgard CB, Cotten CM, Goldberg RN, Muehlbauer MJ, Bain JR, et al. Disrupted maturation of the microbiota and metabolome among extremely preterm infants with postnatal growth failure. *Sci Rep.* (2019) 9:8167. doi: 10.1038/s41598-019-44547-y
55. Gómez M, Moles L, Espinosa-Martos I, Bustos G, de Vos W, Fernández L, et al. Bacteriological and immunological profiling of meconium and fecal samples from preterm infants: a two-year follow-up study. *Nutrients.* (2017) 9:1293. doi: 10.3390/nu9121293
56. Mshvildadze M, Neu J, Mai V. Intestinal microbiota development in the premature neonate: establishment of a lasting commensal relationship? *Nutr Rev.* (2008) 66:658–63. doi: 10.1111/j.1753-4887.2008.00119.x
57. Moles L, Gómez M, Heilig H, Bustos G, Fuentes S, de Vos W, et al. Bacterial diversity in meconium of preterm neonates and evolution of their fecal microbiota during the first month of life. *PLoS ONE.* (2013) 8:e66986. doi: 10.1371/journal.pone.0066986
58. Gregory KE, Samuel BS, Houghteling P, Shan G, Ausubel FM, Sadreyev RI, et al. Influence of maternal breast milk ingestion on acquisition of the intestinal microbiome in preterm infants. *Microbiome.* (2016) 4:68. doi: 10.1186/s40168-016-0214-x
59. Parra-Llorca A, Gormaz M, Alcántara C, Cernada M, Nuñez-Ramiro A, Vento M, et al. Preterm gut microbiome depending on feeding type: significance of donor human milk. *Front Microbiol.* (2018) 9:1376. doi: 10.3389/fmicb.2018.01376
60. Chernikova DA, Madan JC, Housman ML, Zain-ul-abideen M, Lundgren SN, Morrison HG, et al. The premature infant gut microbiome during the first 6 weeks of life differs based on gestational maturity at birth. *Pediatr Res.* (2018) 84:71–9. doi: 10.1038/s41390-018-0022-z
61. Walter J. Ecological role of lactobacilli in the gastrointestinal tract: implications for fundamental and biomedical research. *Appl Environ Microbiol.* (2008) 74:4985–96. doi: 10.1128/AEM.00753-08
62. Pärtty A, Luoto R, Kalliomäki M, Salminen S, Isolauri E. Effects of early prebiotic and probiotic supplementation on development of gut microbiota and fussing and crying in preterm infants: a randomized, double-blind, placebo-controlled trial. *J Pediatr.* (2013) 163:1272–7.e2. doi: 10.1016/j.jpeds.2013.05.035
63. Alcon-Giner C, Dalby MJ, Caim S, Ketskemety J, Shaw A, Sim K, et al. Microbiota supplementation with bifidobacterium and lactobacillus modifies the preterm infant gut microbiota and metabolome: an observational study. *Cell Rep Med.* (2020) 1:100077. doi: 10.1016/j.xcrm.2020.100077
64. Davis EC, Dinsmoor AM, Wang M, Donovan SM. Microbiome composition in pediatric populations from birth to adolescence: impact of diet and prebiotic and probiotic interventions. *Dig Dis Sci.* (2020) 65:706–22. doi: 10.1007/s10620-020-06092-x
65. Radmacher PG, Adamkin DH. Fortification of human milk for preterm infants. *Semin Fetal Neonatal Med.* (2017) 22:30–5. doi: 10.1016/j.siny.2016.08.004
66. Zhang L, van Dijk ADJ, Hettinga K. An interactomics overview of the human and bovine milk proteome over lactation. *Proteome Sci.* (2016) 15:1. doi: 10.1186/s12953-016-0110-0
67. Anil KC, Basel PL, Singh S. Low birth weight and its associated risk factors: Health facility-based case-control study. *PLoS ONE.* (2020) 15:e0234907. doi: 10.1371/journal.pone.0234907
68. Karlberg J, Albertsson-Wikland K. Growth in full-term small-for-gestational-age infants: from birth to final height. *Pediatr Res.* (1995) 38:733–9. doi: 10.1203/00006450-199511000-00017
69. Martin A, Connelly A, Bland RM, Reilly JJ. Health impact of catch-up growth in low-birth weight infants: systematic review, evidence appraisal, and meta-analysis. *Matern Child Nutr.* (2017) 13. doi: 10.1111/mcn.12297
70. Roswall J, Olsson LM, Kovatcheva-Datchary P, Nilsson S, Tremaroli V, Simon MC, et al. Developmental trajectory of the healthy human gut microbiota during the first 5 years of life. *Cell Host Microbe.* (2021) 29:765–6.e3. doi: 10.1016/j.chom.2021.02.021

Permissions

All chapters in this book were first published by Frontiers; hereby published with permission under the Creative Commons Attribution License or equivalent. Every chapter published in this book has been scrutinized by our experts. Their significance has been extensively debated. The topics covered herein carry significant findings which will fuel the growth of the discipline. They may even be implemented as practical applications or may be referred to as a beginning point for another development.

The contributors of this book come from diverse backgrounds, making this book a truly international effort. This book will bring forth new frontiers with its revolutionizing research information and detailed analysis of the nascent developments around the world.

We would like to thank all the contributing authors for lending their expertise to make the book truly unique. They have played a crucial role in the development of this book. Without their invaluable contributions this book wouldn't have been possible. They have made vital efforts to compile up to date information on the varied aspects of this subject to make this book a valuable addition to the collection of many professionals and students.

This book was conceptualized with the vision of imparting up-to-date information and advanced data in this field. To ensure the same, a matchless editorial board was set up. Every individual on the board went through rigorous rounds of assessment to prove their worth. After which they invested a large part of their time researching and compiling the most relevant data for our readers.

The editorial board has been involved in producing this book since its inception. They have spent rigorous hours researching and exploring the diverse topics which have resulted in the successful publishing of this book. They have passed on their knowledge of decades through this book. To expedite this challenging task, the publisher supported the team at every step. A small team of assistant editors was also appointed to further simplify the editing procedure and attain best results for the readers.

Apart from the editorial board, the designing team has also invested a significant amount of their time in understanding the subject and creating the most relevant covers. They scrutinized every image to scout for the most suitable representation of the subject and create an appropriate cover for the book.

The publishing team has been an ardent support to the editorial, designing and production team. Their endless efforts to recruit the best for this project, has resulted in the accomplishment of this book. They are a veteran in the field of academics and their pool of knowledge is as vast as their experience in printing. Their expertise and guidance has proved useful at every step. Their uncompromising quality standards have made this book an exceptional effort. Their encouragement from time to time has been an inspiration for everyone.

The publisher and the editorial board hope that this book will prove to be a valuable piece of knowledge for researchers, students, practitioners and scholars across the globe.

List of Contributors

Pasqua Piemontese, Nadia Liotto, Domenica Mallardi, Valeria Puricelli, Chiara Tabasso, Michela Perrone, Anna Orsi and Orsola Amato
Neonatal Intensive Care Unit, Fondazione IRCCS Ca' Granda Ospedale Maggiore Policlinico (IRCCS), Milan, Italy

Paola Roggero, Maria Lorella Giannì, Daniela Morniroli and Camilla Menis
Neonatal Intensive Care Unit, Fondazione IRCCS Ca' Granda Ospedale Maggiore Policlinico (IRCCS), Milan, Italy
Department of Clinical Sciences and Community Health, University of Milan, Milan, Italy

Manuela Donalisio, Massimo Rittà, Rachele Francese and Andrea Civra
Laboratory of Molecular Virology, Department of Clinical and Biological Sciences, University of Turin, Turin, Italy

Alessandra Coscia
Neonatal Intensive Care Unit, Department of Public Health and Pediatrics, University of Turin, Turin, Italy

Laura Cavallarin
Consiglio Nazionale delle Ricerche-Istituto di Scienze delle Produzioni Alimentari, Bari, Italy
Institute of Sciences of Food Production, National Research Council, Turin, Italy

Marzia Giribaldi
Consiglio Nazionale delle Ricerche-Istituto di Scienze delle Produzioni Alimentari, Bari, Italy
Consiglio per la Ricerca in Agricoltura e l'Analisi dell'Economia Agraria, Centro di Ricerca in Ingegneria e Trasformazioni Agroalimentari, Turin, Italy

Guido E. Moro
Italian Association of Human Milk Banks, Milan, Italy

Elena Sinkiewicz-Darol
Laboratory of Human Milk and Lactation Research at Regional Human Milk Bank in Holy Family Hospital, Department of Neonatology, Medical University of Warsaw, Warsaw, Poland
Human Milk Bank, Ludwik Rydygier' Provincial Polyclinical Hospital in Torun, Torun, Poland

Kamila Strom and Gabriela Oledzka
Department of Medical Biology, Medical University of Warsaw, Warsaw, Poland

Olga Barbarska
Laboratory of Human Milk and Lactation Research at Regional Human Milk Bank in Holy Family Hospital, Department of Neonatology, Medical University of Warsaw, Warsaw, Poland
Department of Medical Biology, Medical University of Warsaw, Warsaw, Poland
First Department of Obstetrics and Gynecology, Medical University of Warsaw, Warsaw, Poland

Malgorzata Rutkowska and Sylwester Rzoska
High Pressure Physics, Polish Academy of Science, Warsaw, Poland

Katarzyna Karzel
Faculty of Psychology, Warsaw University, Warsaw, Poland

Elzbieta Rosiak
Department of Food Hygiene and Quality Management, Faculty of Human Nutrition and Consumer Science, Warsaw University of Life Sciences, Warsaw, Poland

Magdalena Orczyk-Pawiłowicz
Department of Chemistry and Immunochemistry, Wroclaw Medical University, Wroclaw, Poland

Maria Katarzyna Borszewska-Kornacka
Neonatal and Intensive Care Department, University Hospital, Medical University of Warsaw, Warsaw, Polan

Elettra Berti and Anna Ingargiola
Anna Meyer Children's University Hospital, Florence, Italy

Monia Puglia
Health Agency of Tuscany, Florence, Italy

Franca Rusconi
Anna Meyer Children's University Hospital, Florence, Italy
Health Agency of Tuscany, Florence, Italy

Silvia Perugi and Simone Pratesi
Careggi University Hospital, Florence, Italy

Luigi Gagliardi
Versilia Hospital, Viareggio, Italy

Cristiana Bosi
San Giovanni di Dio Hospital, Florence, Italy

Letizia Magi
San Donato Hospital, Arezzo, Italy

Elena Martelli
Santo Stefano Hospital, Prato, Italy

Emilio Sigali
University Hospital of Pisa, Pisa, Italy

Barbara Tomasini
University Hospital of Siena, Siena, Italy

Sertac Arslanoglu
Department of Pediatrics, Division of Neonatology, Istanbul Medeniyet University Goztepe Education and Research Hospital, Istanbul, Turkey

Caroline King
Department of Nutrition and Dietetics, Imperial College Healthcare NHS Trust, London, United Kingdom

Delphine Lamireau
Lactariums de Bordeaux-Marmande, Pôle Pédiatrique, Centre Hospitalo-Universitaire (CHU) de Bordeaux, Bordeaux, France

Paola Tonetto
Neonatal Unit of Turin University, City of Health and Science of Turin, Turin, Italy
Neonatal Intensive Care Unit, Department of Public Health and Pediatrics, University of Turin, Turin, Italy

Debbie Barnett
Greater Glasgow and Clyde Donor Milk Bank, Royal Hospital for Sick Children, Glasgow, United Kingdom

Corinna Gebauer
Abteilung Neonatologie Klinik und Poliklinik für Kinder und Jugendliche, Leipzig, Germany
Department of Neonatology, University Children's Hospital, Leipzig, Germany

Anne Grovslien
Neonatal Unit, Milk Bank, Oslo University Hospital, Oslo, Norway
Breast Milk Bank, Oslo University Hospital, Oslo, Norway

Gillian Weaver
Hearts Milk Bank, Rothamsted Research Institute, Harpenden, United Kingdom
Human Milk Foundation, Harpenden, United Kingdom

Aleksandra Maria Wesolowska
Department of Neonatology, Faculty of Health Science, Medical University of Warsaw, Warsaw, Poland

Caroline Steele
Children's Hospital of Orange County, Orange, CA, United States

Nathalie Kreins
Neonatal Intensive Care Unit, Croix Rousse University Hospital, Hospices Civils de Lyon, Lyon, France

Rachel Buffin
Neonatal Intensive Care Unit, Croix Rousse University Hospital, Hospices Civils de Lyon, Lyon, France
Regional Human Milk Bank, Croix Rousse University Hospital, Hospices Civils de Lyon, Lyon, France
Neonatology Department, Croix-Rousse Hospital, Lyon, France
Régional Rhône Alpes Auvergne Human Milk Bank, Hôpital de la Croix-Rousse, Lyon, France

Diane Michel-Molnar and Veronique Chambon
Centre de Biologie, Hôpital de la Croix Rousse, Hospices Civils de Lyon, Lyon, France

Pierre Pradat
Center for Clinical Research, Croix Rousse University Hospital, Hospices Civils de Lyon, Lyon, France

Jean-Charles Picaud
Neonatal Intensive Care Unit, Croix Rousse University Hospital, Hospices Civils de Lyon, Lyon, France
Regional Human Milk Bank, Croix Rousse University Hospital, Hospices Civils de Lyon, Lyon, France
CarMeN Unit, Inserm U1060, INRA U1397, Claude Bernard University Lyon 1, Pierre Bénite, France
Faculté de Médecine Lyon Sud Charles Merieux, Université Claude Bernard Lyon 1, Pierre Bénite, France
Division of Neonatology, Hôpital de la Croix-Rousse, Lyon, France
Lactarium Auvergne Rhone Alpes, Hospices Civils de Lyon, Lyon, France
Neonatology Department, Croix-Rousse Hospital, Lyon, France
Régional Rhône Alpes Auvergne Human Milk Bank, Hôpital de la Croix-Rousse, Lyon, France

Marie Schreiner and Roland Hentschel
Center for Pediatrics, Department of Neonatology, Faculty of Medicine, Medical Center - University of Freiburg, Freiburg, Germany

Valeria Falcone
Institute of Virology, Faculty of Medicine, Medical Center - University of Freiburg, Freiburg, Germany

Daniel Jonas
Institute for Infection Prevention and Hospital Epidemiology, Faculty of Medicine, Medical Center - University of Freiburg, Freiburg, Germany

Mirjam Kunze
Department of Obstetrics and Gynecology, Faculty of Medicine, Medical Center - University of Freiburg, Freiburg, Germany

Andrea Weber
Institute of Medical Microbiology and Hygiene, Faculty of Medicine, Medical Center - University of Freiburg, Freiburg, Germany

Luigi Corvaglia
Neonatology and Neonatal Intensive Care Unit—S. Orsola-Malpighi Hospital, Bologna, Italy

Anna Giulia Cimatti and Francesca Vitali
Neonatal Intensive Care Unit, S. Orsola-Malpighi University Hospital, Bologna, Italy
Department of Medical and Surgical Sciences, University of Bologna, Bologna, Italy

Silvia Martini, Arianna Aceti and Giacomo Faldella
Department of Medical and Surgical Sciences, University of Bologna, Bologna, Italy
Neonatology and Neonatal Intensive Care Unit—S. Orsola-Malpighi Hospital, Bologna, Italy

Alessandra Munarini and Vilma Mantovani
Department of Medical and Surgical Sciences, University of Bologna, Bologna, Italy
Department of Clinical Medicine, Center of Applied Biochemical Research, S. Orsola-Malpighi University Hospital, Bologna, Italy

Maximilano Zioutas
Pediatric Endocrinology, Department of Pediatrics, S. Orsola-Malpighi University Hospital, Bologna, Italy

Stefania Sbrizzi, Pasqua Anna Quitadamo, Domenico Ravidà, Giuseppina Palumbo, Pier Paolo Cristalli and Massimo Pettoello-Mantovani
NICU, Casa Sollievo della Sofferenza Hospital, San Giovanni Rotondo, Italy

Daniel Klotz, Stefanie Jansen and Hans Fuchs
Department of Neonatology, Center for Pediatrics, Medical Center - University of Freiburg, Faculty of Medicine, University of Freiburg, Freiburg, Germany

Marilyn V. Giorgi, Champa N. Codipilly, Debra Potak, Howard S. Heiman and Richard J. Schanler
Lilling Family Neonatal Research Lab, Division of Neonatal-Perinatal Medicine, Cohen Children's Medical Center, Zucker School of Medicine at Hofstra, Northwell, Feinstein Institute for Medical Research, New York, NY, United States

Lars Bode
Department of Pediatrics and Larsson-Rosenquist Foundation Mother-Milk-Infant Center of Research Excellence (LRF MOMI CORE), University of California, San Diego, La Jolla, CA, United States

Eduardo Villamor-Martínez and Eduardo Villamor
Department of Pediatrics, School for Oncology and Developmental Biology (GROW), Maastricht University Medical Center (MUMC+), Maastricht, Netherlands

Maria Pierro
UOC TIN e Neonatologia, Dipartimento Salute Mamma e Bambino, Fondazione Poliambulanza, Brescia, Italy

Giacomo Cavallaro and Fabio Mosca
Neonatal Intensive Care Unit, Department of Clinical Sciences and Community Health, Fondazione IRCCS Cà Granda Ospedale Maggiore Policlinico, Università degli Studi di Milano, Milan, Italy

Elisa Mariani, Lucia Marvulli and Marcello Stella
Pediatric and Neonatal Intensive Care Unit, M. Bufalini Hospital, Cesena, Italy

Augusto Biasini
Donor Human Milk Bank Italian Association (AIBLUD), Milan, Italy

Silvia Savini
Neonatology and Neonatal Intensive Care Unit—S. Orsola-Malpighi Hospital, Bologna, Italy

Alessandra Sansavini, Francesca Agostini and Erica Neri
Department of Psychology, University of Bologna, Bologna, Italy

Shelley Brandstetter
School of Nursing, University of Washington, Seattle, WA, United States
Maternal Newborn Health and Nutrition, PATH, Seattle, WA, United States
Department of Global Health, University of Washington, Seattle, WA, United States
Seattle Children's Hospital, Seattle, WA, United States

Alessandra DeMarchis
Maternal Newborn Health and Nutrition, PATH, Seattle, WA, United States

Kiersten Israel-Ballard
Maternal Newborn Health and Nutrition, PATH, Seattle, WA, United States
Department of Global Health, University of Washington, Seattle, WA, United States

Kimberly Mansen
Maternal Newborn Health and Nutrition, PATH, Seattle, WA, United States
Seattle Children's Hospital, Seattle, WA, United States

Nga Nguyen Quyhn
PATH Vietnam, Hanoi, Vietnam

Cyril Engmann
Maternal Newborn Health and Nutrition, PATH, Seattle, WA, United States
Department of Global Health, University of Washington, Seattle, WA, United States
Seattle Children's Hospital, Seattle, WA, United States
Department of Pediatrics, University of Washington, Seattle, WA, United States

Claude Billeaud
Neonatology Nutrition, Lactarium Bordeaux-Marmande, CIC Pédiatrique 1401 Children's Hospital, Bordeaux, France

Buffin Rachel
Lactarium Auvergne Rhone Alpes, Hospices Civils de Lyon, Lyon, France

Lukas Christen
CARAG AG, Baar, Switzerland

Diana Escuder-Vieco
Banco Regional de Leche Materna, Hospital Universitario 12 de Octubre, Madrid, Spain

David Lembo
Laboratory of Molecular Virology, Department of Clinical and Biological Sciences, University of Turin, Turin, Italy

Enrico Bertino
Neonatal Intensive Care Unit, Department of Public Health and Pediatrics, University of Turin, Turin, Italy

Gillian A. Weaver
The Milk Bank, Imperial College Healthcare NHS Trust, London, United Kingdom

Ekhard E. Ziegler
The University of Iowa, Iowa City, IA, United States
Department of Pediatrics, University of Iowa, Iowa City, IA, United States

Antoni Gayà and Javier Calvo
Banc de Llet Materna, Fundació Banc de Sang i Teixits de les Illes Balears, Palma de Mallorca, Spain
Terapia Celular e Ingeniería Tisular, Institut d'Investigació Sanitària Illes Balears, Palma de Mallorca, Spain

Riccardo Davanzo
Division of Pediatrics and Neonatology, Department of Mother and Child Health, Ospedale Madonna delle Grazie, Matera, Italy
Task Force on Breastfeeding, Ministry of Health, Rome, Italy

Stéphane Hays
Régional Rhône Alpes Auvergne Human Milk Bank, Hôpital de la Croix-Rousse, Lyon, France

Jocelyne Drai
Biochemistry Laboratory, Lyon-sud Hospital, Pierre-Bénite, France

Marie-Nathalie Sarda
Immunology Laboratory, Lyon-sud Hospital, Pierre-Bénite, France

Radmila Mileusnic-Milenovic
First Serbian Milk Bank, Institute of Neonatology, Belgrade, Serbia

Antoni Gaya
Banc de Teixit, F. Banc de Sang i Teixits de les Illes Balears, Institut d'Investigacio Sanitaria Illes Balears (IdISBa), Barcelona, Spain

Aleksandra Wesolowska
Department of Neonatology, Faculty of Health Science, Medical University of Warsaw, Warsaw, Poland
Laboratory of Human Milk and Lactation Research at Regional Human Milk Bank in Holy Family Hospital, Department of Neonatology, Medical University of Warsaw, Warsaw, Poland
Human Milk Bank, Ludwik Rydygier' Provincial Polyclinical Hospital in Torun, Torun, Poland

Clair-Yves Boquien
INRA, Université Nantes, Centre de Recherche en Nutrition Humaine-Ouest, IMAD, Physiopathologie des Adaptations Nutritionnelles (UMR PHAN), Nantes, France
EMBA (European Milk Bank Association), Milan, Italy

Gérard Demazeau and Adrien Plumecocq
HPBioTECH, Gradignan, France

Philippe Lehours
Laboratoire de Bacteriologie, Centre Hospitalier Universitaire de Bordeaux, Bordeaux, France

Patrice Martin
UMR1313 GABI, INRA, AgroParisTech, Université Paris-Saclay, Jouy-en-Josas, France

Leslie Couëdelo
Department Nutrition-Health & Lipid biochemistry of ITERG, Bordeaux, France

Francesco Cresi, Elena Maggiora and Stefano Sottemano
Neonatology Unit, Department of Public Health and Pediatrics, Università degli Studi di Torino, Turin, Italy

Chiara Peila
Neonatology Unit, Department of Public Health and Pediatrics, Università degli Studi di Torino, Turin, Italy
Department of Maternal, Fetal and Neonatal Health, Azienda Ospedaliera Nazionale SS. Antonio e Biagio e Cesare Arrigo, Alessandria, Italy

Diego Gazzolo
Neonatal Intensive Care Unit, Università degli Studi G. d'Annunzio Chieti e Pescara, Chieti, Italy

Stephanie Fusch
Department of Pediatrics, University Medicine Greifswald, Greifswald, Germany
Department of Pediatrics, Kantonsspital Aarau AG, Aarau, Switzerland

Gerhard Fusch and Efrah I. Yousuf
Department of Pediatrics, McMaster University, Hamilton, ON, Canada

Markus Rochow
Carl-Thiem-Hospital, Cottbus, Germany

Hon Yiu So
Department of Mathematics and Statistics, Oakland University, Rochester, MI, United States

Christoph Fusch
Department of Pediatrics, McMaster University, Hamilton, ON, Canada
Department of Pediatrics, General Hospital, Paracelsus Medical University, Nuremberg, Germany

Niels Rochow
Department of Pediatrics, McMaster University, Hamilton, ON, Canada
Department of Pediatrics, General Hospital, Paracelsus Medical University, Nuremberg, Germany
Department of Pediatrics, Rostock University Medical Center, Rostock, Germany

Safiyyah Abbas
Women's and Children's Health Network, Adelaide, SA, Australia

Andrew J. McPhee
SAHMRI Women and Kids, South Australian Health and Medical Research Institute, Adelaide, SA, Australia

Amy K. Keir
Women's and Children's Health Network, Adelaide, SA, Australia
SAHMRI Women and Kids, South Australian Health and Medical Research Institute, Adelaide, SA, Australia
Adelaide Medical School, The University of Adelaide, Adelaide, SA, Australia
Robinson Research Institute, The University of Adelaide, Adelaide, SA, Australia

Maria Makrides
SAHMRI Women and Kids, South Australian Health and Medical Research Institute, Adelaide, SA, Australia
Robinson Research Institute, The University of Adelaide, Adelaide, SA, Australia

Alice R. Rumbold
SAHMRI Women and Kids, South Australian Health and Medical Research Institute, Adelaide, SA, Australia
Adelaide Medical School, The University of Adelaide, Adelaide, SA, Australia
Robinson Research Institute, The University of Adelaide, Adelaide, SA, Australia

Laura D. Klein
Business Growth and Innovation, Australian Red Cross Lifeblood, Sydney, NSW, Australia

Luke E. Grzeskowiak
SAHMRI Women and Kids, South Australian Health and Medical Research Institute, Adelaide, SA, Australia
College of Medicine and Public Health, Flinders University, Adelaide, SA, Australia

Xifang Ru, Xiaofang Huang and Qi Feng
Department of Pediatrics, Peking University First Hospital, Beijing, China

Miriam Aguilar-Lopez and Sharon M. Donovan
Division of Nutritional Sciences, University of Illinois Urbana-Champaign, Urbana, IL, United States

Christine Wetzel and Alissa MacDonald
Carle Hospital, Urbana, IL, United States

Thao T. B. Ho
Department of Pediatrics, Morsani College of Medicine, University of South Florida, Tampa, FL, United States

Index

www.ingramcontent.com/pod-product-compliance
Lightning Source LLC
LaVergne TN
LVHW080949210926
848485LV00004B/806